HEARING MEASUREMENT
A Book of Readings
SECOND EDITION

edited by

JOSEPH B. CHAIKLIN
Veterans Administration
Medical Center
New Orleans

IRA M. VENTRY
Teachers College
Columbia University

RICHARD F. DIXON
The University of North Carolina
at Greensboro

Addison-Wesley Publishing Company
Reading, Massachusetts

Library of Congress Cataloging in Publication Data

Main entry under title:
Hearing measurement.

  Editors' names in different order in edition for
1971.
  Includes bibliographical references.
  1. Audiometry—Addresses, essays, lectures.
I. Chaiklin, Joseph B. II. Ventry, Ira M.
III. Dixon, Richard Floyd, 1927–   . IV. Ventry,
Ira M. Hearing measurement. V. Title.
RF294.V45 1981   617.8′9′0287   80-28406
ISBN 0-201-01240-5

ISBN 0-201-01240-5
ABDEFGHIJ-AL-8987654321

CONTRIBUTING AUTHORS

Committee on Audiometric Evaluation,
  American Speech-Language-Hearing Association
Donald W. Bell
Robert W. Benson
Bradley L. Billings
Arthur Boothroyd
Robert H. Brey
William Burns
Anthony Canty
Raymond Carhart
Sheila Cawkwell
Joseph B. Chaiklin
R. R. A. Coles
Jesse E. Dancer
Hallowell Davis
Donald D. Dirks
Richard F. Dixon
Allen E. Dugdale
James W. Dunn
Eldon L. Eagles
Elizabeth Eldert
Alan S. Feldman
Cydney M. Fox
Earl R. Harford
George A. Heise
Wathina Hill
Ronald Hinchcliffe
Ira J. Hirsh
Vanja A. Holm
James F. Jerger
Mead C. Killion
E. James Kreul
Sabina A. Kurdziel
Herbert S. Levine
Neil Lewis
William Lichten
Lyle L. Lloyd
Samuel F. Lybarger

Carolyn W. Malmquist
Robert H. Margolis
Max E. McClellan
William Melnick
George A. Miller
Rosemary Morff
Donald E. Morgan
Ralph F. Naunton
David A. Nelson
Hayes A. Newby
James C. Nixon
Douglas Noffsinger
Wayne O. Olsen
Daniel J. Orchik
John P. Penrod
Vilija M. Priede
Michael J. M. Raffin
Scott N. Reger
Quentin R. Remein
Elizabeth G. Reynolds
William F. Rintelmann
Robert E. Roach
Dale O. Robinson
Jay W. Sanders
S. Richard Silverman
F. Blair Simmons
Richard W. Stream
Gerald A. Studebaker
John G. Swindeman
Gary Thompson
Robert M. Thorner
Aaron R. Thornton
Tom W. Tillman
Ira M. Ventry
Wendel K. Walton
Peggy S. Williams
Richard H. Wilson
Wesley R. Wilson

CONTENTS

INTRODUCTION

In a sense, revision of the first edition of this book started before the first edition was in press. The vitality of research and scholarly publication in audiology and related disciplines guaranteed the rapid appearance of new work suitable for a revised edition.

In the decade that has elapsed since the selection process for the first edition, new procedures have been developed and, in some instances, refined with such rapidity that their position has been assured in the basic battery. A parallel phenomenon has been the active research and theoretical formulation that has occurred concerning established basic procedures such as calibration, masking, and speech audiometry. This positive activity broadened our range of choices in almost every section of the book and compounded the difficulty of our task.

The combined effect of new topics and wider range of choices forced us to sharpen our conception of the book's scope and underlying philosophy. This did not produce any radical change from the factors that shaped the first edition, but we did try to achieve a more coherent emphasis on variables that affect basic measurement procedures and on the related process by which research data are used to guide basic measurement methods. Consequently, most of the selections are research reports that illuminate the effects of specific measurement variables on the outcome of basic audiometry. The continuing process of integrating published research data into the clinical process is, in our view, central to obtaining valid audiometric data and may be the most important skill an audiologist must use to remain professionally competent.

The differences between the first and revised editions, therefore, are related more to availability of new articles that expand knowledge on established procedures or illustrate the process of applying research data than to any change in our editorial philosophy. For example, Part III (Speech Audiometry) contains eight new selections, the majority of which concern validity and reliability of speech audiometry, while others represent stimulating new analyses of old problems. Part V on impedance audiometry is completely new and reflects the importance of the impedance battery in basic audiometric assessments.

Our selections are grouped into six parts that are not necessarily mutually exclusive: calibration, pure-tone audiometry, speech audiometry, masking, impedance audiometry, and identification audiometry.

As in the first edition, we have excluded from consideration articles concerning basic anatomy and physiology, hearing pathology, rehabilitation and, to a large extent, pediatric assessment. The scope of the anthology is confined to principles, theories, and methods that the beginning and intermediate student must understand to conduct basic audiometry or progress to advanced procedures. Because of this emphasis, the book should be useful not only to students but to practicing audiologists, otolaryngologists, speech pathologists, and others who may have occasion to conduct or interpret audiometric procedures.

We had to repeatedly remind ourselves that pure-tone and speech audiometry represent the nucleus of the process called basic hearing measurement. Most diagnostic and rehabilitative decisions are based on the outcome of these two procedures, but there is a common tendency to view pure-tone and speech audiometry as rudimentary, simple, and relatively free of technical difficulties.

This may explain why basic hearing measurement is sometimes performed by persons who have no formal preparation. It is probably not an overstatement to observe that more diagnostic and rehabilitative errors result from poorly administered basic audiometry than from poorly administered (or omitted) "advanced" audiometry.

All the selections in this edition were arrived at by the three of us during a long period of deliberation, debate, and consideration of suggestions solicited from reviewers of our prospectus and tentative list of selections. The three basic criteria we used in selecting articles were clinical relevance, quality of research, and timeliness. The readings may or may not be classics, but they do represent, in our present judgment, valuable contributions to the literature on basic hearing measurement. In the final analysis, our selections represent our collective and individual biases. When our work was completed we had selected fifty-four publications. A large percentage of the current selections were published after we completed the first edition.

Each section of the book is prefaced by remarks to place selections in perspective within the section, in relation to other sections, or in relation to the measurement process. Some authors have pro-vided clarifying or interpretive comments that appear as bracketed footnotes. In some instances authors have provided corrections of printers' errors that had appeared in the original published version of their work, or have provided valuable additional data not in their original work. Some figures have been enhanced or recaptioned for clarity. Apart from these corrections or additions, all but two of the selections are reprinted unabridged from their original published versions in journals, books, monographs, or separates. All material has been reset from the originals, but we must accept responsibility for printers' errors introduced by this resetting process and missed by our final proof-reading. We will appreciate readers bringing errors to our attention.

Our deepest gratitude must go to the many authors whose publications make up this collection. Their cooperation, in some cases extraordinary, eased a difficult process. This volume is dedicated to their knowledgeable contributions to enhancing assessment of hearing impaired children and adults.

May 1981   J. B. C.
                                                        I. M. V.
                                                        R. F. D.

CALIBRATION

The first step in obtaining reliable and valid audio-metric data is to make certain that the test equipment complies with appropriate standards. No matter how experienced the clinician or impeccable the clinical technique, faulty calibration will produce faulty results. Thus, equipment calibration is of fundamental importance in all hearing measurement regardless of whether the measurement takes place in a clinic, laboratory, school, or industrial setting. In addition to presenting some recent data on important calibration issues, the articles in this part offer important advice on calibration and calibration problems relevant to students and practicing clinicians.

The first article in this part presents an enlightened discussion of the "missing 6 dB" which, as the reader will learn, really is not missing at all. Killion points out that those who find "a missing 6 dB" in their data should look for measurement and equipment artifacts to account for it because "... nothing is really missing." In addition, Killion's discussion of differences between minimum audible pressure at the eardrum and minimum audible pressure in a coupler alerts us to the fact that pressure at the eardrum is quite different from the zero reference sound pressure levels (coupler pressures) specified in audiometer standards. Finally, Killion supports the notion that audiometer calibration standards "would be substantially simplified if audiometric zero levels were expressed in terms of eardrum pressures instead of coupler pressures corresponding to a specific earphone."

Sound-field audiometry is playing an increasingly important role in audiology clinics. It is used in hearing aid evaluations, and in evaluating patients who will not wear earphones. For example, one of the first measures taken on a difficult-to-test child may be a speech detection threshold in the sound field. Dirks, Stream, and Wilson's article is included here because it directly addresses the problems involved in doing sound-field speech audiometry, and it offers some feasible suggestions for dealing with these problems in clinical settings. For example, Dirks et al. underscore the important effect that loudspeaker placement has on speech thresholds, and they also stress the value of using a speech-spectrum noise, rather than a 1000-Hz pure-tone signal, for calibration purposes. Finally, Dirks et al. describe the interaction between room acoustics and frequency response of loudspeakers, and they urge the use of loudspeakers that have a flat frequency response.

The third selection, by Roach and Carhart, was included in the first edition of this book. We have included it again because the Roach-Carhart method continues to be one of the most widely used behavioral methods for checking the calibration of bone-conduction transducers. Students and practitioners should understand the rationale and evidence underlying the procedure.

Unfortunately, this behavioral approach to bone-conduction calibration has its shortcomings, as Dirks, Lybarger, Olsen, and Billings point out in their article concerning the current status of bone-conduction calibration. Dirks et al describe some of the problems associated with the development of a standard for bone-conduction calibration, and they offer tentative calibration values that appear to hold promise for a future standard. The reader should especially note Table 4-2 showing adjusted RMS force values and the good agreement between air- and bone-conduction thresholds (using the adjusted force values) in a sample of subjects with sensorineural hearing impairment (Figure 4-6).

The widespread use of impedance audiometry has created an urgent need for the development of calibration standards for impedance equipment. The article by Robinson and Brey highlights this need and, perhaps more important, the need for improved quality control of the instruments currently being manufactured. Although their study was limited to equipment produced by two manufacturers, it is sobering to note the frequency with which the equipment failed to perform within reasonable tolerance limits. Robinson and Brey's article is important because it identifies equipment problems and emphasizes the need for careful maintenance and monitoring of impedance audiometers.

Another bleak calibration problem was documented by Walton and Williams in their survey of portable audiometers in use in the Seattle, Washington, area in 1971. Although these audiometers were routinely serviced, 82 percent had one or more calibration problems. Walton and Williams's results might be discounted as atypical were it not for the good agreement between their results and the results of other studies of the calibration problems of portable audiometers. Table 6–3 of the Walton and Williams article shows that their rank order of calibration problems is almost identical to that reported by Thomas et al. (1969). The only conclusion that audiologists and other professionals (and paraprofessionals) can draw from these studies is that time, effort, and money will have to be spent to make certain that portable audiometers meet appropriate calibration standards.

The effect of ambient noise on hearing threshold data is a major calibration issue that confronts personnel working in a variety of settings, especially in schools and in industry. The 1977 ANSI standard that deals with this issue could not be reprinted here, but readers are urged to consult this document because it specifies the maximum allowable background noise levels that permit measurement of thresholds at 0 dB hearing levels re the ANSI 1969 audiometer calibration standard. The Killion and Studebaker article reprinted here is a valuable adjunct to the ANSI 1977 standard in that it provides a rationale for and description of the use of A-scale or C-scale sound level measurements to estimate the lowest threshold levels that can be measured without contamination by ambient noise. For example, an overall sound level reading of 47 dBA would allow threshold measurements down to 25 dB HL from 125 Hz to 8000 Hz. Where 20 dB HL screening levels are used in school screening programs, an overall 42 dBA level would be adequate. The point, of course, is that relatively simple sound level measurements, using an appropriate sound level meter, could substitute, in most cases, for the more complicated and time-consuming octave band analyses specified in the ANSI 1977 standard.

The last article in this part is Harford's nontechnical description of audiometer calibration techniques. This material also appeared in the first edition. While several details may be outdated (e.g., reference to the ASA 1951 standard and cost estimates), the practical suggestions for checking calibration are as useful today as they were in 1965.

REFERENCES AND ADDITIONAL READINGS

American National Standards Institute. *Specifications for audiometers (S3.6-1969)* New York: 1969.

American National Standards Institute. *Criteria for permissible ambient noise during audiometric testing (S3.1-1977).* New York: 1977.

Barry, S. J., and Gaddis, S. Physical and physiologic constraints on the use of bone-conduction speech audiometry. *J. Speech Hearing Dis., 43,* 220–226 (1978).

Melnick, W. Instrument calibration. In *Hearing assessment,* ed. W. F. Rintelmann. Baltimore: University Park Press, 1979, pp. 551–586.

Thomas, W. G.; Preslar, M. J.; Summers, R. R.; and Stewart, J. L. Calibration and working condition of 100 audiometers. *Public Health Reports, 84,* 311–327 (1969).

Wilber, L. A. Calibration, pure-tone, speech and noise signals. In *Handbook of clinical audiology,* 2nd ed., ed. J. Katz. Baltimore: Williams and Wilkins, 1978, pp. 81–97.

1

Revised Estimate of Minimum Audible Pressure: Where Is the "Missing 6 dB"?*

Mead C. Killion, Ph.D.

Senior Engineer, Industrial Research Products, Incorporated, A Knowles Company, Elk Grove Village, Illinois

Eardrum pressures at hearing threshold have been calculated from both earphone data (ISO R389-1964 and ANSI S3.6-1969) and free-field data (ISO R226-1961). When head diffraction, external-ear resonance, and an apparent flaw in ISO R226 are accounted for in the free-field data, and real-ear versus coupler differences and physiological noise are accounted for in the earphone data, the agreement between the two derivations is good. At the audiometric frequencies of 125, 250, 500, 1,000, 2,000, 4,000, and 8,000 Hz, the estimated eardrum pressures at absolute threshold are 30, 19, 12, 9, 15, 13, and 14 dB SPL, respectively. Except for the effects of physiological noise at low frequencies, no evidence of the "missing 6 dB" is seen, an observation consistent with the experimental results of several recent studies.

PACS numbers: 43.66.Cb, 43.66.Sr

INTRODUCTION

The term "Minimum Audible Pressure" (MAP) was first used by Sivian and White (1933) to describe threshold determinations "in terms of the pressure amplitude at the observer's eardrum." Unfortunately, the term MAP has also sometimes been used to mean the *coupler* pressure corresponding to the threshold calibration of a given earphone. To avoid confusion, in this paper the term MAP will be used only with regard to eardrum pressure; the term "Minimum Audible Pressure in a Coupler" (MAPC) will be used when reference to coupler pressures is intended. (MAPC so defined is equivalent to the "reference equivalent threshold sound pressure level" of ISO R389-1964 and the "reference threshold level" of ANSI S3.6-1969.)

Since the Sivian and White study, numerous studies of both earphone MAPC and free-field MAF (Minimum Audible Field, the threshold sound pressure at the listener's position [listener absent] due to a sound source in front of that position) have been made, and international standards exist for both MAPC and MAF (ISO R389-1964 and ISO R226-1961, respectively). In addition, several independent studies of the relationship between free-field pressure and eardrum pressure, and between earphone-coupler pressure and eardrum pressure, have been made. A comprehensive compilation of all available data on the ratio of eardrum pressure to free-field pressure was published by Shaw in 1974, along with a self-consistent set of "best-fit" average curves for both free-field-to-eardrum and earcanal-entrance-to-eardrum transfer ratios.

By combining the available psychoacoustic and physical acoustic data, following the procedure discussed by Pollack (1949), it is possible to arrive at a single estimate of MAP. This paper reports one such estimate. Although the author has found the present estimate quite useful on several occasions, it will un-

*Presented 19 November 1976, at the 92nd meeting of the Acoustical Society of America, San Diego, CA.

Reprinted by permission from *J. Acoust. Soc. Am.,* **63** 1501–1508 (1978).

doubtably require revision as more direct evidence becomes available. The chief purpose of this paper is not to recommend acceptance of the present MAP estimate, but to demonstrate that the apparent differences in commonly accepted threshold values for earphone and free-field listening are easily reconciled.

1. NEW ESTIMATE OF MAP

Figure 1-1 shows the result of the present study as a single estimated eardrum pressure (MAP) curve. Vertical bars at each of the standard audiometric frequencies indicate the differences between the average data derived from earphone MAPC studies and from free-field MAF studies. Agreement between the two approaches is excellent between 1,000 and 3,000 Hz (typically less than 1.5 dB difference between the two determinations), and not as good at lower and higher frequencies. At very low and very high frequencies (below 100 Hz and above 8,000 Hz), the curve of Figure 1-1 was estimated from the studies discussed in Section IC.

The remainder of this paper contains a discussion of the derivation of Figure 1-1 and of possible explanations for the less-than-perfect agreement between the two approaches at both low and high frequencies. The reader uninterested in the details may skip to the Discussion and Recommendations.

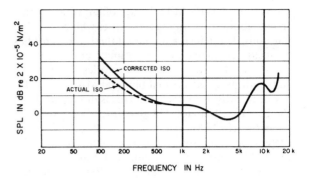

FIGURE 1-2. Binaural Minimum Audible Field (0° incidence) from ISO R226-1961, with low-frequency correction. (See text.)

A. The Estimation of MAP from MAF Data

The sound pressure level in a free field of a sinusoidal, 0°-incident sound wave which is just audible to an observer is usually referred to as his Minimum Audible Field (MAF). The measurement of sound pressure level is made with the subject absent, at a point corresponding to the center of the subject's head. The corresponding eardrum pressure, therefore, will be generally higher due to head and ear diffraction and resonance (see, for example, Wiener and Ross (1946) and Shaw (1974)).[1]

Three important MAF studies cover the audible frequency range: the Sivian and White study (1933), the British study of Churcher and King (1937), and the British National Physical Laboratory (NPL) study of Robinson and Dadson (1956). In addition, the 0-dB-loudness-level curve of Fletcher and Munson (1933) provided an estimate of MAF based on an extrapolation back to zero from suprathreshold loudness measurements performed with field-calibrated earphones.

In the late 1950s, international agreement was reached on a standard curve for absolute binaural threshold (and equal-loudness contours) for normal, young ears. The result was ISO R226-1961, whose threshold values are shown in Figure 1-2.

With the exception of the data at low frequencies, the ISO R226 values appear to represent a reasonable consensus of the available data. At low frequencies, however, the available data suggest that the ISO values are too low. Figure 1-3 shows a comparison of

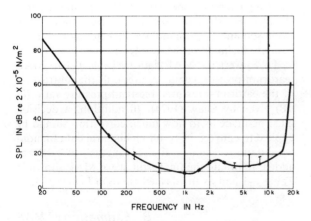

FIGURE 1-1. The present estimate of monaural Minimum Audible Pressure at the eardrum. Vertical bars indicate the difference between the averages of MAF-derived and MAPC-derived data.

the various 100-Hz MAF values obtained at six different laboratories. In the three cases where the original study determined a monaural threshold, 2 dB has been subtracted to obtain an estimate of the binaural threshold.[2] Five out of six laboratories obtained results indicating the normal binaural MAF at 100 Hz is within 2 dB of 33 dB SPL. This is discrepant from the 25 dB SPL at 100 Hz given in ISO R226-1961.[3] (The 100-Hz MAF estimate of 37 dB obtained by Fletcher and Munson (1933) was not included in Figure 1–3 because it was an indirect estimate.)

Since the weight of evidence at 100 Hz is in support of the original Sivian and White and the later Churcher and King studies, it seems reasonable to take an average of their data in the 100–400 Hz region to obtain a "corrected R226 curve." The data shown in Table 1–1 and as the solid curve in Figure 1–2 were obtained in that manner: At 500 Hz and above they are identical with ISO R226, whereas between 100 and 400 Hz they are the average of the (dB) values shown in Figure 10 of the 1933 Sivian and

TABLE 1–1. DERIVATION OF MINIMUM AUDIBLE PRESSURE AT THE EARDRUM FROM MINIMUM AUDIBLE FIELD DATA. DATA ARE IN DECIBELS.

Freq. (Hz)	A MAF (ISO R226 corrected)	B P_D/P_{FF} at $0°$[1]	C MAP (binaural)	D MAP (monaural)
100	33		33	35
150	24		24	26
200	18.5	0.5	19	21
300	12	1.3	13.3	15.3
400	8	1.6	9.6	11.6
500	6	1.7	7.7	9.7
700	4.7	2.8	7.5	9.5
1,000	4.2	2.6	6.8	8.8
1,500	3	5.0	8.0	10.0
2,000	1	12.0	13.0	15.0
2,500	−1.2	16.8	15.6	17.6
3,000	−2.9	15.4	12.5	14.5
3,500	−3.9	14.8	10.9	12.9
4,000	−3.9	14.2	10.3	12.3
4,500	−3	12.8	9.8	11.8
5,000	−1	10.7	9.6	11.6
6,000	4.6	7.4	12.0	14.0
7,000	10.9	4.3	15.2	17.2
8,000	15.3	1.8	17.1	19.1
9,000	17	−0.7	16.3	18.3
10,000	16.4	−1.6	14.8	16.8

[1]P_D/P_H is the ratio of eardrum pressure to free-field pressure as given by Shaw (1974).

A constant 2 dB was added to convert binaural to monaural thresholds; thus, the MAP derived in Column D is the sum of Columns A and B plus 2 dB.

White paper and in Figure 9 of the 1937 Churcher and King paper. (In the 200–400-Hz region, the curve changes less than 0.5 dB at any frequency if the Robinson and Dadson and the Fletcher and Munson data are included in the average.)

To convert the MAF data in Table 1–1 to MAP (eardrum-pressure) data requires only the subtraction of the eardrum-pressure/free-field-pressure ratio (in dB) given by Shaw (1974). In addition, a decision must be made as to how much correction should be applied to convert the resulting binaural data to monaural data. A "monaural disadvantage" of 2 dB was added[2] to obtain the final estimate of MAP shown in Table 1–1 and as the dashed curve in Figure 1–5.

B. Estimation of MAP from Earphone-MAPC Data

Although the term MAP was originally used by Sivian and White to describe threshold "in terms of

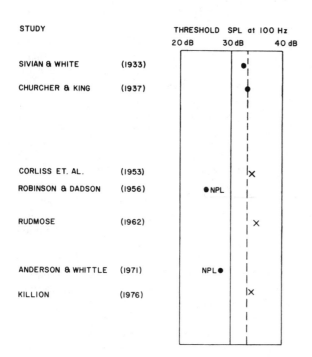

STUDY		THRESHOLD SPL at 100 Hz
		20 dB 30 dB 40 dB
SIVIAN & WHITE	(1933)	
CHURCHER & KING	(1937)	
CORLISS ET. AL.	(1953)	
ROBINSON & DADSON	(1956)	
RUDMOSE	(1962)	
ANDERSON & WHITTLE	(1971)	
KILLION	(1976)	

FIGURE 1–3. 100-Hz free-field thresholds (MAF) obtained at various laboratories: (•) binaural; (x) monaural minus 2 dB.

the pressure amplitude at the observer's eardrum,'' it has since been used by others to refer to earphone thresholds where the pressure developed with the "threshold voltage" applied to the earphone is measured in what was intended to be an ear-like reference coupler such as the NBS-9A. This has been a perversion of the original meaning, since the pressure measured in the reference coupler often bears little resemblance to the pressure at the observer's eardrum. Unfortunately, the term MAP has been used in the latter sense for so long that it now seems to be part of the entrenched jargon of psychoacoustics and audiology.

As the pioneers in audiology quickly discovered, the coupler pressure corresponding to threshold depended on the earphone system used with the audiometer. Moreover, an enormous amount of work went into the determination of the "normal threshold," resulting first in the 1951 ASA standard Z 24.5 and later in the revised values found in the ISO R389-1964 standard. A round robin of loudness balances and threshold comparisons between various laboratories preceded the agreement on ISO R389-1964 (Weissler, 1968), a relatively self-consistent international standard listing the coupler pressures corresponding to threshold for one "standard earphone type" from each of five different countries. The U.S. standard earphone was the Western Electric 705A which, unfortunately, is no longer in production. A substantial additional amount of work within the United States resulted in ANSI Standard S3.6-1969, which included a suggested calibration of four additional earphones; three Permaflux earphones and the Telephonics TDH-39. (Each earphone is to be mounted in an MX41/AR earphone cushion and the reference pressure measured in the NBS-9A coupler.) Additional earphone-coupler combinations are included in the 1975 edition of ISO R389.

Both the TDH-39 and the Beyer DT-48 earphone have MAPCs specified in terms of NBS-9A coupler pressure. By applying the data obtained by Shaw (1966) on the ratio of canal-entrance pressure to NBS-9A pressure for these two earphones, these MAPC values can be converted to represent ear-canal-entrance pressures. By further applying Shaw's 1974 data on the ratio of eardrum pressure to ear-canal-entrance pressure, one obtains the calculated MAP at the eardrum. Table 1–2 shows these calculations for the TDH-39 and the DT-48 earphones.

In addition to these data, a careful study of the thresholds of 25 male and female subjects ranging from 18 to 26 years of age was reported by Albrite et al. (1958) using the WE 705A headphone. In that study, the actual sound pressure level developed in front of the earphone grill was measured with a probe microphone. As would be expected from physical considerations, and as was experimentally verified by Villchur (1969), the pressure measured at that location and the pressure measured at the entrance to the ear canal are essentially identical at 1,000 Hz and below. Thus, at the four audiometric frequencies below 1,500 Hz, the data of Albrite et al. can be converted directly to eardrum pressure, using only the correction given by Shaw (1974). These data are also found in Table 1–2.

1. Potential Errors. For the low-frequency data in Table 1–2, the correction from the NBS-9A coupler to the ear-canal-entrance data of Shaw (1966) represents an average of ten subjects. The value used at 125 Hz was extrapolated (on a 12-dB/oct slope) from Shaw's curve at 200 Hz and above. Even at 250 Hz, however, Shaw found an 18-dB range across the ten subjects due to the well-known cushion-fit variability. Villchur (1970) reported a range of over 25 dB at 125 Hz for the TDH-39/MX41-AR on 13 subjects—a number in substantial agreement with the 27-dB range at 100 Hz previously reported by Burkhard and Corliss (1954) for the PDR-8/MX41-AR combination. It is not too surprising, therefore, that the three estimates of eardrum pressure shown in Table 1–2 have a 16-dB range at 125 Hz, and that even at 250 Hz there is a 7-dB difference between the extremes of the three estimates.

The 125-Hz and 250-Hz thresholds are essentially masked thresholds due to the physiological noise generated under the earphone cushion. Based on the data of Rudmose (1962) at 100, 200, and 400 Hz, an interpolated value of 4.5 dB at 125 Hz and 1 dB at 250 Hz is obtained for the threshold elevation due to the physiological masking when using the TDH-39/MX41-AR earphone. This correction was simply applied to the overall averages in Table 1–2. In light of the variability among estimates at these frequencies, a more elaborate analysis hardly seems justified.[4]

Shaw's data on the ratio of coupler pressure to ear-canal-entrance pressure was obtained with a modified NBS-9A coupler, where the 1-inch-diam-

TABLE 1–2. DERIVATION OF MINIMUM AUDIBLE PRESSURE AT THE EARDRUM FROM MAPC DATA ON THREE EARPHONES. DATA ARE IN DECIBELS; DATA MARKED WITH AN ASTERISK ARE EXTRAPOLATED.

Freq. (Hz)	A P_C[1] (MAPC)	B P_E/P_C[2]	C P_D/P_E[3]	D P_D/P_C	E MAP[4]
TDH-39					
125	45	−19*	0	−19*	26
250	25.5	−7	+0.2	−6.8	18.7
500	11.5	+2.5	+0.7	+3.2	14.7
1,000	7	+3.0	+1.2	+4.2	11.2
1,500	6.5	+2.5	+2.4	+4.9	11.4
2,000	9	+3.5	+3.8	+7.3	16.3
3,000	10	−1.5	+8.5	+7.0	17.0
4,000	9.5	−4.5	+10.2	+5.7	15.2
6,000	15.5	+1.0	+3.7	+4.7	20.2
8,000	13	+4.5	+1.5	+6.0	19.0
DT-48					
125	47.5	−16.5*	0	−16.5*	31
250	28.5	−5.5	+0.2	−5.3	23.2
500	14.5	0	+0.7	+0.7	15.2
1,000	8	0	+1.2	+1.2	9.2
1,500	7.5	+1.5	+2.4	+3.9	11.4
2,000	8	+3	+3.8	+6.8	14.8
3,000	6	+0.2	+8.5	+8.7	14.7
4,000	5.5	0	+10.2	+10.2	15.7
6,000	8	+8	+3.7	+11.7	19.7
8,000	14.5	−3.5	+1.5	−2.0	12.5

Freq. (Hz)		P_E (Probe)	P_D/P_E	MAP from probe measurements	
705-A					
125		42	0	42	
250		26	+0.2	26.2	
500		16	+0.7	16.7	
1,000		7	+1.2	+8.2	

[1] The earphone-MAPC data represent NBS-9A coupler pressure as found in ANSI S3.6–1969 for the TDH-39 earphone in MX41/AR cushion, and from ISO R389–1964 for the Beyer DT-48 earphone in the supra-aural cushion.
[2] Shaw (1966).
[3] Shaw (1974).
[4] The sum of columns A–C.

eter laboratory standard microphone was replaced with a rigid plate containing the small inlet of the same probe tube used for measuring ear-canal-entrance pressures. This had the great advantage of eliminating the possibility of error due to the use of two different microphone setups, with their differing frequency responses, sensitivities, etc. When the frequency is high enough, however, the standing waves set up in any coupler can cause a difference between the pressure in the center of the coupler (at the probe pickup point) and the pressure averaged over the active diaphragm area of standard microphones. An estimate of the possible effect of such standing waves in the NBS-9A coupler indicated that there might be a small effect at the 6- and 8-kHz audiometric frequencies, but that it was unlikely to have altered the data at the lower frequencies. This conclusion was checked experimentally by the author recently, with the finding that the maximum error below 10 kHz is of the order of a few tenths dB as long as the 9A coupler length is increased by the amount necessary (around 2 mm) to compensate for the equivalent volume of the standard 1-inch microphone. (Shaw's data were obtained with such a coupler modification.) Without such a modification, the error can exceed 0.5 dB at low frequencies and 1.0 dB (in the opposite direction) at high frequencies.

The acoustic impedance of the particular TDH-39 and DT-48 earphone samples used at various laboratories might have differed enough to affect the data at high frequencies. Although often ignored, variations in source impedance are always a potential source of error when probe-tube determinations of the real-ear response of one sample of an earphone type are compared to threshold or loudness balance data obtained using a different sample(s). (Note that this error can occur even when the number of human subjects appears adequate to rule out significant real-ear sampling errors in both cases.)

The application of the earphone to the ear changes the dimensions of both the outer ear and the ear canal itself. The change in pinna and concha shape are taken care of automatically in the data since Shaw's sound pressure measurements were made at the ear canal entrance. The constriction of the ear canal, however, can cause changes of up to at least 5 dB in the ratio of eardrum pressure to canal-entrance pressure at frequencies in the 3–6-kHz region, as shown by Villchur (1969).[5]

2. The Final Earphone-Derived MAP Estimate. Figure 1–4 shows the earphone-derived MAP estimates of Table 1–2, with the data derived from each of the three studies plotted separately. The dashed curve below 500 Hz shows the effect of correcting the average

TABLE 1-3. AVERAGE OF THREE EARPHONE-DERIVED MAP ESTIMATES SHOWN IN TABLE 1-2.

Freq. (Hz)	Average	Correction for physical noise	MAP
125	33	−3.5	29.5
250	22.7	−1	21.7
500	15.5	0	15.5
1,000	9.5		9.5
1,500	11.4		11.4
2,000	13.9		13.9
3,000	15.9		15.9
4,000	15.5		15.5
6,000	20.0		20.0
8,000	15.7		15.7

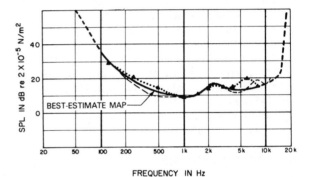

FREQUENCY IN Hz

FIGURE 1-5. MAP estimates derived from earphone-MAPC data corrected for physiological noise (triangles and dotted curve) and free-field MAF data (light dashed curve). Solid curve represents the present estimate of MAP shown in Figure 1–1. The extensions below 100 Hz and above 8,000 Hz (heavy dashed curves) are discussed in the text.

for physiological noise, as discussed above. The close agreement above 250 Hz suggests that earphone-sampling errors were not significant. Because of the other potential errors discussed above, however, one concludes that only in the region between 500 and 3,000 Hz should one expect to find a correspondence between the MAP derived from earphone MAPC data and from free-field MAF data. Nonetheless, the data at all audiometric frequencies have been averaged (the Albrite et al. data were included only at 1,000 Hz and below for the reasons given above) and corrected for physiological noise. The averaged data are shown in Table 1–3 and plotted as the dotted curve in Figure 1–5.

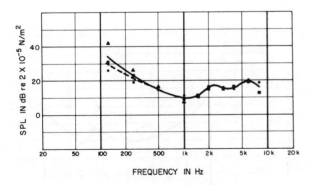

FREQUENCY IN Hz

FIGURE 1-4. MAP calculated from earphone-MAPC data (solid curve) and corrected for the effect of physiological noise below 500 Hz (dashed curve). Data on individual earphones are shown for the TDH-39/MX41-AR(•), DT-48 (■), and 705A (▲).

C. MAP Above 8,000 and Below 100 Hz

For completeness, the present MAP estimate has been extended above 8,000 and below 100 Hz, as shown by the heavy dashed curves in Figure 1–5. These extensions were based directly on the studies described below.

Northern et al. (1972) reported a study of high-frequency audiometric threshold levels in the 8,000–18,000-Hz range. The result of that study was a set of recommended high-frequency threshold values expressed in terms of eardrum SPL. The heavy dashed curve above 8,000 Hz in Figure 1–5 (and the extended solid curve above 8,000 Hz in Figure 1–1) follows their recommendations directly.

Corso (1958) and Yeowart and Evans (1974) reported independent studies of low-frequency thresholds. In both studies, unusual care was taken to avoid contamination of the results due to physiological noise, harmonic distortion, and vibrational artifacts. At most frequencies, the two studies agree within a few dB. The heavy dashed curve below 100 Hz in Figure 1–5 (and the extended solid curve below 100 Hz in Figure 1–1) was drawn smoothly through data points from the two studies.

D. The New Estimate

Figure 1–5 shows a comparison between the calculated MAP derived from free-field MAF data (thin dashed curve) and from earphone MAPC data corrected for physiological noise (dotted curve). There is a difference of 6 dB at 500 Hz, but the rest of the data in the 500–3,000 Hz region—where both transformations are on solid footing—is in excellent agreement: The maximum difference is 1.6 dB, and the average difference is 1.2 dB ignoring sign and 0.4 dB including the sign of the differences. As expected, the data at 4 kHz and above do not agree as well, although even here the average difference is less than 4 dB ignoring sign and less than 2 dB including the sign of the differences. By what must be sheer coincidence, the data at 250 and 125 Hz are also in excellent agreement.[6] The solid curve shown in Figure 1–5 is the (author's) best-estimate MAP curve of Figure 1–1. In arriving at this estimate, little weight was given to the MAPC-derived data in the 3,000–6,000-Hz region for the reasons discussed in Section IB 1. Above 6,000 Hz, the curve was drawn to blend smoothly with the high-frequency MAP recommendations of Northern et al. (1972), which were based on direct measurements of eardrum pressure.

It is interesting to note that the solid curve in Figure 1–5 is not far from the probe-tube MAP data obtained by Sivian on eight ears (1928, unpublished) and reported in a little-noticed series of paragraphs in Sivian and White (1933). The probe tube was located 1–1.5 cm from the eardrum in two sets of experiments they described as follows:

> The results given in Figure 9 represent the average of two determinations. In both, the ear is exposed to a fairly loud tone from a loudspeaker, and the pressure in the ear canal is measured with a search tube.
>
> From the attenuation of the loudspeaker current required to produce threshold, the MAP values are computed. The chief assumption is that the search tube pressures are equal to the drum pressures.
>
> In a second procedure, a telephone receiver is made to produce in the ear a loudness sensation equal to that caused by the loudspeaker. The receiver current is then attenuated to threshold. From this attenuation, and from the above search tube pressure measurement, the absolute MAP value is derived.
>
> Since the attenuation measured by both methods were found to agree fairly well, it was considered justifiable to average the results.

Figure 1–6 shows a comparison between Sivian's data and the MAP curve derived in the present study. Sivian's data are plotted as reported. Correction for the mid-canal location of his probe tube would improve the agreement at high frequencies between Sivian's data and the present estimate.

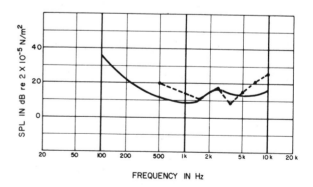

FIGURE 1-6. The 1928 probe-tube MAP data of Sivian (dashed curve) compared to the present MAP estimate (solid curve).

II. DISCUSSION

The comparison of eardrum pressure at absolute threshold derived from available MAF and MAPC data reveals a good agreement. It is no surprise that threshold occurs at a constant eardrum pressure; this has been generally accepted as fact since the so-called "missing 6-dB problem"[7] was put to rest by the studies of Rudmose (1962, 1963), Shaw and Piercy (1962), Shaw (1969), Villchur (1969, 1970, 1972), Anderson and Whittle (1971), Tillman et al. (1973), Morgan and Dirks (1974), and Stream and Dirks (1974). It is somewhat surprising, however, to see such close agreement between two sets of psychoacoustic data, each of which was arrived at in such a roundabout way.

The combined middle- and inner-ear response appears to have a dip in sensitivity (increase in threshold) near 2,700 Hz, where head and ear diffraction effects produce the maximum eardrum pressure (not at 4 kHz as has sometimes been erroneously reported). One wonders if the outer-, middle-, and inner-ear system was simply designed so that all the elements cooperated to produce the best overall performance compromise, or if the 2,500-Hz "hump" seen in the MAP curve of Figure 1–1 is simply an artifact of some sort. The excellent agreement between the two MAP derivations in the 2,500-Hz region lends credence to the former hypothesis, although careful probe-tube monitored threshold measurements performed by the author on one (!) ear showed no signs of such a hump.

One potential explanation for the increased threshold near 2,500 Hz is masking due to the Brownian noise pressure at the eardrum, which exhibits a substantial peak at the 2,700-Hz resonance of the outer ear. Recent estimates by Shaw (1976) of the real part of the acoustic impedance seen looking out from the eardrum permit the estimate of a noise spectrum level of -29 dB SPL at the eardrum at 2,700 Hz. Preliminary noise measurements made with a low-noise XD-985 subminiature microphone (Killion, 1976) at the eardrum position of a KEMAR manikin (Burkhard and Sachs, 1975) appear to confirm this tentative estimate, although a microphone with a substantially lower noise level will be required to obtain precise confirmation. A spectrum level of -29 dB SPL at the eardrum at 2,700 Hz is 24 dB below the approximately -5 dB SPL spectrum level which would be required to explain the 16-dB value for MAP at 2,700 Hz shown in Figure 1–5. The effect

of Brownian noise pressure at the eardrum thus appears inconsequential even for an extremely acute ear, a conclusion consistent with the estimates of other authors. (A somewhat expanded discussion of real-ear noise sources and their effects can be found in Killion, 1976.)

Although no estimate of the noise pressure produced by the damping resistance in the TDH-39 earphone has been attempted, it seems most unlikely that it would be significant. Peaks in noise pressure would be expected at the resonances of the earphone, however, and the primary resonance of the TDH-39 does occur at roughly 3 kHz.

Noise-induced hearing loss might provide an explanation for the reduced sensitivity in the 2,500-Hz region, except such loss normally occurs a half-octave above the frequency of maximum stimulation (Davis et al., 1950). With the typical 2,700-Hz resonance frequency for the outer ear, the greatest noise-induced hearing loss might be expected to occur near 4 kHz. Recent temporary-threshold-shift (TTS) experiments performed by Caiazzo and Tonndorf (1977) appear to confirm the hypothesis that the characteristic 4-kHz notch of noise-induced hearing loss is mainly related to outer ear resonance: By artificially doubling the length of the ear canals of 15 subjects, they found a maximum TTS at 2 kHz under the same noise-field conditions which produced a maximum TTS at 4 kHz with the subjects own (unaltered) ear canals.

Perhaps the 2,500 Hz sensitivity dip will ultimately be explained by the characteristics of the eardrum-to-basilar-membrane transformation. As shown by Dallos (1973), a similar sensitivity dip in the MAP curve for the cat can be nicely explained on the basis of the middle-ear transfer characteristics.

III. RECOMMENDATIONS

Several suggestions previously made by others perhaps bear repeating here. Following the recommendations of Corliss and Burkhard (1953), the standardization of audiometric zero levels would be substantially simplified if audiometric zero levels were expressed in terms of eardrum pressures instead of coupler pressures corresponding to a specific earphone. This would allow use of a relatively simple probe-microphone procedure (such as described by Villchur and Killion, 1975) to establish threshold norms for a new earphone system.[8] The same procedure should also allow validation and/or correction of the MAP estimate given in this paper.

Similarly, anyone contemplating psychoacoustic experiments in which the absolute level of the stimulus (or the relative level between two stimuli having different frequencies) is important would do well to include some means of determining that level on an individual basis. And given the large variations in earphone cushion fit from trial to trial shown by Villchur (1970) for the TDH-39 in either the MX-41/AR or the Zwislocki cushion, a single-sitting determination of the level appears risky if more than one experimental session is contemplated. As Munson and Wiener (1950) observed, many apparently anomalous results in the literature of psychoacoustics can be explained if the failure of the experimenters to obtain real-ear measurements of stimulus levels is taken into account.

Lastly, the overwhelming weight of experimental evidence indicates that anyone finding a "missing 6 dB" in his data would do well to look for (1) inadequate determination of actual stimulus levels, (2) physiological noise, (3) transducer distortion, (4) mechanical vibration coupled to the subject, or one of the several other artifacts which Rudmose (1962, 1963) uncovered in ten years of work on the subject. There *are* very real differences between MAF and MAP—differences which must be taken into account in the calibration of speech audiometers, for example—but they are readily accounted for by the physical factors involved. In short, nothing is really missing.

ACKNOWLEDGMENTS

The author is indebted to Wayne Rudmose for several fascinating discussions on the "missing 6 dB" problem, and to Edgar Villchur and Mahlon Burkhard for extensive suggestions made regarding an earlier draft of this paper.

ENDNOTES

1. Additional variations in eardrum pressure are caused by the exact vertical location of the subject, reflections from the chair, reflections from the subject's shoulders, arms, legs, etc. These have not always been well specified, as discussed by Shaw (1974).

2. Fletcher and Munson (1933) found a 1.8-dB average difference in acuity between the best ear and the average of both ears for frequencies below 2,000 Hz, but only a slight difference between the binaural and best-ear threshold. Assuming Pollack's (1948) finding of an 0.8-dB improvement in binaural versus best-ear threshold when the sensation levels at the two ears differ by 3 dB, one could refine the average-binaural-advantage estimate to approximately 2.6 dB. (The 1.8-dB difference of Fletcher and Munson is equivalent to an average sensation-level-difference of 3.6 dB between ears receiving binaural stimulation at equal intensity levels.) Assuming an across-the-board binaural advantage of 2 dB appears sufficiently accurate for our purposes, however.

3. The ISO standard relied heavily on the Robinson and Dadson study at frequencies below 300 Hz. One explanation for the apparent flaw in the NPL determination may be that vibrations transmitted through the observer's chair caused a reduced "threshold." Rudmose (1962) found that the standard free-field audiometry setup could sometimes produce artificially low thresholds at low frequencies; the summation of the direct airborne stimulus and the tactile stimulus caused by chair vibrations allowed the subject to hear a below-threshold airborne stimulus which he could no longer hear when the chair vibrations were eliminated. One cannot help noticing a similar discrepancy in the earphone study reported by Albrite et al. (1958): Although both NPL and NBS obtain the same "threshold voltage" on a 4026A earphone they exchanged, the probe-tube real-ear average sound pressure measured by NPL was some 12 dB less at 125 Hz than a similar measurement made on the same earphone by NBS (see Figures 4 and 6 of that paper).

4. Other investigators have obtained higher estimates of the masking due to physiological noise. Villchur (1970) obtained 6 dB at 125 Hz and 5 dB at 250 Hz for the MX41/AR cushion. At the same time, Villchur appears to have obtained lower real-ear response levels in his measurements of the TD-39/MX41-AR combination (his Figure 2) than the values used in Table 1-2. The two effects would tend to cancel, i.e., the final threshold estimates based on Villchur's data would be similar to those obtained here. Anderson and Whittle (1971) obtained 11 dB of masking due to physiological noise at 125 Hz, although this estimate was obviously influenced by the unusually low MAF values they obtained (see Figure 1-3, this paper). In any case, only Rudmose (1962) appears to have taken great pains to isolate his subjects from mechanical vibrations, so only his data are used here. It is of some comfort to note that the resulting MAP estimate of 29.5 dB at 125 Hz (Table 1-3) is nearly identical to the 15-subject average of 30.6 dB obtained by Corso (1958) at 125 Hz, since the large-volume construction of Corso's electrodynamic driver should have resulted in greatly reduced physiological noise (see Rudmose, 1962; and Shaw and Piercy, 1962).

5. We assume here that subjects whose canals collapse almost completely under earphones—representing roughly 4 percent of the population according to Hildyard and Valentine (1962)—were excluded from all studies on the basis of audiometric findings.

6. Given the enormous variations in the earphone data at low frequencies, one is reminded of the remark made by Lagrange, the great mathematical analyst, about Newton's treatment of calculus: "All of Newton's ideas were in error; but due to God's infinite kindness, the errors all cancelled!"

7. The term "the missing 6 dB" was apparently first used by Munson and Wiener (1952), who reported the vexing results of nearly twenty years of experiments undertaken to uncover the reason for the apparent difference in earcanal pressure between equally loud earphone-generated and loudspeaker-generated suprathreshold tones at low frequencies; where " . . . a person familiar with Thévenin's theorem but otherwise naive would expect the two pressures to be the same. . . . " Successive experimental refinements produced a progressive decrease in the 100-Hz pressure difference obtained by Munson and Wiener, but it took a substantial amount of additional investigation by Rudmose (1962, 1963) before some of the more subtle experimental difficulties were finally identified. At higher frequencies, of course, the difference has always been of the order of that expected due to diffraction and ear-canal resonance effects; so nothing was generally considered "missing" above a few hundred Hz, although "the missing 6 dB" has occasionally been invoked by writers to explain unusual experimental results.

8. It would not solve the problem of variability due to the age and sex of the subject, as discussed by Erber (1968), of course.

REFERENCES

Albrite, J. P., Shutts, R. E., Whitlock, M. D., Cook, R. K., Corliss, E. L., and Burkhard, M. D. (1958). "Research in normal threshold of hearing," AMA Arch. Octolaryngol. 68, 194–198.

ANSI (1969). "Specifications for audiometers," S3.6-1969 (Am. Natl. Stand. Inst., New York).

Anderson, C. M. B., and Whittle, L. S. (1971). "Physiological noise and the Missing 6 dB," Acustica 24, 261–272.

Burkhard, M. D., and Corliss, E. L. R. (1954). "The response of earphones in ears and couplers," J. Acoust. Soc. Am. 26, 679–685.

Burkhard, M. D., and Sachs, R. M. (1975). "Anthropometric manikin for acoustic research," J. Acoust. Soc. Am. 58, 214–222.

Caiazzo, A. J., and Tonndorf, J. (1977). "Ear canal resonance and temporary threshold shift," J. Acoust. Soc. Am. 61, S78(A).

Churcher, B. G., and King, A. J. (1937). "The performance of noise meters in terms of the primary standard," J. Inst. Electr. Eng. [1889–1940] 81, 57–90. (See their Figure 9.)

Corliss, E. L. R., and Burkhard, M. D. (1953). "Probe tube method for the transfer of threshold standards between audiometer earphones," J. Acoust. Soc. Am. 25, 990–993.

Corliss, E. L. R., Burkhard, M. D. Thompson, R. P., Smith, E. L., Marchetti, A. A., Koidan, W., Dunn, G. H., and Peterson, K. (1953). "Progress on Methods for Calibration of Hearing Diagnostic Instruments," Natl. Bur. Stand. Rep. 2312, 1–33 (Washington, DC).

Corso, J. F. (1958). "Absolute threshold for tones of low frequency," Am. J. Psychol. 71, 367–384.

Dallos, P. (1973). The Auditory Periphery (Academic, New York), pp. 117–126.

Davis, H., Morgan, C. T., Hawkins, J. E., Jr., Galambos, R., and Smith, F. W. (1950). "Temporary deafness following exposure to loud tones and noise," Acta Oto-Laryngol. Suppl. 88.

Erber, N. P. (1968). "Variables that influence sound pressures generated in the ear canal by an audiometric earphone," J. Acoust. Soc. Am. 44, 555–562.

Fletcher, H., and Munson, W. A. (1933). "Loudness, its definition, measurement, and calculation," J. Acoust. Soc. Am. 5, 82–107.

Hildyard, V. H., and Valentine, M. A. (1962). "Collapse of the ear canal during audiometry." Arch. Otolaryngol. 75, 422–423.

International Organization for Standardization (1961). "Normal equal-loudness contours for pure tones and normal threshold of hearing under free-field listening conditions," R226-1961 (available from American National Standards Institute, New York).

International Organization for Standardization (1964). "Standard reference zero for the calibration of pure tone audiometers," R389-1964 (available from American National Standards Institute, New York). Now available as ISO R389-1975 (E).

Killion, M. C. (1976). "Noise of ears and microphones," J. Acoust. Soc. Am. 59, 424–433.

Morgan, D. E., and Dirks, D. D. (1974). "Loudness discomfort level under earphone and in the free field: The effects of calibration methods," J. Acoust. Soc. Am. 56, 172–178.

Munson, W. A., and Wiener, F. M. (1950). "Sound measurements for psychophysical tests," J. Acoust. Soc. Am. 22, 382–386.

Munson, W. A., and Wiener, F. M. (1952). "In search of the Missing 6 dB," J. Acoust. Soc. Am. 24, 498–501.

Northern, J. L., Downs M. P., Rudmose, W., Glorig, A., and Fletcher, J. L. (1972). "Recommended high-frequency audiometric threshold levels (8000–18,000 Hz)" J. Acoust. Soc. Am. 52, 585–595.

Pollack, I. (1948). "Monaural and binaural sensitivity for tones and for white noise," J. Acoust. Soc. Am. 20, 52–57.

Pollack, I. (1949). "Specification of sound-pressure levels," Am. J. Psychol. 62, 412–417.

Robinson, D. W., and Dadson, R. S. (1956). "A re-determination of the equal-loudness relations for pure tones," Br. J. Appl. Phys. 7, 166–181.

Rudmose, W. (1962). "Pressure vs free-field thresholds at low frequencies," Proc. 4th Int. Congr. Acoust., Copenhagen, Paper H52.

Rudmose, W. (1963). "On the lack of agreement between earphone pressures and loudspeaker pressures for loudness balances at low frequencies," J. Acoust. Soc. Am. 35, S1906(A).

Shaw, E. A. G., and Piercy, J. E. (1962). "Audiometry and physiological noise," Proc. 4th Int. Congr. Acoust., Copenhagen, Paper H46.

Shaw, E. A. G. (1966). "Earcanal pressure generated by circumaural and supra-aural earphones," J. Acoust. Soc. Am. 39, 471–479.

Shaw, E. A. G. (1969). "Hearing threshold and earcanal pressure levels with varying acoustic field," J. Acoust. Soc. Am. 46, 1502–1514.

Shaw, E. A. G. (1974). "Transformation of sound pressure level from the free field to the eardrum in the horizontal plane," J. Acoust. Soc. Am. 56, 1848–1861.

Shaw, E. A. G. (1976). "Diffuse field sensitivity of the external ear based on the reciprocity principle," J. Acoust. Soc. Am. 60, S102(A).

Sivian, L. J. (1928) (unpublished.)

Sivian, L. J., and White, S. D. (1933). "On minimum audible sound fields," J. Acoust. Soc. Am. 4, 288–321.

Stream, R. W., and Dirks, D. D. (1974). "Effects of loudspeaker position on difference between earphone and free-field thresholds (MAP and MAF)," J. Speech Hear. Res. 17, 549–568.

Tillman, T., Olsen, W., Killion, M., and Block, M. (1973). "MAP vs MAF for Spondees: Nothing's really missing," presented at Am. Speech Hear. Assoc., Detroit (12 Oct. 1973) (unpublished).

Villchur, E. (1969). "Free-field calibration of earphones," J. Acoust. Soc. Am. 46, 1527–1534.

Villchur, E. (1970). "Audiometer-earphone mounting to improve intersubject and cushion-fit reliability." J. Acoust. Soc. Am. 48, 1387–1396.

Villchur, E. (1972). "Comparison between objective and threshold-shift methods of measuring real-ear attenuation of external sound by earphones," J. Acoust. Soc. Am. 51, 663–664(L).

Villchur, E., and Killion, M. C. (1975). "Probe-tube microphone assembly," J. Acoust. Soc. Am. 57, 238–240.

Weissler, P. G. (1968). "International Standard Reference Zero for Audiometers," J. Acoust. Soc. Am. 44, 264–275.

Wiener, F. M., and Ross, D. A. (1946). "The pressure distribution in the auditory canal in a progressive sound field," J. Acoust. Soc. Am. 18, 401–408.

Yeowart, N. S. and Evans, M. J. (1974). "Thresholds of audibility for very low-frequency pure tones," J. Acoust. Soc. Am. 55, 814–818.

2

Speech Audiometry: Earphone and Sound Field

DONALD D. DIRKS, Ph.D.
Professor, Head and Neck Surgery (Audiology), UCLA School of Medicine, Los Angeles, California

RICHARD W. STREAM, Ph.D.
Associate Professor, Department of Otolaryngology, University of Texas Medical Branch, Galveston, Texas

RICHARD H. WILSON, Ph.D
Chief, Audiology Section, VA Medical Center, Long Beach, California

The relationships between earphone and sound-field speech audiometry have been poorly defined, primarily as a result of the uncertainties of performing sound-field speech testing with precision and validity. This article provides guidelines for specifying the intensity level of spondee words at threshold for loudspeakers at azimuth positions of 0° and 45° from the listener's head. A technique for calibrating the speech stimulus through loudspeakers is suggested. Other related problems, such as the threshold differences between MAP and MAF, and differences in the physical characteristics of loudspeakers and audiometric test rooms are discussed.

Speech audiometry in a sound field* is used extensively in determining performance with a hearing aid and in evaluating the magnitude of hearing loss of children who will not tolerate earphones. The results of such measurements are often suspect due to the lack of a standard specifying the threshold sound pressure level for speech in the sound field. The uncertainty of performing sound-field speech testing with precision and validity has been primarily a result of (1) our limited knowledge of the threshold differences between minimum audible pressure (MAP) and minimum audible field (MAF) for speech, (2) the difficulties of accurately specifying the intensity level of a speech signal, (3) the physical problems created by room acoustics, and (4) the location of the loud-

speakers. This article examines selected aspects of these problem areas and, in some instances, suggests solutions. To facilitate the discussion, representative results from several investigations conducted in the Audiology Research Laboratory at the University of California, Los Angeles, are reported. These results provide guidelines for specifying the intensity level of speech at threshold for loudspeakers located at azimuth positions of 0° and 45° from the listener's head. Since most clinical measurements conducted in the sound field of an audiometric test chamber have been related to earphone results, the difference between sound-field and earphone intensity levels for speech thresholds will be emphasized throughout the paper.

---

*The terms *sound field* and *free field* are used throughout this paper and require brief definition. Free field is here defined as a sound field in which the effects of the boundaries, such as floors, ceiling, and walls, are negligible over the frequency region of interest, in this case, the speech frequency range. A sound field other than the free field refers to those situations in which the field is not free from all bounding surfaces.

Reprinted by permission of the authors from *J. Speech Hearing Dis.*, **37**, 162–176 (1972).

MAP AND MAF THRESHOLD FOR PURE TONES AND SPEECH

To contrast the differences between earphone and free-field listening, it is informative to review briefly some of the relationships between MAP and MAF measurement for pure tones as well as speech. Evidence describing the difference in pure-tone thresholds between MAP and MAF has accumulated from several investigations (Sivian and White, 1933; Munson and Wiener, 1952; Rudmose, 1962). A representative example of this basic relationship is exemplified by recent data collected as part of another study in our laboratory (Stream and Dirks, 1971, unpublished results). The major purpose of the investigation was to determine, particularly for speech, the effects of loudspeaker location on the relationships between free-field and earphone measurements. In the process, however, data were obtained for pure tones as well as spondee words.

Young sophisticated listeners were tested in an anechoic chamber (free field) under loudspeaker (Maximus I) and earphone (TDH-39 encased in MX-41/AR cushions) conditions. For the free-field measurements, the loudspeaker was placed in seven experimental locations in the horizontal plane. These positions were separated by intervals of 30° forming an arc of 180° in the front of the listener. Binaural and monaural thresholds were measured.

Figure 2–1 depicts the effects of earphone and free-field conditions on pure-tone thresholds. The free-field data in this figure are restricted to measurements obtained at 0° azimuth. The graph on the left shows the relationship between the binaural free-field and monaural earphone results. This comparison is identical to that made by Sivian and White in which the classic "6 dB difference" between MAP and MAF was initially described. In the current experiment, the average difference between the two conditions at the test frequencies was 6.9 dB.

Although the left portion of the graph depicts the usual form of listening, binaurally with ears open and monaurally via earphone, a critical comparison between earphone and free-field listening can be made by contrasting parallel listening conditions. Thus, binaural free-field and earphone thresholds are illustrated in the center graph and comparable monaural data are shown in the graph on the right. Notice the similarity in the intensity levels needed to obtain threshold during the MAF and MAP conditions at 500 and 1,000 Hz. This observation is supported by the data of Munson and Wiener and more recently by Villchur (1970). At 250 Hz, however, approximately 8 dB greater intensity is required to obtain threshold by earphone than in the free field. Evidence by Brogden and Miller (1947), Rudmose (1962), and Shaw and Piercy (1962) suggests that the difference between MAP and MAF in the low frequencies may be due partially to physiological noise generated in an enclosed ear canal. To overcome this internal noise factor, it is necessary during earphone conditions to increase intensity to reach threshold. Erber (1968) also reports that an acoustic leak for low and high frequencies may occur due to structural variations in external ears among subjects. Thus, more intensity would be required for real ear as contrasted to artificial ear sound pressure measurement with a constant signal to the earphone. The result is reflected psychophysically in increased intensity required for threshold during MAP conditions. In reviewing the literature neither of these explanations appears to account completely for the difference between the two modes of measurement at low frequencies.

At frequencies above 1,000 Hz, the difference between earphone and free-field thresholds averaged 10 dB. As described by Wiener and Ross (1946), this disparity in the high-frequency region probably reflects free-field enhancement due to a combination of diffraction and resonance effects of the head during MAF and their absence under earphone conditions.

Figure 2–2 illustrates the influence of loudspeaker azimuth position on the monaural free-field threshold. The data were collected with the nontest ear occluded both by a plug (Surg. Mech. Res. #7, 8, or 9) and an earmuff (MSA, Mark II). The combination of these two occluders provided frequency-dependent attenuation of 25 to 45 dB. The decibel difference between the various experimental azimuth positions and 0° is drawn on the ordinate, with the seven loudspeaker positions noted on the abscissa. It is evi-

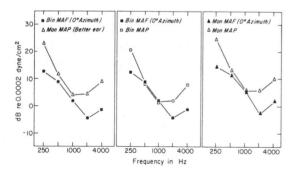

FIGURE 2-1. Comparison of pure-tone MAP and MAF thresholds for binaural and monaural conditions.

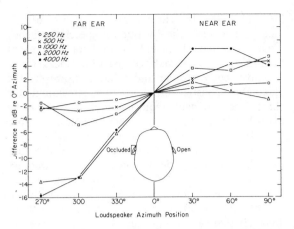

FIGURE 2-2. Average differences in monaural MAF pure-tone thresholds as a function of loudspeaker position.

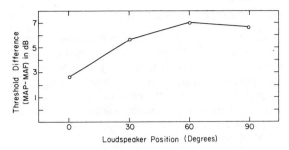

FIGURE 2-3. Spondee threshold differences between MAP and MAF for various loudspeaker positions.

dent that the shadow effects, resulting from the diffraction characteristics of the head, cause an appreciable reduction in the monaural far-ear thresholds, especially for the higher frequencies. In general, thresholds for the monaural near ear improved by 3 to 4 dB as the sound source moved from 0° toward 90°.

Also in the Stream and Dirks study, spondee intelligibility functions were obtained on the same listeners employed in the aforementioned pure-tone investigation. Prior to that investigation, two experiments (Breakey and Davis, 1949; Tillman, Johnson, and Olsen, 1966) had been directed toward the determination of differences between earphone and free-field thresholds for speech. In the Breakey and Davis study, the combined average monaural MAF threshold for spondee words and sentences for normal listeners was 3.4 dB better than comparable earphone results. On the other hand, the normal-hearing and sensorineural hearing loss groups in the Tillman et al. investigation exhibited a 7.5 dB difference between spondee thresholds measured in the free field and those obtained under earphones. The loudspeaker Breakey and Davis used was positioned at 0°, while Tillman et al. collected their data with the loudspeaker 45° from the listener's head. One of the purposes of the Stream and Dirks investigation was to determine whether the comparison of MAP and MAF for speech was altered significantly by changes in the position of the loudspeaker, thereby accounting for the disparity between the two earlier reports.

Figure 2-3 illustrates the difference between earphone and free-field spondee thresholds for monaural near-ear listeners. The data points in the figure were computed by subtracting the earphone thresholds from the free-field monaural near-ear threshold at each azimuth location. Note that the MAP-MAF difference at 0° is 2.8 dB, which compares closely with the 3.4-dB difference between earphone and sound-field thresholds for spondee and sentence materials in the Breakey and Davis report. In the Stream and Dirks data, the largest difference between earphone and free-field listening was 7.0 dB at the 60° azimuth, which is in good agreement with the 7.5-dB difference at 45° reported by Tillman et al. Thus from the data in Figure 2-3 we may conclude that the disparities observed between the earlier studies were due principally to the difference in the location of the loudspeaker. In addition to the loudspeaker location, other parameters of the sound-field environment and calibration of the speech signal need careful consideration.

SPECIFICATION AND CALIBRATION OF SPEECH

Regarding the specification and calibration of speech, three equipment and procedural aspects of the Stream and Dirks experiment and recent investigations in our laboratory are of practical clinical interest—namely, the physical characteristics of the loudspeaker, the method used to calibrate and specify the intensity level of the speech signal, and the relationship between the frequency response of the loudspeaker and the choice of an appropriate calibration signal.

Loudspeaker Characteristics

Figure 2–4 contrasts the frequency response characteristics of a TDH-39 earphone encased in an MX-41/AR cushion (Curve C) and a Maximus I loudspeaker during two physical arrangements (Curves A and B). For the earphone measurement, a constant voltage was maintained across the earphone terminals and the acoustic output, as developed in the NBS 9A coupler, was measured with a condenser microphone (Bruel and Kjaer, 4132) in conjunction with an audio spectrometer (Bruel and Kjaer, 2112). Throughout this paper, unless otherwise specified, all acoustic measurements pertaining to the physical characteristics of the earphone were made in this manner. As shown in Curve C, the output of the earphone is essentially flat below 2,000 Hz, the frequency region wherein the predominant portion of the energy in a speech signal lies. The loudspeaker response was obtained in an anechoic chamber with a constant input of 1.0 volt across the terminals. The condenser microphone (Bruel and Kjaer, 4134), located directly in front of the loudspeaker at a distance of 1 meter, fed its signal to an audiospectrometer (Bruel and Kjaer, 2112). Unless otherwise noted, all subsequent sound-field measurements were made following this procedure. The loudspeaker output (Curve A) exhibits a rather broad spectral response that deviates by no more than ±3 dB between

200 and 7,000 Hz. The frequency response of this loudspeaker is as "flat" within the speech frequency range as we have been able to find for the current experiments. It is a small, compact loudspeaker that is conveniently mobile and reliable; however, the maximum acoustic output is not great enough for clinical measurements requiring levels in excess of 90 dB SPL. While the loudspeaker response is admirably suited for this experiment, the restricted maximum acoustic output of this transducer will reduce its utility in diagnostic and hearing aid evaluatory procedures for individuals with severe hearing loss. Currently it is difficult to find loudspeakers with reasonably flat responses between 200 and 3,000 or 4,000 Hz that can also produce signals of 100 or 110 dB SPL.

Curve B was obtained by the same method as Curve A except that the chair and the head fastener employed to immobilize the listener's head were present. The two curves are shown to demonstrate the minimal changes resulting from the inclusion of the chair and head fastener into the free field. The similarity between Curves A and B indicates the extreme care the investigators took to minimize reflection and baffle effects. This was accomplished by padding all surfaces with two-inch fiberglass insulation covered with muslin.

The comparisons in Figure 2–4 demonstrate two problems inherent in free- or sound-field audiometry: (1) the frequency responses of loudspeakers do not exhibit as flat a response in the speech frequency range as do TDH-39 earphones, and (2) room acoustics and the necessary apparatus, such as chairs, headrests, and tables, may cause further alterations in the sound reaching the ear unless extreme care is taken to provide adequate absorption of reflections from the exposed surfaces. Both of these factors may operate to produce free- or sound-field measurements that are unreliable or invalid.

Intensity Specification of Speech Signals

When using speech as a stimulus, an inherent calibration problem is the difficulty in choosing a method for specifying the intensity level of this rapidly fluctuating signal. According to the American National Standards Institute (ANSI) Specifications for Audiometers (S3.6-1969, p. 15), " . . . the sound pressure level of a speech signal at the earphone is defined as

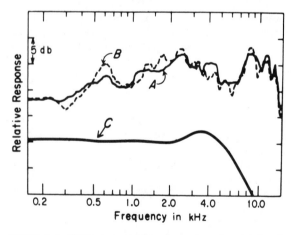

FIGURE 2–4. Frequency response curves for (a) loudspeaker in an empty anechoic chamber, (B) loudspeaker in the experimental arrangement, and (C) TDH-39 earphone encased in an MX 41/AR cushion.

the rms sound pressure level . . . of a 1,000 Hz signal adjusted so that the VU meter deflection produced by the 1,000 Hz signal is equal to the average peak VU meter deflection produced by the speech signal.'' The spondee words in the Stream and Dirks investigation were recorded in this manner. However, the use of a 1,000-Hz tone as the calibrating signal for speech has certain limitations when transducers such as loudspeakers are employed that lack a flat frequency response in the region wherein the predominant energy of the experimental signal (speech) is located. Deviations in the constancy of the output between several loudspeakers will almost always be larger if the calibrating stimulus is a pure tone rather than a wide-band signal. As an illustration of this problem, the following comparison was performed in an anechoic chamber. The electrical signal of a 1,000-Hz tone and the peaks of a speech spectrum noise were individually set at 1.0 volt across the terminals of three loudspeakers of the same model (Maximus I). The levels for each signal were read on the meter of an audio spectrometer (Bruel and Kjaer, 2112) whose speed was set to the slow position. The manufacturer (Bruel and Kjaer Instructions and Application Manual for Model 2112) states that both speeds of meter reaction available on the equipment are in accordance with proposed IEC standards for precision sound level meters. It is, however, practically easier and more reliable to read the level of a fluctuating signal on the slow speed. The physical measurements were conducted in the same manner as described earlier, with the exception that the final read-out was made on a graphic level recorder (Bruel and Kjaer, 2305). The results from the loudspeakers are shown at the left of Figure 2–5. Notice that comparable intensity levels from the loudspeakers differ by a maximum of 5 dB when the 1,000-Hz tone was used. In contrast, the corresponding speech spectrum noise levels are practically identical regardless of

loudspeaker. Our experiences with other loudspeakers indicate that the difference of 5 dB at any one frequency is minimal for these transducers and often much greater when loudspeakers of different manufacturers are compared. Spondee thresholds on several subjects with normal hearing were obtained with each loudspeaker. The voltages required to reach spondee thresholds were essentially the same for each loudspeaker as long as speech spectrum noise was used as the calibration signal. When a 1,000-Hz tone was employed, the voltages required to obtain spondee threshold varied by an equivalent of 6 dB between loudspeakers 2 and 3. Thus, if the 1,000-Hz tone had been used to specify the intensity level of the speech for each loudspeaker, the suggested difference in the threshold between loudspeakers 2 and 3 would have been 6 dB.

A second comparison was undertaken to demonstrate the absence of the foregoing problem with another transducer that had an essentially flat response. A 1,000-Hz tone and speech spectrum noise (peak levels) were again used as calibrating signals, but in this instance delivered to two TDH-39 earphones at a constant voltage. The acoustic outputs were measured in an NBS-9A coupler. The results are shown in the right half of Figure 2–5. Since the earphones are essentially flat below 2,000 Hz, the relative output levels from the two earphones are identical regardless of whether the calibrating signal is a pure tone or speech spectrum noise. As predicted, the empirical results also showed that the voltage levels necessary to reach spondee thresholds were identical for each earphone regardless of whether noise or a pure tone was used. The measurements depicted in Figure 2–5, together with the empirical results, demonstrated forcefully that even minor deviations between loudspeakers that are reasonably flat (± 3 dB) will produce significant differences in the measured intensity level of a speech signal if a pure tone is used to specify the level of the speech.

Choice of Calibrating Signal

The appropriate calibrating signal for speech must now be considered. Since the ANSI Standard for Audiometers (1969) has defined the intensity level of speech in terms of a 1,000-Hz tone for earphone listening, it seems appropriate that this procedure be adhered to unless future evidence indicates otherwise. For the sound-field calibration of a speech

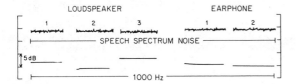

FIGURE 2-5. Output level recordings of three loudspeakers and two earphones for speech spectrum noise and a 1,000-Hz tone.

stimulus, however, the irregularities in the frequency response of loudspeakers obviously does not permit the use of the same procedure as utilized with earphones. For calibration purposes, it seems advisable to enlist a wide-band signal rather than a pure tone in order to minimize the irregularities in loudspeaker response characteristics. Speech spectrum random noise seems desirable, since it approximates the spectral configuration of the stimulus signal and yet does not exhibit the extremely rapid fluctuations of the speech itself. Thus, the calibrating signal can be conveniently read on a VU meter with reliability. For practical purposes, a meter with a speed of reaction time similar to that found on an audio spectrometer (Bruel and Kjaer, 2112), when set to the slow position, or a meter such as found on a Grason-Stadler 162 Speech Audiometer is useful. Lilly (1967) has described some of the problems associated with differences in the ballistics and calibration among commercially available measuring meters. Any final solutions to the present problem of calibrating the speech signal will require strict specification of the ballistics of the meter used to measure the signal as well as in recording the words.

As suggested by Tillman, Johnson, and Olsen (1966), a noise signal produced by a random noise generator (Grason-Stadler, E5539A) has been found useful for specifying the intensity level of speech. This speech spectrum noise has essentially equal energy per cycle up to approximately 1,000 Hz after which it falls at the rate of 6 dB/octave. The choice of signal was somewhat of a compromise, since the spectral characteristics of this noise band represent only a close approximation to reported average speech spectrum curves (Dunn and White, 1940; Rudmose, 1944). Some discrepancies among the speech spectrum curves have been reported, however. Since the noise signal chosen represents an approximation that is close to the described long-term spectral configuration of speech, it seems to be useful. In summary, it is suggested that a noise signal having the spectral configuration of the long-term connected discourse be used as a calibration signal for speech in free- or sound-field environments. The amplitude of the noise should be adjusted so that it produces a deflection on a measuring meter equivalent to the average peak level of the speech. Finally, extreme care must be taken to choose loudspeakers adequate for the desired purpose and to position them in the test room so that the frequency characteristics are not distorted substantially with the described test spectrum.

SPONDEE THRESHOLD IN FREE FIELD

The purpose of the experiment was to determine whether a clinical test procedure administered to unsophisticated listeners would produce an MAF-MAP comparison for spondee words similar to the results of the previous, more rigidly controlled, investigation. The test procedure used by Stream and Dirks for obtaining spondee thresholds required the presentation of ten words at four intensities covering a range of 12 dB. Since this procedure is not easily adaptable to clinic use, a shorter and more direct procedure than used in the previous study was desirable. Initially, subjects heard each of the 36 spondee words at a comfortable listening level. Starting approximately 10 dB above threshold, pairs of words were then presented in a descending manner in 2-dB steps. Thus, two spondee words were administered at each of the 2-dB decrements until five out of six words were missed, at which time the test was terminated and the 50 percent point for threshold was calculated. This procedure is reminiscent of the one suggested for the W-2 spondee word lists.

Nineteen young adults with normal hearing served as listeners. Each subject listened to spondee words during three free-field conditions (at 0° azimuth, and at 45° to either side of center) and via earphone. Speech spectrum noise, used for calibration purposes, was recorded so that its peak amplitude was at a level equivalent to the average peak level of the spondee words. A 1,000-Hz tone was also recorded at the same level as the noise so that it could be used later as a check on our earphone calibration. Earphone and free-field calibration procedures, described earlier, were carried out.

The results from the experimental conditions are shown in Table 2-1. The earphone/0° free-field threshold difference was 3.6 dB, while the difference between earphone and 45° free-field thresholds was 7.5 dB. These findings are in agreement with data

TABLE 2-1. MEAN THRESHOLDS FOR SPONDEE WORDS DURING TEST AND RETEST AT VARIOUS EXPERIMENTAL CONDITIONS (IN dB RE 0.002 DYNES /CM^2).

Condition	Test	Retest	Combined
Earphone	19.2	18.5	18.9
Free Field 0°	15.6	15.1	15.4
Free Field 45°	11.9	10.9	11.4
Difference (1–2)	3.6	3.4	3.5
Difference (1–3)	7.3	7.6	7.5

TABLE 2-2. COMPARISON OF MAP-MAF THRESHOLD DIFFERENCES (SPONDEES) IN DECIBELS (ROUNDED TO NEAREST 0.5 dB) FOR FOUR INVESTIGATIONS.

Investigation	Loudspeaker Location				
	0°	30°	45°	60°	90°
Breakey and Davis, 1949	3.5	—	—	—	—
Tillman et al., 1966	—	—	7.5	—	—
Stream and Dirks, 1977	3.0	5.0	—	7.0	5.0
Current Data 1971					
(Test and Retest)	3.5	—	7.5	—	—
Average	3.5	5.0	7.5	7.0	5.0

from Breakey and Davis, and Tillman, Johnson, and Olsen, as well as from the Stream and Dirks study.

Table 2-2 summarizes the difference in decibel values between earphone and free-field listening for spondee words from four pertinent studies. Of particular interest is the similarity in the results between investigations at the 0° and 45° free-field locations. The relations in the table indicate that for 0 dB HL the intensity level of the spondee words should be 3.5 dB lower than the same signal delivered via an earphone when the loudspeaker is at 0° azimuth. However, if the sound-field measurements are conducted at a 45° azimuth position, the intensity level of the speech signal should be 7.5 dB lower than the equivalent earphone output.

SOUND-FIELD SPEECH AUDIOMETRY

Subsequent to the free-field investigation, it was of interest to determine the utility of the MAF-MAP differences at the 0° and 45° azimuth positions in the sound field of a prefabricated audiometric test room that is used in many clinics. The inside dimensions of the test room (IAC 1200 series) were approximately 7 × 7 × 6.5'. The interior walls of the test room are formed by steel panels perforated with small holes and backed with an acoustic filter. The floor was covered by a commercially available rubber pad. The major acoustic problems encountered in sound field are related to reflections from the boundaries. In this regard, special efforts were made to find the most advantageous location for the loudspeaker in the test room as a means of minimizing the effects of reflections. Selected aspects of this problem are instructive.

Frequency response characteristic curves, shown in Figure 2-6, were obtained for one loudspeaker

(Maximus I) under three room conditions. Curve A was obtained in an anechoic chamber, while Curve B was obtained in the same audiometric test room as Curve C but with the loudspeaker 1.5 feet from the wall with the microphone near the center of the room. The walls of the test room were lined with 1.5-inch thick fiberglass material lined with muslin. The microphone was placed one meter from the loudspeaker in each setting, and the pure-tone input at the terminals of the transducer was held constant at 1.0 volt. The same attenuator-amplifier complex and loudspeaker volume-control settings were used for all frequency-response measurements. Since Curve A was obtained in an empty anechoic chamber, it represents the response of the loudspeaker itself and therefore can be used as a reference.

Curve B shows a large reduction in output at the microphone in the frequency regions around 250–350 Hz and 600–900 Hz, while the intensity level around 350–500 Hz was enhanced. By changing the loudspeaker position, we determined that much of the signal distortion in the low frequencies was due to the sound radiating from the side walls adjacent to the loudspeaker. The reflected sound from these walls either reinforced or interfered with the sound passing directly in front of the loudspeaker and toward the microphone. The results in Curve C demonstrate that positioning the loudspeaker away from and out of the corner resulted in a more favorable response at the microphone, especially in the speech frequency

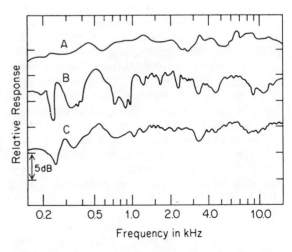

FIGURE 2-6. Frequency response curves for the same loudspeaker (A) in an anechoic chamber, (B) in one corner of an audiometric test room, and (C) 1.5 ft from the wall in an audiometric test room.

range. Felt, fiberglass, or other sound-absorptive materials of this type placed on the walls behind the loudspeaker had little effect on the low frequencies. The principle operating in this instance is that sound absorption depends on the wave length of the signal and the relative thickness of the absorbing materials. Sounds whose wave lengths are not long as compared with the thickness of the material will be readily absorbed and vice versa. Consequently in the higher frequencies, fiberglass or thick curtains may be more effective in reducing reflected energy. The reduction of the peaks and troughs in the high frequencies of Curve C are primarily the result of covering the walls and selected portions of the ceiling with fiberglass materials.

Spondee thresholds were obtained at 0° aximuth in each condition for two sophisticated listeners, to determine the influence of the different frequency response curves on speech thresholds. Repeated spondee thresholds for the listeners in the anechoic chamber were 15 dB SPL. For the environmental condition represented by Curve B the threshold was increased by 4.5 dB to 19.5 dB SPL. When the loudspeaker was moved and selected wall areas covered with absorbing materials, the threshold (Curve C) was 14 dB SPL, which compares favorably with the threshold obtained in the anechoic chamber. From these findings, we conclude that if speech thresholds are desired that can be compared with those in other test rooms, extreme care must be taken regarding all facets of the measurement.

Further measurements of room reflections were carried out in the anechoic chamber, in the test room, and in the test room modified with absorptive material. The oscilloscopic response of the loudspeaker for four cycles of a 1,000-Hz tone (Wavetek Model 116) is shown in Figure 2-7. The time base on the scope was set at 5 msec/cm. The upper response curve in Section A shows the signal as presented to the loudspeaker and the lower response curve is the output of the loudspeaker in an anechoic chamber. As you may observe, the lower response curve shows a brief "after ring" that is common for loudspeakers but minimal in this particular transducer. The response in Section B was obtained from the same loudspeaker located in an empty audiometric test room. The microphone was positioned in the center of the room, and the loudspeaker was set 1.5 feet from the wall. Observe the persistence of energy following the offset of the tone caused by reflections from the different surfaces in the room. Reflected

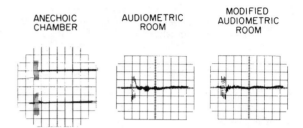

FIGURE 2-7. Oscilloscopic response of the same loudspeaker for 4 cycles of a 1,000-Hz tone (A) in an anechoic chamber, (B) in an empty audiometric test room, and (C) in an empty audiometric test room with walls partially covered by sound absorption materials.

energy extends throughout the period shown on the oscilloscope that is largest during the initial 10–20 msec following the termination of the tone. In Section C, the response was obtained in the same setting as in B, but 1.5-inch thick strips of fiberglass materials were placed on the ceiling, floor, and walls of the room. Notice that some reflections were still present but became minimal shortly after the offset of the tone. Reflection in these rooms is difficult to eliminate even when all major surfaces are covered and the loudspeaker and microphone are placed in the most advantageous positions. Thicker layers of fiberglass may have been advisable but even then all surfaces including the window and lights would have to be covered to eliminate reflections.

Such drastic modifications as employed for these experimental measurements are impractical in clinical settings. Thus, our experience suggests that meaningful results from speech sound-field audiometry on various individuals may be obtained and compared if the measurements are made in the same room. This statement implies that precautions are taken to optimize the frequency response of the loudspeaker by determining the optimal room location of the loudspeaker and the listener, and that efforts are made to eliminate or reduce room reflections. Currently, test rooms and loudspeakers and their locations in the room are so varied that direct test comparisons beyond a particular room environment may often lead to gross errors. The measurement errors inherent in each of the various parameters studied may be considered clinically trivial since most differences between psychophysical measurements do not exceed 6 dB. However, the problems due to changes in the loudspeaker position, the physical characteristics of the loudspeakers, and poor room acoustics may accumulate to produce errors far exceeding 5 to 10 dB. The probable accumulation and often unpredictable nature of these errors make imperative the careful physical evaluation of the test room and equipment used for sound-field measurements. Perhaps our results will encourage further study of these problems and renewed efforts by clinicians, researchers, and manufacturers toward standardization in the area of sound-field speech audiometry.

The results of these experiments indicate that before conducting sound-field audiometry the following points should be considered:

First, two guidelines are now available for specifying the intensity level of speech at threshold for earphones and in the sound field. The ANSI 1969 standard suggested that reference threshold sound pressure level for speech from a TDH-39 earphone is 20 dB above 0.0002 microbar as measured in an NBS 9A coupler. Next, the results of the four investigations reviewed in this paper indicated that the reference sound pressure level for speech threshold in the free field at 0° azimuth is approximately 3.5 dB lower than the same signal via earphones. If the loudspeaker is placed at a 45° azimuth position the dB hearing level for speech is approximately 7.5 dB lower than the same signal via earphone.

Second, the results of a frequency analysis of loudspeaker indicated that the use of a 1,000-Hz tone as the calibrating signal in free or sound field has certain limitations. For precision, it is suggested that the intensity level of the speech signal be specified in terms of a speech spectrum noise adjusted so that its peaks as well as those of a 1,000-Hz tone and the speech stimulus drive a VU meter to the same designated setting.

Third, a loudspeaker should be selected that has a reasonably flat response throughout the frequency range of the test stimulus.

Fourth, the reasonably flat output of the loudspeaker must be maintained at the location where the listener will be positioned. To accomplish this, physical and empirical measurements should be made to determine the optimal location in the test room for the loudspeaker as well as the listener.

ACKNOWLEDGMENT

This research was supported by U.S. Public Health Service Grant NS–5873 and by National Institutes of Health Career Development Award NS 13,341 to Donald D. Dirks. The authors wish to thank Deborah R. Bower for help in data collection and Bruce Walker for assistance in measurements of room acoustics.

REFERENCES

American National Standards Institute. *American National Standards Specifications for Audiometers* (S.3.6–1969). New York, N.Y. (1969).

Breakey, M. R., and Davis, H. Comparisons of thresholds for speech; word and sentence tests; receiver vs field and monaural vs binaural listening. *Laryngoscope,* 59, 236–250 (1949).

Brogden, W. J., and Miller, G. A. Physiological noise generated under earphone cushions. *J. acoust. Soc. Amer.,* 19, 620–623 (1947).

Dunn, H. K., and White, S. D. Statistical measurements on conversational speech. *J. acoust. Soc. Amer.,* 11, 288 (1940).

Erber, N. P. Variables that influence sound pressures generated in the ear canal by an audiometric earphone. *J. acoust. Soc. Amer.,* 44, 555–562 (1968).

Lilly, D. Disc and tape reproduction systems. Paper presented at the Annual Convention of the American Speech and Hearing Association, Chicago (1967).

Munson, W. A., and Wiener, F. M. In search of the missing 6 dB. *J. acoust. Soc. Amer.,* 24, 498–501 (1952).

Rudmose, W. Effects of high altitude on the human voice. Office of Scientific Research and Development Rept. 3106, Washington, D.C. (1944).

Rudmose, W. Pressure vs free field thresholds at low frequency. *Proceedings of the Fourth International Congress on Acoustics.* Copenhagen: Organization Committee of the 4th ICA and Harlang and Toksvig (1962).

Shaw, E. A. G., and Piercy, J. E. Physiological noise in relation to audiometry. *J. acoust. Soc. Amer.,* 34, 745 (1962).

Sivian, L. J., and White, S. D. On minimum audible sound fields. *J. acoust. Soc. Amer.,* 4, 288–321 (1933).

Tillman, T. W., Johnson, R. M., and Olsen, W. O. Earphone versus sound-field threshold sound-pressure levels for spondee words. *J. acoust. Soc. Amer.,* 39, 125–133 (1966).

Villchur, E. Audiometer-earphone mounting to improve inter-subject and cushion-fit reliability. *J. acoust. Soc. Amer.,* 48, 1387–1396 (1970).

Wiener, F. M., and Ross, D. A. The pressure distribution in the auditory canal in a progressive sound field. *J. acoust. Soc. Amer.,* 18, 401–407 (1946).

3

A Clinical Method for Calibrating the Bone-Conduction Audiometer

ROBERT E. ROACH, Ph.D.
Professor of Audiology, and Director, Hearing Clinic, Department of Biocommunication, School of Medicine, University of Alabama in Birmingham
RAYMOND CARHART, Ph.D.
Professor of Audiology, Northwestern University when this article was prepared

The clinician who wishes to make full use of pure-tone audiograms needs a valid and simple method for ensuring that the calibration for his bone-conduction system is adequate. Unfortunately, we lack a standard procedure whereby the physicist can specify for us the vibrational output representing bone-conduction norms (Carlisle and Pearson, 1951; Beranek, 1949). For the time being the clinician must therefore rely upon his own efforts to assure himself that his bone measurements are acceptable. Even after a physical standard is established, the need will remain for an easy and adequate method of checking calibration in a clinical situation.

There are three calibrational methods from which the clinician can choose. The first method utilizes loudness balancing, the second is based on thresholds yielded by normal listeners, while the third relies on the responses of cases with sensorineural (or nerve-type) loss.

The loudness-balance method is advocated by Beranek as a means of transferring air-conduction norms to a bone-conduction system. However, the technique possesses three practical disadvantages. First, the equipment necessary for loudness matching is not available in all clinical situations. Second, recent studies of "on-effect" and "adaptation" (Hallpike and Hood, 1951; Dix and Hood, 1953) clearly imply that very insightful control of the conditions must be maintained for loudness balances to be valid. Lastly, the matching of a bone-conduction sound to the loudness of a monaural air-borne stimulus will be in error because the bone-conduction stimulus will reach both ears unless the contralateral ear is effectively masked (Zwislocki, 1949). Consequently, insofar as the clinical situation is concerned, there is need for a simpler yet valid procedure.

A second approach is to establish the reference values for a bone-conduction system by averaging the bone thresholds exhibited by subjects with normal hearing.[1] This approach has high face validity, and it has been widely accepted. It is, for example, the method which was specified in the American Medical Association requirements for a diagnostic pure-tone audiometer (Council on Physical Medicine and Rehabilitation, 1951). These requirements define the reference threshold, at each test frequency, as the "hearing loss setting of the audiometer" representing the average of the bone thresholds obtained on six subjects with normal acuity. Only measurements on unoccluded ears are to be considered, and all tests are to be conducted " . . . in a room free from extraneous sound of sufficient intensity to vitiate the measurements" (Council on Physical Medicine and Rehabilitation, 1951). Unfortunately, there are numerous clinical situations where this last requirement cannot be easily met. Many audiometric rooms which are adequate for testing normal listeners when they have the extra protection of ear cushions possess ambient noise which is intense enough to mask these same persons when their ears are unoccluded. In other words, a room may be fully usable for air-condition audiometry without being quiet enough to yield uncontaminated measures of normal threshold for bone. In practice, this fact means that the wise clinician will not attempt to calibrate his bone-conduction system on normal ears unless he is certain the noise level in his testing room is so low it will not influence his subjects.

The third method, which utilizes the responses of persons with hearing loss, was described by Carhart as a means of escaping the influences of unavoidable room noise (Carhart, 1950). The method allows the clinician to take advantage of two facts. First, a moderate hearing loss offers protection against the masking effect of mild ambient noise. Second, persons with pure sensorineural loss possess the same impairment whether tested by air or by bone. The procedure involves obtaining both air- and bone-conduction thresholds, in a reasonably quiet room, on a group of ears with impairments of the sensorineural variety. The responses at each test frequency are averaged separately for air and for bone. The clinician must have assured himself in advance that his air-conduction system is in acceptable calibration. This being the case, substantial discrepancies between the two sets of averages represent the corrections required to bring the bone system into calibration. It is a simple matter, once this information is available, to apply these corrections in subsequent clinical testing. Audiometric curves incorporating these corrections should show the proper relation between a patient's loss by bone and the normal reference line on the audiogram chart.

While Carhart's method appears theoretically sound and it is adaptable to most situations, we still need to assure ourselves through appropriate experimentation that it can yield a valid reference level for bone-conduction audiometry. Here, the obvious test of validity is whether normal ears exhibit the anticipated threshold readings for bone when tested with a system calibrated on ears with sensorineural involvement. Validatory measurements must, of course, be made in an environment sufficiently quiet to avoid danger of any masking when testing by either modality. If, under these circumstances, the normal group's average audiogram for air agrees with its average audiogram for bone, Carhart's method will have been shown to be capable of yielding a valid "zero loss" level from which to estimate hearing acuity by bone conduction.[2] In other words, the final criterion for validity of a threshold reference level is that persons without hearing loss shall obtain thresholds which are labeled as normal when they are tested with the system under scrutiny.

The degree to which Carhart's proposal can satisfy this criterion was explored experimentally with a commercial audiometer. The adequacy of this instrument's air-conduction system was first assured through appropriate electroacoustic measurements. Next, a corrected calibration for its bone-conduction system was computed from the responses of 23 ears having sensorineural, or nerve-type, impairments. Thirdly, thresholds for air and bone were obtained on 127 normal ears. Finally, these data were examined statistically to ascertain the adequacy of the corrected calibration assigned to the bone-conduction system.

APPARATUS

The audiometer selected was a Maico E-2.[3] To simplify procedures, only one of the instrument's two channels was employed throughout the study. Both the air- and the bone-conduction receivers were activated through this channel. The air-conduction receiver was a Permoflux PDR-10, in a Maico cushion. The bone-conduction receiver was of the hearing-aid variety.[4]

The physical performance of the audiometer was assessed carefully.[5] The instrument satisfied the requirements for a diagnostic audiometer (Council on Physical Medicine and Rehabilitation, 1951). Test frequencies were within appropriate limits of accuracy. The attenuation system was acceptably linear. Harmonic distortion was adequately controlled. The instrument was suitably free from internal noise, and its bone oscillator did not produce excess sound radiation by air.

The acoustic output of the air-conduction system was measured, in a 6 cc. coupler of the 9A type, with a 640AA microphone. The sound pressure levels for the "zero hearing loss" settings of the audiometer were found to be within 3 dB of the correct value for the earphone involved, except for a discrepancy of 4.6 dB at 8,000 cps. These values are within the limits designated for commercial audiometers (American Standards Association). On this basis we can state that the air-conduction system employed in the present study was correctly calibrated within the accuracy required for clinical audiometry.

The vibrational output of the bone-conduction oscillator was investigated, in relative terms, with an artificial mastoid.[6] The performance of the bone-conduction channel proved quite satisfactory except for some excess harmonic distortion at high output levels for 250 cps.

Special precautions were taken to assure that the audiometer remained stable throughout the entire time span of the study. These precautions involved daily measurement of the acoustic and vibrational outputs of the air and bone channels, respectively. Analysis of these measurements revealed excellent stability in physical performance.

EMPIRICAL CALIBRATION OF THE BONE-CONDUCTION SYSTEM

In order to obtain a group on which to establish an empirical calibration of the bone-conduction system, 23 persons with pure sensorineural losses of intermediate severity were chosen from the case files of the Northwestern University Hearing Clinic. All these persons had been diagnosed by staff otologists as having pure sensorineural (or nerve-type) hearing losses. There were 5 cases of presbycusis, 2 of labyrinthine hydrops, 2 with congenital impairments, and 14 due to miscellaneous or unknown causes. No attempt was made to control the sex or age distribution of the group. The group included 12 men and 11 women. The age range was from 17 to 77 years, with an average age of 50.7 years.

Each subject was given an audiometric test by both air and bone in a room with superior acoustic characteristics. The ascending method, as advocated by Hughson and Westlake (1944), was employed. Only the data for each subject's better ear were used. Consequently, masking was not employed. To obtain bone measurements the oscillator was first positioned at the point on the mastoid yielding maximum sensitivity with 1,000 cps as the stimulus. Thresholds for all frequencies were then determined without shifting the bone unit. Subjects were closely questioned to ascertain whether the sensation was contralateralized. Properly ipsilateralized threshold responses for bone were obtained from 23 subjects at 250 cps, 18 at 500 cps, 21 at 1,000 cps, 18 at 1,500 cps, 16 at 2,000 cps, 13 at 3,000 cps, and 19 at 4,000 cps. These responses, and their comparison responses for air conduction, constitute the data from which the empirical calibration of the bone system was compiled.

Table 3–1 summarizes, in the form of means for the group, the results at each frequency. The table also reports the difference, or discrepancy, at a given frequency between the mean for air thresholds and

TABLE 3–1. MEAN AUDIOMETRIC SETTINGS REPRESENTING THE AIR-CONDUCTION AND THE BONE-CONDUCTION THRESHOLDS OF TWENTY-THREE EARS WITH SENSORINEURAL IMPAIRMENT (EXPRESSED IN DECIBELS RE THE ZERO SETTING OF THE HEARING-LOSS DIAL).

Frequency	Air	Bone	Difference Between Settings
250	13.7	37.2	23.5
500	20.3	46.1	25.8
1,000	39.0	41.9	2.9
1,500	44.7	49.2	4.5
2,000	43.4	49.7	6.3
3,000	42.4	50.0	7.6
4,000	42.9	43.2	0.3

the mean for bone thresholds. These discrepancies, according to Carhart's premise, represent the approximate corrections required to equate the air- and bone-conduction systems.

Higher hearing-loss dial readings were required to reach bone-conduction thresholds than to reach air-conduction thresholds at all frequencies except 4,000 cps. This fact indicates that, at a given dial reading, the bone-conduction system produced a weaker stimulus in the inner ear than did the air-conduction system at the same frequency. Since, in the present instance, the air-conduction system was found to be in satisfactory calibration, the various discrepanceis were judged to reveal the amounts by which bone-conduction reading obtained with this particular audiometer should be reduced in order to yield true indications of the thresholds they represent. In other words, corrected thresholds, estimated to the nearest 5 dB, should be computed by subtracting the following values from the hearing-loss dial readings when testing by bone:

25 dB at	250 cps
25 dB at	500 cps
5 dB at	1,000 cps
5 dB at	1,500 cps
5 dB at	2,000 cps
10 dB at	3,000 cps
None at	4,000 cps

Stated differently, these corrections represent the establishment of empirically revised norms for measuring bone-conduction acuity with the audiometer under study.

VALIDATORY TEST OF EMPIRICAL CALIBRATION

The question which interests us now is whether corrections established by the method just outlined are valid in the sense that they yield the same base of reference as would have been computed directly from the bone-conduction responses of normal ears. This question is easily attacked. One must first administer pure-tone tests to a group of subjects known to have normal hearing. One must then compare the estimate of the group's acuity by air with its apparent acuity by bone. Provided the two estimates of acuity are in close agreement, the bone system may be said to have essentially the same base of reference as the air-conduction system.

In the present instance, 127 college undergraduates constituted the group of normal listeners employed to make this test.[7] The age range of the group was from 17 to 27 years, with the mean age being 18.5 years. The group included 44 men and 83 women.

This phase of the study required a testing room so quiet that its ambient noise would not mask unoccluded normal ears. The room used had a noise level of less than 24 dB when measured with a sound-level meter set to the A scale.

Thresholds for both air and bone were again determined by the ascending method. It had been decided to use data on only one ear per subject. Selection of this ear was random except in those instances where the bone-conduction stimulus appeared to the subject to be contralateralized.[8] When this occurred, the data for the other ear were used unless contralateralization was also evident here, in which event the subject was discarded. The 127 subjects whose thresholds were analyzed each had an ear satisfying this criterion.

The threshold responses for air conduction were recorded without modification, but audiometric readings were corrected by the values mentioned earlier, in order to obtain the estimated thresholds for bone.[9] The criterion by which the validity of the empirical calibration of the bone system was judged was the agreement to be found between the air-conduction thresholds of the 127 normal ears under study and the corrected measures of their bone-conduction acuity.

Table 3–2 summarizes group means for air and for bone. All group means for air conduction are nega-

TABLE 3–2. MEAN ACUITY FOR THE BETTER EAR EXHIBITED BY 127 UNIVERSITY STUDENTS (EXPRESSED AS DECIBELS OF HEARING LOSS RE THE CORRECTED AUDIOMETRIC NORMAL).

Frequency	Air Mean	Bone Mean	Difference*	t-Ratio†
250	−7.3	−5.5	−1.8	5.43
500	−5.9	−6.9	1.0	3.49
1,000	−4.8	−5.9	1.1	3.59
1,500	−4.9	−6.4	1.5	3.90
2,000	−3.9	−3.5	−0.4	1.04
3,000	−3.9	−4.5	0.6	1.38
4,000	−6.7	−4.2	−2.5	6.03

*A negative difference indicates poorer bone-conduction threshold.

†t-Ratio of 1.98 and 2.62 significant, respectively, at 5 percent and 1 percent levels.

tive. This fact indicates that the 127 ears under study were, as a group, slightly hyperacute relative to the "average normal threshold." This result is exactly what would be expected in testing a large group of young college students, and it is consistent with other investigations of undergraduates at Northwestern University.

Group means for bone conduction were also negative to approximately the same degree. As is summarized in Table 3–2, the discrepancy between the means for air and bone conduction is 1.5 dB or less for five of the seven test frequencies. The differences which exceeded 1.5 dB were 1.8 dB at 250 cps and 2.5 dB at 4,000 cps. Even these two latter discrepancies are small enough to be of little importance to the clinician. Moreover, the means for air conduction are not consistently higher or lower than the means for bone.

Despite the fact that the discrepancies just mentioned are too small to have much clinical meaning, most of them were statistically significant. Specifically, five of the seven t-ratios reported in Table 3–2 substantially exceed the 1 percent level of confidence. One may conclude that the discrepancies are a result of a minor yet real margin of uncertainty arising because correction values could be assigned to the bone-conduction system only to the nearest 5 dB interval. For this reason alone, any single correction might deviate by as much as 2.5 dB from the proper value. Fortunately, a systematic calibrational deviation of 2.5 dB or less does not destroy the clinical meaning of a bone-conduction measurement.

In the present instance, there is absolutely no evidence that the method employed for calibrating the bone-conduction system yielded a false base of references. The audiometer labeled normal ears as having, in the aggregate, the bone-conduction acuity which their measured acuity for air conduction required. Thus, calibration of the bone-conduction system on the basis of responses by patients with sensorineural loss has here been demonstrated to yield reference values which are clinically equivalent to those which would have been obtained had the calibration been based on the responses of normal ears.

Further confirmation of the general adequacy of the bone-conduction measurements obtained on the 127 normal ears is found in (1) comparison of population variability for the two stimulus modalities and (2) correlation between the air- and bone-conduction thresholds.

As regards population variability, the two modalities yielded threshold data which were very similar in range and distribution. This fact is illustrated in Table 3–3.

It is particularly instructive to observe the differences between the standard deviations for air and bone which are reported in the sixth column of the table.[10] These differences are all numerically small and do not represent a clinically important distinction in the variability of air- and bone-conduction results for the 127 normal ears under consideration.

The correlation between the air- and bone-conduction thresholds exhibited by individual subjects was found to be very good, as can be seen by noting the product-moment coefficients reported in Table

TABLE 3–4. COEFFICIENTS OF CORRELATION BETWEEN THE THRESHOLDS FOR AIR CONDUCTION AND THE CORRECTED THRESHOLDS FOR BONE CONDUCTION.

Frequency	Product-Moment r
250	0.48
500	0.57
1,000	0.65
1,500	0.58
2,000	0.60
3,000	0.76
4,000	0.64

3–4. The coefficients range between $+0.48$ and $+0.76$. Coefficients of this magnitude indicate a high interdependence, since they were derived from data on normal ears which encompassed relatively narrow ranges. Theoretically, such interdependence should exist if the testing environment and the testing procedures are adequate. Its manifestation in the present instance adds greatly to the confidence we may have in both the air- and bone-conduction measurements obtained on the 127 normal ears. We therefore accept these measurements with greater surety as a means of confirming the adequacy of Carhart's empirical method for establishing the zero reference level for a bone-conduction system.

COMMENT

It has often been emphasized that the median is a more accurate statement of the central tendency of data involving decibel values than the mean (Stevens, 1955). Hence, if the primary interest in the present study had been to express the numerical values of the central tendencies with the greatest precision, medians should have been used. However, the main concern in the present instance was with the discrepancy between the central tendencies in the air- and bone-conduction measures obtained on the 23 cases with sensorineural loss. There is no reason to believe that the span between these central tendencies would have been more accurately expressed by considering medians than means. The same argument applies when comparing the threshold data yielded by the 127 normals. Hence, since tests of statistical significance are more easily applied when means are employed, the latter were chosen as the basis for the analysis reported above.

TABLE 3–3. RANGES AND STANDARD DEVIATIONS OF THRESHOLDS FOR AIR CONDUCTION AND FOR BONE CONDUCTION EXHIBITED BY 127 NORMAL EARS, EXPRESSED IN DECIBELS.

Frequency	Range		Standard Deviation		
	Air	Bone	Air	Bone	Difference*
250	17.5	15.0	3.3	3.9	0.6
500	15.0	17.5	3.8	3.5	0.3
1,000	17.5	17.5	3.9	4.4	−0.5
1,500	22.5	15.0	4.7	4.6	0.1
2,000	20.0	20.0	5.2	5.9	0.7
3,000	42.5	37.5	7.0	6.3	0.7
4,000	25.0	30.0	5.1	5.6	−0.5

*A negative difference indicates that the S.D. for bone is greater than the S.D. for air.

TABLE 3-5. MEDIAN AUDIOMETRIC SETTINGS
REPRESENTING THE AIR-CONDUCTION AND BONE-
CONDUCTION THRESHOLDS OF TWENTY-THREE EARS WITH
SENSORINEURAL IMPAIRMENTS (EXPRESSED IN DECIBELS
RE THE ZERO SETTING OF THE HEARING-LOSS DIAL).

Frequency	Air	Bone	Difference Between Settings
250	15.0	41.3	26.3
500	20.0	45.8	25.8
1,000	38.7	41.2	2.5
1,500	45.0	52.5	7.5
2,000	46.3	53.8	7.5
3,000	47.8	51.8	4.0
4,000	46.3	44.4	−1.9

The propriety of this decision can be easily checked by ascertaining what differences would have resulted had the interpretation been based on medians.

Table 3-5 presents the median audiometric settings for the 23 cases of sensorineural loss and reports the discrepancies between their corresponding air- and bone-conduction medians. Assuming that no correction in the reference for the bone system is necessary until the difference exceeds 2.5 dB, the pattern of correction called for by Table 3-5 becomes 25 dB at 250 and 500 cps; no correction at 1,000 cps; 5 dB at 1,500, 2,000, and 3,000 cps; nothing at 4,000 cps. These corrections are the same as those derived from consideration of means except at 1,000 and 3,000 cps, where in each instance the correction based on medians is 5 dB less than the one based on means.

These two disagreements, while not large, do raise the question as to which criterion of central tendency in this instance yielded the superior calibration. One

method of examining this question is to compute the calibrations which would have been assigned to the bone system if it had been derived from the responses of the 127 normal ears. In this instance the discrepancy between the actual audiometric settings yielding air and bone thresholds of the normal group indicates the magnitude of the correction required by the bone-conduction system. This discrepancy was computed, for each test frequency separately, from the median audiometer readings for the 127 normal ears and, independently, from the mean audiometric readings. The results are reported in Table 3-6. If calibration of the bone conduction had been based on these data, the correction factors reported in Table 3-7 would have applied. Here, too, corrections are in 5 dB steps and differences of 2.5 dB or less have been disregarded. For purposes of comparison the corrections derived from the responses of the 23 cases of sensorineural are also reported in Table 3-7. A "best estimate" is also reported. This estimate is the correction most often called for at each test frequency.

Two generalizations are quickly apparent from Table 3-7.

First, there appears to have been a real discrepancy in the correction required by the two populations at 1,500 cps. The normal group showed such close agreement between the median scores for air and bone, as well as between mean scores, that no correction appears necessary. Both sets of statistics for the hard of hearing population suggest the bone system is 5 dB weak. If one accepts the responses of the normals as the criterion of validity, then the calibration of the bone system based on responses of impaired ears proved at 1,500 cycles to be 5 dB in error. Such a finding should serve as a warning to the

TABLE 3-6. DISCREPANCIES BETWEEN THE CENTRAL TENDENCIES OF THE
UNCORRECTED SETTINGS OF THE HEARING-LOSS DIAL (RAW SCORES) FOR AIR AND
BONE CONDUCTION REPRESENTING THRESHOLD RESPONSES OF 127 NORMAL EARS.

Frequency	Group Median			Group Mean		
	Air	Bone	Difference	Air	Bone	Difference
250	−8.4	18.7	27.1	−7.3	19.1	26.4
500	−6.2	17.1	23.3	−5.9	17.3	23.2
1,000	−5.0	−2.0	3.0	−4.8	−1.6	3.2
1,500	−5.4	−4.2	0.8	−4.9	−3.3	1.6
2,000	−4.9	−0.1	4.8	−3.9	1.1	5.0
3,000	−5.3	−3.0	8.3	−3.9	4.7	8.6
4,000	−8.7	−5.0	3.7	−6.7	−4.2	2.5

TABLE 3-7. THE SUMMARY OF CORRECTIONS IN THE
CALIBRATION OF BONE-CONDUCTION SYSTEM REQUIRED
BY VARIOUS ESTIMATES OF CENTRAL TENDENCY.

Frequency	Normal Ears Median	Normal Ears Mean	Impaired Ears Median	Impaired Ears Mean	Best Estimate
250	25	25	25	25	25
500	25	25	25	25	25
1,000	5	5	0	5	5
1,500	0	0	5	5	0 or 5
2,000	5	5	5	5	5
3,000	10	10	5	10	10
4,000	5	0	0	0	0

clinician, since it indicates that errors can occur even when the calibration of a bone system is based on carefully selected cases of sensorineural loss. Equally important, however, is the fact that only one such error was here observed and that it had a magnitude of only 5 dB. We may retain the conclusion that a bone system can be empirically calibrated on sensorineural losses to a precision which has reasonable clinical accuracy.

Second, the corrections derived from comparison of means, whether for normals or for hard of hearing subjects, are the more defensible in the present study. It would be hazardous to presume that this situation would always apply, but in the present instance the two sets of corrections based on means were in perfect agreement at all test frequencies except 1,500 cps. Concomitantly, at least one of the estimates derived from the comparison of medians was in agreement with the two estimates from means. On the other hand, if either set of medians is used as the basis for calibrating the bone system, the median response of the other population is in disagreement by one correction step (5 dB) at four of the seven test frequencies.

SUMMARY

The present study was undertaken to determine if it is possible to establish a clinically acceptable reference level for bone-conduction audiometry by comparing air- and bone-conduction responses yielded by subjects with sensorineural loss. The study has demonstrated that a clinically acceptable reference level can be achieved in this manner. A commercial audiometer whose air-conduction system met current standards for adequate calibration and performance was used. Standard audiometric tests by air and bone conduction were then administered to 23 cases diagnosed as having pure sensorineural loss. The corrections required by the bone-conduction system of the audiometer were computed to the nearest 5 dB. These corrections were based on the premise that, since the air-conduction system was in calibration, any sizable discrepancy between the group's apparent acuity level by air and bone was due to incorrect calibration of the bone-conduction system.

The adequacy of these corrections was subsequently confirmed by testing 127 normal listeners in a sound-proof chamber of research caliber. Had the original calibration been based on the performance of these normal listeners, exactly the same corrections would have been obtained except at 1,500 cps. Even at 1,500 cps, the error in the calibration based on sensorineural losses was only 5 dB.

Thus a useful set of reference values for the bone-conduction system was here achieved with an empirical procedure utilizing the responses of selected cases with hearing loss. The procedure offers the otologist, the audiologist, and the audiometrician a method for achieving a reasonable calibration of his bone-conduction system which is free from the pitfalls which plague the clinician when he tries to calibrate his bone system on normal listeners in the usual office environment.

ENDNOTES

1. Some workers prefer computing the reference values from medians or modes rather than from means (Harris, 1954). The distinction probably has more theoretical than clinical importance.

2. Even if the method is demonstrated to be valid in the sense that it brings the two systems into calibrational agreement, we must remember that the adequacy achieved in a given clinical situation will depend upon the accuracy with which the air-conduction system has been calibrated.

3. The Maico Company kindly made this instrument available.

4. This bone oscillator was incorporated in the audiometer at our request. So far as we know, the Maico Company has never advocated using this type of receiver with its E-2 audiometer. Therefore, the results we report here do not indicate the performance of the instrument when equipped with the larger bone receiver, which is the standard accessory for the E-2.

5. Details are reported in Roach (1951).

6. The Sonotone Corporation kindly supplied detailed plans for this unit.

7. These cases satisfied Beasley's criterion for normal hearing by air conduction, except for a few subjects with mild high-frequency losses (Beasley, 1935–1936).

8. Masking of the opposite ear was not employed, since Cochran has demonstrated that even a mild noise in one ear may change appreciably the threshold of the other ear (Cochran, 1946).

9. Actually, data from two complete tests on each subject were available. These tests, spaced about a month apart, were administered to gather information on the test-retest reliability of pure-tone audiometry. It was felt that, for present purposes, the average of a subject's two responses for a given test condition would give an improved indication of the subject's acuity. The discussion which follows is based on such an averaging of the test-retest data.

10. The standard deviations were found to be progressively larger as the test frequency became higher. This trend is common to both the air- and the bone-conduction data. It merely indicates that the population of "normal" ears under study possessed greater variability in acuity for higher-pitched tones.

REFERENCES

American Standards Association: Audiometers for General Diagnostic Purposes, Z24:5, New York, 1951.

Beasley, D.: Normal Hearing by Air and Bone Conduction, Hearing Study Series, Bulletin 4, National Health Survey, Washington, D.C., 1935–1936.

Beranek, L.: Acoustic Measurements, New York, John Wiley & Sons, Inc., 1949, p. 370.

Carhart, R.: Clinical Application of Bone Conduction Audiometry, Arch. Otolaryng. 51: 789–807, 1950.

Carlisle, R. W., and Pearson, H. A.: A Strain-Gauge Type of Artificial Mastoid, J. Acoust. Soc. America 23: 300–302, 1951.

Cochran, M.: Masking in Audiometry, M.A. Thesis, Northwestern University, 1946.

Council on Physical Medicine and Rehabilitation: Minimum Requirement for Acceptable Pure Tone Audiometers for Diagnostic Purposes, J.A.M.A. 146: 255–257, 1951.

Dix, M. R., and Hood, J. D.: Modern Development in Pure Tone Audiometry and Their Application to the Clinical Diagnosis of End-Organ Deafness, Proc. Roy. Soc. Med. 46: 992–994, 1953.

Hallpike, C. S., and Hood, J. D.: Some Recent Work on Auditory Adaptation and Its Relationship to the Loudness Recruitment Problem, J. Accoust. Soc. America 23: 270–274, 1951.

Harris, J. D.: Normal Hearing and Its Relation to Audiometry, Laryngoscope 64: 928–957, 1954.

Hughson, W., and Westlake, H.: Manual for Program Outline for Rehabilitation of Aural Casualties Both Military and Civilian, Tr. Am. Acad. Ophth., Supp., pp. 1–15, 1944.

Roach, R. E.: A Study of the Reliability and Validity of Bone Conduction Audiometry, Dissertation, Northwestern University, 1951.

Stevens, S. S.: On the Averaging of Data, Science 121: 113–116, 1955.

Zwislocki, J.: Über die Lautstärkeempfindung bei Knochenleitung, Acta oto-laryng. 37: 239–244, 1949.

4

Bone-Conduction Calibration: Current Status

DONALD D. DIRKS, Ph.D.
Professor, Head and Neck Surgery (Audiology), UCLA, Los Angeles, California
SAMUEL F. LYBARGER, B.S.
an Acoustical Consultant in McMurray, Pennsylvania
WAYNE O. OLSEN, Ph.D.
Consultant in Audiology, Mayo Clinic, Rochester, Minnesota
BRADLEY L. BILLINGS, Ph.D.
Director, Audiology Services, Audiology Center of Redlands Medical Clinic, Inc.

Attempts to specify normal threshold sensitivity by bone conduction have been unsuccessful because of problems in obtaining reliable measurements from commercially available artificial mastoids. Recent design modifications incorporated in the Bruel and Kjaer 4930 artificial mastoids have resulted in greater uniformity among these units. However, the new design has resulted in impedances that are higher than those recommended in current standards. Bone-conduction thresholds referenced to measurements made on B & K 4930 artificial mastoids with the new design were performed on 60 normal listeners by three participating laboratories. The results are reported for consideration in the development of a reference threshold for hearing by bone conduction.

Traditionally, bone conduction vibrators provided with audiometers have not been calibrated to any physical standard maintained by a national laboratory. Manufacturers and clinicians have developed individual standards for bone-conduction audiometry from subjective threshold tests on a group of listeners with normal hearing or sensorineural hearing loss (Carhart, 1950: Roach and Carhart, 1956). The rationale for this method of subjective calibration is based primarily on the theory that air- and bone-conduction thresholds should be essentially equivalent among the population with normal hearing or among patients with pure sensorineural hearing loss. These subjective methods which are time consuming and costly, have not resulted in highly reliable and uniform calibrations. In less rigorous approaches, bone-conduction calibration has been performed by one individual with a golden ear or with a small number of normal listeners. The poor reliability encountered in using small groups of listeners for calibration purposes has been described by Wilber and Goodhill (1967). Thus, the development of a reliable instrument for measurement of the mechanical output of bone vibrators (that is, an artificial headbone or mastoid) is a necessary prerequisite in establishing a uniform reference for specifying threshold sensitivity by bone conduction. This article reviews the problems experienced in obtaining reliable measurements from commercially available artificial mastoids and reports bone-conduction threshold data that may be considered in the development of a reference threshold for hearing by bone conduction.

Reprinted by permission of the authors from *J. Speech Hearing Dis.*, **44**, 143–155 (1979).

During the past 15 years, the physical response of bone vibrators has been reported primarily from measurements on two commercially available artificial mastoids (Beltone Model 5A, Weiss, 1960; and Bruel and Kjaer Model 4930, Stisen and Dahm, 1969). Both the International Electrotechnical Commission (Recommendation 373, 1971) and the American National Standards Institute (S3.13-1972) have recently issued documents recommending identical mechanical impedance characteristics that should be incorporated in the production of artificial mastoids. These specifications were based primarily on the measurement of the mechanical impedance of the human mastoid by Dadson, Robinson, and Greig (1954) and by Corliss and Koidan (1955). Because the coupling force and the dimensions of the vibrators are two critical variables that affect mechanical impedance, the specifications within the standards are limited to use with vibrators having a circular contact tip area of 1.75 cm² and coupled to the head with a static force of 5.4 newtons (N) or ~550 grams/weight.

Although advancement has been made toward specification of the physical characteristics of an artificial mastoid, there is, as yet, no international agreement on a standard for the threshold of hearing by bone conduction. In the United States, calibration of bone vibrators for audiometry was enhanced by the establishment of an interim norm known as the Hearing Aid Industry Conference (HAIC) Interim Bone Conduction Threshold for Audiometry (Lybarger, 1966). The bone conduction threshold data contained in the HAIC norm were referenced to physical measurements made on the Beltone 5A artificial mastoid. Since the Beltone 5A artificial mastoid has a higher mechanical impedance and a different force response than the B & K 4930 artificial mastoid, the HAIC interim threshold data have to be adjusted when the B & K unit is used for calibration (Lybarger, 1971; Wilber, 1972).

In the early 1970s several vibrator-headband assemblies conforming to the standard specification in terms of contact tip dimensions and static force capabilities became available. However, published threshold data with the new vibrators have been limited (Dirks and Kamm, 1975; Sauer and Bellack, 1975; Billings and Winter, 1977). With encouragement and advice from ANSI Working Group S3-43, several investigators in the United States decided to accumulate and pool bone-conduction threshold data

that would be useful in the eventual formulation of a standard. These investigators assumed that the B & K 4930 artificial mastoid would most likely meet the international specifications and therefore that instrument was used for calibration. The participants met at one of the laboratories and agreed on common procedures for making physical measurements of bone vibrators. Measurements of the response of several bone vibrators were then conducted using artificial mastoids available at each laboratory. Figure 4-1 shows the frequency response curves from one vibrator (Radioear B-71, #05906) as measured with the same voltage input on three B & K 4930 artificial mastoids, one from each laboratory. The results from one of the artificial mastoids (Mayo Clinic) differed from the others by as much as 6.0 dB at certain frequencies. Differences of this magnitude were consistently observed while using several other vibrators.

Disparities as large as 7.5 dB between measurements of the same vibrators with constant electrical input on two separate #4930 artificial mastoid have also been reported by Richter and Brinkmann, (1976) in West Germany. Because of the similarities in the results from the laboratories in West Germany and the United States, it was decided to compare bone vibrator responses on several artificial mastoids in both countries. One of the investigators in the United States met with Brinkmann and verified commonality in physical measurement procedures. The frequency responses of the three bone vibrators were then measured at UCLA and subsequently at the PTB.[1] One of these vibrators was also measured by

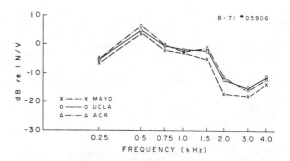

FIGURE 4-1. Frequency response of a Radioear B-71 bone vibrator in dB re 1N/v measured on three B & K 4930 artificial mastoids at three laboratories (Mayo Clinic, University of California at Los Angeles and Audiology Center of Redlands).

the two other participating laboratories in the United States. Figure 4–2 shows the measured vibrator output for the same electrical input to a single Radioear B-71 (#00055) unit. Differences in output levels as great as 10 dB were observed among the five laboratory measurements. Results from one of the artificial mastoids at PTB (#1) agreed closely with those from two of the artificial mastoids in the United States while results from the other PTB mastoid (#2) were closer to those obtained at Mayo Clinic. These large differences in the measured output of the same bone vibrator with the same electrical input suggested that before a threshold standard could be established, tolerances for artificial mastoids would have to be more rigidly controlled.

Inquiry revealed that some changes in the original design of the B & K artificial mastoid had in fact occurred. In particular, the composition of the material used to obtain the desired mechanical impedance had undergone some changes as new batches were used. Furthermore, the two layers of synthetic rubber that were originally cemented together, had been bonded together by a vulcanizing process since the latter part of 1975. Also, a calibration problem, related to resonances in the original bracket system used to hold the shaker and impedance head, had been discovered. The problem was corrected simply by suspending the calibration driver with a coil spring. The upper end of the spring was attached to a 0–1000 gram spring gauge. The height of the spring gauge was set so that the impedance head disc rested on the center of the mastoid pad. In this manner the gauge read the difference between the weight of the

driver unit and the desired contact force of 550 grams weight (5.4N).

To determine the effects of the aforementioned changes, measurements of impedance and vibrator frequency response were conducted on the artificial mastoids used in the participating laboratories.

RESULTS OF PHYSICAL MEASUREMENTS

Impedance Measurements

Mechanical impedance measurements of the artificial mastoids belonging to the participating laboratories were performed prior to and following replacement of the pads on two of the older artificial mastoids (#290073, #21697) and recalibration of the newer (#526228) unit. These measurements[2] were performed with a B & K 8000 Impedance Measuring Head over the frequency range from 100 to 10,000 Hz. The calibration driver was suspended with a relatively soft coil spring, the upper end of which was attached to a 0–1,000 gram spring gauge as described previously. For these measurements the ambient temperature at the test site was maintained at 23°C. Richter and Brinkmann (1977) recently observed changes in the mechanical impedance of the newly designed B & K artificial mastoids with only small variations (±2°C) in the environmental temperature.

Figure 4–3 contains the mechanical impedance curves from the three artificial mastoids with the original pads (top portion of the figure) and those with the new pads (bottom portion of figure). One of the artificial mastoids (#526228) was produced with a new pad, so this unit was only recalibrated. Comparison of the two sets of curves reveals that: (1) the new pads greatly increased the uniformity of the mechanical impedances among the units, (2) the new design has raised the impedance of the artificial mastoids, and (3) the resonance frequency of the impedance has shifted slightly upward toward 3,000 Hz. Inspection of the impedance curves from several other artificial mastoids undergoing calibration by the manufacturer suggested that the uniformity of results apparent in Figure 4–3 was being maintained for other units. These results are in general agreement with the findings of Richter and Brinkmann (1977) who reported frequency response measurements from bone vibrators on five artificial mastoids of the new design.

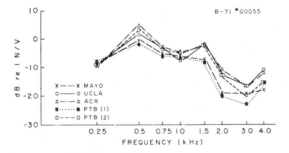

FIGURE 4-2. Frequency response of a Radioear B-71 bone vibrator in dB re 1N/v as measured on five B & K 4930 artificial mastoids at four laboratories in the United States and the Physikalisch-Technische Bundesanstalt in West Germany.

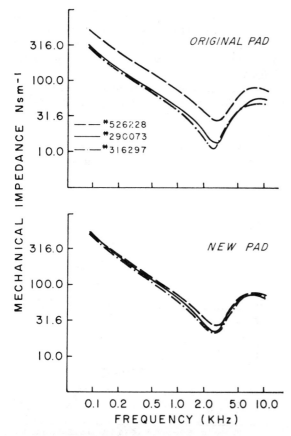

FIGURE 4-3. Mechanical impedance of three B & K 4930 artificial mastoids with the original and new design pads.

same artificial mastoid with the new pads (bottom of Figure 4-4) deviates from the tolerance limits suggested in the standard at most frequencies.

Richter and Brinkmann (1977) have reported individual resistance and reactance curves from five #4930 artificial mastoids with the new pads. Considerably higher impedance values than those specified in S3.13-1972 and IEC 373 were measured except in the frequency region of 4,000 Hz where the impedance values were in closer agreement with the recommended values. If the new design of the #4930 artificial mastoid is considered acceptable for calibration purposes, then it will be necessary either to modify the specified impedance values of S3.13 and IEC 373, or the tolerances currently suggested will have to be increased. Because of the uniformity achieved with the new design, the B & K 4930 artificial mastoid will probably be given strong consideration in developing threshold standards.

The new design of the artificial mastoids resulted in impedances that are somewhat higher than the tolerable limits set forth in ANSI S3.13-1972 or the specification recommended in IEC publication 373. ANSI S3.13-1972 suggested that between 250 and 4,000 Hz the mechanical resistance values specified be held within ± 20 percent and the reactance values within ± 20 percent or ± 4 Nsm^{-1}.

Figure 4-4 shows the impedance curve of one of the older artificial mastoids (#290073), together with the nominal impedance values and the upper and lower tolerance limits (hash marks) suggested in the ANSI standard. The artificial mastoid with the original pads (top of Figure 4-4) falls within the ANSI tolerance limits except for frequencies in the region of 3,000 Hz. However, the impedance of the

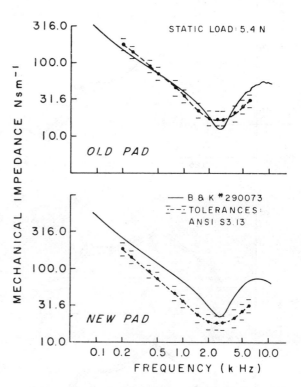

FIGURE 4-4. Mechanical impedance of one B & K 4930 artificial mastoid with the original and new design pad compared with impedance values and tolerances for artificial mastoids as recommended in ANSI S3.13.

Frequency Response of Bone Vibrators

The responses of three commonly used bone vibrator models (Radioear B70AA, B71, and B72) with constant voltage input were measured at each participating laboratory using force sensitivity calibration data appropriate for each artificial mastoid. These force measurements were made before and after replacing the pads. For these measurements the vibrators were coupled to the artificial mastoids with a pressure device supplied with the instruments (similar to Figure 3 of Dirks and Kamm, 1975). The static force was 5.4N. At each laboratory, three separate measurements with each bone vibrator were made and the averaged results are shown in Figure 4–5 A (B70AA), B (B71), and C (B-72).

For each vibrator, the measured output levels are in much closer agreement on the artificial mastoids with the new pads as compared to the original ones. The closest agreement is found with the B-71 vibrator. Some differences in vibrator output continue to be measured at the higher test frequencies (3.0 and

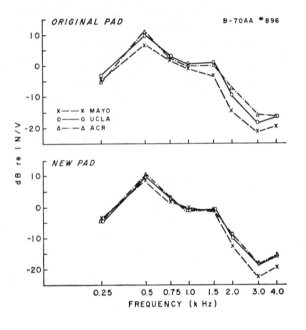

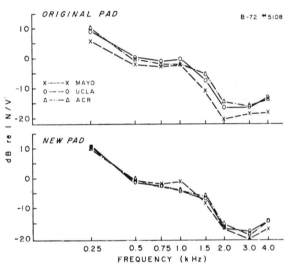

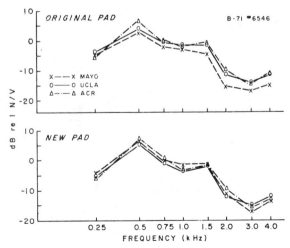

FIGURE 4-5. Frequency response of three bone vibrators as measured on B & K 4930 artificial mastoids. Comparisons are made between responses with the original pads and the new pads for vibrator models a) Radioear B-70AA, b) Radioear B-71 and c) Radioear B-72.

4.0 kHz) even with the new pads. The largest difference in the output level was 2.5 dB at 3.0 kHz for the B-71. However, variations as large as 5.0 dB are observed in this same frequency region for the B-70AA. The B-70AA is the only one of the vibrators measured that had a contact area larger than that recommended in the standards. It may be that the larger differences among the laboratories in the high frequencies are due to variations in positioning this vibrator on the pad. Vibrators with large contact areas may be affected to a greater extent by changes in positioning than those with the smaller recommended contact tip.

RESULTS OF THRESHOLD MEASUREMENTS

Air- and bone-conduction thresholds were collected on 60 young, otologically normal listeners in the three participating laboratories; 24 at Audiology Center of Redlands (ACR), 20 at University of California at Los Angeles (UCLA) and 16 at Mayo Clinic. The results of the bone-conduction thresholds were referenced to measurements made on the B & K 4930 artificial mastoids following installation of the newly designed pads and recalibration of the units by the improved method. Portions of these results have been reported previously (Dirks and Kamm, 1975; Billings and Winter, 1977; Dirks, Kamm, and Gilman, 1976). The original threshold data were corrected by the difference between the measured output level of the artificial mastoids with the new pads and those obtained with the old design. Thus the current threshold values will vary somewhat from the results reported in the original papers because of the changes in the artificial mastoids and because adjustments were not made in all instances for differences between the measured air-conduction thresholds and the ANSI-1969 recommended levels.

The tests were conducted in sound-treated rooms that meet the ANSI S3.1-1977 specification for permissible ambient noise levels. All subjects had hearing thresholds ≤ 15 dB HL re the ANSI-1969 standard at the test frequencies. Each subject was tested under the following conditions: (1) air conduction on each ear via a TDH-39 earphone provided with a MX 41/AR cushion, and (2) bone conduction with a B-71 bone vibrator applied to the mastoid by a headband (Radioear P-3333) that produces a static force close to 5.4 N on adult heads.

Thresholds were obtained with a fixed-frequency Bekesy-tracking procedure using the instructions suggested by Jerger (1960). In one setting (Billings and Winters, 1977) a modified method of limits was used. Short practice sessions preceded each test period. The tonal signals (250, 500, 1,000, 2,000, 3,000, and 4,000 Hz) had a duration of 200 msec, an interstimulus interval of 200 msec and a rise-fall time of 25 msec. The bone vibrator was applied to the mastoid of the subject with the test ear unoccluded, while narrow bands of noise centered on the test tone were presented by way of an earphone to the nontest ear at 30 dB effective level. The effective levels of the masking noise for a subject were determined by the formula and table provided in Appendix A4 of ANSI S3.13-1972. The same earphone used for air-conduction measurement of the nontest ear was used to deliver the masking noise.

The average air-conduction thresholds for the test ear from each laboratory are shown in Table 4-1. Because different numbers of subjects were used by each laboratory, the table contains the weighted average air-conduction thresholds. The air-conduction threshold levels recommended in ANSI-1969 are also shown for comparison. Table 4-2 contains the unadjusted bone-conduction threshold force levels and the threshold levels adjusted by the difference between the ANSI-1969 recommended thresholds and the measured air-conduction thresholds from each laboratory. It is suggested that the adjusted average levels be used for calibration purposes.

During the past year, two of the laboratories (Mayo and UCLA) have accumulated records of air- and bone-conduction hearing levels for persons with otologic and audiologic evidence of pure sensorineural hearing loss. The thresholds in the clinic were obtained using the customary 5 dB steps and narrow band masking in the nontest ear. The bone-

TABLE 4-1. AIR-CONDUCTION THRESHOLDS REPORTED IN dB RE 20 μPa USING A NBS 9A COUPLER.

	Frequency (kHz)					
	0.25	0.50	1.0	2.0	3.0	4.0
UCLA $N=20$	28.5	14.0	8.6	9.5	—	12.9
ACR $N=24$	27.2	11.9	7.8	10.5	12.4	10.5
Mayo $N=16$	26.9	11.8	7.8	9.0	10.2	9.5
Weighted $\overline{X}$	27.6	12.6	8.1	9.8	11.5	11.0

TABLE 4-2. THRESHOLD FORCE CALIBRATION VALUES (B-71 BONE VIBRATOR) FOR THE MASTOID POSITION USING THE 4930 BRUEL & KJAER ARTIFICIAL MASTOID. RMS FORCE LEVELS MEASURED AT THE BONE VIBRATOR TIP FACE, dB RE 1 $\mu N = 0.1$ DYNE. (APPLIES TO B & K ARTIFICIAL MASTOIDS RECALIBRATED WITH NEW PAD DESIGN).

	Frequency (kHz)											
	Adjusted Force Levels						Unadjusted Force Levels					
	0.25	0.50	1.0	2.0	3.0	4.0	0.25	0.50	1.0	2.0	3.0	4.0
UCLA $N=20$	62.5	59.0	38.9	30.3	—	30.2	65.5	60.5	41.5	30.8	—	33.6
ACR $N=24$	57.9	59.5	37.8	31.0	26.4	31.4	59.6	60.3	38.6	32.5	28.8	32.4
Mayo $N=16$	64.3	59.7	39.9	37.5	30.3	32.3	65.7	60.0	40.7	37.5	30.5	32.3
Weighted $\overline{X}$	61.1	59.4	38.7	32.5	28.0	31.2	63.2	60.3	40.1	33.3	29.5	32.8

conduction threshold values reported in Table 4-2 were used for the calibration of the clinic bone vibrators (Type B-71). The air-conduction earphones were calibrated to values specified in ANSI-1969. If the threshold levels described in Table 4-2 reflect 0 dB HL for bone conduction, then the air- and bone-conduction hearing levels should approximate each other. Results from this group of patients are shown in Figure 4-6. The number of subjects tested at each frequency differs because occasionally the maximum output of the bone vibrator was not sufficient to measure threshold and because tests were not routinely performed at 3 kHz. The results indicate

close correspondence between the air- and bone-conduction thresholds on the population tested. Statistical t tests were applied to determine if the difference between the air- and bone-conduction thresholds reached levels of significance at any test frequency. The difference between air- and bone-conduction thresholds of 1.6 dB at 1,000 Hz was the only result that was statistically significant.

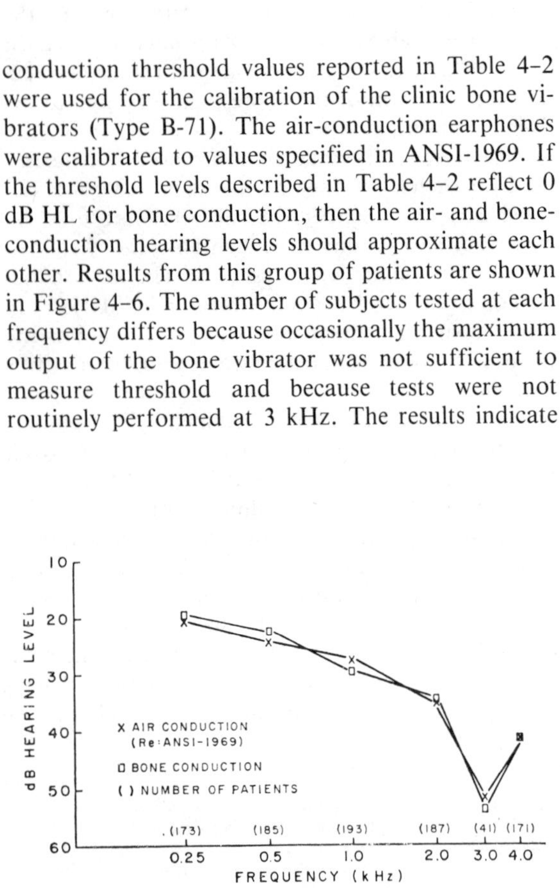

These data indicate that the adjusted threshold levels reported in Table 4-2 are generally acceptable for calibrating bone vibrators for clinical use. Because the suggested values in Table 4-2 are based on only 60 normal listeners and some small differences are still observed between air- and bone-conduction thresholds on sensorineural subjects (Figure 4-6), other investigators are encouraged to accumulate additional threshold results on normal listeners for verification and up-dating of the recommendations in Table 4-2. Such results could then be included in the establishment of even more definitive levels for specifying normal bone-conduction threshold. Individuals currently responsible for the clinical measurement of bone-conduction thresholds may wish to calibrate B-71 vibrators according to the adjusted, average levels reported in Table 4-2, provided the measurements are conducted on B & K 4930 artificial mastoids that incorporate the new design pads and have been recalibrated.[3]

FIGURE 4-6. Mean air conduction and bone conduction thresholds for patients with sensorineural hearing loss. Air conduction referenced to specifications in ANSI S3.6-1969, and bone conduction referenced to Adjusted Force Levels in Table II.

ACKNOWLEDGMENT

We wish to thank Candace Kamm for her assistance in the preparation of the data for this article.

ENDNOTES

1. We wish to express our appreciation to Dr. Klaus Brinkmann of the Physikalisch-Technische Bundesanstalt, Braunschweig, West Germany, who made these comparisons possible.

2. The measurements were conducted at B & K Instruments, Inc., in Cleveland, Ohio on October 1977 by Terry Sparks of B & K, with Sam Lybarger and Wayne Olsen present.

3. Each owner of a B & K 4930 artificial mastoid is encouraged to contact Bruel and Kjaer Inc. to determine whether their artificial mastoid requires installation of a new pad or recalibration.

REFERENCES

American National Standards Institute. *Criteria for permissible ambient noise during audiometric testing.* ANSI S3.1-1977, New York (1977).

American National Standards Institute. *Specification for an artificial head-bone.* ANSI S3.13-1972, New York (1972).

Billings, B. L., and Winter, M. Calibration force levels for bone conduction vibrators. *J. Speech Hearing Res., 20,* 653–660 (1977).

Carhart, R. Clinical application of bone conduction. *Arch. Otolaryng. (Chicago),* 51, 798–807 (1950).

Corliss, E., and Koidan, D. Mechanical impedance of the forehead and mastoid. *J. Acoust. Soc. Am.,* 27, 1164–1172 (1955).

Dadson, R. S., Robinson, D. W., and Greig, R. G. P. The mechanical impedance of the human mastoid process. *British J. of Applied Physics,* 5, 435–442 (1954).

Dirks, D. D., and Kamm, C. Bone-vibrator measurements: Physical characteristics and behavioral thresholds. *J. Speech Hearing Res.,* 18, 242–260 (1975).

Dirks, D. D., Kamm, C., and Gilman, S. Bone conduction thresholds for normal listeners in force and acceleration units. *J. Speech Hearing Res.,* 19, 181–186 (1976).

International Electrotechnical Commission. An IEC mechanical coupler for the calibration of bone vibrators having a specified contact area and being applied with a specified static force, 373 (1971).

Jerger, J. Bekesy audiometry in analysis of auditory disorders. *J. Speech Hearing Res.,* 34, 275–287 (1960).

Lybarger, S. F. Special report-Interim bone conduction thresholds for audiometry. *J. Speech Hearing Res.,* 9, 483–487 (1966).

Lybarger, S. F. Bone vibrator calibration standards. Paper presented at the Annual Convention of the American Speech and Hearing Association, Chicago (1971).

Richter, U., and Brinkmann, K., The sensitivity level of bone-conduction receivers. *J. Audiological Technique,* 15, 2–15 (1976).

Richter, U., and Brinkmann, K. *Messungen an einem "künstlichen" Mastoid.* Bericht Physikalisch-Technische Bundesanstalt (PTB)—Ak—10 (1977).

Roach, R. E., and Carhart, R. A clinical method for calibrating the bone conduction audiometer. *Arch. Otolaryng.* (Chicago), 63, 270–279 (1956).

Sauer, U., and Bellack, D. Zur Eichung von Audiometer—Knochenleitungshören. MDV der DDR, *Verkehrsmedizinisches Zentrum Berlin, Physikalischarbeitsmedizinisches Zentrallabor,* 23, 143–148 (1976).

Stisen, B., and Dahm, M. Sensitivity and mechanical impedance of artificial mastoid type 4930. *Bruel & Kjaer Technical Information (1969).*

Weiss, E. An air damped artificial mastoid. *J. Acoust. Soc. Amer.,* 32, 1582–1588 (1960).

Wilber, L. A. Comparability of two commercially available mastoids. *J. Acoust. Soc. Amer.,* 52, 1265–1266 (1972).

Wilber, L. A. and Goodhill, V. Real ear versus artificial mastoid methods of calibration of bone conduction vibrators. *J. Speech Hearing Res.,* 10, 405–417 (1967).

5

A Study on the Calibration Characteristics of Twenty Impedance Bridges in Clinical Use

DALE O. ROBINSON, Ph.D.
Associate Professor, Department of Audiology, School of Medicine, Wayne State University, Detroit, Michigan

ROBERT H. BREY, Ph.D.
Associate Professor of Audiology, Communicative Disorders Area, Brigham Young University, Provo, Utah

This investigation examines the calibration characteristics as well as real-ear data collected on 20 electroacoustic impedance bridges in clinical use. Calibration data were collected for manometer readings, air-pressure leakage, cavity equivalence, sensitivity, and probe-tone sound pressure level, and harmonic distortion. Real-ear data were gathered for tympanograms and static compliance on all bridges for one otologically normal subject. The results reveal information regarding specific calibration problems that have clinical implications. Recommendations are made for calibration and clinical tympanographic procedures.

Audiologists have been concerned with the calibration of audiometric equipment for many years. This concern is justified because there is a direct relationship between the validity of hearing-test results and the electroacoustic functioning of clinical equipment. Therefore, most university training programs devote a significant amount of time to teaching audiology students the published specifications for calibrating audiometers, as well as acceptable procedures and instrumentation for checking the integrity of their clinical equipment. During recent years, acoustic impedance testing has become a routine procedure in most clinics. Generally, clinical impedance bridges are used in conjunction with either a built-in or an independent audiometer, which is used to elicit the acoustic reflex. It should be expected that those audiometers meet the American National Standards Institute (ANSI) 1969 calibration specifications and be checked for proper functioning as recommended by ASHA's Professional Services Board. However, it is apparent that there has been little, if any, concern

with uniform calibration specifications and procedures for electroacoustic impedance bridges. One possible explanation for this might be the apparent preoccupation of those in our profession with establishing terminology and testing procedures. Yet, it is reasonable to assume that the performance characteristics of impedance bridges are as important to clinical test results as are the performance characteristics of audiometers. To date, our profession has allowed the various manufacturers of acoustic impedance instruments to set their own standards and to determine the performance characteristics of the bridges they manufacture. Emphasis was given to the problem when Feldman and Wilber (1976) pointed out that there is no American National Standards Institute or American Speech and Hearing Association Standard for acoustic impedance meters. Furthermore the authors stated, "Despite the lack of an official standard, it is important that one checks the calibration of certain parameters in any acoustic impedance or otoadmittance device" (p. 378). A lack of calibration standards, of course, raises questions about generalizing from the research findings to the clinical findings obtained with commercially avail-

Reprinted by permission of the authors from *Asha,* **20,** 7–14 (1978).

able instruments. While it is important for the clinician to know that certain test procedures will yield results indicative of particular pathologies or sites of lesions, it is very discouraging for him to know that there are no calibration standards against which to check his bridge. This lack of knowledge concerning the proper functioning of clinical instrumentation must render clinical judgments regarding the validity of any test results equivocal. Therefore, it is reasonable for the clinician to ask whether there are any significant differences in calibration among bridges currently in use, and whether any differences that do exist have a significant effect on test results. This study was undertaken to help answer those questions and to emphasize the need for careful study and decision making in the area of impedance testing.

PROCEDURES

In an effort to acquire information regarding the status of impedance bridges in clinical use, calibration and real-ear test data were collected on 20 electroacoustic impedance bridges in the Detroit metropolitan area. A description of the 20 bridges surveyed is found in Table 5-1, wherein their order, age, frequency of usage, and frequency of calibration are reported. The instruments were selected on the basis of availability and represented approximately 85 percent of the total population of bridges in the area. The study population of bridges consisted of 12 American Electromedics (AE) bridges, and eight Madsen bridges. A control bridge for the study was a Madsen ZO-72. In addition, one normal-hearing male subject, 13 years old, with no history of middle-ear pathology, was used to collect the real-ear impedance data on all study bridges as well as the control bridge.

Calibration Data

Calibration data were collected for manometer readings (air pressure), air-pressure leakage, cavity equivalence, sensitivity, and probe-tone sound pressure level (SPL), and harmonic distortion. Manometer or air-pressure readings were recorded and measured for accuracy with a K.D.G. Model X751338/2 Manometer. Air-pressure leakage was checked by inserting the probe tip into a Madsen Electronics Variables Cavity, and adjusting the pressure reading to +200 mm of H_2O air pressure, while recording the amount of leakage over a 5-minute period on a Hewlett Packard Model 7015A XY recorder. To insure a hermetic seal, a putty substance was used to seal the tip in the variable cavity. In addition, internal air leakage was checked by sealing off the manometer passageway at the back of each instrument while recording.

TABLE 5-1. DESCRIPTIVE INFORMATION ON THE 20 IMPEDANCE BRIDGES
SURVEYED IN THIS STUDY.

Bridge #	Model #	Age	Frequency of Usage	Frequency of Calibration
1	AE-83	1 yr	7–20/day	1/yr
2	Madsen ZO-72	4 yrs	1/day	3/yr
3	AE-81	1 yr	1/day	3/yr
4	AE-83	1 yr	1/day	3/yr
5	Madsen ZO-70	8 yrs	4/day	when not functioning
6	Madsen ZO-72	3 yrs	12/day	1/month
7	AE-83	2 yrs	10–12/day	1/yr
8	Madsen ZO-72	4 yrs	7–10/day	1/yr
9	Madsen ZO-72	3 yrs	10–15/day	1/yr
10	Madsen ZO-72	3 yrs	10–20/day	1 or 2/yr
11	Madsen ZO-72	3 yrs	10/week	1/14 months
12	Madsen ZO-70	6 yrs	20/day	never
13	AE-81	1 yr	8–10/week	never
14	AE-83	3 yrs	2–3/day	1/yr
15	AE-83	2 yrs	daily	1/yr
16	AE-83	2 yrs	15/day	2/yr
17	AE-83	<1 yr	4–8/day	1/yr
18	AE-81	1 yr	2/month	never
19	AE-83	<1 yr	10–20/day	1/yr
20	AE-83	4 yrs	10/day	3/yr

Cavity equivalence measurements were made by sealing the probe in the Madsen Variable Cavity, adjusting the bridge for 0 mm of the H_2O air pressure, adjusting the compliance meter to the balance position, and recording the equivalent cavity size from the cursor scale for 0.5, 2, 4, and 5 cc adjustments of the variable cavity.

Sensitivity was measured for A_D, T, R, and SR settings for AE bridges and 1, 2, 3, and 4 settings for Madsen bridges. This was accomplished by sealing the probe in the Madsen Variable Cavity and adjusting the air pressure to 0 mm of H_2O air pressure. Each sensitivity setting was then measured by recording the cursor scale reading in equivalent volume with the compliance meter set to balance or midscale (S_1). Next, the compliance meter needle was adjusted for maximum scale deflection to the right and a second equivalent volume (S_2) was recorded. The difference was then calculated between the first scale reading (S_1) and the second (S_2), which resulted in the value used for comparison among the bridges (S_3), that is $S_1 - S_2 = S_3$. In other words, the least sensitive settings, A_D or #1, required the greatest equivalent-volume change for the lowest sensitivity setting and progressively less for higher sensitivity settings.

Measurement of the 220 Hz probe-tone SPL was accomplished by use of a 2-cc B & K coupler attached to a 2203 sound-level meter in conjunction with a condenser microphone model 4132 and a 1613 octave band filter centered at 250 Hz. A Madsen probe tip (red) was fitted to the probe and set against the small opening in the 2-cc coupler with earmold canal insert removed. The bridge-compliance meter was balanced to midscale with the cursor knob and the bridge was set for 0 mm for H_2O air pressure. The sensitivity setting was set to T or #1 as used in tympanometry. Thus, the probe tone, in dB SPL relative to 20μ Pascals, could be read on the sound-level meter and recorded for each instrument in the study. Furthermore, the SPL of the second harmonic could be measured using the same procedure and instrumentation simply by switching the octave filter to 500 Hz.

Subject Data

Information regarding real-ear test results was collected on each bridge in the study using the above-mentioned subject. All tests were performed with the same probe tip and employed standard clinical test procedures. Tympanograms were plotted with the use of the Hewlett Packard XY recorder, also mentioned above, which was calibrated for use with 19 of the 20 bridges studied. In one case, the tympanogram was plotted by hand. Tympanograms were plotted first from positive to negative pressure and then from negative to positive pressure. The height of the most compliant point, in millimeters for both traces of the tympanogram, the pressure reading in mm H_2O at the most compliant point of both traces, as well as the point of intersection of the two curves, were recorded as data points.

Static compliance measures were obtained for 19 of the 20 bridges. Equivalent volume measurements in cubic centimeters were made at +200 mm of H_2O pressure (C_1), the pressure at which maximum compliance was obtained (C_2), and at atmospheric pressure (C_3). Two static compliance measurements were then calculated for each bridge, that is $C_2 - C_1$ and $C_3 - C_1$.

No special preparations were made for the 20 bridges under study before measurements were taken except to allow a minimum 15-minute warm-up period and adjustment of the manometer to atmospheric pressure (0 mm of H_2O air pressure).

Real-ear clinical data and calibration measurements as described above were recorded using the control bridge subsequent to collecting data on the 20 bridges used in the study. Prior to its use, the control bridge was carefully calibrated as recommended by the manufacturer for manometer pressure, compliance, sensitivity, and probe-tone sound pressure level.

RESULTS

Manometer Calibration

All 20 bridges were capable of adjustment from +200 to −200 mm of H_2O air pressure without changing the scale, whereas 10 of the AE bridges required switching to an extended range to allow pressure readings beyond ±200 mm of H_2O. Therefore, both normal and extended settings were tested for those instruments. However, we shall first consider ±200 mm of H_2O for all instruments with all the AE bridges set on normal.

Table 5–2 shows the means, standard deviations, and percentages exceeding a 10 percent tolerance limit of the measured values for four manometer settings of the 20 bridges.

TABLE 5-2. MEANS, STANDARD DEVIATIONS, AND TOLERANCES FOR THE 20 STUDY BRIDGES FOR MANOMETER READINGS AT FOUR PRESSURE SETTINGS WITH ALL AE INSTRUMENTS SET TO NORMAL RANGE.

| Item | Pressure in mm H_2O | | | |
	−200	−100	100	200
N	20	20	20	20
Mean	−193.50	−88.00	96.25	200.25
SD	28.98	12.61	12.66	30.80
% Exceeding ± 10%	45%	60%	30%	30%

The manufacturers' recommended tolerance accuracy for bridge manometers is generally ± 10 percent of the meter reading. Applying that criterion, it is apparent that all means are within the tolerance limits except at −100 mm of H_2O air pressure. The mean data, however, provide a false impression because the errors among bridges tend to distribute themselves equally about the mean and thus do not indicate how many bridges do not meet specifications. More interesting and perhaps of more value is the finding shown in Table 5-2 that of 30 to 60 percent of the bridges exceeded the ± 10 percent tolerance limits. A clearer concept of the state of clinical bridges is apparent when viewing the data in this way. It should be noted that fewer bridges were out of calibration at positive pressures than at negative pressures. It should also be noted that 10 bridges needed to be adjusted to 0 mm of H_2O air pressure before manometer readings were taken, and those 10 were greater than ± 10 mm of H_2O relative to atmospheric pressure; they ranged from −140 to +35 mm of H_2O. Obviously, it is wise to check the manometer adjustment before test measures are obtained.

Manometer measurements were also made from −400 to +400 mm of H_2O settings at intervals of 100 mm of H_2O. These measures were taken on all 20 bridges, however, some of the AE instruments required switching to the extended range. For those that did not need switching, the identical values used to compute the means in Table 5-2 were used to compute the means in Table 5-3. Table 5-3 presents the means, standard deviations, and percentages exceeding tolerance for eight pressure settings on all 20 bridges. The small N under −400 mm of H_2O and +400 mm of H_2O was caused by the fact that the meter reading on some bridges yielded pressures beyond the limits of the KDG manometer used to check the calibration of the bridges. It was not capable of reading greater than ± 400 mm of H_2O, therefore, only those bridges whose pressure was ± 400 or less could be measured accurately. Mean values were within the ± 10 percent criterion except at −100 which was 4.25 mm of H_2O greater than the tolerance allowed. Looking once more at the bridges that exceeded the 10 percent tolerance limit, 15 to 60 percent were in fact out of calibration. Again, there was a trend for more bridges to be out of calibration at negative pressures. There did not seem to be any consistent direction to the errors. That is to say, the direction of errors was almost evenly divided between too-much and too-little pressure. A comparison between the normal and extended ranges for the 10 AE bridges revealed a major discrepancy between the two settings. Table 5-4 presents the differences between the two settings; those values in the negative direction indicated the extended setting was worse, those in the positive direction indicated that the extended setting was better, those marked ≠ were just as bad in the extended setting but in the opposite direction, and those with 0 difference were equivalent on either setting. There was a definite trend at −200 and −100 mm of H_2O air pressure for the extended range to be poorer, that is, 60 percent of the bridges were poorer at −200 and 70 percent were poorer at −100 mm of H_2O air pressure.

TABLE 5-3. MEANS, STANDARD DEVIATIONS, AND TOLERANCES FOR 20 BRIDGES FOR MANOMETER READINGS AT EIGHT PRESSURE SETTINGS WITH 10 AE INSTRUMENTS SET TO EXTENDED RANGE FOR ± 300 AND 400 mm H_2O.

| Item | Pressures in mm H_2O | | | | | | | |
	−400	−300	−200	−100	100	200	300	400
N	10	20	20	20	20	20	20	16
Mean	−369.00	−303.75	−192.25	−85.75	98.00	210.00	295.50	372.19
SD	23.78	36.05	34.70	18.23	12.92	24.47	31.16	21.05
% Exceeding ± 10%	30%	25%	60%	55%	25%	20%	30%	15%

TABLE 5-4. DIFFERENCE BETWEEN EXTENDED AND
NORMAL RANGES FOR 10 BRIDGES; EXTENDED WORSE −,
EXTENDED BETTER +, EXTENDED AS BAD BUT OPPOSITE
DIRECTION ≠.

	Pressure in mm H_2O			
Bridge #	−200	−100	100	200
1	+35	+10	−5	≠ 40
2	0	−15	+5	+5
4	−15	−10	0	+35
7	−30	−40	−10	0
13	−30	−10	+30	+20
14	−45	−10	0	−10
16	+5	−10	0	≠ 105
17	−25	−10	+5	−5
19	−25	+30	+5	−5
20	+15	0	+5	+20
% Poorer	60%	70%	20%	40%
% Better	30%	20%	50%	30%
% Same	10%	10%	30%	10%
% Equal but opposite direction	0%	0%	0%	20%

Manometer Circuit Leakage

It was found when measuring the air leakage of the manometer circuits that the 20 study bridges could be divided into four rather distinct groups. The range of air-pressure leakage, such as 0 to 20 mm of H_2O for Group I, is depicted in the top portion of Figure 5-1. Group I consisted of nine bridges that demonstrated a linear loss of pressure when plotted for a 5-minute period. The mean loss for 5 minutes was 7.77 mm of H_2O air pressure with a standard deviation of 7.95. The range of the leakage from the six bridges in Group II, also shown in Figure 5-1, was from approximately 40 to 200 mm of H_2O air pressure in 5 minutes. The mean loss of pressure for this group was 108.83 mm of H_2O air pressure with a standard deviation of 66.66. The pressure drift in this group was also linear across the 5 minutes.

The air-pressure loss individually plotted for bridges in Group III and IV was curvilinear in shape, as seen in Figure 5-2. Group III consisted of two bridges, both of which lost 400 mm of H_2O air pressure during the 5-minute measurement period. This represented a total loss of air pressure, that is, a return to atmospheric pressure. It should be noted that those bridges lost as much as 300 mm of H_2O air pressure in as little as 2.5 minutes. Group IV consisted of three bridges that demonstrated similarly shaped plots for air leakage. They were unique in that they lost 300 mm of H_2O air pressure in less than 1.5 minutes.

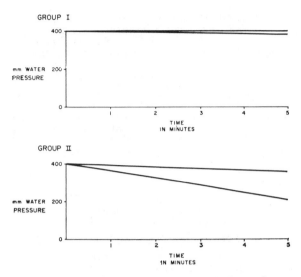

FIGURE 5-1. Range of linear air-pressure leakage. Group I = 9 bridges, Group II = 6 bridges.

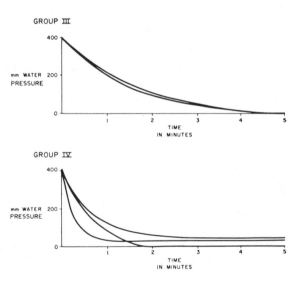

FIGURE 5-2. Individual curvilinear air-pressure leakage. Group III = 2 bridges, Group IV = 3 bridges.

As indicated under Procedures, a second pressure-leakage measurement was made wherein the manometer output at the back of the bridge housing was plugged with a closed tube. Under this condition, all 20 bridges showed essentially no leakage over a 2.5-minute measurement period. This finding serves to emphasize the fact that most of the bridges in this study had some leakage ranging from 1 to 400 mm of H_2O air pressure, and that the pressure loss was due to leaks in the transducer housing, probe tubes, or possibly the tip itself.

Cavity Equivalence

Equivalent cavity size measurements were performed using a Madsen Variable Cavity; the readings were taken from the compliance cursor of each bridge in the study. Measurements were made for 0.5, 1, 2, 4, and 5 cc. Table 5–5 presents the means and standard deviations for the above-mentioned equivalent cavity sizes.

There were only 18 bridges at 4 cc and five bridges at 5 cc that could be measured because cursor readings indicated equivalent volumes larger than 5 cc,—the limit on the cursor scale. If a tolerance criterion of ± 10 percent is once again applied to each individual bridge, 90 percent were out of calibration at 0.5 cc, 35 percent were out at 1 cc, 30 percent were out at 2 cc, 40 percent were out at 4 cc, and none of the five bridges that could be measured were out at 5 cc.

Sensitivity

The sensitivity measurements represent the differences in compliance, as read on the cursor scale, between the equivalent volume required to balance the meter and to adjust it for full-scale deflection to the right. The above-mentioned procedure was carried out for each sensitivity setting in a 2-cc cavity.

The sensitivity measurements indicated that the largest equivalent volume change was required to obtain a full-scale balance meter deflection for the least sensitive settings. The opposite was also true, that is, the most sensitive settings required the least amount of equivalent volume change in cubic centimeters. It is important to restate that there were 12 AE bridges

TABLE 5-6. MEANS AND STANDARD DEVIATIONS FOR SENSITIVITY SETTINGS OF THE AE INSTRUMENTS.

Item	Sensitivity			
	AD	T	R	SR
N	2	11	11	11
Mean	1.90	0.75	0.15	0.05
SD	1.20	0.12	0.06	0.04

TABLE 5-7. MEANS AND STANDARD DEVIATIONS FOR SENSITIVITY SETTINGS OF EIGHT MADSEN INSTRUMENTS.

Item	Sensitivity			
	1	2	3	4
N	8	8	8	8
Mean	0.75	0.53	0.16	0.04
SD	0.14	0.11	0.02	0.02

and eight Madsen bridges. Therefore, data are considered separately for each manufacturer because they have different sensitivity settings. Table 5–6 presents the summary data for the AE bridges.

Data were collected on 11 of the 12 AE bridges for various sensitivity settings. Only two of the 11 bridges could be measured at a sensitivity setting of A_D. It was impossible to make the measurement for the A_D settings because they required adjustments beyond the limits of the cursor scale.

Table 5–7 presents the data collected from the eight Madsen bridges. By comparing Tables 5–6 and 5–7 one observes that the two manufacturers have approximately the same mean values for the settings used to trace a tympanogram, that is, #1 and T. In addition, Madsen settings of #3 and #4 were nearly the same as AE settings R and SR. These settings are, of course, the ones used for acoustic reflex measurements. The small number of bridges measured at A_D rendered meaningful statements difficult.

For all bridges, the standard deviations are relatively small suggesting little variability about the mean. However, there is a trend toward standard deviations being largest at the least sensitive settings of both types of bridges and becoming progressively smaller at the more sensitive settings.

Probe Tone

Eighteen of the bridges studied were calibrated for a probe tone of 220 Hz set for 85-dB SPL in a 2-cc cavity, and the remaining two were older bridges calibrated for 95-dB SPL. The mean level for the 18

TABLE 5-5. MEANS, STANDARD DEVIATIONS, AND TOLERANCES OF EQUIVALENT CAVITY SIZE FOR THE 20 STUDY BRIDGES.

Item	Cubic Centimeters				
	0.5	1	2	4	5
N	20	20	20	18	5
Mean	0.69	1.14	2.12	4.31	4.88
SD	0.25	0.18	0.23	0.27	0.23
% Exceeding $\pm 10\%$	90%	35%	30%	40%	0%

bridges measured 86.22-dB SPL with a standard deviation of 0.84 dB. The largest deviation on either side of the mean was 2.5 dB. The remaining two bridges had output levels of 95.5 and 98.5-dB SPL. Thus, the bridge with the greatest discrepancy between its expected and actual output was one of the older ZO-70 bridges, which was off by 3.5 dB.

The mean of the second harmonic for all 20 bridges was down 29.58 dB from the probe tone with a standard deviation of 2.08 dB. If the ANSI S3.6-1969 standard for the second harmonic of pure tones were applied to the probe tone of each bridge, eight of the 20 bridges (40 percent) would be less than 30 dB down from the fundamental or probe tone.[1]

Tympanographic Characteristics

Real-ear subject data were collected in addition to the above-mentioned calibration data. The two curves shown in Figure 5-3 represent the mean tympanograms run from +200 to −300 mm of H_2O air pressure (left curve), and run from −300 to +200 mm of H_2O air pressure (right curve) on one normal subject with the 20 bridges. The normal range for the relative height of the peaks of the tympanogram shown by the shaded area was from 63.5 mm to 125 mm. The mean height of all tympanograms plotted from study bridges was 100.2 mm. The heights ranged from 75 to 120 mm with a standard deviation of 10.83.

The mean curve, which displays the positive to negative traces, had its peak amplitude at −19.25 mm of H_2O air pressure with a standard deviation of 14.44 mm of H_2O. The mean pressure for the peak of

the curve, plotted negative to positive, in Figure 5-3 was +11.25 mm of H_2O air pressure with a standard deviation of 13.85 mm of H_2O. Plotting the curves in opposite directions produces a hysteresis or difference in pressure between the two maximum peaks, which has been previously reported by Cretan and van Camp (1974), Feldman (1976), and Williams (1976). The mean difference between peaks shown in Figure 5-3 was 30.50 mm of H_2O air pressure.

Static Compliance

Static-compliance measures were made on the subject with 19 of the 20 bridges. This measurement was not possible on one bridge due to its extremely rapid air-pressure leakage, which rendered impossible a measurement of maximum compliance at a negative pressure point at well as at +200 mm of H_2O air pressure. Measurements were made at +200 mm of H_2O air pressure, atmospheric pressure, and at the pressure where maximum compliance was obtained.

The mean compliance at +200 mm of H_2O air pressure was 0.86 cc with a standard deviation of 0.19 cc. At atmospheric pressure the mean compliance was 1.40 cc with a standard deviation of 0.25 cc. The mean compliance of the middle-ear system, as measured by the difference between the compliance at atmospheric pressure minus the compliance at +200 mm of H_2O air pressure, was 0.54 cc with a standard deviation of 0.12 cc. The mean compliance of the middle-ear system as measured by the difference between the value obtained at the point of maximum compliance minus the compliance at +200 mm of H_2O air pressure was 0.60 cc with a standard deviation of 0.11 cc. There was apparently agreement between the measures.

DISCUSSION

The purpose of this study was not to determine specific requirements or tolerance limits for electroacoustic impedance testing devices, rather, to report the everyday characteristics of 20 bridges currently being used in various clinical settings in the Detroit metropolitan area. It is hoped that such a study has pointed out the necessity for developing calibration standards for impedance bridges. We believe establishing standards would allow the audiologist to achieve a higher degree of excellence in providing clinical services.

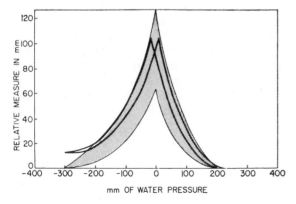

FIGURE 5-3. Mean positive to negative and negative to positive going tympanograms on 20 study bridges.

The first section of this discussion covers the calibration data collected on the 20 clinical bridges studied. The second part of this discussion deals with the real-ear data collected; and finally, the data from the 20 clinical bridges are compared to that obtained on a control bridge (Madsen ZO-72). As stated previously, the control bridge was carefully calibrated according to the manufacturer's specifications, and was used as a standard against which we could compare the data obtained on all clinical bridges.

Calibration Data

The high percentage of bridges (30–60 percent) which exceeded the manometer readings tolerance of ±10 percent generally set by manufacturers leads one to conclude that, not only should clinicians monitor their bridges, but that the manufacturers should attempt to provide more reliable and stable measurement techniques. This problem is compounded by the fact that 20 to 70 percent of the measurements made on bridges which had an extended and normal range switch were poorer in the extended setting.

The amount of air-pressure leakage found in this study was perhaps more an indictment of the clinician than of the manufacturer because with the pressure tube blocked at the rear of the bridge, none of the 20 bridges showed any leakage. However, a great deal of leakage was shown across bridges when the probe tip was sealed in a hard-walled cavity. It must be the responsibility of the clinician to check daily the integrity of the air-pressure system external to the instrument. A clinician must have a thorough understanding of the numerous possibilities where air leakage can occur. This knowledge should include how to check for leaks in the tubing as well as pressure leaks that might occur around the two transducers in the headset.

Some of the leakage problems can be circumvented by using surgical rubber tubing, with an equivalent diameter and length, which is more resistant to puncture than the thin-walled tubing supplied with some bridges. However, one must be certain to duplicate the original equipment if wool has been inserted in the manometer tube. Simply remove the wool from the original manometer tube and insert it in the tube. This is accomplished by pulling it into place with a small piece of wire.

The clinical measurement most susceptible to error when dealing with rapid pressure leakage is the acoustic reflex. Certainly, test data must be questioned when 25 percent of the bridges tested had air-pressure leakages ranging from 200 to 300 mm of H_2O air pressure in the first minute. It is critical that the acoustic reflex be measured at the pressure that produces the maximum compliance for the middle-ear system. Any rapid drift during that test could invalidate the reflex measurements and produce poor reliability.

Equivalent cavity sizes across the bridges showed a wide range of unacceptable values (30–90 percent) based on a tolerance limit of ±10 percent. Measurement of equivalent cavity size is critical when making the static compliance calculations, which is discussed later. In addition, many clinicians rely on equivalent cavity size to help determine the presence of a perforation in the tympanic membrane. Particularly alarming was the number of bridges studied (90 percent), which exceeded the tolerance limits of ±10 percent at 0.5 cc. This should alert the clinician to be cautious about making diagnostic statements regarding cavity size in an infant.

Agreement was found between the Madsen and AE bridges for the sensitivity settings traditionally used for tympanograms (#1 and T) and reflex measures (#3, #4, and S, S.R.), respectively. Standard nomenclature for sensitivity settings would certainly aid in reducing the confusion that arises due to the inconsistencies found among the various bridges on the market.

Sound-pressure levels of the 220 Hz probe tones were amazingly close to the levels specified by the manufacturers. All but one of the 20 bridges were within 2.5 dB of the 85- or 95-dB SPL required. The work *amazingly* is used in this context because this study was initiated due to the difficulties experienced by the investigators in maintaining the proper calibration of the probe tone on a particular bridge. That problem was finally traced to a loose trim pot. Each time the trim pot was adjusted it would turn, causing a solder lug to make contact with an adjacent trim pot, which drastically altered the output of the probe tone. This experience points out the problems that can be encountered by poor quality control and may go unnoticed if the clinician is not monitoring the instrument.

Harmonic distortion of the probe tone was determined by measuring the second harmonic that was approximately 30 dB down from the fundamental. Excessive harmonic distortion could conceivably affect the capability of the bridge to process the signal adequately.

Another parameter that should be checked is the frequency of the probe tone. Although frequency was not measured in this study, personal experience has shown that for bridges with very narrow band-pass filters it is critical that the probe-tone oscillator not drift more than a few Hz.

Real-Ear Data

All of the data mentioned thus far in the discussion were obtained using the calibrating instrumentation describing previously. This portion of the discussion concerns itself with the data obtained by testing one subject on all of the 20 bridges used in the study. As shown by the solid line in Figure 5-4, the mean tympanograms fell within the normal limits (shaded area) for tympanometry. However, due to the variability of the individual tympanograms some of them fell outside the normal limits.

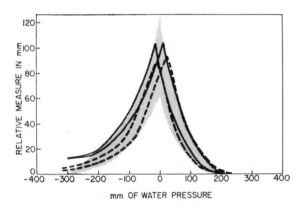

FIGURE 5-4. Comparison of the mean tympanogram obtained from 20 study bridges (solid line) and the tympanogram obtained from the control bridge (hashed line).

The curves obtained on the standard or control bridge, shown by the hashed line in Figure 5-4, indicated that the mean tympanogram curve was slightly higher in relative amplitude. However, because this is a relative measure on this type of impedance bridge there would certainly have been no clinical error in interpretation of such data.

Static compliance, which seems to be struggling to maintain its place in the regimen of clinical impedance tests, is an additional piece of information that can help to verify other test results. The static compliance information obtained on the control bridge when testing the subject was not within one standard deviation of the data obtained on the 20 bridges. The mean values for the 20 study bridges were 0.54 cc and 0.60 cc at atmospheric pressure and the pressure for maximum compliance respectively, whereas they were 0.69 cc and 0.77 cc as measured on the control bridge. Lack of agreement here points out again the necessity for an overall standard and calibration procedure.

It is hoped that those who are presently involved in the development of calibration and standardization procedures for electroacoustic impedance testing devices will continue their efforts in that direction. In the interim, those clinicians who are presently using such instrumentation should do all within their power and knowledge to assure that their equipment is in proper working condition. Only through a concerted effort by all of those involved will the problems and inconsistencies of not only instrumentation but of interpretation be resolved.

ACKNOWLEDGMENT

The authors wish to express their gratitude to the young subject, Christian Omar Robinson, whose patience and tolerance facilitated the collection of our real-ear data.

ENDNOTE

1. Generally, when measuring second harmonics with an octave filter, it is only possible to measure a second harmonic which is approximately 25 dB down from the fundamental. This is due to specifications for filters set by ANSI S1.11–1971 (R–1966). However, this specification refers to a second harmonic one octave from the center frequency of the adjacent octave filters. For the case herein described, the fundamental frequency was 220 Hz which is 280 Hz below the center frequency for the filter centered at 500 Hz which was used to measure the second harmonic. With this configuration, the filter skirts allowed measurement of up to 31 dB down from the fundamental. D.O.R., R.H.B.

REFERENCES

American National Standards Institute. Specifications for audiometers (ANSI S3-1969). New York: American National Standards Institute (1969).

Creten, W. L., and vanCamp, K. J. Transient and quasistatic tympanometry. *Scand. Audiol., 3,* 39–42 (1974).

Feldman, A. S. Tympanometry—procedures, interpretations and variables. In A. S. Feldman and L. A. Wilber (Eds.), *Acoustic Impedance and Admittance—The Measurement of Middle Ear Function.* Baltimore: Williams and Wilkins, 103–155 (1976).

Feldman, A. S., and Wilber, L. A. (Eds.) *Acoustic Impedance and Admittance—The Measurement of Middle Ear Function.* Baltimore: Williams and Wilkins, Appendix I (1976).

Williams, P. S. Effects of rate and direction of air pressure changes on tympanometry. Doctoral dissertation, Univ. of Washington (1976).

6

Stability of Routinely Serviced Portable Audiometers

WENDEL K. WALTON, Ph.D.
Consultant, Connecticut State Department of Education
PEGGY S. WILLIAMS, Ph.D.
Director, Clinic and Hospital Programs, American Speech-Language-Hearing Association, Rockville, Maryland

The need for audiometer maintenance has been emphasized by several authors (Thomas et al., 1969; Eagles and Doerfler, 1961), but only Martin (1968) has reported on the stability of routinely serviced commercial audiometers. Martin calibrated the output levels of 262 audiometers to within plus or minus 2 dB of the British Standard, and then reexamined the same audiometers after six to 12 months of use. Observing that 70 percent of all earphones were within plus or minus 1 dB of the original levels, and 85 percent were within plus or minus 3 dB, Martin concluded that intensity stability was good and advised that audiometers be calibrated at least yearly.

With the adoption by the American National Standards Institute-Specifications S3.6-1969 (1969), interest has been renewed in the general subject of audiometer calibration (Melnick, 1971). With this interest has arisen the question of audiometer stability for factors other than intensity. This study examined how well audiometers receiving routine maintenance and calibration meet specifications for 13 factors.

METHOD

During the winter of 1971, 50 wide-range, portable audiometers representing two makes and nine different models, were borrowed from school districts in the greater Seattle area. Via questionnaire, we learned that all of the audiometers had been purchased between 1957 and 1970, the median purchase year being 1966. Typically, the audiometers received greatest use during the fall months with only occasional use thereafter. Total reported audiometer usage ranged from 15 hours to 640 hours per year, the majority being used approximately 225 hours per year. Typical operators were either school nurses or undergraduates in the Speech Pathology-Audiology Program at the University of Washington. Each of the audiometers had been calibrated to ISO-1964 reference threshold by persons reported to be factory-trained personnel; 96 percent were calibrated during the summer of 1970, and the other 4 percent were calibrated during the preceding summer. All of the audiometers were evaluated following the period of their greatest use.

Equipment. Calibration equipment consisted of a Bruel and Kjaer Type 158 Audiometer Calibration System and a Type 2416 voltmeter, a General Radio 1192 electronic counter, and a Tektronix 564B storage oscilloscope with a 3L5 spectrum analyzer and a 2B67 time base generator.

Procedures. Each of the audiometers was assessed for the following: intensity accuracy, frequency accuracy, tone purity, rise time accuracy, decay time accuracy, shock hazard, signal-to-noise ratio, cross talk, extraneous noise, tonal maximum levels, stability with respect to variations in supply voltage, attenuator linearity, and mechanical condition. Because the audiometers were manufactured prior to the adoption of ANSI Specification S3.6-1969 (1969), the ISO-1964 (1964) reference thresholds—as modified by Cox and Bilger's data (1960) for TDH-39 earphones—were used for intensity assessment, while the applicable sections of ASA Specification Z24.5-1951 (1951) were used for the other assessments.[1]

All output measurements were made acoustically with the earphones on a National Bureau of Standards 9-A coupler. For frequency, purity, rise time,

Reprinted by permission of the authors from *Lang., Speech, Hearing Serv. in Schools,* **3,** 36–43 (1972).

and decay time assessments, the output of the sound level meter was electrically connected to the appropriate analyzing device and the audiometer hearing level attenuator was set for maximum output. All earphones were Telephonics type TDH 39, with 78 percent mounted in MX-41/AR cushions and 22 percent mounted in circumaural housings. Earphones mounted in circumaural units were removed from these and placed temporarily in MX-41/AR cushions for the necessary assessments. Measurements were made at the six-octave test frequencies from 250 through 8,000 Hz. The sound pressure level calibration of the B & K system was checked at least twice daily by pistonphone.

RESULTS

We found results for the percentage of audiometers that had one or more errors for each given type of error; the percentage of errors based on the total possible errors of a given type (for example, with 50 audiometers, and two earphones and six test frequencies per audiometer, there were $50 \times 2 \times 6 = 600$ possible errors of intensity; if 300 such errors were counted, the percentage of errors would equal 50 percent); and the percentage of audiometers failing to meet a given specification at a designated frequency—referred to as "errors-by-frequency."

Intensity. Thirty-four percent of the audiometers had one or more intensity errors and the percent of errors equaled seven. Errors-by-frequency were 8 percent at 250 Hz, 16 percent at 500 Hz, 10 percent at 1,000 Hz, 6 percent at 2,000 Hz, and 1 percent at 4,000 and 8,000 Hz. Without exception, errors of intensity resulted from insufficient energy.

Frequency. The ASA specification (1951) requires that audiometer test frequencies be within plus or minus 5 percent of the nominal values. Twelve percent of the audiometers produced frequencies beyond the 5 percent tolerance, and the percentage of errors equaled two. Errors-by-frequency were 4 percent at 250, 500, and 8,000 Hz, 2 pecent at 2,000 Hz, and 0 percent at 1,000 and 4,000 Hz. There were approximately as many cases of the measured frequency being below the lower-frequency tolerance limit as there were cases of the measured frequency exceeding the upper-frequency tolerance limit.

Purity. Six percent of the audiometers had one or more errors of purity, and the percentage of errors equaled two. Errors-by-frequency were 1 percent at 250 and 4,000 Hz, and 2 percent at 500, 1,000, 2,000, and 8,000 Hz. The ASA specification (1951) requires that all harmonics be more than 25 dB below the level of the fundamental. The excessive distortion we found resulted from the second harmonic being only 18 to 25 dB below the fundamental.

Rise Time. Twenty-eight percent of the audiometers had errors of rise time and the percentage of errors equaled 13. Errors-by-frequency were 5 percent at 250 Hz, 12 percent at 500, 1,000, and 4,000 Hz, 14 percent at 2,000 Hz, and 23 percent at 8,000 Hz. Rise time errors were usually the result of excessively fast rise time, often less than 5 msec.

Decay Time. Only 4 percent of the audiometers had decay time errors, and these audiometers were among the oldest surveyed. The percentage of errors of decay time equaled one-half, and errors-by-frequency were 0 percent at 250, 500, 1,000, and 2,000 Hz, 2 percent at 4,000 Hz, and 1 percent at 8,000 Hz. The few decay time errors resulted from excessively slow decay time, often as long as 700 msec.

Shock Hazard, Signal-to-Noise Ratio, Cross Talk. All of the audiometers met specifications of shock hazard, signal-to-noise ratio, and cross talk.

Extraneous Noise. Thirty-six percent of the audiometers had some type of extraneous noise believed to affect routine use adversely. We examined for the presence of attenuator noise, signal radiation directly from the chassis or some component, and other noise such as mechanical "clicks" from the tone interrupter switch, power supply hum, or vacuum tube or transistor noise. Regardless of the types or source, attenuator and other noises were considered a problem when they were audible through the earphones to examiners with normal hearing sensitivity with the hearing loss attenuator set at 70 dB. Chassis radiation was considered a problem when it was audible to examiners with normal hearing, not wearing earphones, seated in an IAC 1200 series room approximately three feet from the audiometer, and with the attenuator set at 70 dB. The results are shown in Table 6-1.

TABLE 6–1. PERCENTAGE OF AUDIOMETERS HAVING EXTRANEOUS NOISE, BY TYPE.

Type	Percentage of Audiometers Judged Unacceptable (N = 50)	Typical Problem
Attenuator noise	16	Dirt on attenuator
Chassis radiation	8	Components oscillating
Other noise	18	Power supply hum
Combined (one or more of the above)	36	—

Maximum Levels. Four percent of the audiometers had maximum levels less than those recommended. Total possible errors of this type equaled 0.5 percent, and errors-by-frequency were 1 percent at 250, 1,000, and 8,000 Hz, and 0 percent for the other test frequencies.

Stability with Respect to Variation in Supply Voltage. Stability of the audiometers at 1,000 Hz with variation in the supply voltage was determined at three different voltages: 105, 125, and the nominal 117 VAC. We examined the effect on intensity, frequency, and purity. Each audiometer was given a minimum of 30 minutes in which to stabilize at a given supply voltage before any measurements were made. Only two of the audiometers (4 percent) had problems with stability. At 105 VAC, one of the two developed problems with purity and the other had insufficient intensity.

Attenuator Linearity. Attenuator linearity was determined electrically at 1,000 Hz from 15 to 100 dB HL (or 110 dB, where provided) in 5-dB intervals. To account for possible cumulative errors, we also assessed the overall range. Twenty percent of the audiometers had 5-dB interval errors, and 12 percent had errors of overall range. Twenty percent had either or both of the foregoing types of errors of linearity.

Mechanical Condition. We visually examined the condition and apparent operating status of the dials, knobs, switches, power cords, earphone cushions, and earphone cords. We arbitrarily decided whether the observed condition would adversely affect routine usage. Forty-six percent of the audiometers had problems of this type, as shown in Table 6–2.

DISCUSSION

In Table 6–3 the 13 types of errors considered in this study are ranked in decreasing order of frequency of occurrence, together with Thomas et al.'s (1969) findings for the same factors. In every category for which comparative data are available, except decay time, the percentage of audiometers failing to meet specifications is greater for Thomas et al.'s set of audiometers than for those evaluated in this study. Since the audiometers evaluated by Thomas et al.

TABLE 6–2. PERCENTAGE OF AUDIOMETERS HAVING MECHANICAL CONDITION PROBLEMS, BY TYPE.

Type	Percentage of Audiometers Judged Unacceptable (N = 50)	Typical Problem
Dials	14	Loose, misaligned
Knobs, switches	22	Loose, noisy
Earphone cushions	18	Split, material deteriorating
Earphone cords	4	Frayed, partially damaged
Combined (one or more of the above)	46	—

TABLE 6–3. PERCENTAGE OF AUDIOMETERS FAILING TO MEET SPECIFICATIONS FOR EACH OF 13 FACTORS—RANKED IN DECREASING ORDER OF FREQUENCY OF FAILURE—WITH A COMPARISON TO THOMAS ET AL.'S (1969) REPORT ON AUDIOMETER CALIBRATION.

Factor	Walton-Williams Percentage Failure (N = 50)	Rank	Thomas et al. Percentage Failure (N = 100)	Rank
Mechanical condition	46	1	—	—
Extraneous noise	36	2	77–83*	3
Intensity	34	3	89	1
Rise time	28	4	84	2
Attenuator linearity	20	5	24	5
Frequency	12	6	31	4
Purity	6	7	6	7
Decay time	4	9	0	10
Maximum levels	4	9	—	—
Stability with line voltage variation	4	9	12	6
Shock hazard	0	12	2	8.5
Signal-to-noise ratio	0	12	—	—
Cross talk	0	12	2	8.5
Combined (one or more of the 13 types of errors)	82	—	—	—

*Obtained by combining the reported number of audiometers having excessive attenuator noise (77%) with the number having other noise (6%) and allowing for duplications.

had not received the routine maintenance that this set of audiometers had, we expected to find a lower percentage of errors in this study.

As seen in Table 6–3, approximately four out of every five audiometers (82 percent) had at least one of the 13 possible errors. The two most common problems were mechanical condition (46 percent) and extraneous noise (35 percent). When these two factors alone are considered, 32 of the audiometers (64 percent) had one or both of these errors. In other words, of the 41 audiometers (82 percent) having one or more of the 13 possible errors, 32 (78 percent) would have been isolated simply by checking for mechanical problems and noise. These results would indicate that if an audiometer has either of these two types of problems, it probably needs professional service. Only two audiometers had errors of both mechanical condition and extraneous noise, and no other problems. Therefore, if superficial examination reveals that an audiometer has both these types of problems, it has probably other problems as well and should receive immediate attention.

Without question more factors were evaluated in this study than are routinely considered in audiometer calibration. Of the service centers we know, all check intensity accuracy, but few check anything else—yet errors of intensity remain among the most prevalent. Unfortunately, what constitutes a "calibrated" audiometer seems to be determined by the equipment complement of the service center and the user's budget, rather than by the specifications of any national organization.

A comparison of the rank orderings presented in Table 6–3 revealed good agreement between the two studies. When mechanical condition is excluded, extraneous noise, intensity, rise time, attenuator linearity, and frequency were the five most frequently occurring problems in both studies. These five, together with mechanical condition, constitute what we believe to be the minimum set of factors to evaluate routinely in audiometer calibration.

Errors-by-frequency of a given type were essentially the same for the six test frequencies—with the exceptions of rise time and intensity. Rise time errors were fewest (5 percent) at 250 Hz, and most (23 percent) at 8,000 Hz, while the typical error was 12 percent for the other four test frequencies. From 500 through 4,000 Hz, errors of intensity became progressively fewer. Since 500 Hz is frequently included in public school hearing screening programs, and since environmental noise often interferes with testing at this frequency, the finding that intensity errors were greatest at this frequency implies inadvisability of retaining this frequency in routine screening testing. Further, with respect to those frequencies employed in screening programs, 4,000 Hz seemed particularly stable. With the sole exception of decay time, errors at 4,000 Hz were either equal to those found typically at other frequencies, or fewer.

CONCLUSIONS

We evaluated 50 routinely serviced portable audiometers used in public schools after their period of greatest use. The audiometers were of two makes and nine different models with a median age of approximately five years. The performance of the audiometers was determined for each of 13 factors by comparison to the applicable ISO/ASA specification. Eighty-two percent had one or more of the 13 types of errors. The six most frequently encountered problems, in decreasing order of frequency of occurrence, were mechanical condition, extraneous noise, intensity, rise time, attenuator linearity, and frequency. These six factors are proffered as the minimum set for adequate audiometer calibration.

Although the results of this study are more encouraging than those previously reported (Thomas et al., 1969), the situation remains bleak. The audiometers included in this study had been maintained on a routine yearly basis, yet four out of five could not meet specifications. Certainly at least yearly maintenance and calibration are essential for all factors contained within the current specifications for audiometers, but the poor performance we observed in this study suggests a need for improved audiometer circuit design and production quality control.

ACKNOWLEDGMENT

The authors express appreciation to James Labiak for his assistance in the early phases of this work.

ENDNOTE

1. For discussions of the ISO/ASA specifications, consult Thomas et al. (1969), Melnick (1971), and Harford (1971).

REFERENCES

American National Standards Institute. *American National Standard Specifications for Audiometers,* S 3.6-1969. New York (1969).

American Standards Association. *American Standard Specification for Audiometers for General Diagnostic Purposes,* Z 24.5-1951. New York (1951).

Cox, J. R., and Bilger, R. C. Suggestion relative to the standardization of loudness balance data in Telephonics TDH-39 earphones. *J. acoust. Soc. Amer.,* **32,** 1081–1082 (1960).

Eagles, E., and Doerfler, L. G. Hearing in children: Acoustic environment and audiometer performance. *J. Speech Hearing Res.,* **4,** 149–163 (1961).

Eagles, E., Wishik, S. M., Doerfler, L. G., Melnick, W., and Levine, H. S. Hearing sensitivity and related factors in children. Graduate School of Public Health, University of Pittsburgh. *Laryngoscope,* St. Louis, Mo. (1963).

Harford, E. Audiometer Calibration. *Audecibel,* **20,** 80, 82–84 (1971).

International Organization for Standardization. *ISO Recommendation,* R 389-1964, *Standard Reference Zero for the Calibration of Pure-tone Audiometers.* Switzerland (1964).

Martin, M. C., The routine calibration of audiometers. *Sound,* **2,** 106–109 (1968).

Melnick, W. American national standard specifications for audiometers. *Asha,* **13,** 203–206 (1971).

Thomas, W. G., Preslar, M. J., Summers, R. R., and Stewart, J. L. Calibration and working condition of 100 audiometers. *Public Health Reports,* **84,** 311–327 (1969).

7

A-Weighted Equivalents of Permissible Ambient Noise During Audiometric Testing

MEAD C. KILLION, Ph.D.
Senior Engineer Industrial Research Products, Elk Grove Village, Illinois
GERALD A. STUDEBAKER, Ph.D.
Professor of Speech and Hearing Science, Memphis State University

Using the relative octave band levels obtained by Botsford [Sound Vib. 3, 16–28 (1969)] for various noise spectra, it is possible to calculate the A- and C-weighted sound levels of typical noises just meeting the requirements of ANSI S3.1-1977. Such a calculation indicates an A-weighted sound level of approximately 15 dB is required to meet the maximum permissible octave band levels for testing at audiometric zero in the ears-not-covered condition. For the average typical curves shown by Botsford, the calculated A-weighted sound levels range from 14.0 to 16.5 dB. For the case where the ear is covered by an earphone mounted in an MX-41/AR cushion, an A-weighted level of 22 dB or less appears to be required. For applications requiring determination of hearing threshold down to the conventional upper limit of "normal hearing," (25 dB HL) the corresponding A-weighted noise levels are 40 dB for sound field testing and 47 dB for earphone testing.
PACS numbers: 43.66.Cb, 43.66.Yw, 43.66.Sr.

Botsford (1969) studied the octave band analyses of 953 noises which he grouped according to the difference $(C - A)$ between the calculated A- and C-weighted sound levels. He then calculated the Perceived Noise Levels, Speech Interference Levels, Damage-Risk Criteria, etc., corresponding to the octave band analyses of the individual noises. These calculations demonstrated that the A-weighted sound meter readings could provide an accurate gauge of the human response to most noises. Botsford (1973) later presented curves of the average relative octave band levels corresponding to the noises in each of seven $C - A$ groupings.

Following a similar line of reasoning, it is possible to calculate the A- and C-weighted sound levels corresponding to each of Botsford's curves after the values have been adjusted in level to just meet the maximum allowable octave band level requirements of the new standard for audiometer room noise (ANSI S3. 1-1977). Figure 7-1 illustrates the procedure with a range of noise types likely to be encoun-

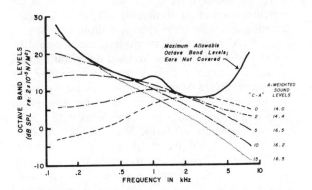

FIGURE 7-1. Estimation of allowable *A*-weighted ambient noise levels for audiometric testing to 0-dB HTL with uncovered ears.

Reprinted by permission of the authors from *J. Acoust. Soc. Am.*, **63**, 1633–1635 (1978). Copyright 1978, Acoustical Society of America.

TABLE 7–1. ALLOWABLE ROOM-NOISE LEVELS FOR "EARS-NOT-COVERED" CONDITION.

C–A (dB)	Allowable A-weighted level (dB)	Allowable C-weighted level (dB)
0	14	14
2	14.4	16.4
5	16.5	21.5
10	16.2	26.5
15	16.5	31.5

TABLE 7–2. ALLOWABLE ROOM-NOISE LEVELS FOR TDH-39/MX-41 AR EARPHONE AUDIOMETRY.

C–A (dB)	Allowable A-weighted level (dB)	Allowable C-weighted level (dB)
0	31.7	31.7
2	27.2	29.2
5	24.5	29.5
10	21.7	31.7
15	21.1	36.1

tered around an audiometric test facility. The solid line represents a smooth curve drawn through the maximum octave band levels permissible when testing at 0-dB hearing threshold level under the ears-not-covered condition. The other curves represent the average octave band levels for Botsford's $C - A$ groupings of 0, 2, 5, 10, and 15 dB. In each case, the vertical position of the curve has been adjusted to just meet but not exceed the curve representing maximum permissible octave band levels. Table 7–1 lists the calculated A- and C-weighted levels for each of the noises. Note that the total range of the A-weighted noise levels is less than 3 dB. It is apparent that an A-weighted noise level below 15 dB will generally meet the requirements of the new standard for the ears-not-covered (field audiometry or un-occluded bone conduction testing) condition.

A similar procedure was carried out for the condition where the ears are covered with an earphone mounted in an MX-41/AR cushion. The results are shown in Table 7–2. In this case, there is a substantially larger spread of values but it appears that an A-weighted sound level of 22 dB or less (or a C-weighted level of 30 dB or less) will generally insure an adequate room for earphone audiometry. Apparently the C scale of the sound-level meter would be more useful for assessing ambient noise during earphone audiometry. This comes about because the noise attenuation of the earphone cushion is greatest in the high-frequency region where the A-weighted response of the sound-level meter is greatest.

The maximum allowable levels in the new standard were designed so that "the average normal hearing listener will produce a threshold free of significant effect from the ambient noise." The allowable effect in this case was a 1-dB increase in threshold above the accepted reference hearing threshold levels. In many cases where the audiometer is to be used for screening purposes or the selection of hear-

ing aids, accurate threshold determinations may not be required below 25-dB hearing threshold level. In such cases, the standard specifies "the maximum allowable ambient noise levels for test conditions which exceed the reference threshold levels may be calculated by arithmetically adding the amount by which the minimum acceptable test hearing threshold levels exceed the reference hearing threshold levels at each test frequency." If the minimum acceptable test hearing threshold levels are set at 25 dB, i.e., at what is normally considered the upper limit of "normal threshold," then the allowable A-weighted noise levels become approximately 40 dBA and 47 dBA for the ears-not-covered and ears-covered conditions, respectively.

Sound level meters of at least type 2 quality (ANSI S1.4-1971) may be used instead of octave or one-third-octave band analyzers to quickly and routinely check the acceptability of an office, classroom, or closet for threshold determinations *at the time of use.*

However, it is emphasized that the use of a sound-level meter for this purpose involves the assumption that the background noise has a reasonably smooth spectrum and that it falls generally within the range of typical noises as illustrated in Figure 7–1. Botsford (1973) states that "These curves can be used to predict the levels of five of eight octave bands within 3 dB for two-thirds of all real noises." This statement indicates that while most environmental noises fall within this range, some do not. In at least half of all cases the effect will be to cause the sound-level-meter reading to read too high. In the remainder, when the sound-level meter underestimates the masking that might be produced by the noise, the error will usually be caused by a concentration of energy in a particular frequency region. In many cases, this energy concentration will be audible as a whistle, screech, hum, or a noise with an identifiable pitch. Such audible concentrations indicate the need for a more detailed narrow-band analysis. If this is not possible, it should be determined whether pure tones with pitches similar to that of the ambient signal are audible to the normal hearing listener at the criterion threshold level in that environment.

All measurments made in bandwidths wider than a critical band are subject to errors caused by concentrations of energy within particular regions in the analysis band width. The magnitude and the likelihood of occurrence of this potential error increases with the analysis bandwidth. Nevertheless, it is felt that the method described herein is adequate for many routine applications such as screening for possible test locations, monitoring test locations where noise levels vary over time, or assessing the adequacy of locations of convenience or necessity such as homes, offices, nursing homes, school rooms, etc., for certain noncritical hearing testing or when no alternatives exist.

The authors believe the following statement is justifiable:

> An ambient noise level of less than 40 dB A will, in most instances, allow accurate sound-field threshold determination down to the upper limit of "normal threshold," i.e., down to a 25-dB hearing level, at the audiometric frequencies of 125–8,000 Hz. This criterion should only be applied when no prominent tonal-like components (whistle, screech, hum, etc.) of the noise are audible. A room just meeting the 40-dB A limit may allow accurate thresholds to be obtained below 25-dB hearing level at some frequencies, depending on the exact spectral characteristics of the noise, but the determination of that fact would require a more sophisticated, narrow-band noise analysis. With unusual distributions of the ambient signal spectrum, thresholds in some frequency region(s) may be elevated above those predicted. Should audible

whistles, screeches, hums, or tonal-like noise suggest the possibility of such an ambient signal, a more detailed analysis should be performed, or the thresholds of normal hearing persons should be ascertained in the presence of that signal.

When earphone audiometry is to be used, the same statement would apply, changing the 40 dBA to 47dBA (or 55 dBC) in each case.

As a check on these results, the authors have calculated the hearing loss—with reference to the ISO R226-1961 recommended values for normal minimum audible field—corresponding to the average 43-dBA residential noise level found by Seacord (1940). The average room-noise spectrum levels (which most nearly correspond to Botsford's $C - A = 5$-dB curve) measured by Hoth (1941) and reported by Fletcher (1953), and the Fletcher critical band levels given in ANSI S1.13-1971, were used for these calculations. The results of these calculations indicate that the masking effect of typical residential room noise produces a nearly uniform 23-dB hearing loss across the 250–4,000-Hz speech frequencies. Thus, the average hearing loss typically produced by the masking effect of a 40-dBA room noise would be 20 dB. Similarly, the calculated loss produced by a typical 40-dBA noise with $C - A = 10$ dB (see Figure 7-1) ranged between a minimum of 17 and 25 dB across the frequencies from the 250 to 4,000 Hz, with an average value of 22 dB.

Subtracting 15 dB from the A-weighted noise level in a room provides a rough estimate of the *maximum* threshold elevation produced by that noise. Alternately, subtracting 20 dB produces a rough estimate of the *average* threshold elevation produced by that noise. The latter is the same rule of thumb suggested earlier by Killion (1976) for assessing the effect of microphone noise levels.

REFERENCES

ANSI (1971*a*), "Specification for Sound Level Meters," S1. 4-1971 (Am. Nat. Stand. Inst., New York).

ANSI (1971*b*), "Methods for Measurement of Sound Pressure Levels," S1.13-1971 (Am. Nat. Stand. Inst., New York).

ANSI (1977), "Criteria for Permissible Ambient Noise During Audiometric Testing," S3.1-1977 (Am. Nat. Stand. Inst., New York).

Botsford, J. H. (1969), "Using Sound Levels to Gauge Human Response to Noise," Sound Vib. 3(10), 16–28.

Botsford, J. H. (1973), "How to Estimate dBA Reduction of Ear Protectors," Sound Vib. 7(11), 32–33.

Fletcher, H. (1953), *Speech and Hearing in Communication* (Van Nostrand, Princeton, NJ), p. 105.

Hoth, D. F. (1941), "Room noise spectra at subscriber's telephone locations," J. Acoust. Soc. Am. **12**, 499–504.

Killion, M. C. (1976), "Noise of Ears and Microphones," J. Acoust. Soc. Am. **59** 424–433.

Seacord, D. F. (1940), "Room noise at subscriber's telephone locations," J. Acoust. Soc. Am. **12**, 183–187.

8

Audiometer Calibration

EARL R. HARFORD, Ph.D.

Professor and Director of Audiology, Department of Otolaryngology, University of Minnesota Medical School, Minneapolis, Minnesota

PART I

Accuracy in audiometry is based upon three important requisites: a competent tester, a controlled acoustic test environment, and accurate test equipment. Too often attention is directed mainly toward these first two requisites, whereas little or no attention is given to the strict calibration and periodic maintenance of test equipment. Satisfaction of these three prime ingredients is as important to the conduct of clinical audiometry as it is to research. It is understandable that the clinician might be inclined to sacrifice rigor in his instrumentation in the face of challenging and difficult clinical problems and a burdensome case load. Yet, as we shall attempt to point out, such neglect is most undesirable and, in fact, a prelude to clinical folly. The word *clinical,* as it is used here, implies any setting where one finds applied audiometry, which includes hearing conservation programs as well as clinics or physicians' offices.

Undoubtedly there are some individuals using audiometers regularly who have little understanding and appreciation for the meaning of the term *calibration.* Consequently, it may be appropriate to begin our discussion of this topic with a brief working definition of this term. A calibrated audiometer is simply one which: (1) emits the signal at the level and frequency it claims to be producing, (2) delivers the signal only to the place (i.e., a specific earphone) it is directed, (3) produces the signal free from contamination by extraneous noises or unwanted by-products of the test signal. For example, when the audiometer is set to deliver a 1,000 cps pure tone signal at 40 dB, re: zero hearing level, to the right earphone, it should do precisely this; instead of, for example, delivering a signal of 1,170 cps at 55 dB to the right earphone with a portion of the same signal to the left phone as well.

Of course, there are recognized tolerances for the important physical characteristics of pure-tone audiometric signals and these should be taken into account in any critical evaluation of the output of one of these units.

The American Standards Association (1952) has a published pamphlet of these specifications including tolerance allowances. These specifications are in the process of revision and a new set should be available in the foreseeable future. Further, there are separate specifications for diagnostic and screening audiometers, which do not, however, differ greatly. We will refer to the diagnostic specifications here.

On the whole, audiometer manufacturers are careful to design and produce audiometers which meet the specifications quoted by the ASA. Unfortunately, once an audiometer is set to these standards of performance, there is no assurance that it will remain in calibration. As a matter of fact, this equipment is sensitive and highly susceptible to unintentional abuse that can result in faulty operation. Recommendations by audiometer manufacturers, personal experience, and published reports (Eagles and Doerfler, 1961) attest to the importance of periodic calibration to assure accuracy of the signal and an overall high level of performance by the audiometer.

The Problem

There are some 50,000 audiometers extant in the United States and probably in excess of 10,000 in active service. The majority are being used in the armed forces, school hearing conservation programs, doctors' offices, industry, speech and hearing centers, and hearing aid dealers' offices. The operators of these audiometers are doctors, nurses, speech clinicians, audiologists, technicians, teachers, parents, high school seniors, and businessmen.

Provided a facility does not conduct its own calibrations, the major source for this service is through the manufacturer or one of his local or re-

Reprinted by permission of the author from *Maico Audiological Library Series,* **3,** Reports 5 and 6 (1965).

gional representatives. A check with two of the leading audiometer manufacturers clearly supports the suspicion that a very small percentage of audiometers receive periodic calibration. In fact, most calibrations are done only after an audiometer has stopped operating completely, or after it becomes noticeably unusable.

One reason for this neglect may be the result of the inconvenience of packing and shipping the instrument as well as parting with a unit that seems to be operating adequately. Regardless of the cause, there appears to be a serious need for a vigorous educational program to draw attention to the importance and value of periodic audiometer calibration.

There are numerous reasons for an audiometer to lose its precision; such as, dropping earphones, overheating (leaving the audiometer turned on after covering it with a dust protector), exposure to excessive dust (transporting an audiometer in the trunk of an automobile over dusty roads), exposure to high humidity and salt-air, excessive jarring, and normal aging of the electrical components. Whenever it is known that an audiometer or the earphones have been subjected to abuse, it should be suspect until proven otherwise.

Let us now examine the nature of inaccurate calibration and the possible sources of error in the signal which an audiometer produces.

Frequency. Most audiometers have little difficulty meeting the ASA ±5 percent specified tolerance for frequency. (The new specifications call for a ±3 percent error.) For example, on the basis of the current standards, this means that an audiometer can produce a signal from 950 to 1,050 cycles per second when set at 1,000 cps or 3,800 to 4,200 cycles when set at 4,000 cps. Of course, the lower the frequency, the less tolerable variance in cycles per second (i.e. 120 to 130 for 125 cps). Even though these tolerances are established, one should strive to maintain as accurate a frequency output as possible. It is obvious what would result if a person with a sharp drop in hearing starting at precisely 1,000 cps would show on two audiometers with considerable variance in frequency output. On one that produces 950 cps at the 1,000 cps setting, threshold could be close to normal, but on another that produces 1,200 cps at the same setting, threshold could conceivably be much poorer than normal. Inaccurate frequency output is a problem chiefly in clinical or diagnostic audiometry. It is of minimal consequence in "field" audiometry.

Harmonics. Even though we are allegedly using pure tones in the basic measurement of hearing, it is possible to have harmonics of the fundamental (test frequency) present in the earphones. The ASA specifications call for the fundamental to be at least 25 dB (30 dB in the new specifications) above the sound pressure level of any harmonic.

A person with a hearing loss in the lower frequencies, with better hearing in the higher frequencies could present optimistic thresholds in the lows if the harmonics are not well below the fundamental. That is, threshold would be obtained for the harmonic instead of the fundamental.

Intensity. In this category we can encounter two problems which may or may not be related. First, the intensity output can be generally too strong or too weak. The ASA standard allows for a ±4 dB variance in intensity over the full range from −10 to maximum output at the test frequency of 2,000 cps and lower, and ±5 dB at the test frequencies above 2,000 cps. It also specifies a ±1.5 dB variation in any 5-dB step throughout the intensity range. The ASA standard notwithstanding, it is important to know whether your audiometer is producing the intensity it claims to be producing on the dial, or if, in fact, it is producing more or less than this reading. For example, if one audiometer is 10–15 dB weak, every person tested on it will show a greater hearing loss than on an accurate audiometer. This can cause such results as an overly optimistic air-bone gap, atypical audiometric configurations in otherwise typical clinical cases (where one or two frequencies are off) and an apparent greater need for amplification or middle-ear surgery than otherwise is the actual case. Further, a person's hearing might be classified as progressive in a case where an audiometer developed this problem between an initial test and follow-up testing. An audiometer that is too strong, however, can present problems similar to those just described, but in an opposite direction.

This problem is probably even more critical in identification audiometry where 5–10 dB one way or the other (strong or weak) can mean the difference between effective screening or an almost complete waste of time. The screening audiometer that is too strong will pass cases that should not have passed. A strong audiometer is a real hazard in an identification audiometry program.

The second problem with intensity is nonlinearity. Figure 8–1 illustrates what happens when an audi-

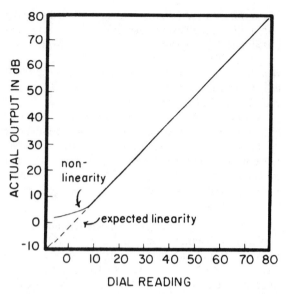

FIGURE 8-1. A graphic illustration of an example of a non-linear auditory test signal. Note, as the dial reading is decreased below 10 dB, the actual output of the signal fails to decrease as the dial reading indicates and then remains constant. In other words, a decrease of the dial does not decrease the output of the signal.

ometer fails to attenuate (decrease output) uniformly below 10 dB. Anyone with an actual threshold of 0 or 5 dB will report hearing a tone when the dial is set at −10 dB. This may be an insignificant problem so far as diagnostic audiometry is concerned, but it does present serious problems in identification audiometry. Audiometers that are non-linear below 15 dB are virtually useless in identification audiometry.

Tone Interruption. Figure 8–2 illustrates the upper-half of a signal on an oscilloscope when it is turned on and then turned off. According to the 1951 ASA specifications, it should rise to its peak within 100 to 500 milliseconds and go off in the same period of time. Actually, it is undesirable to have a rise-decay time more than 200 milliseconds. The audiometer should not present an unusually long rise and decay time (Figure 8–3) and there should be an absence of overshoot in the tone (Figure 8–4). The precision of the signal presentation can be very critical for accuracy in audiometry. The physiological rationale and clinical implications for this are clearly presented by Carhart and Jerger (1959). Briefly a slow rise time may fail to elicit maximum on-effect of the auditory mechanism and result in a poorer threshold than, in

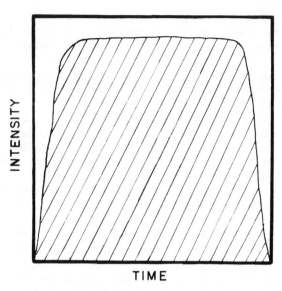

FIGURE 8-2. An illustration of uniform rise (on) and decay (off) times of a pure tone test signal with an absence of undesirable overshoot and uneven plateau.

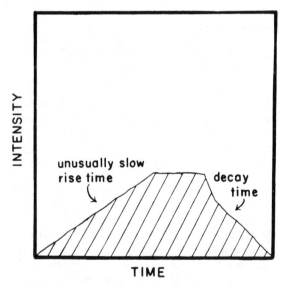

FIGURE 8-3. An illustration of an unusually long rise time and a decay which is unequal to the rise time. A desirable rise and decay time is approximately 100 milliseconds.

fact, is present. On the other hand, overshoot may result in the establishment of better thresholds than are present. Finally, if the rise time is too brief and overshoot is present (Figure 8–5) the result could be

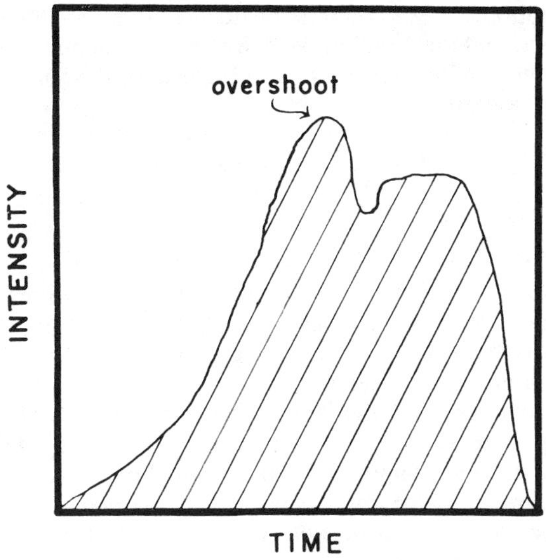

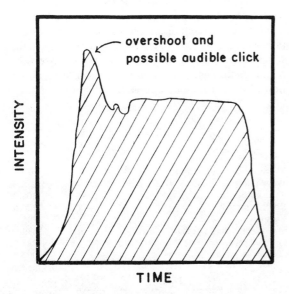

FIGURE 8-4. An illustration of unwanted overshoot in the presentation of a pure-tone test signal.

FIGURE 8-5. An illustration of an undesirably short rise time with overshoot. This situation can lead to an audible click as the tone is presented.

an audible click in the pure tone signal, thus encouraging a threshold for clicks and not for pure tones.

Isolation Between Earphones. Perhaps one of the more subtle and least recognized problems in accu-

rate pure tone instrumentation is a lack of complete isolation between earphones. Ideally, in threshold measurements, when a test signal is delivered to one earphone, nothing should be going to the opposite phone, except, of course, a masking stimulus when desired. Figure 8-6 illustrates what sometimes occurs in an audiometer when complete isolation is neglected. This leakage or cross-talk can be so low in intensity that the average adult ear and even delicate laboratory measuring equipment may not detect the problem. However, we know that children and young adults typically have thresholds somewhat better than −10 dB, re: the USPH norms. Therefore, one could obtain absolutely normal thresholds for both ears in a case where one ear actually has a mild to moderate loss in acuity, because the good ear could have been stimulated when the test tone was delivered to the poorer ear. A quick check of this possibility

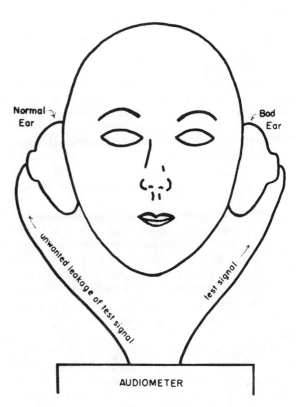

FIGURE 8-6. A schematic showing cross talk or leakage of a test signal from the intended earphone to the opposite phone. This situation could result in an audiogram showing two normal ears, where, in fact, one ear has a hearing loss.

would be the introduction of masking to the good ear, or disconnecting the earphone cord to the good ear, or slipping the non-test earphone away from the ear. Unfortunately, even the alert clinician can err in this situation because children, where slight cross-talk presents the greatest problem, are often unaware of a hearing imbalance between ears. Often, it is not until speech audiometry or other tests are employed that this situation is revealed.

Nevertheless, clinicians should be constantly alert to the possibility of cross-talk and double check clinical cases where bilateral super-normal thresholds are obtained by using low levels of masking in the non-test phone or one of the other two techniques mentioned above.

Other problems. At least the more common shortcomings in audiometer calibration have been discussed above. There certainly are other problems, which are simply listed:

> Audible click in earphone when changing frequency (especially undesirable in screening audiometers).
> Acoustic radiation from audiometer chassis (a serious problem when testing persons with one normal ear or an ear with normal thresholds for a portion of the test frequency range, especially when attempting to establish bone conduction thresholds).
> Erratic earphone response.
> Static or scratching noise with change of hearing level dial.
> External or mechanical click in tone interruptor.
> Noise from other sources (line or power hum) than test signal in earphones. The new ASA specifications state that no noise should be present when audiometer is turned to 50 dB. Above this level, the noise should be 60 dB below the test signal.

Conclusion

Attention to the precision of an audiometer cannot be over-emphasized. Well documented evidence and personal experience attests to the fact that an audiometer can easily fall short of the physical characteristics required as basic requisites to the accurate assessment of auditory function. Audiometers should receive periodic rigorous maintenance and

calibration. Methods and procedures of both laboratory and field calibrations for air conduction and bone conduction receivers will appear in the following Report.

PART II

The previous Report in this two-part series discussed some of the inaccuracies which can affect the precision of an audiometer and stressed the importance of careful periodic maintenance and checks on the calibration of these electroacoustical instruments. This second part of the series will deal with procedures for checking the pure tone signals, both for air and bone conduction. Emphasis will be on non-laboratory procedures, the assumption being that the majority of audiometer users do not have immediate access to specialized technical knowledge and costly measuring equipment.

Accessibility to expensive equipment and special technical knowledge notwithstanding, it is worthwhile to mention at least the equipment necessary to conduct a thorough check on the characteristics of a pure tone signal which were described in Part I of this series. The following is a list and approximate value of the components involved in a laboratory calibration of a pure tone audiometer:

Equipment	Approximate Cost
Condenser microphone	$ 275.00
Microphone complement	875.00
Wave analyzer	1,275.00
Attenuators	200.00
Power amplifier	200.00
Vacuum tube Voltmeter	225.00
Sweep-frequency Oscillator	680.00
Graphic recorder	1,085.00
Oscilloscope	1,000.00
Events per Unit Time Meter	650.00
Total	$6,465.00

Competent assemblage and operation of this equipment is vital to achieve valid measurements and interpretation; consequently, the services of a person well-versed in electroacoustics is essential.

Obviously this array of equipment is more than one could expect to maintain for a small number of audiometers such as often found in the typical school hearing conservation program, a modest speech and hearing center, a doctor's office, or hearing aid dealer's office.

Even so, the absence of such skilled personnel and special equipment is no excuse for neglect of the accuracy of audiometric equipment. It behooves the user to pay strict attention to the operating condition of his unit. Although in some areas laboratory facilities may be readily accessible for periodic calibrations, the operator of the audiometer should be aware of techniques for "spot checks" during those periods between laboratory checks.

The prime objective of this Report will be to discuss procedures and methods for checking accuracy of an audiometer in the absence of special laboratory measuring equipment similar to that listed above. Obviously, precise calibration is not intended, for only sensitive measuring equipment will provide this, but if one follows suggestions cited below he should at least be capable of determining when a laboratory calibration is indicated.

Gross Physical Check and Trouble Shooting

At the start of each day, the operator of an audiometer should examine his unit, both visually and auditorally. He should inspect the earphone cords (the weakest link, incidentally) for worn or cracked insulation, and straighten twisted cords. He should inspect the earphone cushions to be sure they are not cracked or marked with crevices due to shrinkage. The face of the audiometer should be inspected to insure against loose or slipped dials which may have gone out of alignment. Manipulation of the controls will offer a check on mechanical clicks in the attenuators, frequency selector, and interruptor switch. It is wise to vacuum carefully the dust from the inside of an audiometer periodically as it accumulates. Audiometers used in the field are more frequently subject to this need than those used in sound-isolated rooms. Let us now discuss in some detail several problems for which to listen in a gross check.

Following the visual check and after the power on the audiometer has been on for 10–15 minutes, the tester should place the earphones over his ears and listen to the signals as he manipulates the controls on the audiometer. While the pure tone is on continuously in first one phone and then the other at a hearing level high enough to be heard with ease, one should twist first one earphone cord and then the other back and forth a half-turn and jiggle the cord at a place close to the earphone. If the tone goes off and on, either the cord is defective or one or both of the small screws holding the cord plug in the earphone is loose. A small jeweler's type screwdriver should be kept close at hand to tighten these screws periodically. If this does not rectify the problem, chances are good that the earphone cord needs replacement. It is wise always to keep a supply of cords as well as earphone cushions. Defective cords and earphones are the most frequent cause of faulty operating equipment.

Next, with the pure tone signal at a high intensity level, one should listen for a change in the quality of the sound. An earphone which is distorting will frequently be detected by the human ear at high levels whereas such distortion may be inaudible at lower levels of intensity. With the hearing level set high one should interrupt the tone several times and listen for a "click" or "splat" sound just as the tone is turned on followed by the expected pure tone signal. If this is present, there is a good chance of undesirable overshoot or a transient in the rise-time of the signal (refer to Part I of this Series for more details relative to the consequences of this problem).

With the hearing level set at -10 dB and the signal on continuously, the intensity should gradually be increased in steps of 5 dB up to a high level. Each increment must be listened to carefully for a uniform increase in the intensity of the tone. It is not necessary to check this at more than one frequency or for more than one earphone. This provides a gross check on the linearity or uniformity of the attenuator (hearing level control). If a signal does not change in loudness with an increase of the dial, or if it appears to change drastically, it is a clue to a non-linear attenuator.

With the masking signal on in one earphone and the opposite earphone over the cheekbone, one should interrupt the pure tone several times at various intensity levels and listen for a "click" in the masking phone. Such a condition is undesirable for competent testing and can prove to be highly distracting for the person under test when masking is used.

To determine if the loudness varies from presentation to presentation, one should set the hearing level to a comfortable loudness and interrupt the pure tone several times. An audiometer may develop an inconsistency in the actual level of the pure tone signal when it is held at a constant intensity level and interrupted several times.

With the audiometer hearing level control set at about 40 dB, *without presenting the pure tone,* one should increase the intensity to its maximum and listen for the introduction of a hum or any other type of constant random signal. This is especially common in the speech circuit of combination pure tone and speech audiometers. A check for this same noise in the speech network, if it is not found to be present in the pure tone setting, is necessary. If this noise is detected, it is frequently alleviated by running a piece of hook-up wire from a screw on the back of the audiometer chassis to the screw which holds the face plate over a duplex wall power receptacle.

Simultaneously with a check for hum at high intensity levels, it is wise to listen for a static or scratching sound as the hearing level dial is varied. This suggests presence of dust or foreign particles in the attenuator and should be cleaned by a qualified technician if it cannot be alleviated by "working" the hearing level dial back and forth several dozen times.

The frequency selector should be moved through the frequency range with special attention to extraneous noises, such as clicks in the earphones when changing from one frequency to the next. Many audiometers make some noise when changing frequency, but these are external and do not occur in the earphones. Neither mechanical nor electrical noises present a serious problem except in screening audiometers where the frequency is changed more than the hearing level. In this latter case the noises should be alleviated.

"Cross-talk" between earphones can be a very serious problem, as we pointed out in Part I of the Report. Moreover, a couple of methods for checking the presence of "cross-talk" were given in the previous Report. As a last and important step, one earphone should be disconnected and the pure tone signal presented to it with the opposite phone at the ear of the examiner. For example, with the right earphone disconnected and the earphone-selector set to the Right Earphone, the left phone may be placed over the ear of a person with hearing well within normal limits and the pure tone presented. If, under these circumstances, a pure tone signal is heard in the left earphone, there is "cross-talk" in the system. This does not present a problem if the cross-talk occurs only at higher hearing levels starting at 50 or 60 dB because masking is used on the ear of a unilateral under these circumstances (i.e., if the subject has normal hearing in the good ear). It does, however, present a serious problem when the cross-talk is present at lower hearing levels, below 40 dB. Under these

circumstances masking is usually not used because the difference between ears is within the interaural attenuation rate. Nevertheless, cross-talk at low hearing levels should be alleviated as soon as possible after detection.

To summarize, in this section various ways of detecting undesirable elements in the operating characteristics of an audiometer have been discussed. Our comments were limited primarily to the pure tone audiometer. Care should be taken that the person checking the audiometer has normal hearing, at least in one ear. The following section will deal with empirical methods for the calibration of the output level of a pure tone audiometer, both for air and bone conduction.

"Calibration" of the Output Level

We will now address ourselves to the empirical calibration of the accuracy in the output level of the audiometer. That is, is there agreement between what the hearing level dial says is coming out of the earphone and what the earphone *actually* emits? A method for determining this without accessibility to precision measuring equipment will be discussed.

Perhaps the quickest and easiest method is for the operator of the audiometer to keep a record of his own thresholds. He can then check his thresholds with the audiometer in question to determine its accuracy. The shortcomings of this approach are obvious. For one thing, threshold is not a fixed point. Threshold of acuity can be expected to vary within a range of 10 dB from day to day. Slight inconsistency in the location of earphone placement will also have an effect upon the obtained threshold and can cause as much as a 10 dB variance in threshold, especially in the low frequencies. Further, many operators of audiometers have thresholds at or better than -10 dB on our present audiometric scale. Thus, if an audiometer is emitting a signal which is too strong, the person with very acute hearing will have trouble detecting this problem. If the operator has a hearing loss, then this problem does not prevail, however, the possibility of a progressive hearing loss or one which fluctuates must be considered.

Another method was advocated several years ago before some of the valuable research had been reported on age and hearing level. In recent years we have come to appreciate some of the shortcomings in the 1951 ASA audiometric standard for threshold and the strong influence of age upon the average thresholds of groups.

The method advocated was to run threshold measurements on 10 or so young persons with "healthy normal ears." The persons in the group should be chosen carefully to avoid a history of familial hearing loss, ear problems, or noise exposure. The idea was to take an average of the thresholds obtained from the group and correct the audiometer to the amount which this average at each frequency deviated from zero. The problem with this approach is that a young healthy group of normal ears will present an average threshold at most frequencies of −10 dB on an audiometer with accurate output calibration. Unfortunately, they will also present a −10 dB average threshold if the audiometer is emitting a signal which is too strong. This method will isolate the audiometer which is too weak, provided the interpretation takes into account the 10 dB better sensitivity of young healthy ears. In brief, this method of employing a "group of normals" can be very risky.

If it is used, one should insert an attenuator in the line of the earphone which will decrease the output of the pure tone a known amount at each frequency. This will avoid the problem of obtaining a −10 dB average and the amount of this intended attenuation can be subtracted from the mean thresholds for the corrected value. However, the final interpretation will still have to take into account the 10 dB better sensitivity of the young normal group.

An approach which seems to be practical and void of serious shortcomings is a loudness balance method. In this case, the output from an audiometer known to be accurate is matched against an audiometer under question of accuracy. The mechanics of this procedure are simple, as illustrated in Figure 8–7. One earphone is detached from the headband of the accurate audiometer and placed on the headband of the "unknown" audiometer after removing one of its phones. The earphones should be placed on the ears of a young listener with healthy normal ears and with negligible difference in sensitivity between ears. Each audiometer is then set to the same frequency and the known audiometer is set to present a 40 dB interrupted-train of signals from 1 to 1½ seconds duration for each toneburst. When the signal is off in the "known" earphone, it should be presented in the unknown earphone. While this presentation of signals continues, the hearing level of the unknown audiometer is varied until the point is reached where the signals in each earphone are equal in loudness. Simultaneous presentation of the signals from both audiometers should be carefully avoided.

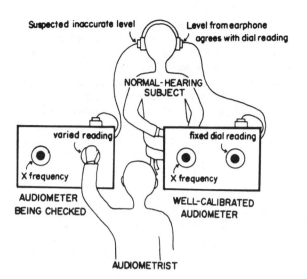

FIGURE 8-7. An illustration of a loudness balance method for checking an audiometer suspected of being inaccurate with one that is well-calibrated. The "tester" alternately operates the interruptor switches manually by first depressing one and then the other. At the same time, he varies the hearing level of the "unknown" audiometer until the subject reports that the signals delivered to each ear are equal in loudness.

At least three observers should be used when checking an audiometer with this method. It is worthwhile to balance at three hearing levels (20, 40 and 60 dB) at each frequency. Also, an average of three judgments should be obtained at each level for each frequency. A loudness-matching procedure can be very accurate, provided the subject is careful and well trained. Further, this approach is not nearly as time consuming as it may appear. Three subjects could be run through this procedure in one hour.

If a well-calibrated audiometer is available, this loudness balance procedure need not be used. Instead, thresholds can be obtained for ten hearing-impaired ears (one ear per subject) with both the "known" and "unknown" audiometers. The average threshold obtained at each frequency with the "unknown" audiometer can be compared with the "known" audiometer. Any difference between mean thresholds is probably due to an error in the unknown audiometer and can be corrected by this amount. That is, if a mean threshold of 40 dB is obtained with the accurate audiometer at a particular frequency, and a 50 dB mean threshold with the suspected audiometer at the same frequency, it might be assumed that the suspected audiometer is weak by 10 dB.

At least one obvious problem with these procedures is accessibility of the "known" audiometer. If one is available, it can certainly be used to check others that are unknown. When errors are found, it is not necessary to retire the audiometer until it is correctly adjusted at the source of trouble.

Instead, a simple correction notation can be attached to control panel in view of the tester. A sample of such a correction chart is shown in Figure 8-8. This chart can be used until the audiometer is calibrated by a service laboratory.

If funds are available it is wise to procure a simplified "artificial ear." A variety of these instruments are usually exhibited at the national meetings of the American Speech and Hearing Association and the American Academy of Ophthalmology and Otolaryngology. An accurate and a stable artificial ear is a valuable asset to a facility engaged in the measurement of hearing.

Let us now turn our attention to the calibration of the bone conduction system on an audiometer.

There is an artificial mastoid now commercially available for approximately $3,000.00 which is stable and has very promising potential. Unfortunately, at the time of this writing, there is no standard bone threshold, thus this mastoid has limitations for clinical application. Moreover, the cost is rather high so that most clinicians are left with empirical bone calibration for the present time. Because of the problems

of isolating a bone-conducted signal to a specific ear, loudness matching is perforce an undesirable technique for calibrating a bone vibrator.

Over the years, the method which has probably best stood the test of time as the most accurate approach is the one advocated by Roach and Carhart (1956). Their method utilizes a group (ten persons will suffice) of individuals with otologically-diagnosed sensorineural hearing impairment. From our present-day experiences, the hearing loss should be of moderate degree and bilaterally symmetrical, but persons with presbycusis should be avoided.

Only one ear from each subject should be used; and masking should not be necessary if air thresholds are nearly identical in both ears. Of course, the ears should be unoccluded when making the bone measurements. The subjects should first have their hearing tested with a well-calibrated air conduction system. Then the bone conduction thresholds are obtained using the vibrator in question. Average air and bone thresholds are obtained for each frequency. The bone threshold is corrected to the air threshold at each frequency. For example, if the average air conduction threshold is found to be 40 dB at 1,000 cps and the average of the bone thresholds for the group is 30 dB, one can assume that the bone system is too strong and optimistic bone thresholds are being obtained at this frequency. Therefore, a notation should be made on the correction card indicating that obtained bone thresholds at 1,000 cps should be made 10 dB poorer. The reverse situation exists when the average bone threshold is found to be greater (poorer) than the air threshold. In this case, the correction should instruct the tester to make the obtained bone threshold better by a specified amount.

These empirical calibration checks should be made if an earphone or bone vibrator is dropped or receives a hard blow. There is a good chance that other problems, such as distortion, also are present. Under current conditions, it is not uncommon to find a bone vibrator to deviate 10 to 20 dB from air conduction "norms." Such deviations in the bone system do not necessarily suggest other problems. Consequently, it is probably safe simply to be aware of the deviation in the bone system and make the necessary corrections when recording the audiometric results.

Replacing the bone vibrator with a new one of the same make may not alleviate the error. However, in the air conduction channel, if it is discovered that

Corrections			date:						
	125	250	500	1K	2K	3K	4K	6K	8K
right									
left									
bone									
Red: make hearing poorer by above amounts									
Black: make hearing better by above amounts									

FIGURE 8-8. An example of a calibration correction card which can be mounted on the control panel of an audiometer. A color code reduces the confusion created by + or − signs. For example, black numbers could mean, "make hearing level better by the designated amount," and red numbers could mean, "make hearing level poorer by the designated amount." These corrections can be posted for b/c as well as a/c and can be changed when necessary.

rather large (more than 5 dB) corrections are necessary for an earphone at more than one or two frequencies, the earphone should be replaced.

SUMMARY

Consistent attention to the accuracy of an audiometer should not be taken lightly. Validity and reliability of hearing tests rest heavily upon the accuracy of the audiometer being used. Part I of this Series describes the problems which can develop in an audiometer. Part II offers suggestions for checking some of these problems in the absence of costly laboratory measuring equipment and specialized technical knowledge. Errors in the intensity level of pure tone signals can be noted on the face of an audiometer and be made in the recording of audiometric thresholds. However, when other problems are detected, arrangements for competent service should be made to correct the situation as quickly as possible. It is important that the operators of audiometric equipment should recognize that these units cannot be used ad infinitum without service.

REFERENCES

American Standards Association, Z24.5–1951, approved March 21, 1951. See Hirsh, I., *The Measurement of Hearing.* McGraw-Hill, New York, 1952, pp. 321–327.

Carhart, R., and Jerger, J. F., Preferred Method for Clinical Determination of Pure-Tone Thresholds. *Journal of Speech and Hearing Disorders,* **24,** 1959, 330–345.

Eagles, E., and Doerfler, L. G., A Study of Hearing in Children: Acoustic Environment and Audiometer Performance. *Transactions of the American Academy of Ophthalmology and Otolaryngology,* May–June, 1961, 283–296.

Roach, R., and Carhart, R., A method for calibrating a bone-conduction audiometer, *AMA Archives of Otolaryngology,* **63,** 1956, 270–278.

part **II**

PURE-TONE AUDIOMETRY

Although the clinical audiologist has many tests available to determine degree and type of hearing impairment, the air- and bone-conduction audiogram furnishes the best single description of auditory function. Results of other measurements are usually interpreted in conjunction with the pure-tone audiogram.

Carhart and Jerger, in one of the most frequently-cited articles concerning pure-tone audiometry, make a plea for universal acceptance of a modified Hughson-Westlake method for determining air- and bone-conduction thresholds. They compare this ascending technique with other methods of determining threshold and present theoretical bases and practical considerations in support of the proposed method. Carhart and Jerger's recommendations have received wide acceptance among professionals who recognize the need for standardization of test methods.

The next two readings in this section are "guidelines" designed to promote uniform procedures for measuring and recording pure-tone thresholds. The first of these two guidelines, both published by the American Speech-Language-Hearing Association (ASHA), is, in many respects, an endorsement of the Carhart-Jerger method. It includes, however, additional detail about measurement method, as well as discussion of monitoring techniques, masking, bone-conduction, and symbols used in recording results. The other set of guidelines, which is devoted entirely to audiometric symbols, is included here to foster standardization, even though we recognize that much variation probably still exists in the symbols used by professionals.

Methods for determining absolute pure-tone thresholds are not limited to variations of the so-called "conventional" method. One of the most

commonly-used alternatives to conventional pure-tone audiometry is Békésy audiometry, which requires the test subject to track his or her own thresholds by means of a subject-controlled attenuator. In addition to its use as a threshold-estimating procedure, Békésy audiometry is used for screening, monitoring, and specialized diagnostic audiometry. We have selected a brief research report by Burns and Hinchcliffe because it documents the equivalence of discrete-frequency pure-tone thresholds measured by conventional audiometry and by Békésy audiometry. Both methods yielded similar thresholds and had comparably good reliability.

Another alternative to conventional pure-tone audiometry is pulse-counting audiometry, a procedure validated by Gardner in 1947 but developed at Bell Telephone Laboratories. Unlike conventional audiometry, which is a constant vigilance task, pulse-counting audiometry requires the subject's attention only during clearly identified intervals; no attention is required during the intervening silent periods. We have included an abridged version of an early article by Reger because it describes clearly the rationale and technique of pulse-counting audiometry. Reger notes that the pulse-counting paradigm is more accessible to standardization than conventional audiometry, less susceptible to examiner error, and more attractive to the subject. Portions of the Reger selection apply to the variables that must be controlled in order to obtain valid and reliable thresholds regardless of measurement format. Reger's observations and advice are as relevant today as they were thirty years ago.

The audiologist must be prepared to deal with the difficult-to-test listener who may be unwilling or unable to follow verbal instructions. Lloyd presents a summary of techniques that employ features of operant conditioning; the imaginative audiologist may select from these, or devise variations of them, to obtain thresholds on a particular subject. For more comprehensive discussion of this topic, the reader should refer to Fulton (1974, 1978).

The next four articles highlight selected problems encountered during pure-tone audiometry. A recent study by Dancer, Ventry, and Hill investigates the false-alarm response, which is a response that occurs when no signal is present. The type of instructions given to the listener was found to affect the number of false-alarm responses; the lowest number occurred when listeners were told to respond only when they were sure they heard a tone. In addition, fewer false-alarms occurred when subjects were required to count pulsed tones than when a continuous tone was used. The absolute thresholds, however, did not change with type of instruction or signal mode. The authors emphasize the desirability of controlling false-alarm responses and question the advisability of instructing a listener to respond when he or she "thinks" a tone is present.

The reading by Chaiklin and McClellan is included to alert professionals to errors produced when standard supra-aural earphone cushions cause partial or complete closure of the external auditory meatus. This article describes the nature of such errors, but is primarily concerned with the relative efficiency of various methods for reducing or eliminating the effects of collapsible ear canals.

Boothroyd and Cawkwell, among others, recognize that some responses to air- and bone-conducted stimuli represent tactile rather than true auditory sensation. They show typical audiometric levels for tactile sensation and emphasize the considerable intersubject variability that characterizes responses mediated by tactile sensation during audiometry. They suggest that the clinical audiologist should be alert to the invalidating effects of such responses during routine audiometry, particularly during evaluations of persons with severe hearing losses.

Simmons and Dixon also caution against the tendency of audiologists to assume that the physical characteristics of a signal are always closely related to what a subject hears. They provide evidence to indicate that the sensation experienced by the listener may be quite different from the usual sensation elicited by the input signal. They also suggest that, in some cases, it is necessary to ask the listener to describe the sensation that produced the response.

Three articles are presented concerning some crucial variables that affect measurement and interpretation of bone-conduction thresholds. The first, by Studebaker, is included to demonstrate, particularly for beginning clinicians, that bone-conduction thresholds may sometimes be appreciably poorer than air-conduction measurements, and that some bone-conduction thresholds better than air-conduction thresholds may not be indicative of conductive pathology.

The Dirks and Swindeman and the Dirks and Malmquist articles, both frequently cited, concern some of the factors that affect bone-conduction thresholds. The Dirks and Swindeman selection should make the student aware of the magnitude and intersubject variability of the occlusion effect under usual test conditions. More specifically, the article compares the variability of the occlusion effect with two types of earphone cushions. Dirks and Malmquist present evidence regarding mastoid versus forehead placement of the bone-conduction vibrator. After a summary of arguments in favor of forehead placement, they present evidence that a comparison of thresholds obtained at both sites may be diagnostically valuable, particularly in subjects with conductive pathology.

We regret that space restrictions prevented us from including articles concerning other aspects of bone conduction. Information about the physiology of bone conduction is available in Tonndorf (1966), about noncochlear effects on bone conduction in Carhart (1962), and about general problems of measurement in Dirks (1964).

REFERENCES AND ADDITIONAL READINGS

Carhart, R. Effects of stapes fixation on bone-conduction response. In *International Symposium on Otosclerosis*, ed. H. Schuknecht. Boston: Little, Brown, 1962, pp. 175–197.

Dirks, D. D. Factors related to bone-conduction reliability. *Arch. Otolaryng.*, **79**, 551–558 (1964).

Fulton, R. T. Auditory stimulus-response control. Baltimore: University Park Press, 1974.

Fulton, R. T. Pure tone tests of hearing—Age one year through five years. In *Pediatric Audiology*, ed. F. Martin. Englewood Cliffs, N.J.: Prentice-Hall, 1978.

Gardner, M. B. A pulse-tone technique for clinical audiometric threshold measurements. *J. Acoust. Soc. Amer.*, **19**, 592–599 (1947).

Hirsh, I. J. Békésy's audiometer. *J. Acoust. Sec. Amer.*, **34**, 1333–1336 (1962).

Tonndorf, J. Bone conduction: Studies in experimental animals. *Acta Otolaryng.*, Suppl. 213 (1966).

9

Preferred Method for Clinical Determination of Pure-Tone Thresholds

Raymond Carhart, Ph.D.
Professor of Audiology, Northwestern University when this article was prepared
James F. Jerger, Ph.D.
Professor of Audiology, Baylor College of Medicine

Confusion and disagreement exist as to the preferred method for clinical determination of pure-tone thresholds. The procedures described in the literature are contradictory and sometimes quite complicated (Bunch, 1943; Heller, 1955; Newby, 1958; Watson and Tolan, 1949). Moreover, as Hirsh emphasizes, "Since there is still no accepted standard technique, the clinician must be warned that the differences among these techniques may be responsible for differences among the thresholds that result from their use" (Hirsh, 1952). Not only does this uncertainty distress the conscientious audiometrist, but he often feels uneasy because necessary simplifications of routine cause him to deviate from full adherence to recognized methods for psychophysical measurement.

The purpose of the present paper is to urge that clinicians standardize their practices by adopting the basic features of the Hughson-Westlake (1944) technique.[1] Both theoretical and practical considerations make this procedure logical for routine use when testing is done with a conventional pure-tone audiometer. This technique was accepted in 1944 by the Committee on Conservation of Hearing of the American Academy of Ophthalmology and Otolaryngology. In slightly revised form, it has since been advocated in various publications sponsored by the Committee (Newhart and Reger, 1951, 1945). Clinicians who have used the method have found it to be straightforward and satisfactory.

The discussion which follows (1) gives a brief description of an improved version of the Hughson-Westlake technique, (2) reviews those features of auditory behavior which determine the suitability of this method and (3) reports an experimental comparison between this method and two other procedures.

Reprinted by permission of the authors from *J. Speech Hearing Dis.*, **24**, 330–345 (1959).

HUGHSON-WESTLAKE METHOD

The fundamental feature of the Hughson-Westlake procedure is that *minimum audibility is measured only by progressively increasing the stimulus intensity.* In other words, presentations always progress from levels where the sound is inaudible to the first level where perception of the stimulus occurs. As soon as the stimulus is heard, a new ascent is initiated. When using this procedure, *the clinical threshold is defined as the minimal level at which perception is achieved in more than half of the ascents.* In consequence, the Hughson-Westlake technique is sometimes called "the ascending method."

Obviously, the specific exploratory procedure just described cannot be undertaken until the subject has been appropriately prepared for it. Consequently, the total process of administering an audiometric test is more involved than the preceding paragraph implies. The important thing, from the clinician's standpoint, is to keep the preparatory phases clearly separate in his own thinking from the procedures of threshold exploration *per se.*

The first step in preparation is to assure that the subject is fully aware of the experience for which he is to listen. The audiometrist, therefore, begins by presenting to the subject a tone of sufficient intensity to evoke a clear and concise response. This tonal presentation, as is also true of all subsequent ones, should be one or two seconds in duration. A particularly easy way of evaluating the subject's response is to have him raise his finger whenever he hears the stimulus. The audiometrist must, of course, estimate the presentation level which is required and must be prepared to use more intense levels if a clear and concise response is not evoked at the outset. The only purpose here is to be certain that the subject understand fully the task expected of him.

It has proved practical, when testing by air conduction, to administer the first tonal presentation at a hearing level of 30 to 40 dB if the subject appears to have approximately normal acuity, and at a hearing level of 70 dB if only a moderate impairment seems to be present. Provided these levels are inadequate, subsequent presentations are increased in steps of 15 dB until the subject's response is positive. In any event, at least one definitive practice response should be elicited before proceeding to the next step in the procedure.

The second step is to decrease the tonal level until the stimulus is definitely inaudible. The only purpose here is to prepare for the first exploratory ascent. An efficient method for reaching the level of inaudibility is to drop the intensity of successive presentations in steps of 10 or 15 dB. This sequence is carried through rapidly. A single response at one level is the cue to decrease to the next lower level. The advantage of such a sequence, in contrast to the process of dropping immediately to a hearing level of zero dB or weaker, is that the subsequent ascent will usually be started closer to the level at which the threshold lies. The saving in time is important to the clinician.

Once the level of inaudibility has been reached, the exploration for threshold begins. This exploration is carried out with a series of short tonal presentations. So long as the subject does not respond, each presentation is made five decibels stronger than its predecessor. However, as soon as a response occurs, the level of the next stimulus is dropped 10 to 15 dB and another ascent in five-decibel steps is begun. The clinician keeps track of the levels at which responses occur. He designates the intensity at which the majority of responses appear as the threshold level for the test tone. Experience has shown that a practical criterion is to accept three responses at a single intensity as the threshold. This criterion is often achieved in three or four ascents.

The clinician must remember always to present successive stimuli as discrete events separated by completely toneless intervals. Moreover, each tonal burst should be not less than one second and not more than two seconds in duration. This requirement is easily achieved. The clinician merely adjusts the audiometer while the instrument is set so that no signal is being emitted. He then presses the "tone-on" switch to produce the next stimulus presentation.

All other details of procedure, such as the choice of the ear to be tested and of the progression of frequencies to be employed, are flexible. Moreover, the revised Hughson-Westlake technique is applicable to both air-conduction and bone-conduction explorations. The only restrictions in the latter instances are those imposed by the reduced range of hearing levels which are testable through bone conduction.

In summary, the critical features of the revised Hughson-Westlake technique are (1) that only ascending series of tonal stimuli are used, (2) that successive stimuli are separated by toneless intervals and (3) that each ascending run is terminated as soon as the subject responds. The technique is easy to employ when the subject is properly indoctrinated. The question which remains to be answered is whether the Hughson-Westlake technique is defensible from the standpoint of audiological theory.

ADAPTATION AND ON-EFFECT

It is a fundamental fact, as the statement quoted earlier from Hirsh implies, that an individual's auditory sensitivity can be modified substantially by the conditions of stimulus presentation. This fact imposes a responsibility on the clinician to select test conditions which encourage consistency in the subject's momentary acuity and which explore a precise boundary of sensitivity. In other words, since arbitrary decisions regarding procedure are unavoidable, it is the clinician's duty to choose reasonable stimulus conditions and to understand why he has chosen them.

Our knowledge of two auditory phenomena, on-effect and adaptation, makes it possible to state categorically that relatively brief tonal presentations must be used in conventional pure-tone audiometry. Such presentations enhance the reliability of the measured threshold. They also encourage response at the minimal intensity level to which the subject is ordinarily sensitive, thus giving an estimate of his best practical acuity. Stated conversely, continuous stimuli are clinically unacceptable because they induce variability in the intensity levels at which responses occur. This problem arises because prolonged stimuli produce temporary and progressive desensitization of the auditory system. Such desensitization become particularly pronounced with some kinds of hearing impairment.

To explain: the initial response of the auditory system at the onset of stimulation is its most vigorous response. This initial reaction is termed the on-effect. When the stimulus is sustained, the on-effect is followed by a reduction in responsiveness even though the stimulus is too weak to produce fatigue. This change is known as auditory adaptation.

On-effect and adaptation have been demonstrated through animal experimentation. Derbyshire and Davis (1935) observed the two phenomena of on-effect and equilibration in the action potentials recorded from the eighth nerve of the cat. Galambos and Davis (1943) found both rate-adaptation and amplitude-adaptation in the impulse trains carried by second order neurons of the cat's auditory system, while Tasaki (1954) noted gradual decrease in the frequency of impulses elicited in response to sustained tones within first-order nerve fibers of the guinea pig.

The features of on-effect and adaptation, as exhibited by both subjects with normal hearing and with auditory impairments, were discussed by Hood (1950) when he reported his studies on perstimulatory fatigue. Normal adaptation has subsequently been explored extensively (Egan and Thwing, 1955; Jerger, 1957). However, it was Hallpike and Hood (1951) who highlighted the clinical implications of the two phenomena by their suggestion that "on-effect normality" may be combined with susceptibility to extreme adaptation, called relapse. This combination, they claim, characterizes not only the adapted normal ear, but also the "recruiting sense organ of Ménière's disease." In both instances, there is an initial burst of auditory response at the onset of stimulation, provided, of course, that the threshold intensity is exceeded. This state is manifest to the listener as an initial maximal loudness. It is followed, if the stimulus is sustained, by a rapid deterioration in the response. This deterioration is the manifestation of relapse. Hallpike and Hood emphasize that recovery occurs quickly. The full on-effect may be elicited anew provided the listener is allowed a brief respite from stimulation.

The existence of individuals who undergo relapse and yet preserve the capacity for strong on-effect responses has been demonstrated repeatedly and in various ways (Jerger et al., 1958; Jerger, 1955; Lierle and Reger, 1955; Palva, 1955). One must now recognize that relapse at threshold is not restricted to cases with cochlear lesion, but that this phenomenon can at times be encountered with neural lesions. One must also recognize that details such as the speed of relapse, the rapidity of recovery, and the variation of effect with frequency differ from one case to another. The unescapable fact, from the standpoint of deciding on a routine for clinical audiometry, is that subjects are encountered whose momentary responsiveness is radically affected by exposure to sustained tones.

A critical point here is that both the normally adapted auditory system and the relapsed auditory system regain responsiveness after a brief resting period. Full recovery ordinarily occurs in a second or two. Consequently, the audiometrist may have confidence that he is exploring his subject's maximal acuity at each test frequency if every stimulus is preceded by a toneless interval of several seconds. Moreover, since the on-effect will be elicited at the outset of stimulation, there is no value in prolonging any tonal presentation more than a couple of seconds. When the audiometrist does prolong the tone, he merely initiates a process of normal adaptation or one of relapse, depending upon the case being tested.

The foregoing considerations lead to the conclusion that, provided one wishes to measure the subject's unadapted threshold (his on-effect responsiveness) by conventional audiometry,[2] each audiometric stimulus should be one or two seconds long and should follow a silent interval of at least three seconds. One is not justified in conducting a routine clinical test by presenting a clearly audible tone and then decreasing its intensity without interruption until the tone becomes inaudible. Such a procedure produces an unknown amount of adaptation. The amount depends upon the speed of stimulus transitions, upon the susceptibility of the subject to abnormal adaptation and, since higher intensities produce greater adaptation, upon the starting level of the sequence. The only thing one can be certain about is that such a procedure will usually give a pessimistic impression of the subject's acuity.

Evidence supporting this last statement was obtained by Miller and Rosenblith. These investigators, according to Hirsh (1952), found that "descending" thresholds obtained on normal hearers with continuous tones of 4,000 cps required as much as 15 dB more sound pressure than did the analogous "ascending" thresholds. They also found that the magnitude of the discrepancy increased as the starting level of the descending sequence was raised. Only when the descending sequence was begun essentially at threshold was acuity as good with it as with the ascending progression. Furthermore, Rosenblith and Miller obtained better thresholds for both ascending and descending progressions when the 4,000-cps stimulus was interrupted than either progression yielded when the stimulus was continuous. One would expect the differences to be more dramatic in cases where relapse operates.

The clinician must recognize one further characteristic of any procedure which uses discrete tonal presentations separated by substantial intervals of time. Such a test situation is not even analogous to one wherein a train of successive pulses is changing continuously in intensity. In the former case each tonal presentation is an event sufficiently isolated in time so that it is independent of its neighbors. The subject will respond if his momentary sensitivity in relation to the stimulus intensity is sufficient for the on-effect to be evoked. Since each event is independent, it is theoretically irrelevant whether the clinician has patterned the succession of stimuli in a descending, in an ascending, or in a combined sequence. One is not justified in thinking of this procedure as constituting a form of the method of limits simply because he decides to vary presentation levels progressively. Therefore, one need not feel any responsibility to combine sequences of ascending and descending "crossings" of the threshold. Instead, the audiometrist may choose whichever sequence has the greatest practical advantage. Hence, it is legitimate to adopt the revised Hughson-Westlake technique. This method has the practical advantages of simplicity and of high economy in clinical effort.

FIVE-DECIBEL STEP

The traditional concept of a threshold rests on the premise that the subject is continually undergoing fluctuations in sensitivity (Stevens, 1951). According to this view, the subject's minimal response level at any given instant is determined by his status at that instant. Therefore, a series of measurements must be made in order to obtain a statistical estimate of his threshold, which is usually defined as the stimulus value at which there is a 50 percent chance that he will perceive the stimulus. This estimate is derived from a finite series of measurements. The series is obtained according to one of the standard psychophysical methods.

A critical requirement, which applies to all psychophysical methods, is that it must be possible to present a reasonable array of stimulus values which actually lie within the subject's range of moment-to-moment variability. Stated conversely, if the steps between stimulus levels are too large, a precise estimate of the threshold will be impossible because information which contributes to the estimate is not obtainable at enough levels. Under such circumstances, some levels will be useless in threshold computation because they always evoke response, whereas others will be analogously useless because they never evoke response. The most extreme case, of course, is the situation where the size of the interval between successive stimulus levels is greater than the range of the subject's moment-to-moment variability. When this situation exists, all that can usually be determined is that response never occurs at one presentation level and always occurs at the next higher level. Here, even in those fortuitous instances where one stimulus level happens to probe the subject's moment-to-moment variability, the none-and-all pattern will characterize responses at the two flanking levels. Again, a precise estimate of threshold is impossible, and the investigator must still be satisfied with designating one presentation level at which responses seldom or never occur and a second level, immediately higher, at which responses usually occur. Such information may be highly useful, but it is not threshold determination according to the traditional premises of psychophysical exploration.

There exists substantial evidence, some of which is reviewed below, that moment-to-moment fluctuations in auditory sensitivity are often encompassed within a range which is less than the five-decibel step used in conventional audiometry. Since such is the case, the audiometrist should recognize that he cannot define an individual's threshold in precise statistical fashion so long as he varies stimulus intensity in five-decibel steps. Hence, the audiometrist need not feel impelled to structure his testing technique according to one of the classical methods of psychophysics, and he need not feel guilty if he does not do so. Instead, the clinician should choose his audiometry technique to take advantage of the high consistency of response which may be expected from most subjects during single tests when the five-decibel step is used. He should adopt a procedure which quickly gives the dichotomous information to which the five-decibel step restricts him.

Several studies supply evidence supporting the premise that the moment-to-moment variability of the individual is not large in relation to the five-decibel step of conventional audiometry. These studies help one answer the question, "What is the moment-to-moment stability in the auditory sensitivity in the ordinary listener?"

Ward (1957a, 1957b), while developing his technique of "single descent" group audiometry, obtained two kinds of information which are pertinent.

For one thing, Ward tested 12 enlisted men repeatedly at both 500 and 4,000 cps. The stimulus was a continuously changing train of pulses. Ward combined two pulse rates (1.5 and 2.25 pps) with two attenuation speeds (1.5 and 3.0 dB). Each of the four resulting conditions was presented five times to every subject. Subjects were instructed to report "just when the beats disappeared." Ward found his four parameters of stimulus descent to be essentially equivalent in reliability as gauged by the standard deviation of repeat judgments. Moreover, he comments, ". . . the standard deviation of repeat judgments (earphones not moved) is 1.7 dB . . ." (Ward, 1957b).

Secondly, Ward used his 2.25 pps and 3 dB/sec. parameter of descent to study the test-retest consistency exhibited at 2,000 and 8,000 cps by 1,200 naval personnel. He remarks, "The median difference, disregarding sign, is 2.4 dB for both 2,000 and 8,000 cps. This implies that the median SD of repeat judgments is 1.7 dB" (1957a). It is also evident from Ward's data that almost 50 percent of the test-retest discrepancies were less than 2.5 dB and about 80 percent were smaller than five dB.

One may interpret Ward's findings as indirect evidence that the short-term physiological fluctuations in the auditory acuity of ordinary listeners (as exemplified by Ward's subjects) are generally of the same order of magnitude as the five-decibel step employed in clinical audiometry. If this had not been the case, test-retest differences would have emerged as much larger in Ward's study—since physiological fluctuations constitute only one of several factors contributing to the variability he observed.

Of course, since Ward used only descending series of pulses, one wonders whether the consistency he found in repeat judgment was thereby spuriously improved. In one sense it is irrelevant to raise this question, because any method which induces consistency in human response demonstrates the reliability which it is possible to achieve if one structures the test situation properly. In another sense, however, the question is highly pertinent when one is inquiring into the moment-to-moment fluctuations of human listeners. Hence, the findings of other workers are *apropos*.

Wertheimer (1955) investigated the stability of the threshold for 80-msec. clicks by the method of constant stimuli. Three subjects were used. Wertheimer found ". . . that the average sigma of measurement

of the auditory threshold within one session was .69 dB. . . ." This value is astonishingly small, and it indicates short term stability in auditory acuity which is much better than clinicians usually assume. Interestingly, Wertheimer found that the average sigma of 10 thresholds obtained within a single day was only .87 dB, while the sigma of thresholds obtained daily over a period of 23 successive days was only 1.22 dB. Hence, he demonstrated that consistency of auditory acuity can persist over relatively long periods of time.

Munson and Wiener (1950) investigated the differences between successive thresholds at 1,000 and 6,000 cps as obtained by the "ABX" method. They reason, "Within the framework of the limited tests reported here, it can be concluded that the variance σ^2 of the threshold determinations . . . is about 1.5 (dB)^2 if a good method is used for measuring the stimulus. This variance is believed to be primarily a measure of the variability of the observers' sensory system." Harris and Myers (1952) add the comment that each threshold obtained by Munson and Wiener was roughly an average of the status of sensitivity over a five-minute interval. Even as such, the Munson-Wiener findings bespeak greater stability of auditory sensitivity than many would expect.

The investigation conducted by Myers and Harris (1949) on the inherent stability of auditory thresholds is a most provocative exploration of short-term fluctuations in auditory sensitivity. Myers and Harris measured the auditory acuity of three young men at each of 11 frequencies. The procedure used was the serial method of limits. Five descents and five ascents were employed at each test frequency. Stimuli were presented at five-sec. intervals. Every stimulus was a .75-sec. pulse of the test tone. Successive pulses differed in intensity by one dB. A point of "threshold crossing" was computed independently for each descent and for each ascent. The exploration was conducted not only by air conduction but, in duplicate, by bone conduction. Myers and Harris summarize their basic finding as follows, "The typical short-term threshold fluctuation was of the order of less than a decibel. This is the total fluctuation as the result of instability in the subject's attending and responding systems as well as in his auditory system proper."

The minimum standard deviation exhibited by a single subject for a single frequency is .34 dB and the maximum is 1.68 dB. Considering individual subjects and each frequency separately, the standard deviation is under one dB in exactly half of the instances. Moreover, Myers and Harris (1949) conclude that, "There is no difference in threshold fluctuation between air and bone conduction or among frequencies." They also state, "Inexperienced subjects are not troubled with the 'zone of detectability,' a region within which an experienced subject is uncertain whether the stimulus is an indefinite noise or is actually a pure tone."

Two further points are important:

1. Myers and Harris (1949) report, "There is a tendency for a descending series to yield a somewhat better threshold than an ascending series." They add, however, "No completely reliable difference (between the two sequences) exists at any frequency for any subject . . . At most . . . (the difference) . . . amounts to little more than one decibel . . ." Actually, the average superiority of the descending thresholds over the ascending thresholds is .16 dB when computed for all subjects at all frequencies by both air and bone conduction. Obviously, from the practical point of view, .16 dB is an infinitesimal difference which is completely negligible. Hence, the Myers and Harris data support the expectation, which derives from recognition of on-effect, that a single tone of short duration is a sufficiently discrete entity that the listener's response to each presentation is essentially independent of the sequence in which it is placed.

2. Myers and Harris (1950) found, "Four crossings of the threshold (two ascending and two descending) are a sufficient number to produce a reliable threshold." Actually, in only five comparisons out of 66 does the threshold as estimated from the first four crossings differ by a decibel or more from the threshold as estimated from all 10 crossings. Furthermore, the mean difference for all 66 comparisons is .35 dB. Such results are encouraging to the clinician because they add to the assurance with which he can accept a threshold based on a few trials, provided, of course, he employs a method which has the requisite inherent reliability.

All the foregoing findings give one confidence in the validity of the Hughson-Westlake technique as a method for assessing the maximal acuity of clinical subjects. The moment-to-moment variability which typifies the normal hearing subject is sufficiently small so that the five-decibel step employed in conventional audiometry is too large to allow effective exploration of this variability. In other words, when the five-decibel step is used, any technique which excites on-effect may be expected to yield essentially equivalent findings for subjects with normal hearing. All that one can do under such circumstances is to ascertain the five-decibel step which separates the minimum hearing level at which responses always or usually occur from the maximum level at which responses are evoked only occasionally or not at all. Moreover, one is restricted to the same kind of information when testing cases with conductive impairments, since these people possess normal sensori-neural systems and hence will exhibit moment-to-moment variability similar to that of persons without hearing impairment.

The situation is less certain when dealing with sensori-neural losses. Many such cases, particularly those whose involvements have stabilized, probably also undergo restricted fluctuations in acuity. True, this expectation awaits experimental test. The important point, for the moment, is that the Hughson-Westlake method is justified even in instances where this expectation is not realized. To explain: when testing patients who undergo abnormal moment-to-moment variability in acuity, it is particularly important to use a technique which evokes on-effect, because many, if not all, of these patients will be prone to relapse. Testing such patients with sustained stimuli will increase their variabilities by evoking responses while they are in various stages of relapse. Exploration with short-duration tones will counteract this difficulty by eliciting on-effect. Such exploration has the further advantage of yielding estimates of unadapted acuity. These estimates are more valid criteria of each subject's capacity to react to transient sounds, like speech, than are measures of their sensitivities while relapsed. Therefore, the Hughson-Westlake method is appropriate even when testing subjects whose transient fluctuations in acuity are abnormally large. The method's simplicity recommends it over other procedures which evoke on-effects but which embody more complicated exploratory sequences.

EXPERIMENTAL COMPARISON

Theoretically, the Hughson-Westlake method will yield thresholds which are equivalent to those obtained with other clinical techniques that also excite on-effect responses. This premise required experimental scrutiny. Therefore, the investigation reported below was undertaken. Its purpose was to evaluate the extent to which different sequences of stimulus presentation affect the level that is designated as threshold. Specifically, thresholds were obtained by the ascending method of Hughson-Westlake, by an analogous descending sequence of isolated tones, and by a combined ascending-descending sequence.

All testing was done with a commercial audiometer (ADC-50-E) which activated a PDR-1 earphone mounted in an MX41/AR cushion. An auxiliary 20-dB pad was inserted between the audiometer and the earphone to provide the range of low intensities required to test normal hearing subjects, some of whom could be expected to exhibit hyperacute auditory sensitivity.

The acoustic output of the audiometer was measured daily by means of a 6-cc coupler (ASA Type 1), a calibrated condenser microphone (Western Electric, 640 AA), a cathode follower (ADC, D5153) and a vacuum-tube voltmeter (Hewlett-Packard, Model 400A). The pure-tone thresholds obtained during the study could consequently be reported in terms of the sound pressure level developed in the ASA Type 1 coupler.

The clinical room employed was one constructed for psychoacoustic research. The ambient noise level in the room was 30 dB, as measured on the C scale of a sound level meter (General Radio, Type 759).

The subjects used in the study were 36 students at Northwestern University. Their ages ranged from 18 to 24 years. Half were males and the other half females. Each was required to exhibit normal hearing as evidenced by the ability to pass an audiometric screen at a hearing level of 10 dB re the USPHS norm. This screening test was administered at the octave frequencies from 125 through 8,000 cps. In addition, only subjects whose history indicated freedom from ear pathology and from excessive noise exposure were accepted.

Each subject was seen for a single experimental session, during which thresholds at 250, 1,000 and 4,000 cps were established by each of the three clinical methods under investigation. The order of presentation of these three frequencies was counter-balanced with the three testing methods through the use of a Graeco-Latin Square design. One ear per subject was tested and the earphone was not moved once the test sequence had begun.

The following instructions were read to each subject at the outset of the experimental session:

> The purpose of this test is to see how well you can hear some faint tones. Each tone will be quite short. Some will be easy to hear. Others will be very faint. Whenever you hear one of these tones, no matter how faint it is, raise your finger. As soon as the tone goes off, lower your finger.

The experimenter assured himself that these instructions were understood and then the threshold testing was begun.

The three methods of threshold determination were designed to be as parallel as possible except for the progression of intensity changes:

1. The ascending method was the Hughson-Westlake procedure. Specifically, the following sequence was employed. The pure-tone stimulus was first presented 30 dB above the subject's presumed threshold. The purpose was to obtain a positive and decisive response. Attenuation was next introduced in 10-decibel steps until the subject failed to react. Only one stimulus per level was presented. Both during this downward progression and in subsequent ascents, each stimulus was a tonal pulse lasting between one and two seconds. After the subject failed to respond, the first ascent was initiated. Successive increments were in five-decibel steps. The first ascent was stopped as soon as the subject reacted to a stimulus. The signal was next attenuated 10 to 15 dB, and a new ascent was begun at this latter level. Ascending trials were continued until the subject had responded three times at one level. It was not required that these three responses be consecutive. The level eliciting these three reactions was recorded as the threshold.

2. The descending method was patterned analogously. Again, the exploration was initiated by presenting the pure-tone stimulus 30 dB above the subject's presumed threshold. Again, too, all stimuli were tonal pulses of a second or two, and only one stimulus was presented per audiometric level. Here, however, the second step was to descend in five-decibel intervals until the subject failed to respond. The level was then increased 10 to 15 dB and a new descent was initiated. This process was repeated until three failures to respond were obtained at a single audiometric level. The next higher hearing level, i.e., the last level at which response was noted in these three instances, was designated as the threshold.

3. The third method combined descending and ascending progressions. After an initial presentation at approximately 30 dB above the subject's threshold, a descent like those just described was performed. The lowest intensity at which response persisted was recorded. Next, an additional attenuation of 10 to 15 dB was introduced and then an ascent such as used in the Hughson-Westlake method was initiated. The level at which reaction first appeared was recorded. The hearing level was increased 10 or 15 dB and a second descent was conducted, following which a second ascent was, in turn, completed. After a third descent and a third ascent, the average for the six measures of minimum audible levels was computed as representing threshold.

Table 9-1 summarizes the results obtained when the foregoing methods were administered to the 36 university students. The table reports both mean thresholds and standard deviations for the group. One notes that the mean threshold for the descending method is slightly better at every frequency than for either of the other two methods. Its maximum superiority occurred at 1,000 cps where the mean threshold for the combined method was 1.7 dB higher. The means of descending thresholds were .6, 1.5 and 1.3 dB better than the means of ascending thresholds at 250, 1,000 and 4,000 cps, respectively. Interestingly enough, the combined method yielded poorer mean thresholds than did the ascending method at 250 and 1,000 cps.

The superiority of the descending method over the other two methods might be argued from the results reported in Table 9-1. However, the magnitude of the mean advantage achieved by the descending thresholds over the ascending thresholds falls far short of the 10 to 15 dB differential which clinicians often assume to exist. Moreover, the present results fail to confirm the commonly held hypothesis that a combination of ascending and descending series will

yield threshold values intermediate between those which either type of run will yield if employed alone. Thus, as one contemplates the present results, he is impressed by the fact that the mean thresholds obtained here by the three methods are indistinguishable, from the practical point of view.

Further confidence in the general equivalence of the three methods is found in the standard deviations reported in Table 9-1. Considering each test frequency separately, the three standard deviations were highly similar. Thus, one concludes that the variability among subjects remained the same from one method to another.

The data at hand may be summarized in another way. One may ask how closely each subject agreed with himself when tested by the three methods. Such a comparison gives a particularly provocative picture of the findings because it highlights the practical equivalence which the three test methods exhibit.

The procedure for making the comparison was simple. All thresholds first had to be designated on a five-decibel scale. The original data from both ascending and descending techniques were already aligned in five-decibel intervals. It was therefore only necessary to assign each original threshold for the combined sequence to the closest five-decibel step on the audiometric scale. When the original measure was equidistant between steps, the better hearing level was selected. In other words, the data for the combined method were recast in the form that would logically be used in recording routine findings on an audiogram.

Differences among thresholds obtained by the three test procedures were then compared for each subject separately. Tables 9-2, 9-3, and 9-4 summarize the tabulations of these differences. One notes that within each table the distribution of differences is sufficiently similar for the three test frequencies so that only the totals of differences for all frequencies need be discussed in comparing methods. There is *no*

TABLE 9-1. MEANS AND STANDARD DEVIATIONS OF THRESHOLD SOUND PRESSURE LEVELS* YIELDED BY 36 NORMAL HEARING SUBJECTS UNDER THREE MEASUREMENT TECHNIQUES.

Technique	250 cps		1,000 cps		4,000 cps	
	Mean	S.D.	Mean	S.D.	Mean	S.D.
Ascending	24.7	4.0	9.3	4.6	16.8	7.2
Descending	24.1	4.3	7.8	4.8	15.5	8.4
Ascending-Descending	25.1	4.0	9.5	4.0	16.4	7.5

*dB re: .0002 microbar in ASA Type 1 Coupler.

TABLE 9-2. DISTRIBUTION OF DIFFERENCES IN CLINICAL THRESHOLDS YIELDED BY 36 NORMAL HEARING SUBJECTS WHEN TESTED BY ASCENDING AND BY DESCENDING SEQUENCES.

Ascending Minus Descending	Test Frequency			Total	
	250	1,000	4,000	N	%
−5	3	0	2	5	4.6
0	25	26	23	74	68.5
5	8	9	11	28	25.9
10	0	1	0	1	.9
Total	36	36	36	108	

TABLE 9-3. DISTRIBUTION OF DIFFERENCES IN CLINICAL THRESHOLDS YIELDED BY 36 NORMAL HEARING SUBJECTS WHEN TESTED BY ASCENDING AND BY COMBINED ASCENDING-DESCENDING* SEQUENCES.

Ascending Minus Combined	Test Frequency			Total	
	250	1,000	4,000	N	%
−5	5	2	2	9	8.3
0	24	31	28	83	76.9
5	7	3	6	16	14.8
Total	36	36	36	108	

*Nearest 5-dB step designated as clinical threshold for combined sequences with better level selected when the mean of six runs was equidistant between two audiometric levels.

TABLE 9-4. DISTRIBUTION OF DIFFERENCES IN CLINICAL THRESHOLDS YIELDED BY 36 NORMAL HEARING SUBJECTS WHEN TESTED BY DESCENDING AND BY COMBINED ASCENDING-DESCENDING* SEQUENCES.

Descending Minus Combined	Test Frequency			Total	
	250	1,000	4,000	N	%
−5	6	10	10	26	24.2
0	27	26	21	74	68.4
5	3	0	5	8	7.4
Total	36	36	36	108	

*Nearest 5-dB step designated as clinical threshold for combined sequences, with better level selected when the mean of six runs was equidistant between two audiometric levels.

difference between the individual thresholds in 74 (68.5 percent) out of the 108 comparisons involving the ascending and descending methods. In all but one of the remaining comparisons the difference in threshold is a single audiometric step (five dB). The agreement is even better between ascending and combined methods. Here, 83 subjects (76.9 percent) yielded identical thresholds; all of the 25 differences (23.1 percent) were discrepancies of only five dB. Finally, the parallelism between descending and combined methods was almost identical to the parallelism between descending and ascending procedures. Again, 74 (68.5 percent) of the comparisons represented complete equivalence. All of the remaining 34 comparisons yielded a discrepancy of one audiometric step. Thus, Tables 9-2, 9-3, and 9-4 may be summarized by the statement that in approximately seven out of every 10 comparisons, audiometric results were identical when designated in a conventional clinical manner, and (with only one exception in the 318 comparisons) the remainder yielded differences of only one interval on the recording scale.

Two further factual items have some interest: (1) Identical thresholds for a single subject were obtained by all three methods in 62 (57.4 percent) out of a possible 108 instances. Thus, more than half the time there was absolutely no deviation of one method from the other two. (2) In 45 of the 46 remaining instances, two of the three thresholds were the same. Here the distribution was as follows: the descending and the ascending thresholds were alike 12 times, the descending and the combined 13 times, while the ascending and the combined thresholds were equal 20 times. Thus, if one were using the results for the combined method as a criterion, he would observe that the ascending thresholds agree with this criterion better than do the descending ones. However, since there is really no way in the present instance of selecting a particular threshold as the more valid in each specific incident of discrepancy, one must reach the conclusion that the three methods under study emerge as clinically indistinguishable when the five-decibel step is the unit of testing and of threshold recording. Therefore, the choice among methods may rest on practical considerations rather than theoretical imperatives.

DISCUSSION

The failure of the present study to demonstrate clinically important differences between procedures is merely evidence that the five-decibel step employed in routine pure-tone audiometry is too large to yield measurements which distinguish the subtleties of the listener's auditory variability. This outcome is to be expected when one remembers the nature of the on-effect and the small range of momentary fluctuations in auditory sensitivity which normal hearers undergo.

The clinician must be clear on the implications of these facts. He must distinguish between the reliability of reaction he may expect from an individual subject during a single audiometric test and the day-to-day consistency he may assume for re-tests performed in the clinical situation. The reliability of the former can be very good, as the foregoing discussion has demonstrated, while the repeatability of measurement from one clinical examination to the next can be relatively poor. The latter fact has been amply demonstrated in many studies, ranging from the investigation by Witting and Hughson (1940) to the one by Roach and Carhart (1956). These studies supply the clinician with information on the precision with which he may accept any particular test as illustrative of the audiometric level which characterizes the patient's everyday hearing. These studies do not tell the clinician anything about the precision of measurement within a single test. In other words, such factors as difference in adjusting the earphones, other changes in the test situation, and true shifts in

the hearing of the patient are responsible for the discrepancies which appear from one day's test to another. The clinician must make allowances for the unreliability which such factors produce, but he must not make the mistake of presuming that comparable variability is inherent in the patient's acuity from one moment to the next.

The alert clinician will bear in mind Hirsh's comment, "The sources of . . . threshold variability are numerous and are not necessarily related to the variability of the observer's physiological threshold" (1952). He will choose a technique for testing which is parsimonious of his own effort, which is simple for the subject and which gives an estimate of the observer's physiological threshold that satisfies clinical requirements for intra-test reliability.

The Hughson-Westlake technique meets these three criteria. Clinicians who have used it found it to be highly satisfactory because of the rapidity with which a skilled tester can obtain threshold and because of the easy task it imposes on the subject. Moreover, as demonstrated above, the Hughson-Westlake technique is equivalent, within reasonable clinical margin, to other techniques which also excite on-effect and which also employ the five-decibel step of traditional pure-tone audiometry. The procedure has the added merit of having been recommended for many years to audiometrists by the Committee on Conservation of Hearing of the American Academy of Ophthalmology and Otolaryngology. Therefore, the Hughson-Westlake method can quite properly be adopted by clinicians throughout the world as the preferred technique for determining thresholds for pure tones when using the conventional audiometer.

One thing must be remembered by the reader as he contemplates the recommendation, which is here renewed, that he use the Hughson-Westlake method. Every clinician has habituated a procedure which is now so comfortable for him that he finds it hard to believe another method could be as good. Despite his feelings of comfortableness with it, his technique has theoretical and practical limitations if it does not elicit on-effect. However, if he uses a technique which does elicit on-effect, his method is as good in seeking out the unadapted physiological threshold as is the Hughson-Westlake technique. Under such circumstances, choice between methods cannot be resolved by the criteria of simplicity and of parsimony. For one thing, habituation regarding these matters influences belief. In addition, there are other methods, such as the analogous descending exploration, which are equally fast and precise. The only way of choosing between clinical procedures which are fundamentally equivalent in seeking out the unadapted threshold is to make an arbitrary selection. In the writers' opinion, the reason favoring arbitrary selection of the Hughson-Westlake technique is found in the long-term sponsorship which has been given to the method by the Committee on Conservation of Hearing. This sponsorship should encourage clinicians to adopt the method for the purpose of achieving widespread uniformity of routine audiometric procedures. Obviously, there will continue to be specific instances in which other audiometric methods are preferable, but audiology will achieve new maturity if clinicians employ these other techniques as conscious variations from a standardized practice.

formed with a five-decibel intensity interval. The procedure, which presents stimuli for a second or two so as to elicit on-effect responses from the subject, encourages stability of reactions and yields measurement of the unadapted level of acuity. According to the theory of on-effect, the Hughson-Westlake method should yield thresholds which are clinically equivalent to those obtained by similar short tonal presentations patterned in descending or "threshold crossing" sequences. Experimental exploration with 36 normal hearing subjects confirmed this expectation. Adoption of the Hughson-Westlake method is recommended over the other methods which also elicit on-effect for the purpose of gaining uniformity of procedure throughout the field of clinical audiometry.

SUMMARY

The Hughson-Westlake ascending method for establishing pure-tone auditory threshold is recommended for general clinical use when audiometry is per-

ACKNOWLEDGMENTS

The authors acknowledge the helpful assistance of Earl R. Harford, Bud D. Kimball and Robert J. Harrison in the successful completion of this study.

ENDNOTES

1. This research was supported by the United States Air Force under Contract AF 41(657)-185, monitored by the School of Aviation Medicine, USAF, Randolph Air Force Base, Texas.

2. Various techniques of pulse-tone audiometry are justifiable in terms of the considerations reviewed here. However, discussion of these techniques is beyond the scope of the present paper, which is concerned exclusively with an analysis of the traditional audiometric methodology.

REFERENCES

Bunch, C. C., *Clinical Audiometry*. St. Louis: Mosby, 1943.

Derbyshire, A. J., and Davis, H., The action potentials of the auditory nerve. *Amer. J. Physiol.,* 113, 1935, 476–504.

Egan, J. P., and Thwing, E. J., Further studies on perstimulatory fatigue. *J. Acoust. Soc. Amer.,* 27, 1955, 1225–1226.

Galambos, R., and Davis, H., The response of single auditory nerve fibers to acoustic stimulation. *J. Neurophysiol.,* 6, 1943, 39–57.

Hallpike, C. S., and Hood, J. D., Some recent work on auditory adaptation and its relationship to the loudness recruitment phenomenon. *J. Acoust. Soc. Amer.,* 23, 1951, 270–274.

Harris, J. D., and Myers, C. K., Experiments on fluctuation of auditory acuity. U.S. Navy Med. Res. Lab. Rep. No. 196, 1952, 2–29.

Heller, M. F., *Functional Otology.* New York: Springer, 1955.

Hirsh, I. J., *Measurement of Hearing.* New York: McGraw-Hill, 1952.

Hood, J. D., Studies in auditory fatigue and adaptation. *Acta Otolaryng., Stockh., Suppl.,* 92, 1950, 1–57.

Hughson, W., and Westlake, H., Manual for program outline for rehabilitation of aural casualties both military and civilian. *Trans. Amer. Acad. Ophthal. Otolaryng. Suppl.,* 48, 1944, 1–15.

Jerger, J. F., Auditory adaptation. *J. Acoust. Soc. Amer.*, 29, 1957, 357–363.

Jerger, J. F., Differential intensity sensitivity in the ear with loudness recruitment. *J. Speech Hearing Dis.*, 20, 1955, 183–193.

Jerger, J. F., Carhart, R., and Lassman, J., Clinical observations on excessive threshold adaptation. *Arch. Otolaryng., Chicago*, 68, 1958, 617–623.

Lierle, D. M., and Reger, S. N., Experimentally induced temporary threshold shifts in ears with impaired hearing. *Ann. Otol., etc., St Louis*, 64, 1955, 263–277.

Munson, W. A., and Wiener, F. M., Sound measurement for psychophysical tests. *J. Acoust. Soc. Amer.*, 22, 1950, 382–386.

Myers, C. K., and Harris, J. D., Variability of the auditory threshold with time. U.S. Navy Med. Res. Lab. Rep. No. 165, 1950, 230–257.

Myers, C. K., and Harris, J. D., The inherent stability of the auditory threshold. U.S. Naval Med. Res. Lab. Progress Rep. No. 3, Bu Med Project NM-003-021, April, 1949.

Newby, *H. Audiology*. New York: Appleton-Century-Crofts, 1958.

Newhart, H., and Reger, S., Manual for a school hearing conservation program (revised 1951, C. E. Kinney, G. D. Hoople, S. R. Guild and S. N. Reger, eds., for Committee on Conservation of Hearing). *Trans. Amer. Acad. Ophthal. Otolaryng. Suppl.*, 1951.

Newhart, H., and Reger, S. N. (eds.), Syllabus of audiometric procedures in the administration of a program for the conservation of hearing of school children *Trans. Amer. Acad. Ophthal. Otolaryng. Suppl.*, April 1945, 1–28.

Palva, T., Studies on per-stimulatory adaptation in various groups of deafness. *Laryngoscope, St Louis*, 65, 1955, 829–847.

Roach, R. E., and Carhart, R., A clinical method for calibrating the bone-conduction audiometer. *Arch. Otolaryng., Chicago*, 63, 1956, 270–278.

Stevens, S. S. (ed.), *Handbook of Experimental Psychology*. New York: John Wiley and Sons, 1951.

Tasaki, I., Nerve impulses in individual auditory nerve fibers of guinea pig. *J. Neurophysiol.*, 17, 1954, 97–122.

Ward, W. D., Method of "single descent" in group audiometry. *J. Acoust. Soc. Amer.*, 29, 1957a, 371–376.

Ward, W. D., The single-descent group audiometer. *Noise Control*, 3, 1957b, No. 3, 15–18.

Watson, L. A., and Tolan, T., *Hearing Tests and Hearing Instruments*. Baltimore: Williams and Wilkins, 1949.

Wertheimer, M., The variability of auditory and visual absolute thresholds in time. *J. Gen. Psychol.*, 52, 1955, 111–147.

Witting, E. G., and Hughson, W., Inherent accuracy of a series of repeated clinical audiograms. *Laryngoscope, St Louis*, 50, 1940, 259–269.

10

Guidelines for Manual Pure-Tone Threshold Audiometry

COMMITTEE on AUDIOMETRIC EVALUATION, AMERICAN SPEECH-LANGUAGE-HEARING ASSOCIATION

The set of *Guidelines for Manual Pure-Tone Threshold Audiometry* is the third of a series developed by the Committee on Audiometric Evaluation, under the office of Vice President for Clinical Affairs of the American Speech and Hearing Association (ASHA). The first in the series was the *Guidelines for Audiometric Symbols* (1974), adopted by ASHA in December 1973. The second was the *Guidelines for Identification Audiometry* (1975), adopted by the Association in November 1974.

Each of the guidelines presents a recommended set of procedures based on existing practice and research findings. The spirit of these guidelines is not to mandate a single way of accomplishing a clinical process; rather, they suggest standard procedures that, in the final analysis, will benefit the persons we serve. The intention is to improve interclinician and interclinic comparison of data, thereby allowing for a more effective transfer of information.

The ASHA *Guidelines for Manual Pure-Tone Threshold Audiometry* presents procedures for accomplishing hearing threshold measurement with pure tones that are applicable in a wide variety of settings. Diagnostic pure-tone threshold audiometry, used most often in clinical settings, includes manual air-conduction measurements at octave intervals from 250 Hz (125 Hz under some circumstances) through 8,000 Hz plus bone-conduction measurements at octave intervals from 250 Hz through 4,000

Hz as needed. Also, when required, masking is used. Monitoring pure-tone threshold audiometry, used most often in industrial settings, includes manual air-conduction measurements at the frequencies of 500, 1,000, 2,000, 3,000, 4,000, and 6,000 or 8,000 Hz.

SCOPE

Pure-tone threshold audiometry is the measurement of an individual's hearing sensitivity for calibrated pure tones. Two general methods are employed (1) manual audiometry, also referred to as conventional pure-tone audiometry; and (2) discrete-frequency or sweep-frequency testing by automatic audiometry referred to as Bekesy-type audiometry. The guidelines presented in this document relate only to manual pure-tone audiometry.

The historical antecedents of pure-tone audiometry were the classical tuning fork tests. The development of the audiometer made it possible to control signal intensity and duration in ways that were not possible with tuning forks. One cannot assume, however, that calibrated equipment insures that valid measurements are always obtained. Differences among measurement methods may affect validity and reliability in significant ways as pointed out by a number of authors (Hughson and Westlake, 1944; Reger, 1950; Watson and Tolan, 1949; Hirsh, 1952; Carhart and Jerger, 1959; Price, 1971; and Newby, 1972).

These guidelines present a standard set of procedures that will minimize interest differences. These guidelines represent a consensus of recommendations found in the literature, with particular emphasis on the suggestions of Carhart and Jerger (1959) and Reger (1950). The American Speech and Hearing Association does not intend to imply that only one method is correct; variations in procedure may be

ASHA Editor's Note: The set of "Guidelines for Manual Pure-Tone Threshold Audiometry" was approved by the ASHA Legislative Council in November 1977. The following members of the ASHA Committee on Audiometric Evaluation developed these guidelines: Vincent Byers, Joseph B. Chaiklin, James T. Graham, Norma T. Hopkinson, Z. G. Schoney, Francis L. Sonday, and Wesley R. Wilson, Chairman. ASHA encourages the professional community to use these guidelines.

Reprinted by permission of the American Speech-Language-Hearing Association from *Asha*, **20**, 297–301 (1978).

demanded by special clinical problems. For example, special populations such as very young children, severely mentally-retarded persons, severely hearing-impaired persons, uncooperative persons, or neurologically handicapped persons may require modifications of the guideline procedures if the audiologist is to develop sufficient information for case management. When variations in procedure are necessary, they should be noted in a manner that allows other testers to understand how thresholds were obtained. The pure-tone guidelines are presented in three sections (1) determination of pure-tone thresholds, (2) standard procedures for monitoring and diagnostic air-conduction measures, and (3) standard procedures for bone-conduction measures.

DETERMINATION OF PURE-TONE THRESHOLDS

Some of the factors that influence the manual assessment of pure-tone thresholds are (1) the instructions to the individual, (2) the response task required of the individual, and (3) the examiner's interpretation of the individual's response behavior during the test.

Instructions. The instructions shall be phrased in language appropriate to the listener and shall indicate

1. the response task,
2. that the person is to respond whenever the tone is heard, no matter how faint it may be,
3. the need to respond as soon as the tone comes on and to stop responding immediately when the tone goes off,
4. that each ear is to be tested separately.

Response Task. Overt responses are required from the listener to indicate when the tone goes on and off. Any response task meeting this criterion is acceptable. Examples of commonly used responses are (1) raising and lowering the finger, hand, or arm and (2) pressing and releasing a signal light switch.

Interpretation of Response Behavior. The primary parameters used by the tester in determining threshold are latency of response, presence of on- and off-responses and number of false responses.

1. The latency of the on-responses should be consistent. If the first response to a tone in an ascending series is slow, present a 5-dB higher tone and the response should be without hestitation.
2. Each suprathreshold presentation should elicit two responses—an on-response at the start and an off-response at the end of the tone. Listeners who are unable to signal correctly the termination of the tone, following proper instruction and reinstruction, may be demonstrating auditory problems and be in need of more detailed testing.
3. False responses may be of two types (1) a response when no tone is present (false-positive), or (2) failure to respond when a tone that is audible to the listener is present (false-negative). Either type complicates the measurement procedure. Reinstruction may reduce the rate of either type. The rate of false-positive responses may also be reduced by such techniques as varying the time between audible tones, pulsing or warbling of the signal, or using pulse-counting procedures.

Determination of Threshold

The basic procedure for threshold determination consists of (1) familiarization with signal and (2) threshold measurement. The procedure is the same regardless of frequency, output transducer, or ear under test.

Familiarization. The listener should be familiarized with the task prior to threshold determination by presenting a signal of sufficient intensity to evoke a sharp and clear response. The step of familiarization assures the examiner that the listener understands and can perform the response task. The following two methods of familiarization are commonly used:

1. Beginning with the tone continuously on but completely attenuated, gradually increase the sound-pressure level of the tone until a response occurs.
2. Present the tone at a hearing level of 30 dB. If a clear response occurs, begin threshold measurement. If no response occurs, present the tone at 50 dB HL and at successive additional increments of 10 dB until a response is obtained.

Neither method requires the tester to make a prior assumption about the listener's threshold, in contrast with some methods in common use. The American Speech and Hearing Association recommends a method not requiring such an assumption.

Threshold Measurement. The method described is recommended as a standard procedure for manual pure-tone threshold audiometry.

1. *Tone Duration.* Threshold exploration is carried out by presenting continuous tones of 1–2 sec in duration.
2. *Interval Between Tones.* The interval between tone presentations shall be varied but not shorter than the test tone.
3. *Level of First Presentation.* The level of the first presentation of tone for threshold measurement is 10 dB below the level of the listener's response to the familiarization presentation.
4. *Levels of Succeeding Presentations.* The tone level of succeeding presentations is determined by the preceding response. After each failure to respond to a signal, the level is increased in 5-dB steps until the first response occurs. After the response, the intensity is decreased 10 dB and another ascending series is begun. (Note: An exception is as explained previously under Interpretation of Response Behavior —Latency.)
5. *Threshold of Hearing.* Threshold is defined arbitrarily as the lowest level at which responses occur in at least half of a series of ascending trials with a minimum of three responses required at a single level.

When variations in the standard method are used, the audiogram form shall indicate the nature of the variation. Examples of variation to be noted are

1. Threshold determined by descending presentations method,
2. "Pulsed tone substituted," and
3. "Warbled tone substituted."

STANDARD PROCEDURES FOR MONITORING AND DIAGNOSTIC AIR-CONDUCTION MEASURES

Instrumentation and Calibration. Air-conduction audiometry shall be accomplished with an audiometer and earphones that meet the specifications of the American National Standard Specifications for Audiometers S3.6–1969, and appropriate to the technique being used—monitoring or diagnostic.

Test Environment. The test environment shall meet the specifications for allowable ambient noise detailed in *The American National Standard Criteria for Permissible Ambient Noise During Audiometric Testing S3.1–1977.* When the ambient noise exceeds the allowable value for a specific frequency, the threshold for that frequency may be recorded if the obtained threshold exceeds by 10 dB the difference between the ambient noise level and the allowable ambient level.

In the interest of listener and examiner comfort, the test room and examiner's work area should provide for proper control of temperature, air exchange, and humidity. In the interest of listener and examiner safety, sound-isolated areas must be provided with either or both visual and auditory warning systems. These warning systems should be connected to the building warning system (fire, civil defense).

Earphone Placement. The ear canal should be checked for blockage by cerumen or for collapse of canal without or with earphones. The earphones should be held in place by a headband with the earphone grid directly over the entrance to the ear canal. The earphones should be placed by the tester, not the listener. Long hair and other obstacles should be clear of the space under the earphone.

Frequency. The frequencies tested differ, depending on the technique used.

1. *Monitoring Technique.* Threshold assessment shall be made at 500 Hz, 1,000 Hz, 2,000 Hz, 3,000 Hz, 4,000 Hz, and 6,000 or 8,000 Hz.
2. *Diagnostic Technique.* Threshold assessment shall be made at octave intervals of 250 Hz to 8,000 Hz, except when a low frequency hearing loss exists, in which case threshold shall be assessed at 125 Hz, as well. When the difference between the values at any two adjacent octave frequencies from 500 Hz to 8,000 Hz is 20 dB or more, intraoctave measurements should be completed.

Order. When appropriate information is available, the better ear should be tested first. The initial test frequency should be 1,000 Hz, and then either higher or lower frequencies shall be assessed sequentially followed by a retest of 1,000 Hz and the remaining frequencies. Selection of 1,000 Hz as the initial test frequency rests largely on past convention rather than on substantial research evidence. Until evidence is developed in support of a different initial frequency, no persuasive reason exists to change past convention except for special populations (for example, severely hearing impaired) which may require a different initial frequency.

Masking for Diagnostic Audiometry. When the air-conduction threshold obtained in one ear exceeds the apparent bone-conduction threshold in the contralateral ear by 40 dB or more, appropriate masking shall be applied to the nontest ear. Since the procedures for masking are not confined to pure-tone measures, these procedures are not discussed in this set of guidelines.

Recording of Results. Results may be recorded in graphic or tabular form or both. Separate forms to represent each ear may be used.

1. *Audiogram Form.* When the graphic form is used, the audiogram shall be on cross-section paper, with the abscissas being frequencies on a logarithmic scale and the ordinates being hearing levels in decibels on a linear scale. It is recommended that one octave on the frequency scale be linearly equivalent to 20 dB on the hearing level scale. The vertical scale is to be designated hearing level (Decibels); the horizontal scale is to be labeled Frequency in Hz.

2. *Audiogram Symbols.* When the graphic form is used, the symbols presented in ASHA's *Guidelines for Audiometric Symbols* (1974) should be used (see Figure 10–1 for sample).

Other pertinent information describing the test situation should be reported on the audiogram or test results form.

STANDARD PROCEDURES FOR BONE-CONDUCTION MEASURES

Instrumentation and Calibration. The testing should be accomplished with a wide-range audiometer as defined by ANSI specification S3.6–1969. The bone-conduction vibrator is to be calibrated to the Interim-Threshold Calibration Values (Appendix A, Table A4) of the American National Standard

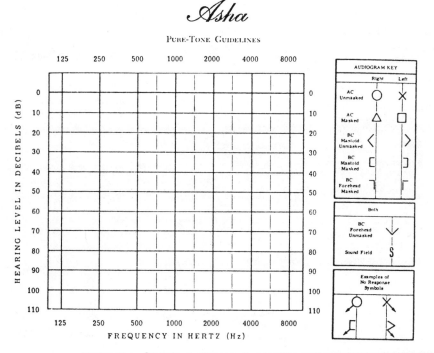

FIGURE 10–1. Sample audiogram form with symbols.

Specifications for Artificial Head-Bone for the Calibration of Audiometer Bone Vibrators S3.13–1972 and should incorporate the appropriate calibration for either frontal or mastoid placement. NOTE: In addition to this standard, one may use comparison values for other artificial mastoids (Wilber, 1972).

Standard bone-conduction vibrator placement should allow mastoid or forehead placement. The test ear should never be covered for standard bone-conduction measurements. The contralateral ear will be covered when masking is being used. The tester is to place the transducer(s) not the listener.

Frequencies. Thresholds should be obtained at octave intervals of 250 Hz to 4,000 Hz. Testing at frequencies below 500 Hz demands excellent sound isolation for cases with normal or near normal sensitivity, but may be accomplished when such an environment is available.

Order. The initial frequency tested shall be 1,000 Hz and then either higher or lower frequencies shall be tested sequentially followed by the remaining frequencies.

Masking. If the unmasked bone-conduction threshold is 10 dB better than either air-conduction threshold at the frequency, masking must be used. Since the threshold values on which the calibration of bone vibrators is based were measured with masking noise in the contralateral ear, the tester may prefer always to use masking in the testing procedure.*

Recording of Results. Results may be recorded in graphic or tabular form. A standard set of symbols has been delineated in *Guidelines for Audiometric Symbols* (1974) and is to be used with the graphic form (audiogram). See Figure 10–1 for an example of recommended bone-conduction symbols.

CONCLUSIONS

The guidelines for manual pure-tone threshold audiometry are

---

*(Editors' note: There is divided opinion about the merit of routine masking in bone-conduction audiometry. Other selections (Studebaker, reading 19; Coles and Priede, reading 36) contain further discussion of this issue.)

1. *Instructions.* Indicate response task in language appropriate for the listener.
2. *Response Task.* Use any overt response signaling both tone on and tone off.
3. *Determination of Threshold:*
   A. Familiarization is accomplished by presentation of a signal at suprathreshold level.
   B. Threshold exploration involves ascending presentations of short-duration tones with level based on response to preceding presentation. After each failure to respond, the level is raised 5 dB until a positive response is obtained. After a response, the intensity is decreased 10 dB and another ascending series initiated.
   C. *Threshold* is defined as the lowest level at which responses occur in at least half of the ascents with a minimum of three responses required at a single level.
4. *Frequencies:*
   A. Monitoring audiometry includes air-conduction thresholds at the frequencies of 500, 1,000, 2,000, 4,000, and 6,000 or 8,000 Hz.
   B. Diagnostic audiometry includes both air-conduction and bone-conduction thresholds.
      i. Air-conduction threshold is measured at the octave intervals of 250 Hz to 8,000 Hz (plus 125 Hz in the case of low frequency hearing impairment) and at intraoctave intervals of any two successive octaves between 500 and 8,000 Hz that differ by 20 dB or more.
      ii. Bone-conduction threshold is measured at the octave intervals of 250 Hz to 4,000 Hz.
5. *Instrumentation and Calibration.* Audiometers are to be maintained to the current ANSI specifications.

Note: When the following guidelines and standards referred to in this document are superseded by an approved revision, the revision shall apply

1. American Speech and Hearing Association Guidelines for Audiometric Symbols (1974);
2. American National Standard Specifications for Audiometers S3.6–1969 (R 1973);
3. American National Standard Specifications for Artificial Head-Bone for the Calibration of Audiometer Bone Vibrators S3.13–1972; and
4. American National Standard Criteria for Permissible Ambient Noise During Audiometric Testing S3.1–1977.

REFERENCES

American National Standards Institute. *American National Standard Specifications for Artificial Head-Bone for the Calibration of Audiometer Bone Vibrators* (S3.13–1972). New York: American National Standards Institute (1973).

American National Standards Institute. *American National Standard Specifications for Audiometers* (S.3–1969 [R 1973]). New York: American National Standards Institute (1970).

American National Standards Institute. *American National Standard Criteria for Permissible Ambient Noise During Audiometric Testing* (S3.1–1977). New York: American National Standards Institute (1977).

American Speech and Hearing Association. *Guidelines for Audiometric Symbols.* Washington, D.C.: American Speech and Hearing Association (1974).

American Speech and Hearing Association. *Guidelines for Identification Audiometry.* Washington, D.C.: American Speech and Hearing Association (1975).

Carhart, R. and Jerger, J. F. Preferred method for clinical determination of pure-tone thresholds. *J. Speech Hearing Dis., 24,* 330–345 (1959).

Hirsh, I. J. *The Measurement of Hearing.* New York: McGraw-Hill Book Co., Inc. (1952).

Hughson, W. and Westlake, H. D. Manual for program outline for rehabilitation of aural casualties both military and civilian. *Trans. Am. Acad. Ophthal. Otolary., Suppl.* **48,** 1–15 (1944).

Newby, H. A. *Audiology* (Third ed.). New York: Appleton-Century-Crofts (1972).

Price, L. L. Pure-tone audiometry. In *Audiological Assessment,* Rose, D. E. (Ed.). Englewood Cliffs, N.J.: Prentice-Hall, Inc. (1971).

Reger, S. N. Standardization of pure-tone audiometer testing technique, *Laryngoscope, St. Louis,* **60,** 161–185 (1950).

Watson, L. A. and Tolan, T. *Hearing Tests and Hearing Instruments.* Baltimore: Williams and Wilkins (1949).

Wilber, L. A. Comparability of two commercially available artificial mastoids. *J. acoust. Soc. Am.,* **52,** 1265–1266 (1972).

11

Guidelines for Audiometric Symbols

COMMITTEE ON AUDIOMETRIC EVALUATION, AMERICAN SPEECH-LANGUAGE-HEARING ASSOCIATION

The set of *Guidelines for Audiometric Symbols* is the first of a series developed by the Committee on Audiometric Evaluation under the Vice-President for Clinical Affairs of the American Speech and Hearing Association.

Each of the guidelines presents a recommended set of procedures based on existing clinical practice and research findings. The spirit of these guidelines is not to mandate a single way of accomplishing the clinical process; rather, the intent is to suggest standard procedures that, in the final analysis, will benefit the patients we serve. The intention is to allow for a more efficient and uniform transfer of information.

Audiometric symbols used to record the results of conventional pure-tone threshold audiometry have never been standardized by the American Speech and Hearing Association. A wide variety of symbols and symbol systems is in use for recording data on audiograms, as has been demonstrated most recently by Martin and Kopra (1970) and by Sweetman and Miller in an ASHA convention paper (Chicago, 1969). Although certain audiometric symbols are in almost universal use, others are employed in widely disparate ways by different clinicians. Widespread use of unstandardized, idiosyncratic symbol systems increases the possibility of a misinterpretation of data when records are exchanged between clinical services. In addition, such use impedes the orderly exchange of information with other professions, in both clinical practice and published reports.

The purpose of these guidelines is to detail a set of standard audiometric symbols for recording graph-

ically the results of pure-tone audiometry. From this set of symbols the clinician may select those necessary to record the information collected. Presentation of these guidelines does not imply that the audiogram is the only appropriate means of recording audiometric results;[1] however, when an audiogram is used, these symbols should be used.

THE AUDIOGRAM

As recommended in the ANSI S3.6–1969 *Specifications for Audiometers,* the audiogram shall be shown as a grid with test frequencies, in Hertz (Hz), represented on the abscissa by means of a logarithmic scale and the hearing level (HL), in decibels (dB), represented on the ordinate by a linear scale. One octave on the frequency scale shall be equivalent in span to 20 dB on the HL scale. The horizontal scale shall be labeled *Frequency in Hertz* and the vertical scale shall be labeled *Hearing Level in dB.* The zero reference threshold level should be shown prominently.

Grid lines of equal darkness and thickness are recommended at octave intervals on the frequency scale and at 10-dB intervals on the HL scale. Grid lines used for interoctave frequencies should be finer and lighter in hue than those for octave frequencies.

The audiogram form is illustrated in Figure 11–1. Specific recommendations on the type and amount of additional information to be included on the audiogram form, such as client identification, tester identification, results of speech audiometry, and results of tuning fork tests, are not included in these guidelines since they more appropriately are specified by individual clinics.

THE AUDIOMETRIC SYMBOLS

Any effort to modify behavior through the establishment of guidelines must consider current practices. One of the most recent sources used by the Com-

ASHA Editor's Note: The "Guidelines for Audiometric Symbols" was approved by the ASHA Executive Board in December 1973. Members of the ASHA Committee on Audiometric Evaluation, which developed the guidelines, are F. L. Sonday, W. R. Wilson, J. B. Chaiklin, J. T. Graham, Z. G. Schoeny, and N. T. Hopkinson, Chairman. ASHA encourages the professional community to use these guidelines in clinical practice and in publications.

Reprinted by permission of the American Speech-Language-Hearing Association from *Asha* **16**, 260–264 (1974).

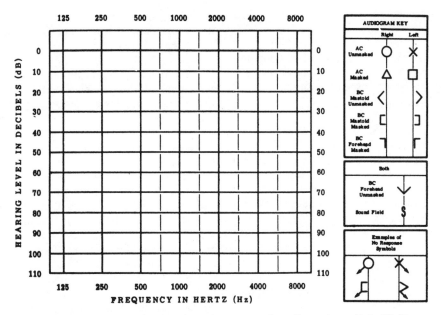

FIGURE 11-1. The audiogram form, showing appropriate dimensions. Note 20 dB on the ordinate equals an octave on the abscissa.

mittee on Audiometric Evaluation is Martin and Kopra's (1970) survey of audiometric symbols used by ASHA-certified audiologists. Although the Committee considered the apparent popularity of certain symbols, all symbols considered had to meet four basic criteria. Each symbol had to be

1. Simple in design, easily drawn, and sharply reproducible by xerography or other reproduction methods.
2. Mutually exclusive from and internally consistent with other symbols in the system.
3. Capable of delineating, without recourse to color coding, the following distinctions:
   a. left ear from right ear,
   b. air conduction from bone conduction,
   c. unmasked from masked results,
   d. response from no response, and
   e. the transducer (phone, vibrator, or speaker) used to present signals.
4. Designed to permit multiple notation at a single level on the audiogram.

Based on these four criteria, the Committee on Audiometric Evaluation recommends the set of symbols presented in Table 11-1.

TABLE 11-1 RECOMMENDED SYMBOLS FOR THRESHOLD AUDIOMETRY. UNLESS OTHERWISE SPECIFIED, SYMBOLS ARE TO INDICATE THAT TEST SIGNALS USED WERE PURE TONES. THE SAME SYMBOLS MAY BE USED FOR WARBLE TONES AND NARROW-BAND NOISE, IF SO NOTED ON THE AUDIOGRAM.

MODALITY	EAR[+]		
	RIGHT	BOTH	LEFT
AIR CONDUCTION - EARPHONES			
UNMASKED	O		X
MASKED	△		□
BONE CONDUCTION - MASTOID			
UNMASKED	<		>
MASKED	⊏		⊐
BONE CONDUCTION - FOREHEAD			
UNMASKED		∨	
MASKED	⌐		⌐
AIR CONDUCTION - SOUND FIELD		S	

[+] The fine vertical lines represent the vertical axis of an audiogram.

Further Specifications

Air-Conduction Symbols. The air-conduction symbols should be drawn on the audiogram so that the midpoint of the symbol centers on the intersection of the vertical and horizontal axes at the appropriate HL (shown in Figures 11–2 through 11–8).

Bone-Conduction Symbols. The bone-conduction symbols, with one exception, should be placed adjacent to, but not touching, the frequency axis and centered vertically at the appropriate HL. The symbol for the left ear should be placed to the right of the frequency axis and that for the right ear to the left of the frequency axis (Figures 11–2, 11–3, 11–5, 11–7, and 11–8).* The symbol for unmasked forehead bone conduction should be centered on the vertical axis at the appropriate HL (Figure 11–5).

Multiple Notation. When the left ear unmasked air-conduction threshold is the same as the right air-conduction threshold, the left air-conduction symbol should be placed inside the right air-conduction symbol (Figures 11–3, 11–4, 11–5, 11–7, and 11–8). When bone-conduction thresholds (except unmasked forehead bone conduction) occur at the same HL as air-conduction thresholds, the bone-conduction symbols should be placed adjacent to, but not touching, the air-conduction symbols (Figures 11–2, 11–3, and 11–8). The midline bone-conduction symbol in this circumstance should be placed with the point of the carat barely entering the region of the air conduction symbols (Figure 11–5).

When bone conduction is measured at the mastoid with unmasked and masked thresholds occurring at the same HL, the unmasked symbol should be placed

closest to the frequency axis. The masked symbol should surround, but not touch, the unmasked symbol (Figures 11–2 and 11–3).

No Response. To indicate "no response" at the maximum output of the audiometer, an arrow should be attached to the lower outside corner of the appropriate symbol and drawn downward and at about 45° outward from the frequency axis—to the right for left-ear symbols and to the left for right-ear symbols. The arrow for sound-field or unmasked forehead bone-conduction symbols should be attached at the bottom and drawn straight downward.

The "no response" symbol should be placed on the audiogram at the HL representing the maximum output limit for the particular test frequency, test modality, and audiometer. Each of the "no response" symbols is shown in Table 11–2. Appropriate usage is illustrated in Figures 11–4, 11–6, and 11–8.

When a patient has many "no responses," notation other than by symbol may be used to conserve time and to avoid unnecessary cluttering of the audiogram, as shown in Figure 11–4. For example, when a patient fails to hear by bone conduction at maximum audiometric output, this finding may be

TABLE 11–2 RECOMMENDED "NO RESPONSE" SYMBOLS FOR THRESHOLD AUDIOMETRY.

MODALITY	EAR[+]		
	RIGHT	BOTH	LEFT
AIR CONDUCTION - EARPHONES			
UNMASKED			
MASKED			
BONE CONDUCTION - MASTOID			
UNMASKED			
MASKED			
BONE CONDUCTION - FOREHEAD			
UNMASKED			
MASKED			
AIR CONDUCTION - SOUND FIELD			

+ The fine vertical lines represent the vertical axis of an audiogram.

---

*Although the Committee favored placing the bone-conduction symbols to the right of the frequency axis to indicate the right ear and to the left to indicate the left ear, which was the most common preference reported by the Kopra and Martin (1970) survey, it adopted the reverse format, which is right of the frequency axis for the left ear and left of the frequency axis for the right ear. This decision was made, partly, on arbitrary bases and, partly, in deference to the preferences expressed by representatives of the American Academy of Ophthalmology and Otolaryngology (AAOO). The rationale for the second most common system reported by Martin and Kopra is that the BC symbol should represent the patient's ears from perspective of the otolaryngologist facing the patient (Fowler, 1951) and the prevalence of similar notation systems depicting the human form found in medical records and medical examination forms.

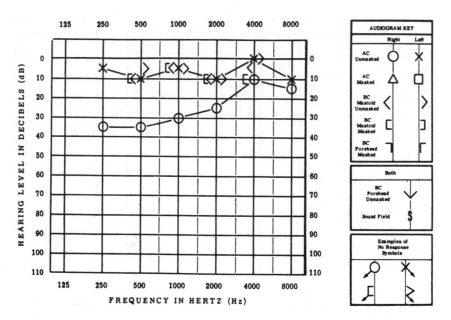

FIGURE 11-2. The use of symbols for masked bone-conduction (BC) thresholds for the right ear at 500 Hz, 1,000 Hz, and 2,000 Hz. Note that the BC brackets for the right ear are to the left of the ordinates and that the masked BC symbols are to the left of the unmasked symbol.

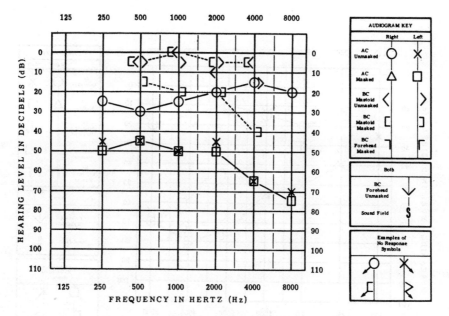

FIGURE 11-3. The use of masked bone-conduction (BC) symbols for the left and right ears and masked air-conduction (AC) symbols for the left ear. Note that the left ear BC symbols are to the right of the ordinates and the right ear BC symbols are to the left of the ordinates.

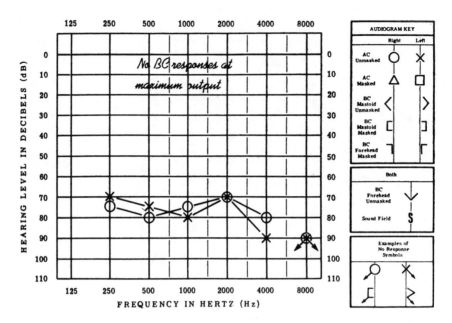

FIGURE 11-4. Air-conduction (AC) "no response" symbols (8,000 Hz) and use of written "no response" notation.

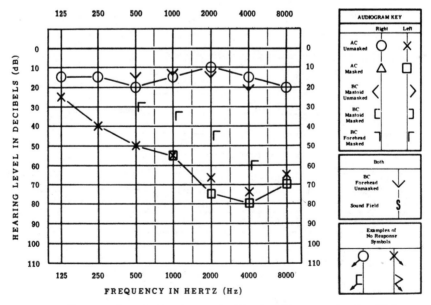

FIGURE 11-5. The use of masked and unmasked forehead bone-conduction (BC) symbols.

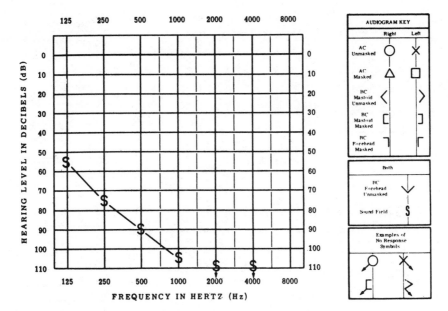

FIGURE 11-6. The use of air-conduction (AC) sound field symbols.

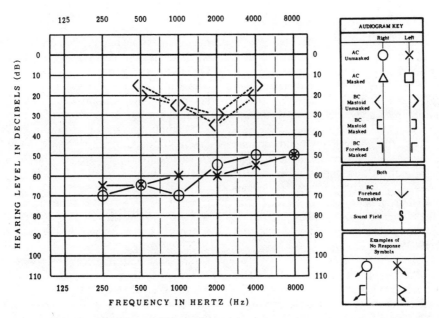

FIGURE 11-7. Air- and bone-conduction (AC and BC) symbols when bone-conduction thresholds were lower than air conduction.

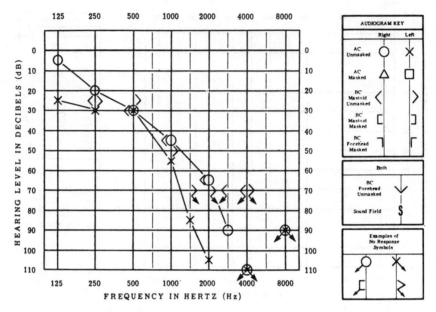

FIGURE 11-8. Air- and bone-conduction (AC and BC) symbols when thresholds were similar. The option was taken not to connect bone-conduction symbols because of the similarity. Symbols are shown for AC and BC when no response was obtained at high frequencies.

expressed on the audiogram by writing "No BC responses at maximum output," rather than drawing a series of "no response" symbols on the audiogram. Another example is the patient who responds only at low frequencies. This may be summarized by writing "No responses obtained above 500 Hz at maximum output."

Responses to tactile sensation should not be plotted on an audiogram. If it is not possible to determine whether the patient's responses reflect tactile sensation or auditory sensation (or both), the examiner should make a prominent notation on the audiogram to alert the viewer to the possibility that the responses were confounded with vibrotactile sensation (Nober, 1964; 1967).

Lines Connecting Symbols. Lines may be used to connect the symbols on an audiogram. When used, a solid line should connect the air-conduction threshold values (Figures 11-2 through 11-8). Bone-con- duction symbols may be connected by a dashed line when an air-bone gap exists (Figures 11-3 and 11-7). Otherwise, bone-conduction symbols should not be connected (Figures 11-2 and 11-8). The clarity of the audiogram will be improved if connecting lines approach, but do not touch or pass through symbols.

Symbols representing "no response" for air conduction or bone conduction should not be connected to each other or to any of the response symbols (Figures 11-4, 11-6, and 11-8).

Color Coding. Color coding is not necessary to transmit information about sidedness in this symbol system. In practice it may be desirable to avoid color coding because of the increasing use of multiple-copy audiograms and photoduplication of audiograms. However, if color is employed, red should be used for the right-ear symbols and connecting lines and blue for the left-ear symbols and connecting lines, with a third color used for the "both ears" symbols.

ENDNOTE

1. In many clinics numerals are used to record the results of air-conduction and bone-conduction measurements. Examples of this form of reporting data are included in Newby (1972). Some clinicians choose to collect their data in numerical form and then transfer the results to an audiogram, using symbols for their reports. Others collect the raw data on audiogram forms, using symbols, and transfer numbers to a block form for reports. Still others collect and report clinical data consistently using either symbols or numbers.

REFERENCES

American National Standard Specifications for Audiometers (ANSI S3.6-1969). New York: American National Standards Institute, Inc. (1970).

Fowler, E. P. Signs, emblems and symbols of choice in plotting threshold audiograms. *Arch. Otolaryng.,* **53,** 129–133 (1951).

Martin, F. N., and Kopra, L. L. Symbols in pure-tone audiometry. *Asha,* **12,** 182–185 (1970).

Newby, H. A. *Audiology.* (3rd ed.) New York: Appleton-Century-Crofts, 71–115 (1972).

Nober, E. H. Pseudoauditory bone conduction thresholds. *J. Speech Hearing Dis.,* **29,** 469–476 (1964).

Nober, E. H. Vibrotactile sensitivity of deaf children to high intensity sound. *Laryngoscope,* **77,** 2128–2146 (1967).

Sweetman, R. H., and Miller, M. L. What's the symbol? Paper presented at the Annual Convention of the American Speech and Hearing Association, Chicago (1969).

12

Comparison of the Auditory Threshold as Measured by Individual Pure Tone and by Békésy Audiometry

WILLIAM BURNS
Emeritus Professor of Physiology, University of London, London, England

RONALD HINCHCLIFFE
Professor of Audiological Medicine, Royal National Nose, Ear and Throat Hospital, London, England

Twenty subjects, age 20 to 58 years, were clinically screened to exclude gross otological pathology. Their auditory thresholds were then determined both by Békésy audiometry and by conventional individual pure-tone audiometry by the method of limits, in 2 dB steps. Measurement of the threshold of hearing by either method gave essentially similar results, and the reliabilities of the methods were of the same order for all frequencies tested. When both tests were repeated after an interval of one week, mean improvements of 1 to 2 dB were found at all frequencies by the Békésy method, and in all but one by the individual pure tone method. In both methods, however, improvements were significant only at 1,000 and 3,000 cps.

I. INTRODUCTION

The conservation of hearing in occupational noise is an important part of industrial medicine. The application of hearing-conservation programs requires audiometric screening, perhaps on a large scale, with subsequent examinations at intervals. The attractions of some form of simplified audiometry for this purpose are obvious. The method of Békésy[1] is potentially suitable, since it requires a less skilled operator than conventional audiometry, and provides a standard procedure, with a graphic record for each audiogram. The conventional methods of clinical pure-tone audiometry are, however, so well established that any suggested alternative must be compared with them, particularly with regard to threshold values and to the possible effects of learning. One study has been made by Corso[2] on the effects of testing methods on hearing thresholds. He found that conventional clinical pure-tone audiometry gave lower threshold values than the "midpoint" audiogram readings obtained by Békésy-type audiometry. With regard to the possibility of learning affecting thresholds, Maire and Zwislocki[3] have shown an improvement of 4 dB in the auditory threshold at 100 cps after 6 weekly tests, using the Békésy method; most of the improvement occurred at the second test. Zwislocki and Feldman,[4] however, with the same method, failed to find improvement after five weekly tests at 1,000 cps. It has been suggested that learning effects at particular frequencies might be partially responsible for the disparities between the British and American standard for the auditory threshold, since, in the work of Dadson and King[5] and of Wheeler and Dickson[6] on which the British standard[7] is based, all subjects received an initial screening audiogram.

The experiments here described were therefore designed to try to answer the following questions:

1. Does the auditory threshold as measured by clinical audiometry correspond to that given by Békésy audiometry?

Reprinted by permission from *J. Acoust. Soc. Amer.*, **29**, 1274–1277 (1975).

2. How do the test-retest reliabilities of the two methods compare?
3. Does any alteration occur in the auditory threshold when measured a second time, by both methods, one week after the first examination?

II. APPARATUS

The audiometer used has already been described.[8] It provided continuous variation of frequency, and for Békésy audiometry the intensity was variable in steps small enough to be subjectively equivalent to a continuous change. For clinical audiometry, steps of approximately 2 dB were used. By the use of the same oscillator and attenuator system for both types of audiometry certain instrumental variables were eliminated. Both the electrical output of the oscillator and the acoustic output of the telephone (Standard Telephones Model 4026) were approximately constant over the frequency range used in the investigation. In order to yield values relative to any particular curve of auditory thresholds, corrections are normally applied to the attenuator readings of this audiometer. For Békésy operation the rate of change of intensity, both increasing and decreasing, was approximately 2 dB/sec. The frequency range of 500–6,000 cps was swept in 7 min 55 sec, with a paper speed of 1 cm/min.

The equipment is normally satisfactorily stable in output and frequency, and since the procedure was intended to simulate field use, calibration was performed only before and after the investigation. The output intensity was found to have remained within limits of less than 0.5 dB, but some change of frequency did occur. This ranged from 2½ percent to 5 percent approximately. Due to the design of the experiment and the fact that both techniques of audiometry utilized the same oscillator and attenuator, we do not consider it likely that significant errors have been introduced into the mean results by this variation in frequency.

III. PROCEDURE

The subjects, whose ages ranged from 20 to 58 years, were either medical students or university teachers. None had previously had an audiometric test, and they were all screened to exclude gross ear defects, such as severe hearing losses, perforations or marked

scarring of the tympanic membrane, but minimal tympanic membrane scarring or subclinical hearing losses did not exclude a subject. With these criteria we expected that our sample would more nearly resemble otologically the type of population to which a hearing conservation program would be applied.

The sequence of testing these subjects was determined by a Latin square design. This gave four possibilities, according to the order in which the two ears and the two methods of audiometry were used. The first four subjects were used to obtain experience in the procedure, and these results were not included in the analysis. Each subject was tested on two occasions, one week apart, by both techniques, and the entire investigation was spread over six weeks.

For the purposes of individual pure-tone audiometry the classical psychophysical method of limits was used. At each frequency the threshold value taken was the mean of the thresholds for ascending and descending intensities, employing steps of 2 dB. The frequencies used were 1,000, 2,000, 3,000, 4,000, 6,000, and 500 cps in this order.

The Békésy audiometry covered the same frequency range, starting at 500 cps and terminating at 6,000 cps. The first minute of the Békésy test was at a fixed frequency of 500 cps in order to familiarize the subject with the procedure. The tone was continuous.

In instructing the subjects on their procedure during the tests, the directions were kept as simple as possible. An indication of the pitch of the tones to be heard, particularly with regard to the order, was given, and the main emphasis was placed on the fact that in either method of audiometry, the signal switch was to be pressed down immediately when a tone was heard, and released immediately when the tone was no longer heard. It was thus intended that repeated definite crossings of the auditory threshold should occur in the Békésy method as originally described by Békésy.

We did not measure the threshold of hearing below 500 cps, since we were primarily interested in the region where noise-induced hearing losses, either temporary or permanent, would occur.

IV. RESULTS

The cursive threshold, i.e., the line joining the midpoints of the excursions on the tracing, was drawn on each Békésy audiogram and the auditory threshold noted at frequencies of 500, 1,000, 2,000, 3,000, 4,000, and 6,000 cps. Comparative values of the threshold of hearing were then available for the two procedures at these six frequencies, for a total of forty ears, together with complete duplicate values for the procedure done one week later.

The data were then analyzed in the following ways:

1. Student's *t* test was applied to the results of the two methods at each frequency and on each occasion of testing. The statistical values so derived are shown in Table 12–1.
2. Product-moment correlation coefficients were calculated for the first and second test results at each frequency and for both audiometric procedures. These values are shown numerically in Table 12–2, graphically in Figure 12–1.
3. Student's *t* test was applied to the results obtained on the first and second occasion at each frequency and for both methods. These values are shown in Table 12–3.

In Figure 12–2 is shown the arithmetic mean of the difference in threshold at the first and second tests for both Békésy and pure-tone methods at each frequency.

TABLE 12-2. TEST-RETEST RELIABILITY IN TERMS OF PRODUCT-MOMENT CORRELATION COEFFICIENT.

Audiometric method	Frequency (cps)					
	500	1,000	2,000	3,000	4,000	6,000
Békésy	0.68	0.80	0.92	0.82	0.87	0.80
Pure tone	0.77	0.86	0.84	0.86	0.77	0.83

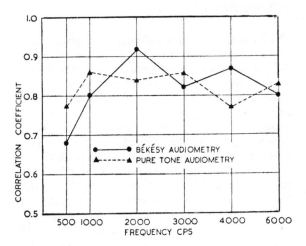

FIGURE 12-1. Test-retest reliabilities of the two audiometric methods.

V. DISCUSSION

Table 12–1 shows that there is a highly significant difference between the thresholds measured by the Békésy and by the pure-tone procedure only at 1,000 cps. This difference was demonstrable at both the

TABLE 12-1. COMPARISON OF BÉKÉSY AND PURE-TONE RESULTS ON FIRST TEST.*

Statistical value	Frequency (cps)					
	500	1,000	2,000	3,000	4,000	6,000
$\bar{x}$	1.1	−3.2	−1.3	−1.6	−1.2	0.5 dB
σ	5.5	5.1	4.7	6.0	7.1	9.2 dB
t	1.27	*−3.92*	−1.77	−1.73	−1.02	0.34

Comparison of Békésy and pure-tone results on second test.

$\bar{x}$	1.1	−3.0	−0.8	−1.9	−0.9	−2.0 dB
σ	5.7	4.7	5.0	5.3	7.0	7.6 dB
t	1.22	*−4.0*	−0.99	−2.27	−0.84	−2.41

*$\bar{x}$ = mean difference between the results by the two methods. A negative value indicates that the Békésy threshold is lower. The values of *t* in italics are significant at the level $p < 0.01$.

first and the second tests, the Békésy technique giving the lower threshold by about 3 dB. This we attribute to the fact that we started the individual pure tone audiometry at 1,000 cps. This would support the recommendation of Watson and Tolan[9] that, in clinical audiometry, the threshold at the first frequency tested should be checked later in the course of the test.

A significant ($p < 0.05$) value of *t* also occurred for the results at 3,000 and 6,000 cps on the second test. We infer that there is a trend towards a lower threshold by the Békésy method but, since this is less than 3 dB for frequencies other than 1,000 cps, it may be neglected. Therefore, it seems likely that, if the frequency at which one starts the procedure in pure-tone audiometry is checked at the end of the test, one can accept that these two techniques essentially measure the same thing.

This finding is not immediately reconcilable with that of Corso,[2] who found that conventional pure-tone audiometry gave, in general, lower threshold

TABLE 12-3. COMPARISON OF FIRST AND SECOND RESULTS:
BÉKÉSY METHOD.*

Statistical value	Frequency (cps)					
	500	1,000	2,000	3,000	4,000	6,000
$\bar{x}$	1.0	2.0	1.0	2.1	1.2	1.7
σ	6.4	5.2	3.8	6.2	6.4	10.4 dB
t	1.01	*2.39*	1.69	*2.15*	1.19	1.04

Comparison of first and second results: Pure-tone method

$\bar{x}$	1.0	2.2	1.5	2.0	1.4	−1.7
σ	4.9	4.2	4.7	4.7	4.7	7.6dB
t	1.32	*3.22*	1.99	*2.74*	1.91	−1.44

*$\bar{x}$ = mean difference between the results for the first and second tests. A negative value indicates that the second test gave a higher threshold. The values of t in italics are significant at the level $p < 0.05$.

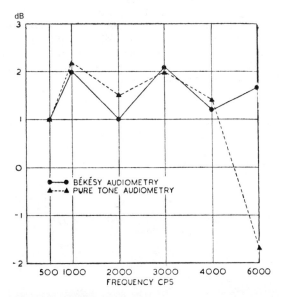

FIGURE 12-2. Mean improvement at second test for twenty subjects (40 ears).

Table 12-2 and Figure 12-1 show that the test-retest correlation coefficients are of the same order for both audiometric methods. The poorest correlation occurred at 500 cps but, for frequencies of 1,000 cps and above, a coefficient of the order of 0.8 or more was found, so that, in the range where noise-induced threshold shifts might occur, both methods are statistically reliable.

Table 12-3 and Figure 12-2 show that improvements at the second test, with significant values ($p < 0.05$) of t, occur at 1,000 and 3,000 cps and at these frequencies only. Moreover, this applies to the results for both audiometric methods. This finding is contrary to Zwislocki and Feldman's[4] statement that there is no significant improvement from session to session at 1,000 cps. However, these investigators employed fewer subjects and their procedure was somewhat different. Our results, however, agree with Zwislocki and Maire[10] in that any improvement which does occur is not specific for the Békésy method.

We do not attach very much importance to the finding that significant improvement at the second test occurred only at 1,000 and 3,000 cps. Figure 12-2 shows that the graph of mean improvement as a function of frequency fluctuates between 1 and 2 dB, with the exception of the single value at 6,000 cps for the pure-tone method, for which there is no obvious explanation. Only the two peaks on this graph attain significance level. We might therefore conclude that the "learning" factor which occurs between the first and second hearing test is of the order of 1–2 dB for the range 500 cps to 6,000 cps. We can therefore probably discount learning as a factor in the discrepancy between the British and the American standards for the threshold of hearing.

VI. CONCLUSIONS

It would appear from the results of this series that measurement of the threshold of hearing either by the Békésy technique or by pure-tone audiometry gives essentially similar results.

The reliability of both audiometric methods was of the same order at all frequencies. The reliability would be considered satisfactory at all frequencies examined except possibly at 500 cps.

A second audiogram, performed one week after the first, appears to yield, in general, a lowering of

values than the midpoint values in his Békésy audiometry. The differences were statistically significant at 2,000 cps and below. However, Corso's and our own subjects used different criteria in judging the threshold for Békésy audiometry; his were instructed to keep the tone always just audible, whereas our subjects allowed the tone to diminish to complete inaudibility in each cycle of operations. This would tend to produce apparent differences in the thresholds in the sense that our midpoint figures should be lower than those of Corso.

threshold of 1 to 2 dB only, but the improvements are of marginal significance value.

It seems justifiable to conclude, therefore, that the employment of the Békésy technique, within the limits used in this study, is a satisfactory alternative to conventional pure-tone audiometry.

ACKNOWLEDGMENTS

We wish to acknowledge our indebtedness to the subjects in this investigation, and to Dr. T. S. Littler of the Wernher Research Unit on Deafness, for helpful discussion and criticism.

ENDNOTES

1. G. v. Békésy *Acta Otolaryngol.,* Stockholm **35,** 411 (1947).

2. J. F. Corso, *Arch. Otolaryngol.* **63,** 78 (1956).

3. F. Maire and J. Zwislocki, Periodic Status Report XXVII, Harvard University Psycho-Acoustic Laboratory, Cambridge, Massachusetts (1956), p. 8.

4. J. Zwislocki and A. S. Feldman, Periodic Status Report XXVII, Harvard University Psycho-Acoustic Laboratory, Cambridge, Massachusetts (1956), p. 8.

5. R. S. Dadson and J. H. King, *J. Laryngol.,* London **66,** 366 (1952).

6. L. J. Wheeler and E. D. D. Dickson, *J. Laryngol.,* London **66,** 379 (1952).

7. British Standard Specification B. S. 2497, British Standards Institution, London (1954).

8. W. Burns and G. A. Morris, *J. Physiol.* **131,** 4 (1956).

9. L. A. Watson and T. Tolan, *Hearing Tests and Hearing Instruments* (Williams and Wilkins, Baltimore, 1949), p. 36.

10. J. Zwislocki and F. Maire, Periodic Status Report XXVIII Harvard University Psycho-Acoustic Laboratory, Cambridge, Massachusetts (1956), p. 7.

13

Standardization of Pure Tone Audiometer Testing Technique*

SCOTT N. REGER, Ph.D.
Emeritus Professor of Audiology, Department of Otolaryngology, University of Iowa Hospitals, Iowa City, Iowa

Among the factors which influence the reliability of pure tone audiometer test results are the following: (1) the accuracy of the calibration of the audiometer; (2) the magnitude of the masking effect of ambient noise in the testing environment, which includes noise produced by the audiometrist, the patient, and any sound in the receiver resulting from operation of the audiometer other than the desired test tone; (3) position and pressure (coupling) of the sound reproducer in relation to the auricle or bones of the head; (4) physical conditions within the test room which influence body comfort, such as temperature, humidity, barometric pressure, altitude, and time of day; (5) age, intelligence, reaction time and previous test experience of the patient; (6) physiologic condition and mental attitude of the patient (alert, interested, relaxed, cooperative, indifferent, lethargic, depressed, fatigued, tense, apprehensive or antagonistic). Patients who experience tinnitus or auditory after-images, malingerers and those with hysterical perceptual abnormalities present additional test difficulties; (7) training experience, insight and personality of the audiometrist; and (8) the complexity of the stimulus presentation technique used in the determination of the auditory threshold. Ambiguity of response instructions to the patient and the use of complex recording methods may be responsible for occasional errors in the patient's response or in the recording of the test data.

It is merely a matter of time until one or more of several nationally recognized professional groups or committees interested in the accuracy and reliability of audiometric measurements will recommend that certain aspects of manual audiometry be standardized. For example, general agreement on whether the auditory acuity should be ascertained by means of an ascending or descending intensity series (or a combination of both), the number of correct responses that should be required to indicate the threshold out of a given number of stimuli presentations at near the threshold level, and possibly the order in which the various test frequencies should be presented are questions about which there should be no uncertainty. Certainly the more uniform the test procedure, the less the confusion in the teaching and the practice of audiometry, with a resultant increase in the accuracy and reliability of test results.

Due to the fact that the presentation of the test tones (the measuring stick) of the usual clinical audiometer is under the manual control of the audiometrist, there are as many variations in testing procedure (as many different ways of applying the yardstick) as there are audiometrists. As indicated previously, no two competent audiometrists could possibly test a given patient in precisely the same way, nor could a given audiometrist test the same patient twice in exactly an identical manner. If similar audiograms are obtained in either instance the skill of the audiometrist is principally responsible—not the naive assumption that since the audiometer is a precision instrument for the accurate testing of auditory acuity, hearing tests made with an audiometer are correspondingly precise. So long as every operational step in the testing procedure is dependent upon the manual control of the audiometrist, audiometry is and will remain principally an art rather than a science. Consequently an effective testing procedure can be acquired and applied only through practice. No one can make accurate hearing tests with the usual clinical audiometer until he is so familiar with the mechanical operation of the instrument and an adequate tone presentation sequence

---

*This article has been abridged from the original with the author's permission. The portions retained are concerned primarily with pulse-counting audiometry and sources of error in conventional audiometry.

Reprinted in abridged form by permission of the author and *Laryngoscope*, **60**, 161–185 (1950).

that his attention is focused on the patient's response rather than the manipulation of the instrument's controls during the testing procedure.

A second factor which supports the viewpoint that present day audiometry is more an art than a science is the fact that the evaluation of the patient's responses often is a matter of subjective judgment, especially when the patient makes frequent incorrect or haphazard responses during the testing procedure. When the response of such a "difficult" patient is synchronized with a tone presentation the audiometrist often wishes he knew if the response were merely chance coincidence or a significant response. If patients responded only during the presentation of tones and never made haphazard judgments, audiometry would be very simple indeed. It is a certainty that Bunch (1943) was concerned less with the difficulties inherent in the mechanics of the operation of the audiometer than with the problem of the evaluation of the patient's responses when he wrote: "The reliability of an audiogram is directly proportional to the skill of the examiner."

The writer does not wish to foster the impression that the art of audiometry is inherently a grossly inaccurate and unreliable test procedure. A certain amount of skill necessarily always will be required to manipulate the controls of equipment which require frequent adjustment or attention from the operator. Obviously any decrease in the amount of manual control needed for the effective operation of a given instrument will result in more uniform and exact performance of that instrument. Audiometry will more nearly approach the scientific goal of measurement in proportion to the degree that the tone presentation technique attains invariable uniformity and the evaluation of the patient's responses becomes subject to quantitative verification.

Unfortunately the belief is all too prevalent that since the audiometer is a so-called "precision" instrument designed for the scientific measurement of auditory acuity, the results of hearing tests made with the audiometer are correspondingly precise and accurate. Nothing could be further from the truth. Few will deny that most of the functional and operational features embodied in the modern clinical audiometer are based on considerable research and engineering skill; however, present day use of the audiometer leaves much to be desired from the scientific point of view. One of the most fundamental and elementary tenets of science is the application of an exact measurement technique under carefully controlled conditions. The "measuring stick" itself must remain an invariable factor and must be applied and evaluated in precisely the same way each time it is used. Its limits of accuracy (error of measurement) also must be known.

It is obvious that a type of audiometer which would facilitate the production of test tones in a predetermined reproducible sequence or pattern, which did not present clues that would enable the patient to make correct responses when the tone was presented but not heard, and which permitted an objective quantitative evaluation of the patient's responses would possess certain definite advantages. Among these advantages are the following: (1) Any given patient could be retested any desired number of times with an identical tone presentation technique; (2) any desired number of individuals could be tested with the same invariable reproducible tone presentation sequence; (3) if sufficiently simple to operate mechanically, an individual with very little training in audiometry could obtain results as reliable as an expert audiometrist and different audiometrists would obtain more nearly the same results on the same patient; and (4) if generally adopted, such an instrument would make possible the standardization of audiometer technique with increased universal accuracy of test results. Such an instrument is highly desirable from the research point of view. And to the extent that the tone presentation technique attained invariable reproducibility and the evaluation of the patient's responses approached objectivity, the testing of auditory acuity with such an instrument would be less an art and a skill and become a more scientific procedure.

An instrument constructed by the writer in 1944 meets the criteria suggested above in a reasonably satisfactory manner. As is often the case, since building this instrument, Gardner (1947) pointed out that practically an identical design was suggested by Munson in a Bell Telephone Laboratories memorandum, which to my knowledge was not published in accessible literature until 1947. The first description of the mechanical tone interrupter devised by the writer is contained in a Master of Arts thesis by Bartell, placed in the State University of Iowa Medical School Library in August, 1945. Bartell (1945) states: "The purpose of this thesis, then, is twofold: first, to describe a technique by means of which individuals can be tested and retested in an exactly reproducible manner, and second, to investigate the variability of normal bone conduction measurements in comparison to normal air conduction measurements. . . . The major apparatus consisted of an audiometer and an automatic stimulus interruption device.'' The instrument consists essentially of a motor-driven tone interruption device which can be attached to a commercial audiometer. Functionally, the gadget is used to produce one of four stimulus patterns as one, two, three or four dashes or tone pulses coincident with the presentation of an attention light . . . for a time interval of six seconds. The light, of course, is off the following four seconds. During the four second interval the light is off, the patient indicates the number of tone pulses heard and the audiometrist selects the desired frequency, intensity and pulse pattern which he desires to present next. A time interval of 0.1 second for both the attack and release of the pulses has been found satisfactory. The minimum duration of the ''steady state'' presentation of each pulse should exceed 0.2 second, since Munson (1947) reports that: ''Full loudness is not reached until over 0.2 second has elapsed.'' As indicated previously, the duration of the pulses of the present interrupter is 0.8 second. Further experimentation with the device is to be undertaken to ascertain the optimum relations between the duration of the pulses and intervening silent intervals in order to learn the minimum time required for reliable pulse pattern audiometry.

Very little more time is required to test the acuity by means of the pulse tone audiometer than is expended in manual audiometry. It may be found advantageous to combine the usual manually controlled audiometer tone presentation and the mechanically (or electronically) controlled pulse tone techniques in certain clinical applications as follows: first, determine the approximate threshold level according to one of the manual approaches described earlier; then employ the pulse tone presentation technique. The patient is instructed to listen for one, two, three or four tone pulses or dashes each time the light is on and to indicate the number of pulses heard immediately after the light goes off. Needless to say successive pulse patterns must be presented in random order.

The first pulse pattern may be presented 10 or 5 dB above the approximate threshold. Each succeeding pattern is attenuated 5 dB until either an incorrect or no response is obtained. Then increase the intensity of the next pattern 5 dB. If the pulse pattern is heard correctly at this level, present a second pattern at the same level. If the second pattern also is heard correctly, attenuate 5 dB and note the response. Determine the lowest intensity level at which at least two out of three patterns are recognized correctly. Due to the fact there are no defined criteria of correctness of response in terms of pulse tone audiometry, the writer, at the present time, arbitrarily regards the correct clinical threshold value as the lowest intensity level at which at least two of three pulse patterns are recognized correctly, assuming two out of two correct responses for the adjacent 5 dB higher level.

As previously intimated, the technique of pulse tone audiometry includes an objective evaluation of the mathematical probability of the accuracy of the patient's response. In order to ascertain the probability of a repeated or combined event, the probabilities of the single events are multiplied. Assuming haphazard or chance presentation of any one of four different pulse patterns, the patient's chance of guessing correctly the single inaudible pattern is one in four, of guessing correctly two successive inaudible patterns is one in sixteen, of guessing correctly three successive inaudible patterns, one in sixty-four and so on. Application of the terms of the *binomial expansion* shows that the patient has nine chances in sixty-four (approximately one in eight) of guessing correctly any two inaudible patterns out of three, and 27 in 64 of guessing correctly any one pattern out of three. (For a discussion of probability statistics, see Guilford (1936) or any standard text of statistical methods.)

Since the patient has an almost 50–50 chance (27 in 64) of guessing correctly one out of three inaudible patterns, the writer believes it is reasonable to require two correct responses out of three pattern presentations, in spite of the fact the patient has only nine chances in sixty-four (approximately one in eight) of guessing correctly any two inaudible patterns out of three inaudible pattern presentations. This requirement may seem excessively cautious in view of the fact that the auditory threshold is defined in terms of the minimum intensity at a given frequency level that has a probability of 0.50 of producing a response; however, as indicated previously, this 0.50 value is ascertained by means of a psychophysical technique which presupposes the presentation of a sufficient number of stimuli to amass sufficient data for statistical computation and analysis—a procedure requiring radical modification for clinical application. Additional clinical use and research with pulse tone audiometry are needed to determine the most effective testing procedures and to evaluate the usefulness of the pulse tone technique.

Pulse tone audiometry is ideally suited for certain research applications. For such use, it may be advisable to construct a table or key to indicate the intensity levels and pulse tone patterns to be presented at each frequency level. The observer's responses, recorded on an appropriate blank, constitute a permanent record for subsequent analysis. Various types of stimulus keys—ascending, descending or haphazard intensity series—may be devised to meet the requirements of the experiment. In any given key it is essential that the same number of one, two, three and four pulse patterns be used and that the order of presentation of the patterns be due to chance. Of course, keys with more or less than four different pulse patterns may be found advisable for certain experimental purposes.

Gardner (1947), reported the results of several clinical threshold measurements as made with an electronically generated pulse tone audiometer. He found that ". . . the pulse-tone test procedure gives threshold results which are somewhat more reproducible than results obtained with the standard test procedure, although the time required to make the former is slightly longer. In terms of the attractiveness of the tests for the operator and for the listener, the pulse-tone test appears to be at an approximate three to one advantage. The normal threshold intensity calibrations of the two tests are in good agreement, so that either test may be used interchangeably with the other. For the very young subject, the pulse-tone test appears to be preferable in the majority of cases and tends to lower the age limit at which threshold measurements can be made. . . ."

The attention lights used in connection with the Burr and Mortimer and the mechanical and electronic pulse tone audiometers, and the varying frequency of the Békésy instrument are devices which enable the patient to exert maximum attention during the presentation of the test stimuli. Conventional audiometer technique requires that the patient be listening intently with no relaxation of his attention during the critical part of the testing procedure, since he must not know just when a tone at or near the threshold level will be presented. Also he is attempting to indicate the instant the tone is presented and

the instant it is terminated. This is expecting a higher order of attention over a longer period of time than can reasonably be expected. Fluctuation in the patient's attention is responsible for much of his erratic response and variability. If by coincidence he happens to be attending at the instant a near threshold level tone is presented, he may hear it; otherwise he may not. Stevens and Davis (1938) make an interesting comment on a well-known psychological observation: "The inherent variability of the observer himself can be easily demonstrated by presenting him with a steady tone at an intensity very near threshold and requiring him to press a button during all the time that he hears the tone. Almost without exception observers press the button intermittently."

SUMMARY

1. Many factors influence the accuracy of clinical audiometric measurements among which are the differences in tone presentation techniques used by various audiometrists and the difficulties inherent in evaluating the patient's responses.

2. Auditory threshold acuity measurements of the maximum accuracy are obtained by means of psychophysical techniques which necessitate securing a sufficient quantity of data under carefully controlled conditions to enable significant statistical analysis and evaluation of the data.

3. Due to "certain" practical considerations (such as limitations on time, personnel, equipment and testing environment), the testing techniques generally employed in clinical audiometry at best must be regarded as exceedingly abbreviated and modified versions of the psychophysical method of limits.

4. Variations in test results between different audiometrists will be minimized by the general adoption of a uniform tone presentation technique, including emphasis on the approach to the threshold (ascending or descending or mixed intensity series), the number of required synchronized responses to the stimulus at a minimum intensity level 5 dB below which there is uncertain or no response, the sequence of presentation of the different test frequencies and possibly the duration of the response the patient is instructed to make to the audible test stimuli.

5. At the present time clinical audiometry is more an art than a science.

6. Although the audiometer is generally regarded as a precision instrument for the clinical testing of auditory acuity, the accuracy of the results obtained with the audiometer are limited principally by factors extraneous to the instrument itself.

7. Pulse tone audiometry introduces a testing procedure which possesses the following advantages: (a) a method of retesting a given patient any desired number of times with an automatically controlled, exactly reproducible, tone presentation technique; (b) a means of testing any desired number of individuals in an invariable manner; (c) a technique by means of which a relatively untrained examiner can obtain results as accurate as those of the skilled audiometrist; (d) the type of tone presentation makes possible an objective evaluation of the mathematical probability of the accuracy of the patient's response with relatively few data (responses); (e) the stimuli are presented while the patient is alerted by a signal light to give maximum attention to the stimulus; (f) there is little or no ambiguity of patient response; and (g) pulse tone audiometry presents many features which can be standardized.

8. Pulse tone audiometry makes possible a practical group pure tone hearing test.

9. The audiometers described by Burr and Mortimer (1939) and Békésy (1947) possess desirable self-administering and self-recording features, and constitute uniform testing procedures.

10. Standardization (general acceptance of uniform technique) of manual audiometry and/or of electromechanically controlled audiometers will introduce more science into the art of audiometry.

BIBLIOGRAPHY

Bartell, B. R. Variability of Air Conduction and Bone Conduction Measurements in Individuals with Normal Air Conduction Acuity. M.A. Thesis, State University of Iowa, 1945.

Békésy, G. V. A New Audiometer. *Acta Otolaryngol.,* **35:** 411–422, 1947.

Brogden, W. J., and Miller, G. A. Physiological Noise Generated Under Earphone Cushions. *Jour. Acoust. Soc. Amer.,* **19:** 620–623, 1947.

Bunch, C. C. Clinical Audiometry. St. Louis: C. V. Mosby Co., 1943, 186 pp.

Burr, E. G., and Mortimer, H. Improvements in Audiometry at the Montreal General Hospital. *Canad. Med. Assn. Jour.,* **40:** 22–27, 1939.

Gardner, M. B. A Pulse-Tone Clinical Audiometer. *Jour. Acoust. Soc. Amer.,* **19:** 592–599, 1947.

Garrett, H. E. Great Experiments in Psychology. New York: The Century Co., 1930, 337 pp.

Guilford, J. P. Psychometric Methods. New York: McGraw-Hill Book Co., Inc., 1936, 566 pp.

Hughson, W., and Westlake, H. D. Manual for Program Outline for Rehabilitation of Aural Casualties, Both Military and Civilian. Supp. to *Trans. Amer. Acad. Ohpthal. and Otolaryngol.,* 15 pp., 1944.

Munson, W. A. The Growth of Auditory Sensation. *Jour. Acoust. Soc. Amer.,* **19:** 584–591, 1947.

Myers, C. K., and Harris, J. D. Detection Thresholds and Pure Tone Thresholds in Auditory Acuity. U. S. Naval Med. Research Lab., U. S. Naval Submarine Base, New London, Conn., 7 pp., 1948.

Myers, C. K., and Harris, J. D. The Emergence of a Tonal Sensation. U. S. Naval Med. Research Lab., U. S. Naval Submarine Base, New London, Conn., 15 pp. 1948.

Pollack, I. The Atonal Period. *Jour. Acoust. Soc. Amer.,* **20:** 146–149, 1948.

Reger, S. N., and Newby, H. A. A Group Pure Tone Hearing Test. *Jour. Sp. Disor.,* **12:** 61–66, 1947.

Riesz, R. R. Differential Intensity Sensitivity of the Ear for Pure Tones. *Phys. Rev.,* **31:** 867–875, 1928.

Stevens, S. S., and Davis, H. Hearing—Its Psychology and Physiology. New York: John Wiley and Sons, Inc., 1938, 489 pp.

Thurstone, L. L Psychophysical Methods, Chapter 5 of Methods of Psychology, edited by T. G. Andrews. New York: John Wiley and Sons, Inc., 1948, 716 pp.

Westlake, H. The Reality of the Zero Reference Line for Pure Tone Testing. *Jour. Sp. Disor.,* **8:** 285–288, 1943.

Woodworth, R. S. Experimental Psychology. New York: Henry Holt and Co., 1938, 889 pp.

14

Behavioral Audiometry Viewed as an Operant Procedure

LYLE L. LLOYD, Ph.D.

Professor of Audiology, Purdue University, West Lafayette, Indiana

Behavioral audiometry as defined by Frisina (1963, p. 137) is based on the principle of reinforcement. The essence of behavioral audiometry is to bring operant responses of the subject under stimulus control and then use such responses to obtain a reliable index of some aspect of the subject's hearing. This generalization is true in the case of both threshold and suprathreshold measures. The purpose of this paper is to discuss the more frequently used forms of pure-tone behavioral audiometry in terms of reinforcement and other operant principles.

THE CONVENTIONAL OR STANDARD METHODS

Conventional or standard pure-tone audiometry, where the subject is asked to raise his hand or press a signal button when he hears a sound, uses verbal reinforcement. Frequently the subject's first appropriate response is followed by the examiner's statement of "good," "that's fine," or some other statement which serves as social reinforcement. The verbal forms of social reinforcement are usually paired with, or in some cases supplemented by, other forms of social reinforcement such as a smile or nod of the head. Throughout the testing session the astute examiner administers additional social reinforcement as frequently as he thinks is appropriate. For example, when testing an intelligent, motivated, and cooperative adult, verbal reinforcement may be provided after the first appropriate response and then

only an additional time or two throughout the testing session. However, when testing a suspicious, uncooperative, or poorly motivated young child, the examiner will initially follow each of the child's appropriate responses with social reinforcement. With a child of this type the social reinforcement will probably include a "pat on the back," "hand clapping," or some other animated actions indicating approval and fun. Actually such overt behavior by the clinician is the main form of social reinforcement paired with verbal forms of social reinforcement. As the child's response is strengthened, e.g., it has shorter latency and is more decisive, the examiner will reduce the reinforcement schedule from 100 percent reinforcement. Although the schedule may be reduced, the frequency, either variable ratio or fixed ratio, will probably be higher at the end of the test session in the latter case than in the previous case of the adult.

Once the pattern of responding to sound is established, the clinician usually reduces the frequency and amount of reinforcement. This reduction during the testing session results in greater testing efficiency. The skilled audiologist attempts to apply a sufficient schedule and amount of reinforcement to maintain a high rate of responding but does not waste time administering excessive reinforcement, which is not only inefficient in terms of measurements per unit of test time but which also increases the chances that the subject will become satiated and cease responding.

A typical example of the intrasession reduction in reinforcement may be observed in the example mentioned above of the doubtful, suspicious child. The clinician reduces the schedule from reinforcement once every appropriate response to every several responses. In addition to this reduction in the schedule

Reprinted by permission of the author from *F. Speech Hearing Dis.*, **31**, 128–136 (1966).

of reinforcement, the clinician would probably reduce the amount of time and energy in the reinforcement. Initially, the reinforcement which includes overt, animated approval behavior paired with verbal praise is reduced to less overt behavior and verbal output. On the basis of clinical observation the reinforcement with such a child is frequently reduced to an occasional nod of the head or smile.

Since reinforcement increases the frequency of the subject's responses, the audiologist makes the reinforcement contingent upon the desired behavior or responses, usually raising a hand or pressing a button when the auditory signal is heard. The audiologist knows only when the signal is presented, not when the subject hears the signal. Therefore, the initial signal presentations are usually at levels assumed, upon the bases of clinical observation and case history data, to be above the subject's threshold. These suprathreshold presentations afford the opportunity to administer reinforcement for appropriate responses. When reinforcement principles are applied in behavioral audiometry the primarily descending, and the descending-ascending or bracketing, methods over the ascending methods are apparently advantageous. The threshold searching methods that include suprathreshold presentation offer more opportunity to administer reinforcement when the subject has met the appropriate response contingency. Although such methods do not automatically eliminate the possible error of reinforcing a subject for responding when he did not hear the sound, they do reduce such errors. The primarily descending methods allow the audiologist better control of the delivery of reinforcement under the appropriate contingencies.

One minor problem in the use of reinforcement with a primarily descending threshold searching method is the danger of administering reinforcement only at suprathreshold levels, and thereby training the subject to respond at these levels but not near threshold. This danger is reduced by the instructions and demonstrations given to the subject. The effectiveness of typical instructions depends primarily upon the subject's ability to understand the audiologist's verbal communication system. Dependence on the subject's understanding of verbal instructions is reduced by demonstration of the task. By using reinforcement principles the subject is taught to respond to lower and lower signals during the instruction and demonstration phase of the test session. During the

threshold searching phase the reinforcement of responses to various levels of signal presentations further strengthens the response to signal at any level.

The use of partial reinforcement schedules was discussed as a testing efficiency measure, but partial reinforcement is also useful in maintaining response patterns. In general, partial reinforcement schedules may result in learning a given task more slowly, but when a task is learned the use of partial reinforcement tends to result in a response more resistant to extinction. The use of partial reinforcement is one of the clinician's best safeguards against failure of the subject to respond to the signal control as a result of satiation.

EAR CHOICE METHODS

Once the most conventional forms of behavioral audiometry, use of standard hand raising or button pressing response, are viewed as operant procedures, the application of these principles in other forms of behavioral audiometry becomes apparent. In the original Curry and Kurtzrock (1951) ear choice technique and the modified ear choice technique (Lloyd, 1965a), the application of reinforcement is almost identical to that described above for the conventional or standard method. The same forms of verbal and nonverbal social reinforcement are used in the same schedules for reinforcing appropriate responses. In applying reinforcement principles to the ear choice methods the only thing that has changed is what is considered an appropriate response. In the standard methods either raising a hand or finger or pressing a signal button is defined as the response. In the ear choice methods the appropriate response is pointing to the ear in which the signal is presented.

PLAY METHODS

When confronted with young children, especially those between 2 and 6 years of age, many audiologists employ various forms of play audiometry (e.g., Barr, 1955; Donnelly, 1965; Frisina, 1962; Lloyd, 1965a; Lowell and others, 1956; O'Neill and others, 1961; Utley, 1949). Play audiometry has involved a number of responses such as putting rings on a peg, putting pegs in holes, hitting a peg board, hitting a drum, stacking blocks, putting marbles in a box, and putting blocks in a box. In this paper the block dropping, putting blocks in a box, response will be used to illustrate the various play audiometry techniques. The child is taught through verbal instruction and demonstration to drop a block in a box when and only when the auditory signal is presented.

It is assumed that the child's play activity is of interest to him and that completion of the response is rewarding. The child's block dropping behavior may be considered as high probability behavior, and the proper structuring of such as a play activity is an extremely useful operant technique. High probability behavior may be used to increase low probability behavior. However, in the typical application of play audiometry the clinician simply uses the child's high probability behavior by structuring the contingencies which allow the child to respond with such behavior.

Although the child's block dropping response may in itself be reinforcing, the skilled clinician usually pairs the inherent reinforcement of the play response with considerable social reinforcement. Actually with some children the play activity may be of only limited interest; it may be a relatively weak reinforcer. In such cases, the verbal and nonverbal behavior of the clinician may be the more powerful reinforcer and the block dropping response a secondary reinforcer. In some cases the game played alone is not reinforcing but with a partner, such as a lively clinician, it is extremely reinforcing. The social reinforcement used in play audiometry is similar to the verbal and nonverbal reinforcement discussed above for other forms of behavioral audiometry. The clinical application of a variation in the amount and schedule of social reinforcement is also similar.

In general, a combination of the high probability behavior of the child and the social behavior of the clinician provides a powerful reinforcer for testing most young children, although obviously what is reinforcing for one subject may not be for another. The novice clinician frequently makes the mistake of assuming that because a given method or procedure was successful with several subjects, it is infallible. The experienced clinician recognizes individual differences and exercises ingenuity in finding an appropriate reinforcer for each subject.

What may be reinforcing for a subject at the beginning of the test session may be a relatively weak reinforcer by the end of the session. Such subject satiation can be extremely perplexing to the audiologist. It is easy to observe satiation in experimental animals when food is the reinforcer, but it takes a keenly observant clinician to recognize the early signs of a client's satiation in the audiometric testing session.

The individuality of reinforcers and the problem of satiation in play audiometry can be illustrated by the following two cases. The first is a relatively negative and extremely aggressive six year old boy seen in a university out-patient clinic. During the day he failed to cooperate on the psychological tests and in the speech and language examination. He showed no interest in several forms of play audiometry using blocks, rings on a peg, or various toys, but did indicate interest in playing with a drum. High probability drum beating behavior was therefore structured into the test. The boy's drum beating was put under stimulus control. Approximately fifteen minutes and two broken drumsticks later an entire air conduction threshold test was completed.

The second example is a relatively cooperative five year old girl, who quickly conditioned to play audiometry using a block dropping response paired with a social reinforcer. She responded quickly while the first three frequencies were tested, but when the fourth frequency test was begun her responses were slower. When this change in response pattern was observed, the clinician increased his verbal and nonverbal behavior in an attempt to increase social reinforcement. The girl's responses again were sharp and quick. Four additional frequencies were tested with short latency reponses but again the responses slowed down; consequently, the clinician increased his verbal and nonverbal behavior to increase the reinforcement. This change in the clinician's behavior did not, however, bring the girl's block dropping under sharp stimulus control as it did earlier. Therefore, the clinician, enthusiastically changed the game and had the girl stack the blocks as a response to the auditory stimulus, which, once more brought the response under good stimulus control. Before the test was completed two additional responses—putting rings on a peg and hitting a toy xylophone—were used. Although the reinforcer varied slightly during the test, it was basically the same reinforcer; namely, a combination of some form of high probability play behavior of the girl and the social reinforcer of the clinician's contingent behavior.

VISUAL REINFORCER METHODS

Since the successful use of audiometric tests with visual reinforcers was first described (Evans, 1943; Dix and Hallpike, 1947), numerous variations of these instrumental or operant conditioning methods have been employed to test young children. Basically, the child's responses to auditory signals are increased by reinforcing his pressing of a button when the signal is presented and not reinforcing his button pressing when no signal is presented. The multitude of visual reinforcement methods previously described by audiologists are enumerated below under the five main types of visual reinforcers utilized.

1. *Pictures* (Dix and Hallpike, 1947; Evans, 1943; Kaplin, 1957; Lloyd, 1965a, 1965b; Miller, 1962; Miller, 1963; Shimizu and Nakamura, 1957; Weaver, 1965).
2. *Miniature Scenes* (Statten and Wishart, 1956).
3. *Animated Toy Animals or Puppets* (Cotton and Hall, 1939; Green, 1958; Guilford and Haug, 1952; Miller, 1962; Sullivan and others, 1962; Waldrop, 1953).
4. *Toy Trains* (Ewing, 1930; Gaines, 1961; Ishisawa, 1962; Keaster, 1951).
5. *Other Mechanical Toys* (Denmark, 1950; MacPherson, 1960; Schwartz, 1952).

Typically, the visual reinforcers are presented on a 100 percent reinforcement schedule. In the clinical application of these visual reinforcer methods, social reinforcers are also employed. In most behavioral audiometry methods, regardless of response method and the kind of reinforcer, verbal and nonverbal social reinforcers are important. The prominent role may be related to the universality of this type of verbal and nonverbal behavior as a positive reinforcer. The generalized reinforcement value of much of the clinician's behavior is apparent when one considers that a smile is usually associated with pleasurable experiences. The same is true of many other types of clinical behavior such as a nod of the head, a pat on the back, clapping of hands, the word "good," or even the expression "oh boy!" Such behavior is a powerful tool when used with proper contingencies, i.e., when it occurs immediately after the child's appropriate response.

Two findings are of interest in the literature on visual reinforcement audiometric methods. First, the study by Statten and Wishart (1956) demonstrated superiority of the operant conditioning procedure with visual reinforcers over the classical conditioning psychogalvanic skin response (GSR) procedure. A second finding was the relative lack of success with the early use of the tunnel test (Ewing, 1930, p. 51) and the toy dog test (Cotton and Hall, 1939). The reinforcers were strong in these two unsuccessful attempts to use visual reinforcement. The childen engaged in high probability behavior of playing with the objects intended as reinforcers and did not attend to the listening task because the contingencies were not properly structured. The children were allowed considerable access to the reinforcers for a minimal amount of responding. By restructuring the contingencies later investigations have eliminated the difficulty and have found the test quite useful. Gaines (1961) has even reported success in using the train test with institutionalized moderately retarded subjects. More recently Lloyd (1965a, 1965b) and Weaver (1965) have reported the successful use of the slide show type of visual reinforcers with institutionalized retardates.

A variation of the button pressing procedure is the conditioned orientation reflex (COR) previously described by Suzuki and Ogiba (1960, 1961). The COR reinforces a localization response and does not require the child to make a button pressing response to receive visual reinforcement. If the child looks at the appropriate loudspeaker when an auditory signal is presented, a doll located near that speaker is illuminated as a form of visual reinforcement. MacPherson (1960) and Fulton (1962) in their doctoral dissertations reported on the use of COR procedures with severely retarded subjects. Fulton's (1962) data indicated greater success with the behavioral conditioning (COR) procedure than with the classical conditioning (GSR) procedure. This basic procedure of reinforcing the location of the signal has been modified by several audiologists who use lights rather than an illuminated doll (Houston Speech and Hearing Center, 1964; Kimball, 1964; MacPherson, 1960).

TANGIBLE REINFORCER METHODS

Relatively intangible reinforcers have been used in the forms of behavioral audiometry mentioned above. Such intangible reinforcers as the word "good," a smile, a pat on the back, or the opportunity to see a picture function as reinforcers for many children, but for some subjects such behaviors or consequences are relatively ineffective. More tangible reinforcers have been used with operant conditioning procedures to obtain audiometric data on retardates (Meyerson and Michael, 1960; LaCrosse and Bidlake, 1964; Spradlin and Lloyd, 1965).[1] Edible items such as candy, popcorn, sugar coated cereal, crackers, dietary supplements, and various fluids as well as nonedible objects such as miniature toys or trinkets have been used in various forms of tangible reinforcement operant conditioning audiometry (TROCA).

In some cases the examiner decided that a single tangible item would be given to each subject. In other cases each subject was given a variety of these tangible items as selected by the examiner. With others, the experimenter has attempted to determine which items are effective reinforcers before starting the audiometric test; then that reinforcer is used during the test. Spradlin and Lloyd (1965) have described one procedure for determining which tangible items are effective reinforcers for a given subject. Since the only reason for using tangible reinforcers is that the other more conventional forms of reinforcement were not effective, it would seem that the audiologist using TROCA should attempt to determine an effective, tangible reinforcer for each subject rather than use an arbitrarily determined reinforcer. It should be noted that a reinforcer is defined in terms of its functional relationship to the behavior being reinforced and is not some item or event that the experimenter or clinician has predesignated as a reinforcer.

One of the TROCA reports (LaCrosse and Bidlake, 1964) did not give details on their procedure; however, the other two (Meyerson and Michael, 1960; Spradlin and Lloyd, 1965) did describe their procedures. These investigations were designed to test the retarded child who did not respond to verbal instructions. After using a variety of procedures Meyerson and Michael (1960) concluded by suggesting that the most effective procedure involved two responses. When there was no auditory signal present, the response of pressing one button was reinforced on a partial schedule, and when the signal was present the response of pushing a second button was reinforced on a similar schedule. They also provided extra reinforcement for appropriate quick switches.

Spradlin and Lloyd (1965) also tried various procedures, but they reported that a single response system which reinforced pressing the button when the auditory signal was present was the most efficient for clinical testing. They used a 100 percent reinforcement schedule with the single response system. This TROCA procedure is similar to the operant audiometry procedures which use visual reinforcers. The primary difference is in the reinforcers.

Both investigations (Meyerson and Michael, 1960; Spradlin and Lloyd, 1965) used automated programs of signal presentation. The programming equipment also reduced the latency of reinforcement delivery. Some of the visual reinforcer operant procedures involved immediate (automated) reinforcement, but most of the behavior audiometry procedures considered were not automated for reinforcement delivery. In the typical audiometric test an extremely small latency in reinforcement delivery is of relatively little consequence, but in some cases the reinforcement latency may be an extremely critical factor. With the more difficult cases special attention should be afforded the reinforcement timing. The reinforcement should be presented immediately after an appropriate response.

SUMMARY AND CONCLUSIONS

Several behavioral audiometry methods are reviewed in terms of operant conditioning principles. A primary focus of the paper is upon reinforcement principles. The importance of stimulus control is obvious in all forms of audiometry. The obtaining of stimulus control is related to factors such as simplicity of response, selection of an appropriate reinforcer, reinforcement contingencies, immediate reinforcement, reinforcement schedules, and reinforcement shifting. Sensitivity in the use of these variables frequently marks the difference between the skilled and the unskilled clinician. Many of the rather vague clinical qualities considered under the term "rapport" may also be analyzed in terms of operant principles.

ACKNOWLEDGMENTS

Preparation of this paper was partially supported by a National Institute of Mental Health Grant No. MH-01127. The author is grateful to his friend and colleague Joseph E. Spradlin, Coordinator of Research, Bureau of Child Research, University of Kansas and Parsons State Hospital and Training Center, for his review and constructive criticism of the manuscript.

ENDNOTE

1. Spradlin and Lloyd (1965) made their preliminary report of the TROCA procedure developed at Parsons in a monograph publication of limited printing. However, Lloyd, Spradlin, and Reid have recently published a more complete description of the TROCA procedure in *F. Speech Hearing Dis., 33,* 236–245 (1968). Lloyd *et al* (1968) describe the TROCA procedure in five interrelated phases: (1) determining the reinforcer, (2) initial training, (3) stimulus generalization, (4) sound field screening, and (5) bilateral screening and threshold testing.

They report the results of the first fifty (50) profoundly retarded patients they attempted to test with TROCA and the initial results obtained from three normal infants (5, 15, and 18 mos. old) to demonstrate some of the potential of this procedure with non verbal and difficult-to-test-patients. The validity of the procedure was demonstrated by reasonable audiometric configurations, agreement with other data, and three cases of unilateral hearing impairment. Masking and bone-conduction testing were briefly considered.—LLL

REFERENCES

Barr, B., Pure tone audiometry for pre-school children. *Acta-Otolaryng.,* Suppl. 121 (1955).

Cotton, J. C., and Hall, Jayne, Administration of the 6-A audiometer test to kindergarten and first grade children. *Volta Rev., 41,* 291 (1939).

Denmark, F. G. W., A development of the peep-show audiometer. *J. Laryng. Otol., 64,* 357–360 (1950).

Curry, E. T., and Kurtzrock, G. H., A preliminary investigation of the ear-choice technique in threshold audiometry. *J. Speech Hearing Dis., 16,* 340–345 (1951).

Dix, Mary R., and Hallpike, C. S., The peep show: A new technique for pure tone audiometry in young children. *Brit. Med. J., 2,* 719–723 (1947).

Donnelly, K. G., A vibro-tactile method of conditioning young children for hearing tests. In Lloyd, L. L., and Frisina, D. R. (Ed.), *The Audiologic Assessment of the Mentally Retarded: Proceedings of a National Conference,* Parsons, Kansas: Speech and Hearing Dept., PSH&TC (1965).

Evans, Mary L., An adaptation of the audiometric technique for use with small children. Masters thesis, Univ. Illinois (1943).

Ewing, A. W. G., *Aphasia in Children.* London: Oxford Medical Publication (1930).

Frisina, D. R., Audiometric evaluation and its relation to habilitation and rehabilitation of the deaf. *Amer. Ann. Deaf, 107,* 478–481 (1962).

Frisina, D. R., Measurement of hearing in children. In Jerger, J. (Ed.), *Modern Developments in Audiology,* N.Y.: Academic Press (1963).

Fulton, R. T., Psychogalvanic skin response and conditioned orientation reflex audiometry with mentally retarded children. Doctoral dissertation, Purdue Univ. (1962).

Gaines, Judy A. L., A comparison of two audiometric tests administered to a group of mentally retarded children. Masters thesis, Univ. of Nebraska (1961).

Green, D. S., The pup-show: a simple, inexpensive modification of the peep-show. *J. Speech Hearing Dis., 23,* 118–120 (1958).

Guilford, R., and Haug, O., Diagnosis of deafness in the very young child. *Arch. Otolaryng., 55,* 101–106 (1952).

Houston Speech and Hearing Center, Audiometric assessment technique. *Asha, 6,* 261 (1964).

Ishisawa, H., A study on play audiometry. (Japanese text) *Otol. Fukuoka,* 6 (Supp. 7), 397–415 (1960). From: *dsh Abst., 2,* 201 (1962).

Kaplin, Harriet, A comparison of picture response and hand raising technique for pure tone audiometry with young children. Masters thesis, Penn. State Univ. (1957).

Keaster, Marjorie J., A pure-tone audiometric test for pre-school children. Masters thesis, Univ. of Wisc. (1951).

Kimball, B. D., Addendum to previous article. *Asha, 6,* 500 (1964).

LaCrosse, E. L., and Bidlake, H., A method to test the hearing of mentally retarded children. *Volta Rev., 66,* 27–30 (1964).

Lloyd, L. L., A comparison of selected auditory measures on normal hearing mentally retarded children. Doctoral dissertation, Univ. of Iowa (1965*a*).

Lloyd, L. L., Use of the slide show audiometric technique with mentally retarded children. *Exceptional Children, 32,* 93–98 (1965*b*).

Lowell, E., Rushford, Georgina, Hoversten, Gloria, and Stoner, Marguerite, Evaluation of pure tone audiometry with pre-school age children. *J. Speech Hearing Dis., 21,* 292–302 (1956).

MacPherson, J. B., The evaluation and development of techniques for testing the auditory acuity of trainable mentally retarded children. Doctoral dissertation, Univ. of Texas (1960).

Meyerson, L., and Michael, J. L., *The Measurement of Sensory Thresholds in Exceptional Children: An Experimental Approach to Some Problems of Differential Diagnosis and Education with Special Reference to Hearing.* U.S. Office of Education, Cooperative Research Project No. 418, Univ. of Houston, Houston, Texas (1960).

Miller, A. L., The use of reward techniques in testing young children's hearing. *Hear. News, 30,* 5–7 (1962).

Miller, A. L., The use of slide projectors in pure tone audiometric testing. *J. Speech Hearing Dis.*, **28**, 94–96 (1963).

O'Neill, J., Oyer, H., and Hillis, J., Audiometric procedures used with children. *J. Speech Hearing Dis.*, **26**, 61–66 (1961).

Shimizu, H., and Nakamura, F., Pure-tone audiometry in children: lantern-slides test. *Ann. Oto. Rhino. Laryng.*, **66**, 392–398 (1957).

Spradlin, J. E., and Lloyd, L. L., Operant conditioning audiometry (OCA) with low level retardates: a preliminary report. In Lloyd, L. L., and Frisina, D. R. (Ed.), *The Audiologic Assessment of the Mentally Retarded: The Proceedings of a National Conference,* Parsons, Kansas: Speech and Hearing Dept., PSH&TC (1965).

Statten, P., and Wishart, D. E. S., Pure tone audiometry in young children: Psychogalvanic-skin-resistance and peepshow. *Ann. Oto. Rhino. Laryng.*, **65**, 511–534 (1956).

Schwartz, A., Supplementary pure tone audiometric screening test for pre-school children. Masters thesis, Univ. of Wisconsin (1952).

Sullivan, R., Miller, M. H., and Polisar, I. A., The portable pup-show: A further modification of the pup-show. *Arch Otolaryng.*, **76**, 49–51 (1962).

Suzuki, T., and Ogiba, Y., A technique of pure tone audiometry for children under three years of age: Conditioned orientation reflex (COR) audiometry. *Rev. Laryng.*, Paris, **1**, 33–45 (1960).

Suzuki, T., and Ogiba, Y., Conditioned orientation reflex audiometry. *Arch. Otolaryng.*, **74**, 192–198 (1961).

Utley, J., Suggestive procedures for determining auditory acuity in very young acoustically handicapped children. *Eye, Ear, Nose, Thr., Mon.*, **28**, 590–595 (1949).

Waldrop, W., A puppet show hearing test. *Volta Rev.*, **55**, 488–489 (1953).

Weaver, R. M., The use of filmstrip audiometry in assessing the auditory sensitivity of mentally retarded children. In Lloyd, L. L., and Frisina, D. R. (Ed.), *The Audiologic Assessment of the Mentally Retarded: The Proceedings of a National Conference,* Parsons, Kansas: Speech and Hearing Dept., PSH&TC (1965).

15

Effects of Stimulus Presentation and Instructions on Pure-Tone Thresholds and False-Alarm Responses

Jesse E. Dancer, Ph.D.
Assistant Professor of Audiology, University of Arkansas at Little Rock, University of Arkansas Medical Sciences Campus
Ira M. Ventry, Ph.D.
Professor of Audiology, Teachers College, Columbia University
Wathina Hill, Ed.D.
Professor of Speech Pathology and Audiology, William Paterson College, Wayne, New Jersey

The effects of three instructional sets (conventional Carhart-Jerger, strict, and lax) and of two stimulus presentation methods (continuous tones, pulsed tones) on pure-tone thresholds and false-alarm responses were determined for 20 male subjects. False alarms were tallied during hearing measurement periods and during 30-second time-out periods totaling nine minutes of time-out per subject. Results showed that 50 percent of the subjects made false-alarm responses to some extent at 250, 1,000, and 4,000 Hz. Instructions and stimulus mode, along with frequency, affected the number of false alarms, but thresholds under the experimental conditions were unchanged. It is suggested that a method for assessing and controlling false alarms is an important clinical consideration.

Pure-tone thresholds in clinical audiometry are obtained by eliciting a behavioral response, such as raising a finger, from the subject each time a tone is heard. A false-alarm response is defined as the occurrence of the specified response in the absence of a pure-tone stimulus. A false-alarm response in contiguity with a pure-tone stimulus cannot be distinguished from a true response, and the determination of valid thresholds is jeopardized if false alarms are uncontrolled or unrecognized.

Although the importance of controlling false-alarm responses is well recognized in electrophysiologic techniques for testing hearing (Price, 1969; Goldstein, 1973; Ventry, 1975), there is no procedure in general use for evaluating the false-alarm response and its effect upon threshold in conventional pure-tone testing. Signal detection theory has developed methods for estimating and eliminating the effect of false alarms (Clark and Bilger, 1973), but the methods are time-consuming and as yet do not lend themselves to clinical use.

In clinical testing, the audiologist does have a degree of control over such factors as instructions and the manner in which tones are presented; however, little experimental attention has been given to determining the effects of instructions and stimulus presentation methods on false-alarm responses and thresholds in clinical audiometry. The present study will investigate the effects of three instructional sets and two stimulus presentation methods on false alarms and thresholds within a conventional hearing testing situation.

PURPOSES OF STUDY

Instructions. Conventional instructions for pure-tone threshold testing have been proposed by Carhart and Jerger (1959). Alterations in these instructions are often used clinically when either the false-alarm rate is too high or the obtained threshold is poorer than anticipated. If the false-alarm rate is unacceptably high, then instructions which discourage guessing (strict instructions) may be given. If the obtained

Reprinted by permission of the authors from *J. Speech Hearing Dis.*, **41**, 315–324 (1976).

threshold is considered too poor, then instructions which encourage guessing (lax instructions) may be given.

It is reasonable to assume that such altered instructions in the clinical setting do have some effect upon both false alarms and thresholds. However, the use of altered instructions is presently unstandardized and their effects are unknown. Individual clinicians must decide when and how to change instructions. One purpose of the present investigation is to determine the differential effects of three sets of instructions on false alarms and thresholds in a clinical testing situation.

Stimulus Presentation Methods. When false-alarm rates are unacceptably high to single-tone presentations (continuous mode), alternative methods of stimulus presentation are available and may be used to measure threshold. For example, pulsed tones, most often used with Bekesy audiometry, have been recommended by Veniar (1965) for routine testing and have been compared favorably to the continuous method (single-tone presentations) by Hochberg and Waltzman (1972). However, it would appear that a pulsed-tone technique would make the detection of false-alarm responses even more difficult than the continuous-tone technique. With a single-tone presentation, latency factors help to validate a response; if the response occurs too early or too late, it is unacceptable. A pulsed-tone technique which requires the same response as the continuous-tone technique (that is, a single finger raised to a series of pulses) obscures latency information by increasing the amount of time the stimulus is on. From the standpoint of false-alarm detection and control, therefore, a pulsed-tone technique which requires the same response as the continuous-tone technique is unacceptable.

A pulse-counting technique described for screening programs (Reger and Newby, 1947; Gardner, 1947) appears attractive as an alternative to the conventional (continuous-tone) method for threshold testing. In the pulse-counting technique, the listener is required to report not only the presence of a series of pulses, but also the number of pulses which occur within a specific time period. The pulse-counting technique requires information from the listener (a number) which is quantifiably different from that obtained with the continuous stimulus mode (raising a finger or saying "yes"). A comparison of false-alarm rates and thresholds under the continuous stimulus mode (single-tone presentations) and under

the pulsed stimulus mode (pulse-counting) has not been reported. The second purpose of this investigation is to use a continuous-stimulus mode and a pulse-stimulus mode and to compare their effects upon false alarms and thresholds.

PROCEDURES

Subjects. Twenty male subjects were used in the present investigation. They ranged in age from 21 to 64, with a mean age of 48.5. All subjects had normal hearing at 250 and 1,000 Hz (thresholds no greater than 15 dB HL re: ANSI, 1969) and at least a mild sensorineural hearing loss at 4,000 Hz (hearing levels no better than 30 dB, with no greater than a 5 dB air-bone gap). Subjects had no medical or emotional complaints that would interfere with the experimental tasks.

Environment. The testing environment was an IAC booth with visual communication between the subject's chamber and the control room through a two-way window. The subject was seated in a straight-back cushioned chair with arm rests; he was unable to observe the experimenter during testing.

Instrumentation and Calibration. The pure-tone stimuli were generated by a Maico (Model 24) audiometer and were delivered to the subjects via TDH-39 earphones in MX-41/AR cushions. Pure-tone air-conduction stimuli were calibrated to ANSI, 1969 standards and were checked periodically with an artificial ear.

Experimental Session

Prior to earphone placement, all subjects were read the instructions for pure-tone testing from Carhart and Jerger (1959), which will be designated as the conventional instructions for threshold testing. Following instructions, pure-tone thresholds were determined under two stimulus modes: (1) the continuous mode, to which the listener responds to single-tone presentations, and (2) the pulsed mode, to which the listener counts the number of tone pulses occurring in succession.

Verbal responses were used for both stimulus modes: "yes" for the continuous mode and a specific number for the pulsed mode. The subject was told under the pulsed condition to listen for pulses ranging from one to four in succession and to report the number heard. Under both stimulus modes, the lowest hearing level at which three correct responses were obtained (not necessarily consecutive) was defined as threshold.

The presentation of the two stimulus modes was randomized among the conditions. Pure-tone thresholds were measured at 250, 1,000, and 4,000 Hz in the left ear of each subject. The Carhart-Jerger ascending measurement method was used for both stimulus modes.

Following the determination of pure-tone thresholds under the conventional instructions for the two stimulus modes, thresholds were redetermined under the following experimental conditions: (1) lax instruction condition—subjects here were encouraged to guess, even if they only thought they heard the tone; and (2) strict instruction condition—subjects here were told to respond only when they were certain they heard a tone. Thus, all subjects served under the following three conditions:

Condition I. Subjects were given conventional Carhart-Jerger (1959) instructions and thresholds were determined by a continuous-stimulus mode (single-tone presentations) and a pulsed-stimulus mode.

Condition II. Subjects were given lax instructions and thresholds were determined by the continuous- and pulsed-stimulus modes.

Condition III. Subjects were given strict instructions and thresholds were determined by the continuous- and pulsed-stimulus modes.

The experimental conditions (II and III) were counterbalanced to distribute practice effects. All subjects were used in all three conditions, which were all completed within one experimental session.

False-alarm rates were determined for the three instructional sets and the two stimulus modes by imposing a 30-second time-out interval at each of the three test frequencies. Time-out intervals could occur at any time in the determination of a threshold, and the time-outs were varied to keep the subject from knowing when time-outs were in effect. Subjects were not told that time-outs would occur.

Time-out periods contained no tones, and the experimenter determined the number of false alarms by tallying the number of "yes" responses during the continuous-mode technique and the number of numerical responses during the pulsed-mode technique. The number of false-alarm responses during hearing

measurement periods were also tallied. A response was classified as a false alarm if, in the clinical judgment of the examiner, it was not paired closely enough with the stimulus presentation. For each subject, a total time-out period of nine minutes provided ample opportunity for false alarms.

RESULTS

False Alarm Distribution among Subjects

There was a total of 97 false-alarm responses, 67 during the time-out periods and 30 during hearing measurement periods. Ten of the 20 subjects did not make false-alarm responses at any time or under any condition. Of the 10 subjects with false-alarm responses, two subjects accounted for 61 false alarms and were the major contributors to the statistics on the number of false alarms. Thus, data on false alarms are skewed to represent primarily the responses of only 10 percent of the total number of subjects. This must be considered in any interpretation of the data. Because of the markedly skewed distribution, inferential statistics were not used in the data analysis.

Overall Effects of Instructions, Stimulus Frequency, and Stimulus Mode on False Alarms

Table 15–1 shows the overall effects of instructions, stimulus frequency, and stimulus mode on the number of false alarms in the 10 subjects who showed such responses. The number of subjects with false-alarm responses within each condition is also indicated. The major findings are:

1. False alarms were affected by instructions, with the fewest false alarms under strict instructions and the most under lax instructions. Conventional and lax instructions produced a similar number of false alarms.

2. The number of false alarms was greater at 4,000 Hz than at the other two frequencies. A similar number of false alarms was obtained at 250 and 1,000 Hz.

3. False alarms occurred more often to the continuous stimulus presentations than to a pulse-counting procedure.

TABLE 15-1. NUMBER OF FALSE ALARMS AS A FUNCTION OF INSTRUCTIONS, STIMULUS FREQUENCY, AND STIMULUS MODE. A TOTAL OF 97 FALSE ALARMS WAS PRODUCED; NUMBER OF SUBJECTS WAS 20.

	Number	
Variable	False Alarms	Subjects*
Instructions		
Conventional	36	8
Strict	18	7
Lax	43	9
Frequency (Hz)		
250	17	5
1,000	20	7
4,000	60	9
Mode		
Continuous	60	10
Pulsed	37	6

*Indicates number of subjects who made false-alarm responses at least once under that condition.

Thus, false alarms were minimal when instructions were strict, when the stimulus frequency was 250 Hz, and when the stimulus mode was pulsed. False alarms were maximal when instructions were lax, when the frequency was 4,000 Hz, and when the stimulus mode was continuous. The number of subjects whose responses included false alarms within each condition followed these general trends. For example, there were 10 subjects with at least one false alarm when the stimulus mode was continuous (Table 15-1), but only six subjects with false-alarm responses when the stimulus mode was pulsed.

Combined Effects of Frequency, Instructions, and Stimulus Mode on False Alarms

Tables 15-2, 15-3, and 15-4 show the combined effects of instructions and test frequency, instructions and stimulus mode, and test frequency and stimulus mode, respectively on false alarms. These major effects are:

1. Lax instructions produced more false alarms at each stimulus frequency than did strict instructions, and more false alarms occurred at 4,000 Hz than at the other two frequencies regardless of instructions. Conventional and lax instructions tended to yield similar false-alarm rates, especially at 4,000 Hz; and 250 and 1,000 Hz were similar in false-alarm rates under all instructions (Table 15-2).

2. Conventional instructions combined with the continuous-stimulus mode (Carhart-Jerger's "preferred clinical method") gave the greatest number of false alarms in the instructions-stimulus mode pairings (Table 15-3), while strict instructions combined with a pulsed-stimulus mode gave the fewest false alarms. Differences in false alarms under the two stimulus modes were greatest under conventional instructions and are less apparent under strict and lax instructions, but there was a trend for the pulsed-stimulus mode to yield fewer false alarms under all instructions.

3. A pulsed-stimulus mode tended to give fewer false alarms at all frequencies than the continuous-stimulus mode (Table 15-4), but differences in the continuous and the pulsed modes were most apparent at 4,000 Hz.

In summary, false alarms were affected by instructions, by stimulus frequency, and by stimulus mode. These effects, however, could not be demonstrated in half the subjects who did not manifest false alarms.

TABLE 15-2. NUMBER OF FALSE ALARMS UNDER COMBINED EFFECTS OF STIMULUS FREQUENCY AND INSTRUCTIONS.

Frequency	Instructions		
(Hertz)	Conventional	Strict	Lax
250	6	2	9
1,000	5	3	12
4,000	25	13	22

TABLE 15-3. NUMBER OF FALSE ALARMS UNDER COMBINED EFFECTS OF INSTRUCTIONS AND STIMULUS MODE.

	Stimulus Mode	
Instructions	Continuous	Pulsed
Conventional	25	11
Strict	12	6
Lax	23	20

TABLE 15-4. NUMBER OF FALSE ALARMS UNDER COMBINED EFFECTS OF FREQUENCY AND STIMULUS MODE.

Frequency	Stimulus Mode	
(Hertz)	Continuous	Pulsed
250	11	6
1,000	11	9
4,000	38	22

TABLE 15-5. MEAN THRESHOLDS IN HEARING LEVEL (HL) FOR TWO STIMULUS MODES (CONTINUOUS AND PULSED) AND THREE INSTRUCTIONAL SETS (CONVENTIONAL, STRICT, LAX) AT THREE FREQUENCIES.

Instructions	Continuous Mode Frequency (Hz)					
	250		1,000		4,000	
Conventional	8.5	(5)*	8.2	(3)	41.0	(17)
Strict	8.2	(2)	8.1	(1)	40.7	(9)
Lax	7.5	(4)	6.8	(7)	40.0	(12)
	Pulsed Mode					
Conventional	10.0	(1)	9.3	(2)	41.4	(8)
Strict	8.8	(0)	7.2	(2)	41.0	(4)
Lax	7.8	(5)	7.5	(5)	40.7	(10)

*Numbers in parentheses indicate the number of false alarms within that condition.

Effects of Instructions and Stimulus Mode on Thresholds

Table 15-5 shows mean thresholds at three frequencies for both stimulus modes under the three instructions for all 20 subjects. The number of false alarms within each condition is noted. Neither instructions nor stimulus mode has any important effects on thresholds at any frequency; that is, the great majority (86 percent) of repeat thresholds were grouped within the 5-dB range usually thought to represent the variability in good clinical test-retest situations. The largest mean difference between any of the six repeat threshold measurements at each frequency was only 2.5 dB. All repeat threshold measurements were within 10 dB.

Although thresholds did not vary importantly with instructions or stimulus mode, note that false alarms varied within the measurement conditions. False alarms ranged from 0 (250 Hz, strict, pulsed) to 17 (4,000 Hz, conventional, continuous). Such variations underline the effects of instructions, stimulus frequency, and stimulus mode on false alarms.

DISCUSSION

The Effects of Instructions, Stimulus Frequency, and Stimulus Mode on False Alarms

It was anticipated that instructions encouraging and discouraging guessing would affect the number of false alarms, with strict instructions suppressing such

responses in comparison to the conventional and lax instructions. The similarity of the number of false alarms in the conventional and lax conditions indicates that conventional instructions are not the most effective instructions in controlling false-alarm responses. This point is discussed in more detail under the section on clinical implications.

The greater frequency of false alarms at 4,000 Hz in comparison to 250 and 1,000 Hz is subject to two possible interpretations: (1) false alarms are a function of stimulus frequency, with higher frequencies producing more false alarms, or (2) false alarms are a function of the severity of hearing loss. In the present study, these two effects of frequency and hearing loss are confounded by the required 30 dB or more sensorineural hearing loss at 4,000 Hz, while thresholds at 250 and 1,000 Hz were normal. Further study is necessary to determine the independent effects of stimulus frequency and of hearing loss in influencing false alarms.

The pulse-counting stimulus mode produced fewer false alarms than the continuous stimulus mode for nine out of 10 subjects showing false alarms. It is possible that the pulse-counting technique reduces false alarms by requiring more information than does the continuous mode. That is, the continuous stimulus mode requires a categorical "yes" decision, while the pulse-counting technique requires one decision for the presence of the stimulus and another decision for the number of stimulus pulses.

In terms of information theory, one bit of information (presence-absence) is necessary for a response to the continuous-stimulus mode, while two bits of information (presence-absence, number) are necessary for a response to the pulsed-stimulus mode. Within certain limits, as information necessary for a response increases, equivocal responses (loosely translated, false alarms) decrease (Miller, 1956; Frick 1959). Response requiring increased information thus tend to be more precise and certain. The pulsed-stimulus mode requires that the listener be quantitative rather than qualitative in his judgments.

Effects of Instructions and Stimulus Mode on Thresholds

In the present study, threshold measurements were not importantly affected clinically by instructions or stimulus mode. These findings are rather surprising, since some changes at least as a function of instructions were anticipated. One possible factor in leading to the present results is the 5-dB measurement interval used in clinical audiometry, which tends to produce all-or-none threshold decisions. In the conventional testing method, threshold is defined as three responses, not necessarily consecutive, at the lowest hearing level. A significant proportion of those individuals tested clinically show three consecutive responses at a given hearing level and no responses below this level. This is especially noted in patients with sensorineural hearing losses; such threshold certainty may be less characteristic in patients with conductive hearing losses. More study is necessary to determine whether instructions or stimulus mode might affect thresholds in conductive hearing losses or whether the results of this study (no effects on threshold) may be generalized to all types of hearing losses.

Implications for Clinical Hearing Measurement

The findings of this study suggest that the clinician may minimize false alarms without affecting threshold measurements. That is, false alarms are least when instructions are strict and when a pulse-counting technique is used, but thresholds are unaffected. It would appear that as long as the subject is instructed to respond to the faintest tones, it is not critical to encourage the subject to guess. Such encouragment may ultimately affect the validity of thresholds by increasing false alarms.

It is noteworthy that among the subjects whose responses included false alarms, the "preferred clinical method" of Carhart-Jerger (conventional instructions, continuous-stimulus mode) produced the greatest number of false alarms in comparison with the other pairings of instructions and stimulus mode (Table 15-3). Since conventional instructions were always used first, it is possible that fatigue effects per se served to reduce false alarms under the other two instructional sets. However, strict instructions always produced the fewest number of false-alarm responses regardless of its order among the three conditions.

False-alarm responses were not a consideration in the Carhart-Jerger (1959) recommendations for pure-tone threshold determinations. However, since 50 percent of the subjects within this investigation evidenced false-alarm responses to some extent, a method for assessing and controlling false alarms is an important clinical consideration.

REFERENCES

Carhart, R., and Jerger J. Preferred method for clinical determination of pure-tone thresholds, *J. Speech Hearing Dis.*, **24,** 330–345 (1959).

Clarke, F., and Bilger R. The theory of signal detectability and the measurement of hearing. In J. Jerger (Ed.), *Modern Developments in Audiology.* New York: Academic, 437–476 (1973).

Frick, F. Information theory. In S. Koch (Ed.), *Psychology: A Study of a Science* (Vol. 2). New York: McGraw-Hill, 611–636 (1959).

Goldstein, R. Electroencephalic audiometry. In J. Jerger (Ed.), *Modern Developments in Audiology.* New York: Academic, 407–435 (1973).

Gardner, M. A pure tone technique for clinical audiometric measurement. *J. acoust. Soc. Am.,* **19,** 592–599 (1947).

Hochberg, I., and Waltzman, S. Comparison of pulsed and continuous tone thresholds in patients with tinnitus. *Audiology,* **II,** 337–342 (1972).

Miller, G. The magical number seven, plus or minus two. *Psychol. Rev.,* **63,** 81–97 (1956).

Price L. Cortical evoked response audiometry. In R. Fulton and L. Lloyd (Eds.), *Audiometry for the Retarded.* Baltimore: Williams and Wilkins, 210–237 (1969).

Reger, S., and Newby, H. A group pure-tone hearing test. *J. Speech Hearing Dis.,* **12,** 357–362 (1947).

Veniar, F. Individual masking levels in pure tone audiometry. *Archs. Otolar.,* **82,** 518–521 (1965).

Ventry, I. M. Conditioned galvanic skin response audiometry. In L. Bradford (Ed.), *Physiological Measures of the Audio-Vestibular System.* New York: Academic, 215–248 (1975).

16

Audiometric Management of Collapsible Ear Canals

JOSEPH B. CHAIKLIN, Ph.D.
Supervisor, Audiology Section, Veterans Administration Medical Center, New Orleans
MAX E. MCCLELLAN, Ph.D.
Chief, Audiology Section, Veterans Administration Hospital, Albuquerque

The audiometric management of collapsible ear canals was investigated by performing pure-tone audiometry under six conditions with 12 subjects having normal hearing and normal ear canals and 12 subjects with collapsible ear canals. Sound-field audiometry provided valid and reliable threshold estimates. With appropriate calibration, a circumaural earphone assembly provided valid and reliable results between 125 and 3,000 hertz but produced large intersubject differences above 3,000 Hz. A hand-held supra-aural earphone was effective above 1,000 Hz but grossly unreliable below 1,500 Hz. A small ear insert was relatively ineffective in neutralizing the effects of collapsible ear canals. It was concluded that sound-field audiometry or a circumaural earphone are useful for assessing patients with collapsible ear canals and that earmolds, ear inserts, or polyethylene tubing are inappropriate solutions to the problem.

Some external ear canals collapse under pressure of supra-aural earphone cushions causing elevated air-conduction (AC) thresholds, intertest and intratest variability, and other audiometric errors. Relative bone-conduction (BC) and sound-field thresholds are unaffected because the pinnae are not compressed by earphones for these tests. A collapsible ear canal collapses only when pressure is applied to the pinna. An ear canal that is collapsed in its normal state is called a prolapsed ear canal. Failure to identify and resolve the effects of collapsible ear canals can lead to inappropriate medical, surgical, and audiological decisions.

Collapsible ear canals may be more common in people with small or narrow canals, the elderly, and people with protruding pinnae. The problem has been observed in adults and children (including siblings) of both sexes. The prevalence of collapsible canals is not known.

The largest effects of collapsible canals usually occur above 1,000 hertz but there is great intersubject variability in magnitude of effects and frequency range affected. Significant threshold elevations may occur above 1,000 Hz before complete closure of the canal; as closure increases threshold shifts increase, eventually affecting the entire audiometric range. The effect is similar to the attenuation provided by an ear plug, although the dynamics of collapsible canals are probably much more complicated.

Collapsible ear canals were first described in 1961 by Ventry et al. (1961) who reported test-retest variability and threshold shifts attributable to collapse of the ear canal and suggested that the prevalence of callapsible ear canals is unknown. They speculated that the magnitude of threshold shift should be related to degree of collapse, probably requiring complete or nearly complete closure to cause significant effects. The possibility of stable threshold shifts without interest or intratest variability was also sug-

Reprinted by permission of the authors from *Arch. Otolaryng.*, **93**, 397–407 (1971). Copyright 1971, American Medical Association.

gested. The following year Hildyard and Valentine (1962) emphasized that in their experience a positive Rinne test in the presence of an audiometric AC-BC gap occurs frequently in patients whose external canals collapse under earphone pressure.

Hildyard and Valentine reported that 4.5 percent of their clinical sample had collapsible canals but mean effects were so small (11.4 dB maximum at 2,000 Hz), that we have reservations as to whether all of their subjects had audiometric effects large enough to define the presence of collapse. Creston (1965) studied the prevalence of collapsible canals in 282 school children, and concluded that 3.5 percent of his sample had collapsible canals. The "average error" reported by Creston was only 13 dB; he did not report mean effects at specific frequencies.

Chandler's (1964) investigation of earmolds with progressively smaller bores provides indirect evidence on the effects of degrees of canal collapse. Chandler's largest earmold bore, which was presumed to represent 80.5 percent canal occlusion, caused a mean AC threshold increase of 13 dB at 2,000 Hz, 14 dB at 4,000 Hz, and 20 dB at 8,000 Hz. Progressively smaller bores caused greater threshold shifts, eventually affecting the entire audiometric range. For a variety of reasons the effect of Chandler's earmolds is not directly analogous to the effect of a collapsed ear canal. For example, his earmolds occupied portions of the concha and external canal that are not occupied when a canal collapses.

Previous articles have advocated various types of ear inserts, polyethylene tubing, and stock earmolds to counteract the effects of ear canal collapse (Ventry et al., 1961; Hildyard and Valentine, 1962; Creston, 1965; Creston and Tice, 1964; Ross and Tucker, 1965; Smith, 1966; Stark, 1966; Rupp et al., 1968; Juers, 1969; Lynn, 1969). Our experience with these devices has persuaded us that they introduce too much error for routine clinical use despite the fact that they work in individual cases. Too often they cause poorer thresholds in the range most affected by collapse of the canal. Since the physical characteristics of the normal pinna and external ear canal enhance auditory sensitivity at frequencies above 1,000 Hz (Shaw, 1966; Teranishi and Shaw, 1968; Bauer et al., 1967; Erber, 1968; Villchur, 1969; Berland and Nielson, 1969) it follows that any object introduced into a normal canal may negate these enhancing effects.

Intersubject variability is a prominent problem associated with using stock earmolds to overcome the effects of collapsible canals. In 1968 Rupp et al. (1968) recommended that median attenuation values produced by stock earmolds may be used as corrections to offset the attenuation introduced when the molds are used with patients who have collapsible canals. While Rupp et al. did not discuss intersubject variability, data provided by Rupp in a personal communication show attenuation ranges of 25 dB or more at the six frequencies tested and ranges exceeding 35 dB at two frequencies. Individual attenuation values ranged from 0 dB to 45 dB.

Sometimes the medial opening of a stock insert, earmold, or polyethylene tube becomes blocked as it butts against a turn in the canal wall, or the external opening of the insert may be blocked by the tragus thus causing higher thresholds than those found in the collapsed state without an insert (Ventry et al., 1961). Tubing tends to be uncomfortable and may be hazardous if it is too long (Creston, 1965). Stock inserts can also be uncomfortable and have the additional potential for measurement error caused by expanding the meatus beyond its resting dimensions, especially in prolapsed or partially prolapsed ear canals.

Another method that can be used to overcome the effects of collapsible ear canals (Ventry et al., 1961) is to hold the MX-41/AR cushion and phone assembly in light contact with the skin of the pinna at the pinna's natural angle. This method is tedious, difficult to use with small children, and must be confined to measurements above 1,000 Hz (see Results and Comment).

There appears to be a need for further assessment of the collapsible ear canal phenomenon and a related need for an evaluation of methods to overcome its effects. Until valid and reliable methods exist for assessing the hearing of persons with collapsible ear canals it will not be possible to provide reasonable prevalence estimates.

This study investigated sound-field audiometry, a circumaural cushion, a hand-held supra-aural cushion, and a stock insert as approaches to improving the validity of audiometry with patients who have collapsible ear canals. We did not use polyethylene tubing or stock earmolds because of the problems described above. The stock insert was studied mainly for illustrative purposes.

METHOD

Subjects

There were two groups of subjects—a collapse group comprised of people with physical and audiometric evidence of collapsible ear canals and a comparison group with no obvious signs of narrow or collapsible ear canals. All subjects were inspected for narrow canals and were checked for collapsible canals by manual pressure on the auricles to simulate supra-aural earphone pressure.

Comparison Group. Comparison group subjects were four male and eight female normal-hearing adults between the ages of 22 and 54 (mean = 30 years). They had negative otologic histories and pure-tone thresholds of 10 dB or better (re ISO 1964) at most frequencies in the audiometric range, but a few had thresholds higher than 10 dB at some of the higher frequencies. No subject in the comparison group had narrow or collapsible ear canals on visual inspection. Comparison group subjects were university faculty, graduate students, and VA employees.

Collapse Group. Collapse group subjects were 11 males and one female. They ranged from 8 to 74 years of age (mean = 42.5 years) and were free from active middle ear disease. Eight subjects in this group evidenced collapsible canals on previous audiometric tests and two were found to have collapsible canals when screened for inclusion in the comparison group. Eight had bilateral sensorineural loss, one had a stable bilateral conductive loss, and three had bilateral normal hearing.

Subjects in the collapse group were VA and university employees, patients from a county hospital and VA patients. Only one of the VA patients was eligible for disability compensation for hearing loss. Functional hearing loss was ruled out through interest comparisons.

Equipment

The measurement system consisted of an Allison 22 audiometer equipped with 16-ohm loudspeakers (Electrovoice, Model SP 12), TDH-39 earphones (10 ohms), and a Radioear B-70A bone receiver. Air-conduction measurements employed only one earphone and one channel of the audiometer. Attenuation range was −10 to 110 dB (re ISO 1964) with line attenuators available for measurements below −10 dB HL. Sound-field tones were frequency-modulated 3.6 times per second at 1 percent of the base frequency.

The audiometer was in one room and the transducers were in the second room of a single-walled, double-room audiometric test suite (Industrial Acoustics Co., Model 40), which met the ANSI standard (1960) for noise levels in audiometric test environments.

Calibration. The calibration of the earphone was checked periodically with a Bruel and Kjaer (B & K) artificial ear (Type 4152) in conjunction with a microphone amplifier (B & K Model 2603), microphone (Model 4132), and a cathode follower (Model 2613). Over the 12-month period in which data were gathered, the earphone calibration varied 0.5 dB or less between 125 and 3,000 Hz and in the 4,000–8,000 Hz range variation was between 0.75 and 1.0 dB.

The B & K system was used to check calibration of the warble-tone signals in the sound field. The listener's chair faced the loudspeaker in a position which placed the average listener's head on the zero axis approximately 3 feet from the loudspeaker grill. Chair position was marked on the floor to permit accurate repositioning during the experiment, and the microphone was positioned on a microphone stand approximately at the point where the seated listener's head would be. The microphone face was placed at a 90° angle relative to the loudspeaker face.

The sound-field output was adjusted to produce the sound pressure levels prescribed in the instruction manual for the Allison 22 audiometer. These values were used as reference points for periodic evaluation of sound-field calibration. The final calibration check revealed that seven of the nine test frequencies were within ± 3 dB of the original calibration values and two were within ± 5 dB. Small differences in microphone placement may explain part of this variation since near-field measurements are particularly susceptible to this type of error. Empirical calibration on normal ears throughout the study showed that sound-field thresholds agreed well with thresholds obtained under earphones.

Test Conditions

Sound-Field Warble Tone. All subjects in both groups were tested by sound-field warble-tone audiometry at nine audiometric frequencies between 250 and 6,000 Hz. The nontest ear was covered with a sound-attenuating muff and headset (David Clark Co. Model 19A). The muff on the test-ear side was removed and its mounting was covered with foam rubber. Eleven comparison group subjects received a sound-field retest, usually within two months of the original test (average = eight weeks). The comparison group mean sound-field thresholds were used as biological calibration for sound-field comparisons in the collapse group.

The attenuating characteristics of the muff in the modified headset were determined by sound-field warble-tone testing of three unilaterally-deaf subjects, first with and then without the muff covering the normal ear. Retest data were obtained after the headset was removed and replaced. Mean attenuation ranged from 36 to 48 dB between 500 and 4,000 Hz, and was approximately 28 dB at 250 and 6,000 Hz. Test-retest differences did not exceed 5 dB.

A head restraint was not used but subjects were asked to sit erect and look straight ahead at an object centered on top of the loudspeaker. The subject's chair was a conventional office side chair with arm rests and a lightly padded back.

Air Conduction. All subjects in both groups were tested by AC audiometry at 11 audiometric frequencies (125–8,000 Hz) using the TDH-39 earphone mounted in the MX-41/AR supra-aural cushion. Eleven of the 12 comparison group subjects were retested by AC, usually within two months (average = eight weeks).

Bone Conduction. All subjects were tested by BC audiometry at eight frequencies (250 to 4,000 Hz). Contralateral masking was not used during BC testing but the small error from possible participation of the nontest ear was considered acceptable particularly since prior audiometry had demonstrated that the test ear of most collapse group subjects had better BC sensitivity than the nontest ear. The mean BC thresholds of comparison group subjects were compared to their mean AC thresholds and corrections corresponding to the differences between these means were used as a biological calibration to correct the BC thresholds of Collapse Group subjects.

Hand-Held Phone (Hand-Held MX). In the hand-held condition AC thresholds were measured at 11 frequencies (125 to 8,000 Hz) using the TDH-39 earphone mounted in the MX-41/AR cushion. One experimenter held the phone-and-cushion assembly in light contact with the pinna of the test ear while the other experimentor measured thresholds. Care was taken not to displace the pinna from its resting position.

Phone + Insert (MX + Insert). In the phone + insert condition, AC thresholds were measured at 11 frequencies (125 to 8,000 Hz) using the TDH-39 earphone and MX-41/AR cushion plus one of the small rubber-tipped inserts used by Ventry et al. (1961) in the canal of the test ear. Two subjects' ear canals were so small that a smaller insert of a similar type had to be used, and one subject's ear canals were too small for any of our inserts.

Circumaural Cushion (NAF). Pure-tone AC thresholds were measured twice at 11 frequencies (125 to 8,000 Hz) with the TDH-39 earphone mounted in a circumaural "doughnut" cushion (NAF-48490-1, Grason Stadler Co.). After the first set of threshold measurements the earphones were removed and then repositioned by a second tester who repeated the test.

Mastoid-Helix Distance. The distance between the mastoid and helix of the test ear was measured for all subjects to determine whether the auricles of subjects with collapsible ear canals protruded more than those of comparison group subjects.

Test Order and Threshold Method

In all conditions testing was in the following order: 1,000, 1,500, 2,000, 3,000, 4,000, 6,000, 8,000, 1,000, 750, 500, 250, and 125 Hz. All thresholds were measured with a modification of Carhart and Jerger's (1959) ascending method.

The initial plan called for counterbalancing conventional AC and BC audiometry and sound-field warble-tone audiometry. Shortly after the experiment began, the hand-held phone and phone + insert conditions were added. Both always followed the first three conditions and with few exceptions the hand-held condition followed the insert condition. The hand-held phone was used with ten comparison group subjects and ten collapse group subjects and the insert was used with 11 comparison group and ten collapse group subjects. Still later, evaluation of the circumaural cushion was added, always in last position, for nine comparison and six collapse group subjects. After all tests were completed the mastoid-to-helix distance was measured.

Investigator bias during retests and between conditions was minimized by alternating testers (J.B.C. and M.E.M.) and by using a random variable attenuator (RVA) (Chaiklin and Ventry, 1964) which allowed various amounts of attenuation to be introduced into the earphone or BC receiver line. The amount of attenuation introduced was determined only after each threshold was measured. The power needed to drive the loudspeaker exceeded the design limits of the RVA, so it was necessary for a second tester to do sound-field audiometry unless sound-field audiometry occurred first. When only one experimenter was available (three instances) sound-field or hand-held tests were done by a third tester who had no knowledge of previous test results.

A 20 dB pad in the loudspeaker line permitted measurement to −30 dB (re ISO 1964). Since the RVA was used for all other measurement conditions there was usually sufficient attenuation in the line to permit measurement below −10 dB HL. If there was not, a different RVA option was selected.

RESULTS

Comparison Group

Table 16-1 presents mean comparison group thresholds (re ISO 1964) and standard deviations (SD) for all test conditions. Negative values indicate that the average hearing level was lower (better) than 0 dB HL. For example, in the MX condition (line 1, Table 16-1) the −1.70 dB mean threshold at 1,000 Hz was 1.70 dB lower than 0 dB HL.

It can be observed in Table 16-1 that SDs for all conditions are relatively small, most ranging between 3 and 6 dB. For all of the devices under study variability was greatest above 3,000 Hz.

Table 16-2 shows selected intertest and intratest mean differences and ranges of individual differences for comparison group subjects. A threshold difference was computed by subtracting an individual's threshold for one test condition from his threshold for another test condition. A negative difference indicates that the mean for the second condition was higher than the mean for the first condition. For example, in the MX vs sound-field comparison of

TABLE 16-1. COMPARISON GROUP MEAN THRESHOLDS* AND STANDARD DEVIATIONS FOR FIVE TEST CONDITIONS: †MX-41/AR CUSHION (MX), NAF-48490-1 CUSHION (NAF), SOUND FIELD, MX + INSERT AND HAND-HELD MX.

Condition	125	250	500	750	Frequency (Hz) 1,000	1,500	2,000	3,000	4,000	6,000	8,000
MX(12)‡	6.70	−0.40§	0.80	2.10	−1.70	−2.50	−1.70	1.30	5.80	10.00	7.90
SD	5.09	4.77	4.94	4.76	2.33	4.79	6.23	5.81	7.89	5.77	11.09
SF(12)	...	−7.10	−3.30	0.40	−2.90	−5.00	0.40	0.00	7.10	11.30	...
SD	...	3.16	4.74	4.77	4.32	5.40	6.60	6.77	6.89	3.45	...
NAF(9)	18.90	13.90	11.10	10.60	8.90	7.80	5.60	9.40	10.60	12.20	10.60
SD	3.08	4.55	7.39	6.36	5.65	4.74	5.94	5.58	7.91	11.11	7.18
MX + insert(11)	5.00	−0.90	−0.50	−0.90	−3.20	−2.30	3.20	11.80	13.20	20.00	14.50
SD	3.69	5.14	5.41	3.58	3.84	4.44	6.82	5.38	7.44	7.07	8.98
Hand-held MX(10)	30.80	25.00	17.80	11.10	4.40	1.50	2.00	2.00	6.00	18.00	6.70
SD	5.53	4.71	5.25	3.96	2.90	5.02	8.12	6.40	6.63	4.00	3.67

*re Zero HL, ISO 1964.

‡Numbers in parentheses indicate number of subjects who contributed data to the mean for the indicated test.

§Negative values indicate that the average hearing level was lower (better) than 0 dB HL.

TABLE 16-2. COMPARISON GROUP MEAN THRESHOLD DIFFERENCES* BETWEEN AND WITHIN CONDITIONS AND RANGES OF INDIVIDUAL DIFFERENCES FOR FIVE TEST CONDITIONS: †SOUND FIELD (SF), MX-41/AR CUSHION (MX), NAF CUSHION (NAF), HAND-HELD MX-41/AR CUSHION (MX), AND MX + INSERT.

Comparisons	Frequency (Hz)										
	125	250	500	750	1,000	1,500	2,000	3,000	4,000	6,000	8,000
MX vs SF(12)‡	...	6.7	4.2	1.7	2.1	2.5	-2.1	1.3	-1.3	-1.3	...
Range		5 to 15	0 to 10	-10 to 5	-10 to 5	-5 to 10	-10 to 10	-10 to 10	-10 to 5	-10 to 5	...
NAF$_1$ vs MX$_1$(9)§	12.2	14.4	9.4	8.9	11.7	10.6	6.7	8.3	5.6	0	1.7
Range	10 to 20	10 to 20	0 to 15	5 to 15	0 to 20	0 to 20	0 to 10	0 to 15	0 to 30	-15 to 20	-20 to 15
MX + insert vs MX$_1$(11)	-0.9	0	-0.9	-2.7	-3.6	0.9	4.6	10.5	6.8	9.6	12.3
Range	-5 to 5	-5 to 5	-5 to 5	-5 to 5	-15 to 0	-5 to 15	0 to 15	5 to 15	0 to 15	0 to 25	-20 to 25
Hand-held MX vs MX$_1$(10)	24.2	27.2	17.2	10.0	8.9	4.0	4.0	0.5	1.0	8.0	2.5
Range	10 to 35	20 to 35	15 to 20	0 to 20	5 to 15	-5 to 10	0 to 10	-5 to 10	-10 to 10	5 to 15	-5 to 5
MX$_1$ vs MX$_2$(11)§	0.9	-0.5	1.8	1.8	4.5	-0.9	-0.5	-0.5	1.8	0.9	-0.9
Range	-5 to 10	-5 to 5	-5 to 5	-5 to 10	-5 to 15	-5 to 5	-5 to 5	-5 to 10	-5 to 15	-10 to 10	-10 to 15
SF$_1$ vs SF$_2$(11)	...	0.9	1.4	0	0.5	-0.9	-2.3	1.8	0	2.3	...
Range		-5 to 10	-5 to 10	-5 to 15	-5 to 15	-5 to 5	-5 to 5	-5 to 10	-5 to 10	-5 to 10	...
NAF$_1$ vs NAF$_2$(9)	-0.6	1.1	0.6	-2.2	0.6	-1.1	-1.1	1.1	2.2	0.6	4.4
Range	-5 to 5	-5 to 5	-5 to 5	-10 to 0	-5 to 15	-10 to 5	-10 to 15	-10 to 10	-5 to 20	-20 to 20	-5 to 15

*A negative difference indicates that the second threshold of a comparison pair was poorer than the first. The same TDH-39 earphone was used with the NAF and MX cushions.

‡Numbers in parentheses indicate the number of difference scores and the number of subjects for each mean difference.

§Subscript 1 indicates first test and subscript 2 indicates retest.

Table 16-2 the mean threshold difference at 4,000 Hz was −1.3 dB indicating that the average sound-field threshold was 1.3 dB poorer than the average threshold obtained with the earphone and MX assembly. Similarly, the range of differences (−10 to 5 dB) shows that individual sound-field thresholds ranged from 10 dB poorer to 5 dB better than thresholds obtained with the earphone and MX assembly. Intermodality comparisons used the first set of thresholds obtained in each mode.

MX vs. Sound Field. The small mean differences shown in Table 16-2 for the MX vs Sound-field comparison indicate close correspondence between thresholds obtained in the two conditions for comparison group subjects. Except for 250 Hz, mean differences did not exceed 4.2 dB, and six of the nine were positive indicating lower sound-field thresholds, probably because of small calibration artifacts.

Of the 108 individual threshold differences computed for the MX vs sound-field comparison, 92 (85.2 percent) were 0 to 5 dB, and 15 (14 percent) were 10 dB. Only one difference (at 250 Hz) was 15 dB. On the basis of these results it was decided that a sound-field threshold for an experimental group subject had to be at least 15-dB lower (better) than the corresponding threshold under the MX cushion to be considered indicative of ear canal collapse.

NAF vs. MX. The mean threshold differences between the NAF and MX conditions shown in Table 16-2 for the comparison group ranged from 0 to 14.4 dB; between 125 and 4,000 Hz all differences were positive, indicating that a stronger signal was required at threshold with the NAF cushion. The largest intercondition mean differences were between 125 and 1,500 Hz. The sensitivity loss caused by our NAF cushion agrees well with data reported by Jerger and Tillman (1959) for a PDR-10 earphone in an NAF cushion.

Individual intercondition threshold differences were similar for most subjects but there was greater intersubject variability above 3,000 Hz. This is reflected in the 30 to 35 dB ranges of differences above 3,000 Hz. Although the range of individual differences for the NAF vs MX comparison exceeds the range of differences for the MX vs sound-field comparison, appropriate calibration corrections for the NAF cushion result in reasonably accurate threshold estimates in the 125 Hz to 3,000 Hz range.

Consequently the mean NAF vs MX differences, rounded to the nearest 5-dB interval, were used as corrections for audiometric zero for collapse group comparisons involving the NAF condition.

MX + Insert vs. MX. The ear insert had generally little effect on thresholds between 125 Hz and 1,500 Hz, but between 2,000 and 8,000 Hz, mean thresholds were 4.6 to 12.3 dB poorer with the insert than without it. The range of effects above 1,000 Hz was large—as great as 25 dB at 6,000 Hz and 45 dB at 8,000 Hz. These results are consistent with previous data (Chandler, 1964; Rupp et al., 1968) which show that an insert in the external ear canal attenuates high frequencies more than low frequencies. This underscores the problems associated with using inserts or earmolds to neutralize the attenuating effects of a collapsed ear canal.

Hand-Held MX vs. MX. Table 16-2 shows that at all frequencies the hand-held phone and MX cushion assembly produced poorer mean thresholds than the conventional arrangement. Intercondition mean differences below 1,500 Hz were especially large, ranging from 8.9 dB at 1,000 Hz to 24.2 dB at 250 Hz, but above 1,000 Hz all but one of the mean differences were less than 5 dB. Similarly, intersubject variability was relatively large below 1,000 Hz and relatively small at most frequencies above 1,000 Hz. These data suggest that a hand-held phone provides useful data above 1,000 Hz but causes gross threshold errors and larger intersubject variability below 1,500 Hz.

MX Test-Retest. Test-retest mean differences for the comparison group ranged from 0.5 to 4.5 dB for the MX condition. The close test-retest agreement is even more impressive if one considers that ten of the mean differences were between 0.5 and 1.8 dB and the 11th (1,000 Hz) was 4.5 dB. Of the 121 individual threshold differences reflected in these mean differences, 110 (91 percent) were 5 dB or less, nine (7.4 percent) were 10 dB, and two (1.7 percent) were 15 dB.

Sound Field Test-Retest. Test-retest mean differences for sound-field audiometry ranged from 0 to 2.3 dB in the comparison group. Of the 99 individual differences, 89 (90 percent) were 5 dB or less, eight (8 percent) were 10 dB, and two (2 percent) were 15 dB. At five of the nine test frequencies reliability was as good or better than reliability under the MX cushion and at the other four frequencies it was only slight poorer. If the data from one particularly variable subject are excluded, then 95 percent of the individual differences would be 5 dB or less and the other 5 percent would be 10 dB.

NAF Test-Retest. Table 16–2 shows that the comparison group's mean test-retest differences with the NAF cushion ranged from −2.2 dB to +2.2 dB in the 125 to 6,000 Hz range; at 8,000 Hz the mean difference was 4.4 dB. Of the 99 individual threshold differences, 86 (87 percent) were 5 dB or less, seven (7 percent) were 10 dB, three (3 percent) were 15 dB, and three (3 percent) were 20 dB. The six individual threshold differences that were greater than 10 dB were between 3,000 and 8,000 Hz and were assignable to three subjects. In the speech range, therefore, an NAF cushion permits reasonably good test-retest reliability even when the cushion and phone are removed and repositioned.

Collapse Group

Table 16–3 shows selected collapse group mean differences and ranges of individual differences between thresholds for various test conditions, with particular emphasis on differences between sound-field thresholds and thresholds for other conditions. In effect, sound-field thresholds (recomparison group performance) were used as a validity standard. After correction for calibration error all comparison group sound-field thresholds were within 10 dB of conventional thresholds (108 comparisons). It was assumed, therefore, that sound-field audiometry would provide valid resolution of the effects of collapsible canals. Test-retest data for sound-field audiometry were not obtained for the collapse group. However, the reliability of the sound-field procedure was amply demonstrated by the test-retest performance of the comparison group.

MX vs. Sound Field. The mean differences between the sound-field and MX conditions shown in Table 16–3 for the collapse group reflect the threshold decrement caused by collapse of the ear canal when the MX cushion was used. Mean differences range from 9.7 dB at 500 Hz to 33.8 dB at 3,000 Hz. Generally, the effect was greatest between 1,500 and 6,000 Hz, but the range of effects was wide at all frequencies, varying from insignificant 5-dB shifts to 40-dB and 50-dB shifts. There was wide intersubject variability in the frequencies affected and in magnitude of effects. One subject showed a 20-dB effect at only one frequency (6,000 Hz) while several had 20- to 45-dB shifts at almost all frequencies in the 250 to 6,000 Hz range.

NAF vs. Sound Field. Thresholds obtained in the sound field and under the NAF cushion were compared for six subjects. Six of the nine mean differences shown in Table 16–3 did not exceed 5 dB and the other three ranged from −6.7 to +9.2 dB. Of the 54 individual threshold differences, 51 (94.4 percent) did not exceed 10 dB and the remaining three (5.6 percent) were 15 and 20 dB. These data indicate the two measurement systems produced highly equivalent thresholds for most of the measurement range.

MX + Insert vs. Sound Field. Mean differences between sound-field thresholds and thresholds obtained with an ear insert ranged from 1.0 to 22.5 dB for the collapse group, indicating residual overestimates of thresholds at all test frequencies when the insert was used. At five of the nine frequencies the mean for the insert condition was more than 11 dB poorer than the sound-field mean. For one subject the insert resolved the effects of collapse almost as well as the sound-field procedure, but for most other subjects the insert provided only partial resolution at selected frequencies. In fact, two of the three subjects with the most collapse experienced negligible resolution with the insert.

Hand-Held MX vs. Sound Field. Table 16–3 shows that mean differences between sound-field thresholds and thresholds obtained with a hand-held phone and MX cushion assembly ranged from 1.4 to 28.6 dB. Sound-field means were better at all frequencies, but at lower frequencies the hand-held phone introduced large errors similar to those demonstrated with the comparison group.

Sound Field vs. BC. Table 16–3 shows mean threshold differences between sound-field and BC thresholds for the 11 collapse group subjects with pure sensorineural loss or normal hearing. This comparison was made to determine whether BC thresholds predict sound-field thresholds accurately when no conductive impairment exists. By operational definition

TABLE 16-3. COLLAPSE GROUP MEAN THRESHOLD DIFFERENCES* BETWEEN AND WITHIN CONDITIONS AND RANGES OF INDIVIDUAL DIFFERENCES FOR FIVE TEST CONDITIONS: †SOUND FIELD (SF), BONE CONDUCTION (BC), NAF CUSHION, HAND-HELD MX-41/AR CUSHION (MX) AND MX + INSERT.

Comparisons	\multicolumn{11}{Frequency (Hz)}										
	125	250	500	750	1,000	1,500	2,000	3,000	4,000	6,000	8,000
MX vs SF$_1$(12)‡§	...	12.9	9.7	12.1	15.4	21.7	24.2	33.8	25.8	25.4	...
Range	...	0 to 30	0 to 30	–5 to 25	–15 to 35	5 to 40	–5 to 40	10 to 50	5 to 45	5 to 45	...
NAF$_1$ vs SF$_1$(6)	...	–2.5	–0.8	–1.7	–6.7	0	0.8	5.0	6.7	9.2	...
Range	...	–5 to 0	–10 to 5	–10 to 5	–15 to 5	–5 to 5	–5 to 5	0 to 10	–5 to 15	0 to 20	...
MX + insert vs SF$_1$(10)	...	7.5	2.0	4.0	1.0	11.5	13.5	22.5	16.5	21.0	...
Range	...	–5 to 30	–10 to 25	–5 to 30	–20 to 30	–5 to 40	0 to 40	10 to 45	0 to 45	5 to 40	...
Hand-held MX vs SF$_1$(10)	...	28.6	17.1	9.3	1.4	5.5	3.5	6.5	7.5	10.5	...
Range	...	15 to 40	5 to 30	5 to 20	–10 to 15	–5 to 15	0 to 10	0 to 15	0 to 15	5 to 20	...
SF$_1$ vs BC(11)	...	–2.3	9.5	4.5	3.6	0	0.5	–3.0	4.5	...	...
Range	...	–10 to 5	0 to 35	–5 to 20	–10 to 15	–15 to 10	–10 to 15	–10 to 20	–15 to 15	...	...
NAF$_1$ vs NAF$_2$(6)§	–0.8	–0.8	0	–0.8	–4.2	–2.5	0.8	0	0.8	4.2	0
Range	–5 to 5	–5 to 5	–5 to 5	–5 to 5	–10 to 0	–5 to 0	–5 to 5	–5 to 5	–5 to 10	–5 to 10	–5 to 5

*A negative difference indicates that the second threshold of a comparison pair was poorer than the first. The same TDH-39 earphone was used with the NAF and MX cushions.
‡Numbers in parentheses indicate number of difference scores and the number of subjects for each mean difference.
§Subscript 1 indicates first test and subscript 2 indicates retest.

BC thresholds are accurate predictors of AC thresholds for individuals with no conductive pathology.

The largest mean difference between sound-field and BC thresholds for the collapse group was 9.5 dB at 500 Hz but at all other frequencies mean differences were 5 dB or less. It should be noted that prior audiometry demonstrated that the ear selected for study had BC sensitivity better than or equal to the BC sensitivity of the ear not under test.

Although there were individual comparisons in which sound-field thresholds were as much as 15 dB better or poorer than BC thresholds, 78 (91 percent) of the 86 sound-field thresholds were within ± 10 dB of the BC thresholds. Thus, when there is no conductive component BC thresholds are good predictors of the AC thresholds that should be obtained when the effects of collapse are overcome.

NAF Test-Retest. Table 16-3 shows test-retest data for the NAF condition for the six collapse group subjects on whom such data were gathered. Mean test-retest differences ranged from −4.2 to +4.2 dB; 61 (93.8 percent) of the 65 individual differences were 0 to 5 dB and the other four (6.2 percent) were 10 dB. These test-retest data equal or exceed comparison group performance at all frequencies.

Bilateral vs. Unilateral Effects. One subject in the collapse group had no hearing in one ear, hence it was not possible to determine whether the deaf ear was affected by collapse of the ear canal. Ten of the other 11 collapse group subjects had bilateral collapsible canals and all of the ten had more effect in one ear. Thus, all subjects with collapsible canals had more demonstrable effect in one ear, but there was no apparent predilection for right or left ears to be affected differentially: the left ear had larger effects in six subjects and the right had more effect in the other six. In all instances the ear with the larger effect was studied.

Mastoid-Helix Distance. The distance between the mastoid and helix of the test ear was measured for all subjects. The mean distance for the comparison group was 1.25 cm with individual values ranging from 0.9 to 1.7 cm. The mean for the collapse group was 1.76 cm with distances ranging from 1.1 to 2.8 cm. Seven subjects in the collapse group had mastoid-to-helix distances exceeding the largest value

in the comparison group (i.e., 1.7 cm for one subject). Although these data indicate that the auricles of subjects with collapsible canals tended to protrude more than those of comparison group subjects, it is not possible to say how many subjects were identified on the basis of their protruding ears. Further research is needed to resolve this question.

COMMENT

There are a number of problems involved in audiometry with patients who have collapsible external ear canals. Resolution of collapse effects is obviously far easier for threshold audiometry than for suprathreshold audiometry. Our data indicate that sound-field audiometry, under proper test conditions, is a valid and reliable method for overcoming collapsible canals. An NAF cushion with appropriate calibration corrections also provides valid and reliable results in the range most crucial for many clinical decisions.

Sound-field audiometry has the advantage of being applicable to a wide variety of patients, but some patients' thresholds are not measurable in the sound field unless special precautions are taken. For example, when one ear is normal, the other has a severe loss, and both canals are collapsible, the intense sound-field signals required to test the poorer ear may stimulate the normal ear by BC even when the better ear is maximally blocked by a solid ear insert and an attenuating muff. One solution to this dilemma is to mask the normal ear (using a circumaural cushion and phone assembly) while the poorer ear is tested in the sound field. Another alternative is to use circumaural cushion and phone assemblies for test and masking signals if the patient's ears are small enough to fit under the circumaural muff without being compressed or distorted.

We believe that some type of circumaural earphone assembly may ultimately be the most versatile approach to resolving the effects of collapsible ear canals for most patients. Procedures like Stenger tests, SISI, tone decay, ABLB, and masking are not adaptable to sound-field audiometry but could be accomplished with circumaural earphones. While there have been thoughtful reservations expressed about the limitations and calibration problems of circumaural earphones (Benson et al., 1967; Harris, 1968) there have also been encouraging reports by Atherley and his colleagues (Atherley et al., 1966, 1967) concerning a new circumaural earphone assembly that permits test-retest reliability in the 1,000 to 8,000 Hz range equivalent to or superior to results produced with a supra-aural device. Data for the lower frequencies were not reported. Shaw (1966) has commented on the theoretical advantages of a circumaural earphone assembly that would preserve a pressure distribution at the ear similar to that existing in a free field. His comments appear particularly relevant to the collapsible ear canal problem.

While the major emphasis of our study has been the accurate assessment of hearing in patients with collapsible external ear canals, an important prior concern is the determination of whether an ear canal collapses sufficiently to invalidate audiometry with supra-aural cushions. The literature on collapsible ear canals reflects an apparent widespread belief that visual inspection of the external ear is an efficient method for determining whether a significant effect exists.

We have found that visual inspection is subject to an unacceptable amount of error. In some instances visual inspection leaves no question about the existence of an effect, but in other instances it is difficult to visualize the extent of collapse.

We are not suggesting that visual inspection be abandoned. On the contrary, it seems prudent to inspect every patient's ears for narrow canals and closure caused by collapse. One way to accomplish this is to press the auricle against the head with a finger and observe the degree of closure. Another visual method is to apply pressure to the auricle with an empty MX-41/AR cushion and observe the degree of closure through the cushion aperture. These methods have limitations but they are useful adjuncts to the diagnostic process.

Lynn (1967) has proposed a related screening test for collapsible canals: an empty MX-41/AR cushion is placed over the ear in question and the stem of a vibrating tuning fork is placed on the patient's skull to see whether an occlusion effect is induced by collapse of the canal. Lynn points out that his technique is valid only for normal ears and ears with pure sensorineural loss. Unfortunately, the absence of a conductive component is sometimes difficult to establish until collapsible canals have been ruled out. Furthermore, patients with conductive impairment may be as likely to have collapsible canals as other patients.

Our data indicate that screening for collapsible canals can probably be accomplished efficiently by testing at 2,000, 3,000, and 4,000 Hz in the sound field, with a hand-held phone, or with a circumaural phone assembly. The best single frequency for screening might be 3,000 Hz since the largest mean effect we observed was at 3,000 Hz. Unless audiometry is used to screen for collapsible canals it may not be possible to make a positive judgment about whether an apparently collapsible ear canal collapses enough to produce significant audiometric error. It should be noted that the use of a hand-held phone is tedious, requires extreme care and usually requires a competent assistant.

There are certain audiometric relationships which can aid in evaluating the collapse phenomenon. For example, a conductive loss confined to frequencies above 1,000 Hz is reason to suspect the presence of collapsible canals. One group of investigators (Rupp et al., 1968) recommends that all patients with apparent AC-BC gaps should be suspected of having collapsible ear canals, a recommendation based on the earlier observation by Hildyard and Valentine (1962) that a patient with an AC-BC gap and a positive Rinne may have collapsible ear canals.

Available data do not permit refined statements about the prevalence of collapsible canals. For example, we do not know whether collapsible canals are more frequent in the elderly than in the young (Creston and Tice, 1964) even though we find this an attractive and testable hypothesis. It is possible that Hildyard and Valentine's (1962) 4 percent prevalence estimate is not a representative figure, even for a clinical sample. Their sampling procedure did not exclude collapsible canals in all patients but focused on those who satisfied one or more of three criteria (AC-BC gap in presence of positive Rinne, audiometric inconsistency, and discrepancy between ability to communicate and audiometric findings). Hildyard and Valentine's small average effects—6.9 dB at 4,000 Hz and 6.2 dB at 500 Hz—are inconsistent with our data which show appreciably more effect at 4,000 Hz than at 500 Hz. Creston's (1965) prevalence data for children must also be viewed cautiously. The details of his procedure were not spelled out and no subject was included unless he had 20 dB (re ASA 1951) or greater "loss" at two frequencies or 30 dB at one frequency. Furthermore, repeat audiograms conducted to resolve the problem were accomplished with ear inserts or by simply repositioning the earphones. Creston's (1965) data were gathered by people described only as "experienced audiometrists." On the other hand, both of these studies were valuable because they emphasized that collapsible ear canals may be far more common than clinicians had imagined a decade ago.

We believe that studies on the prevalence of collapsible ear canals should take account of test-retest errors that occur when earphones are positioned and repositioned on normal listeners. Atherley and Dingwall-Fordyce (1963) and Atherley and Lord (1965) have published estimates of test-retest differences which must be exceeded in normal ears before the differences can be considered statistically significant. At 4,000 and 6,000 Hz the difference must exceed 12.5 dB to be significant at the 0.05 level and at 8,000 Hz the difference must exceed 15 dB. At frequencies below 4,000 Hz the criterion value ranges between 7.5 dB and 10 dB. The extreme changes cited by Atherley and Dingwall-Fordyce are very close to the small number of extreme test-retest changes observed in a few of our comparison group subjects (Table 16–2, MX_1 vs MX_2). Consequently, it may be hazardous to identify a collapsible ear canal on the basis of threshold shifts smaller than 15 dB.

Further research is needed on the relations among collapsible ear canals, protruding auricles and other anatomical features. For example, the size and position of the tragus may be crucial. We have seen some tragi large enough to cover the canal orifice. A large tragus, an anterior meatus opening (Creston, 1965) and a collapsible canal may interact to produce maximum audiometric error. It remains to be seen whether most patients with collapsible ear canals have normal-appearing ears (Creston, 1965) or whether many have ears with identifying characteristics.

Finally, there should be additional work on test-retest variability related to collapsible canals. We did not study test-retest error under the MX cushion in the collapse group, but we did observe substantial differences between the identifying audiograms and the MX study data of some collapse group subjects. In fact, the collapse group subject with the least demonstrable effect demonstrated more effect on an earlier test. Many of the identifying audiograms of subjects in the collapse group were very similar to their experimental MX data. Headset tension, earphone placement, and the presence of cerumen in a canal may influence the magnitude of test-retest errors. We have suspected each of them in specific cases.

EDITORS' ENDNOTE

(Our continued experience has produced numerous examples of diagnostic and rehabilitative errors that may occur when routine screening is not conducted to identify collapsible ear canals. Clinicians who claim that they hardly ever (even never) encounter collapsible canals tend not to screen for the problem and may not be inclined to consider it as a possible cause of test-retest inconsistency and unexplained conductive loss (not just high-frequency conductive loss). Articles that have appeared since 1970 suggest that polyethylene tubing or plastic ear inserts continue to be used to maintain a canal lumen during audiometry with patients who have collapsible ear canals. Reported success with such devices can't be discounted; in a significant number of cases a patent canal may be maintained and result in significant, even complete, resolution of audiometric artifacts caused by a collapsible canal. The results of our study suggest that such apparent success may be offset by the fact that many collapsible ear canals have unusual characteristics (e.g., smallness, slit-like or anteriorly-placed openings, abrupt changes of direction and very large tragi) that can cause partial or complete obstruction of either end of the device, apart from the variable effects inserts may have on canal resonance. Errors in such cases may be particularly difficult to identify when there is significant middle ear pathology. The NAF cushions that were demonstrated so effective in our study are to the best of our knowledge no longer manufactured, but there is a clinical need for a circumaural cushion comparable to the NAF cushion (manufactured by Telephonics Corporation for Telephonics earphones) or for a new circumaural assembly like the one developed by Villchur (1969). In our opinion, future audiometer standardization should be directed to adopting a circumaural earphone assembly that does not compress the pinnae uncomfortably against the head. If such a device were adopted, collapsible ear canals would be eliminated as an audiometric problem and patients would be relieved of the discomfort associated with MX-41/AR cushions. Meanwhile, clinicians will have to employ devices and calibration methods that minimize calibration error. J.B.C., M.E.M., April 1981.)

REFERENCES

Atherley, G.R.C., and Lord, P. A preliminary study of the effect of earphone position on the reliability of repeated auditory threshold determination. *Int. Audiology* 4: 161–166, 1965.

Atherley, G.R.C., and Dingewall-Fordyce, I. The reliability of repeated auditory threshold determination. *Brit. J. Industr. Med.* 20: 231–235, 1963.

Atherley, G.R.C.; Hempstock, T.I.; Lord, P.; et al. Reliability of auditory threshold determinations using a circumaural-earphone assembly. *J. Acoust. Soc. Amer.* 42: 199–203, 1967.

Atherley, G.R.C.; Lord, P; and Walker, J.G. Basis for the design of a circumaural earphone suitable for MAP determinations. *J. Acoust. Soc. Amer.* 40: 607–613, 1966.

Bauer, B.B.; Allan, J.R.; and Abbagnaro, L.A. External-ear replica for acoustical testing. *J. Acoust. Soc. Amer.* 42: 204–207, 1967.

Benson, R.W.; Charan, K.K.; Day. J.W.; et al. Limitations on the use of circumaural earphones (LTE). *J. Acoust. Soc. Amer.* 41: 713–714, 1967.

Berland, O. and Nielsen, E. Sound pressure generated in the human external ear by a free sound field. *Audecibel* 18: 103–109, 1969.

Carhart, R. and Jerger, J.F. Preferred method for clinical determination of pure-tone thresholds. *J. Speech Hearing Dis.* 24: 330–345, 1959.

Chaiklin, J.B. and Ventry, I.M. Spondee threshold measurement: A comparison of 2- and 5-dB methods. *J. Speech Hearing Dis.* 29: 47–59, 1964.

Chandler, J.R. Partial occlusion of the external auditory meatus: Its effect upon air and bone conduction hearing acuity. *Laryngoscope* 74: 22–54, 1964.

Creston, J.E. Collapse of the ear canal during routine audiometry. *J. Laryng. and Oto.* 79: 893–901, 1965.

Creston, J.E., and Tice, R.E. Collapse of the ear canal during audiometry: Observation in siblings. *Arch. Otolaryng.* 79: 389–392, 1964.

Erber, N.P. Variables that influence sound pressures generated in the ear canal by an audiometric earphone. *J. Acoust. Soc. Amer.* 44: 555–562, 1968.

Harris, J.D. *The Use of Circumaural Earphones in Audiometry.* Report No. 540, Groton, Conn. US Naval Submarine Center, July 15, 1968, pp. 1–13.

Hildyard, V.H., and Valentine, M.A. Collapse of the ear canal during audiometry: A further report. *Arch. Otolaryng.* 75: 422–423, 1962.

Jerger, J.F., and Tillman, T.W. Effect of earphone cushion on auditory threshold (LTE). *J. Acoust. Soc. Amer.* 31: 1264, 1959.

Juers, A.L. Pure tone-speech hearing discrepancy. *Eye Ear Nose Throat Monthly* 48: 28–31, 1969.

Lynn, G.E. A test to detect collapse of the external ear canal during audiometry. *J. Speech Hearing Dis.* 32: 273–274, 1967.

Lynn, G.E. Effects of collapsed auditory canals during audiometry. *Maico Audiological Library Series,* report 8, 1969.

Ross, M., and Tucker, C.A. A case study of collapse of the ear canal during audiometry. *Laryngoscope* 75: 65–67, 1965.

Rupp, R.R.; Milinsky, L.; and Jackson, P. The identification and resolution of audiometrically induced hearing loss due to collapsed canals. Read before the convention of the American Speech and Hearing Association, 1968.

Shaw, E.A.G. Ear canal pressure generated by circumaural and supra-aural earphones. *J. Acoust. Soc. Amer.* 39: 471–479, 1966.

Shaw, E.A.G. Ear canal pressure generated by a free sound field. *J. Acoust. Soc. Amer.* 39: 465–470, 1966.

Smith, C.R. Collapsing ear canals (LTE). *J. Speech Hearing Res.* 9: 317, 1966.

Stark, E.W. Collapse of the ear canal during audiometry: A case report. *J. Speech Hearing Dis.* 31: 374–376, 1966.

Teranishi, R., and Shaw, E.A.G. External-ear acoustic models with simple geometry. *J. Acoust. Soc. Amer.* 44: 257–263, 1968.

Ventry, I.M.; Chaiklin, J.B.; and Boyle, W.F. Collapse of the ear canal during audiometry. *Arch. Otolaryng.* 73: 727–731, 1961.

Villchur, E. Free-field calibration of earphones. *J. Acoust. Soc. Amer.* 46: 1527–1534, 1969.

17

Vibrotactile Thresholds in Pure Tone Audiometry

ARTHUR BOOTHROYD, Ph.D.
*Director of Research and Clinical Services,
The Clarke School for the Deaf,
Northampton, Massachusetts*
SHEILA CAWKWELL, B.A.
*a degree candidate at the University of
Manchester, Manchester, England, when this
study was conducted*

*Research into vibrotactile sensations at the ear is complicated by the problem of
distinguishing them from auditory sensations. Normal hearing subjects may have
difficulty in dissociating the two sensations while profoundly deaf subjects may
never have experienced an auditory sensation. This paper describes experiments
with unilaterally deaf subjects. It was found that they could consistently distinguish between the two sensations and could therefore give a measure of vibrotactile
threshold. The results indicated that vibrotactile responses are very probable when
testing profoundly deaf subjects with a standard clinical audiometer, and that individuals vary considerably in their vibrotactile sensitivity. It was not found possible
to predict vibrotactile sensitivity at the ear from that at the fingertips.*

It has long been known that when sound vibrations
reach a sufficiently high intensity, they may be perceived through the sense of touch. The relationship
between this vibrotactile sensitivity and auditory sensitivity has been studied by a number of writers, but
the implications of their findings in clinical audiology
have not, in general, been widely recognized.

It is important in testing severely or profoundly
deaf subjects to know at what levels one should
expect responses to vibrotactile stimulation. To
report vibrotactile air conduction thresholds may
lead to the assumption of residual hearing when, in
fact, none exists, while reporting similar thresholds
in bone conduction testing may lead to the faulty
diagnosis of a middle ear condition through the presence of an apparent air/bone gap.

In Figure 17–1 are shown the thresholds for vibrotactile sensitivity to air-borne sounds which have
been reported by various workers. The data of Wegel
(1922, 1932) and of Fletcher (1953) were obtained
from normal listeners reporting "feeling" sensations
as a result of high energy stimulation. It will be seen
that these thresholds are generally higher than those
given for deaf subjects. An early determination of
vibrotactile thresholds of "deafmutes" was made by
Schindler (1936) and the values found by him are
very similar to those given by more recent workers
(Groen, 1950; Langenbeck, 1965; Barr, 1954; Nober,
1967). The results which show the most disagreement
with the general trend are those of Barr who indicates
vibrotactile thresholds at levels of 100 dB for frequencies of 1 and 2 kHz. It should, however, be
pointed out that Barr's results show the lowest
thresholds of 38 "totally deaf" children and Barr
himself felt that these responses could equally well
have been to vibrotactile or auditory stimulation.

In bone conduction audiometry, the problem of
vibrotactile stimulation becomes more acute. This is

Based on "Vibrotactile Thresholds in Pure Tone Audiometry"
by S. Bayne, (now Cawkwell) Diploma Dissertation, Manchester University.
Reprinted by permission from *Acta Otolaryng.*, **69**, 381–387
(1970).

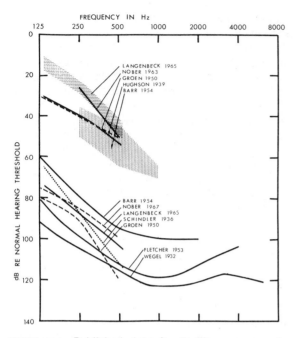

FIGURE 17-1. Published data for tactile responses to sound by bone conduction (*upper curves*) and by air conduction (*lower curves*). As far as we know, all the air conduction data were obtained using earphones. The data published with reference to physical zero has been corrected to the ISO (1964) threshold values. Data published in Europe prior to 1964 and expressed with reference to clinical zero has been left unchanged. All the bone conduction data are given as published. In view of the difficulties of international standardization of bone conduction thresholds, it is probable that the reference levels vary from writer to writer.

because the vibrator is specifically designed to transmit mechanical vibrations to the mastoid region. In consequence of this, the phenomenon has been more widely recognized in relationship to bone conduction testing. In a survey of the population of a school for the deaf, Hughson et al. (1939) felt that the bone conduction thresholds obtained at 128 and 256 Hz were definitely the result of vibrotactile stimulation, although they were satisfied that the higher frequency thresholds were auditory. Many writers have referred to this aspect of bone conduction audiometry without giving quantitative data. For example, Newby (1964) has said, ". . . at 250 Hz the patient may respond to the vibrations of the oscilla-

tor without actually hearing the tone" (*Audiology,* p. 81). Similarly, Portmann & Portmann (1961) say, "one must explain (to the patient) that with the low tones, for example, it is the threshold of auditory sensation which is being looked for (sonorous) and not the threshold of tactile sensation (vibratory)" (*Clinical Audiometry,* p. 11). More recently, Reger (1965) has stated ". . . patients with severe hearing losses for bone conducted sounds may respond to the vibrator with the vibration sense (pallesthesia) before the bone conduction threshold is stimulated, thereby giving a false result" (*Audiometry: Principles and Practices,* ed. Glorig, "Pure Tone Audiometry," p. 120).

Quantitative data on vibrotactile thresholds in bone conduction testing have been given by Groen (1950), Langenbeck (1965), and Barr (1954) and are illustrated in Figure 17-1. Also shown in the figure are the results of Nober (1963, 1964) who has carried out perhaps the most extensive work on this aspect of the problem.

Several workers have referred to the possibility of other types of response to sound vibration. For example, Bocca & Perani (1960) have suggested that the bone conduction thresholds of severely deaf patients may represent "vestibular hearing." Similarly the "feeling" thresholds for air borne sounds found by Wegel (1932) were reported by his subjects to produce sensations which could be related to vestibular disturbance, and Schindler (1936) quotes threshold results for "influence of the vestibular apparatus" which are different from those produced by vibrotactile stimulation of the ear. Nober (1964) does not accept the theory of vestibular hearing, however, one of his strongest arguments being based on the similar configuration of bone conduction thresholds of profoundly deaf subjects and their vibrotactile thresholds at the fingertips.

While many educators may have acclaimed the discovery of "residual hearing" in a large percentage of the deaf population without a critical examination of the possible interpretations of the experimental evidence, others have recognized the possibility that much, so-called residual hearing may be tactile. Several, however, have proceeded to use vibrotactile sensitivity as a possible channel of communication. For example, van Uden (1958) has stated, ". . . all deaf children can react to sound in the ears . . . in a certain percentage of our deaf children these reactions seem to be very similar to vibration feeling. It seems to be probable that these children have only vibration feeling in the ears." He has, however, developed educational techniques to make maximum use of this sensitivity.

Emphasis on the vibrotactile sense has also been placed by Guberina (1963) who has transmitted information through vibrators placed on various parts of the body. He has stated ". . . it is not by pure chance that a deaf person remains sensitive to the low frequencies which are commonly called 'vibrations'." It is not clear why Guberina should put vibrations in quotes. The point in question is not the physical nature of the stimulus, which is undoubtedly vibratory, but of the sensory modality through which it is perceived. Possibly, Guberina feels it unnecessary to make a distinction between the auditory and tactile sensations and wishes to emphasize the communication value of the tactile sense.

The relevance of vibrotactile sensitivity to the fitting of hearing aids has been discussed by Bellefleur & Smith (1967). Again, these writers have made the point that perception through the tactile sense does not necessarily imply the inability of deaf people to benefit from amplified sound.

In examining the thresholds quoted in the literature for responses to vibrotactile stimulation, two points should be borne in mind. Firstly, normal hearing subjects must experience a simultaneous auditory sensation when exposed to sound intensities sufficient to produce vibrotactile stimulation within the usual frequency range of pure tone audiometry. Under these conditions, the two are perceived as a whole and unless the observer is able to dissociate the sensations he may be unaware of the vibrotactile element until it is well above threshold levels. This may account for the higher thresholds found by Wegel and Fletcher. Secondly, when using profoundly deaf subjects it is difficult to decide whether they are responding to an auditory or a vibrotactile sensation, since a person who is sufficiently deaf as to have no experience of auditory sensations will be unable to make the subjective distinction. Those with true residual hearing may be able to do this, however. Barr (1954) quotes the case of a deaf boy who, after many years of testing, informed the tester that his responses to air conduction testing were to an auditory sensation while his responses to bone conduction testing were to a tactile sensation. Because of their inability to give a reliable subjective report as to the

nature of the sensation it has generally been necessary, in interpreting the results of tests on profoundly deaf subjects, to infer this from such features as air/bone gaps in populations with no middle ear disorders, the similarity of threshold configurations with those obtained from vibrotactile stimulation of non-auditory areas, the uniformity of threshold curves among populations having various causes of deafness, and the differential reaction to masking of the auditory and vibrotactile thresholds (Nober 1963–1964 and 1967). Recent work by Risberg (1968) however, indicates that it may be possible to reliably distinguish auditory from tactile responses in terms of the discrimination of periodic and aperiodic sounds.

It has apparently been overlooked that a ready source of experimental material exists in the form of subjects with profound unilateral deafness. Such subjects have virtually normal auditory perception, but at the same time, it is possible to investigate their responses to high intensity stimulation of the deaf ear. The present paper describes the results of a pilot study carried out on unilaterally deaf subjects and although the sample was small, it was felt that the results were sufficiently definitive to warrant publication at this stage.

Aims of the Experiment

The aims of the experiment were as follows:

1. to determine whether unilaterally deaf subjects could reliably distinguish between vibrotactile and auditory sensations at the deaf ear;
2. to determine the range of vibrotactile threshold responses to be expected in air conduction and bone conduction testing;
3. to see whether vibrotactile thresholds of a region remote from the ear could be used in predicting thresholds at the ear.

Subjects

Nine subjects aged between 10 and 15 years were used in the experiments. Each had previously been diagnosed as having a profound unilateral deafness with normal or near normal hearing in the better ear. Seven of the subjects were boys and two were girls. Choice of age range and individual subjects within this range were determined by accessibility in a school population close to the University of Manchester, the setting for this research.

EQUIPMENT

A Peters Audiometer Type AP6 was used for all threshold measurements. This was fitted with a 20 dB booster to permit air conduction testing at levels above those normally available on clinical audiometers. Thresholds for vibrotactile stimulation of the fingertips were determined with the bone conduction vibrator of the audiometer, the reference level being that of the auditory thresholds for mastoid placement in normal hearing subjects. Pressure at the fingertips was applied by a device designed for earlier research by Wilson (1967), which was arranged to apply a force of 300 g weight. This is approximately equal to the force applied by the headband in normal bone conduction testing.

PROCEDURE

The frequencies used for threshold determinations were 250, 500, 750, 1,000 and 2,000 Hz. Under all test conditions, it was necessary to mask the better ear of the test subject. That this should be necessary in both air and bone conduction testing is obvious, but even when measuring thresholds at the fingertips sufficient sound was radiated from the vibrator and heard by the subject through the better ear to make the distinction between auditory and tactile sensations extremely difficult. In the bone conduction tests, measurements were also made at 4,000 Hz, but no responses were obtained at the maximum level available. The required masking levels were too high to permit air conduction tests at this frequency. Narrow band masking was used throughout and the shadow technique of Hood (1960) was employed. This involved determining threshold levels for increasing levels of masking, it being assumed that sufficient masking was employed when the measured threshold was independent of masking level for a range of 20 dB of masking. Throughout the testing, the subject was questioned as to the nature of the sensation to which he was responding, and he was instructed to respond regardless of the nature of this

sensation. Care was taken not to influence his answers by such questions as "Can you feel it yet?," but rather "Tell me whether you hear it or feel it."

RESULTS

Figure 17–2 shows the median values and ranges of vibrotactile thresholds determined in the experiment. All of the subjects were able, without difficulty, to distinguish between auditory and tactile sensations. At the fingertips and at the mastoid, all nine subjects reported that the threshold levels finally determined were of a tactile sensation. However, one of the nine subjects reported that the masked air conduction threshold was that of an auditory sensation. The threshold levels of this ninth subject are shown in Figure 17–3, and it will be seen that the air conduction threshold was well outside the range of vibrotactile thresholds obtained from the other eight subjects.

No evidence was found of a positive correlation between sensitivity at the ear and at the fingertips.

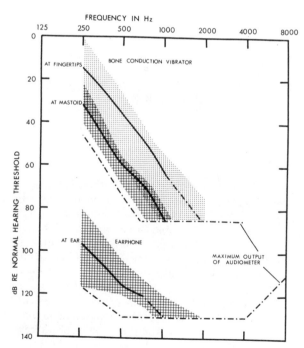

FIGURE 17-2. Heavy lines show the median values of vibrotactile thresholds found in the experiments. The ranges of threshold values are indicated by the shaded areas.

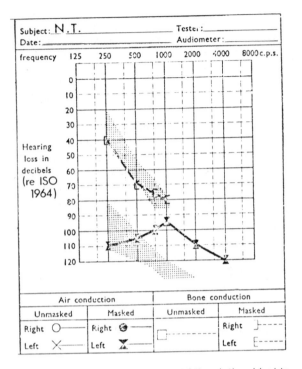

Subject: N.T. Tester:
Date: Audiometer:

FIGURE 17-3. Threshold responses of the ninth subject to stimulation of the "deaf" ear. His subjective report was that the bone conduction thresholds were to vibrotactile stimulation while the air conduction thresholds were to auditory stimulation. A comparison with the thresholds of the other eight subjects is given.

DISCUSSION

A striking feature of the results is the wide range of vibrotactile thresholds, particularly at the fingertips and for low frequency earphone stimulation. Had more consistent thresholds been found, it might have been possible to indicate a line on the audiogram form below which vibrotactile sensations would almost certainly be experienced by a test subject. However, one can say that within the shaded areas shown in Figure 17-3, there is a strong possibility of the occurrence of vibrotactile stimulation, and that a deaf subject whose air and bone conduction thresholds fall within or below these areas might well be totally deaf.

It was hypothesized that the sensitivity at the fingertips of an individual subject might be used to predict his vibrotactile sensitivity at the ear. How-ever, no correlation was found and such prediction does not appear possible.

It will be seen from Figures 17–1 and 17–2 that the vibrotactile thresholds found in this experiment are similar to those found by other researchers, the most noticeable exceptions being the high frequency air conduction thresholds given by Barr. On the basis of the present findings one would assume that thresholds of 100 dB at 1 and 2 kHz most probably indicate the presence of true residual hearing.

It is important to examine the vibrotactile thresholds in relation to the maximum output of standard clinical audiometers. Without the 20 dB booster available on the machine used in this experiment, air conduction thresholds would have been measurable only at frequencies of 500 Hz and below, and then only for two or three subjects. Similarly an audiometer whose bone conduction output is limited to 65 dB would not have been able to produce vibrotactile stimulation of the mastoid area in any of the nine subjects at frequencies above 500 Hz. However, even with a standard clinical audiometer there is a possibility that reported thresholds will be those of a vibrotactile sensation in a certain percentage of profoundly deaf subjects for frequencies of 500 Hz and below.

It is not surprising that the sensitivity of test subjects was generally better at the fingertips than at the mastoid. This has a direct implication for the use of hearing aids with certain profoundly deaf subjects, however, since those with particularly low sensitivity at the ear may benefit more from amplification by stimulation of the hand. Experiments along these lines have been begun by one of us (A.B.), in which a bone conduction vibrator is attached to a high power hearing aid and worn in the hand, using a specially designed mitten. With this device several children have demonstrated improved voice control and are now able to participate in sound perception activities along with their classmates.*

*(After several years of trial, I discontinued the use of vibrotactile hearing aids with totally deaf children. Although it was possible to demonstrate improved aided thresholds and discrimination of time envelope patterns in a clinical setting, the problems of signal to noise ratio and low information content were considerable. The practical benefits in terms of language and speech development were therefore very small and did not appear to justify the inconvenience. Other researchers have studied the potential role of frequency transposition and vocoding in both vibrotactile and electrotactile devices, but the educational potential of these techniques is still uncertain. January 7, 1980.)

Further research is required into the influence of transducer design, age of subject and cause of hearing loss on measured vibrotactile thresholds, the development of reliable methods of distinguishing vibrotactile from auditory responses in individual subjects and on the perceptual possibilities of the vibrotactile response in profoundly deaf subjects.

CONCLUSION

The following conclusions were drawn from the findings of this experiment:

1. that subjects with profound monaural hearing losses can consistently distinguish vibrotactile from auditory sensations and may therefore be used in experiments on vibrotactile sensitivity at the ear.

2. that individuals may differ considerably in their vibrotactile sensitivity.

3. that if an individual gives audiometric thresholds within the shaded areas shown in Figure 17–3, there is a strong possibility of their being the thresholds of a vibrotactile sensation.

4. that vibrotactile sensitivity at the ear could not be predicted from that at the fingertips.

ACKNOWLEDGMENTS

The authors wish to thank Professor Taylor of the University of Manchester for permission to publish this material. Thanks are also due to the children who acted as experimental subjects, to their parents, and to Mr. G. Hart, peripatetic teacher of the deaf for the County of Lancashire, who made his files available and assisted with the selection of test subjects.

REFERENCES

Barr, B. 1954. Pure tone audiometry for pre-school children. *Acta Otolaryng* (Stockh.) Suppl. **110.**

Bellefleur, P. A. & Smith, S. 1967. Audition or vibration. *Hearing Dealer* **17,** 11.

Bocca, D. & Perani, G. 1960. Further contributions to the knowledge of vestibular hearing. *Acta Otolaryng* (Stockh.) **51.**

Fletcher, H. 1953. *Speech and Hearing in Communication,* chap. 8. Van Nostrand, New York.

Groen, J. J. 1950. Electrische Verstärker für Taubstummen. *Int Cong on the Care of Deafmutes,* Groningen.

Guberina, P. 1963. Verbotonal method and its application to the rehabilitation of the deaf. *American Instructors of the Deaf Forty-first Convention,* Gallaudet College, p. 275.

Hood, J. D. 1960. The principles and practice of bone conduction audiometry. *Laryngoscope* **70,** 1211.

Hughson, W., Ciocco, A. & Palmer, C. 1939. Studies of the pupils of the Pennsylvania School for the Deaf. *Arch Otolaryng* (Chic.) **29,** 403.

Langenbeck, B. 1965. *Textbook of Practical Audiometry.* Williams and Wilkins, Baltimore.

Newby, H. A. 1964. *Audiology.* Appleton-Century-Crofts, New York.

Nober, E. H. 1963. Pure tone air conduction thresholds of deaf children. *Volta Rev* **65,** 229.

— 1964. Pseudo auditory bone conduction thresholds. *J S H Dis* **29,** 469.

— 1967. Vibrotactile sensitivity of deaf children to high intensity sound. *Laryngoscope* **78,** 2128.

Portmann, M. & Portmann, C. 1961. *Clinical Audiometry.* Thomas, Illinois.

Reger, S. N. 1965. Pure Tone Audiometry. In *Audiometry: Principles and Practices* (ed. Glorig). Williams and Wilkins, Baltimore.

Risberg, A. 1968. Periodic-nonperiodic test of hearing capacity. Speech Transmission Laboratory. *Quarterly Progress and Status Report. 2–3,* April–September, 1968, p. 19.

Schindler, B. 1936. Das Schallfühlen der Taubstummen und Seine Praktische Bedeutung. *Arch Ohrenheik* **39,** 431.

Van Uden, A. 1958. A sound perceptive method. In *The Modern Educational Treatment of Deafness* (ed. Ewing). Manchester University Press.

Wegel, R. L. 1922. Physical examination of hearing. *Proc Nat Acad Sci U.S.A.* **8,** 7.

— 1932. Physical data and physiological excitation of the auditory nerve. *Ann Otol* **41,** 740.

Wilson, G. E. 1967. *Comparisons of forehead and mastoid thresholds in bone conduction audiometry.* Diploma Dissertation, Manchester University. Unpublished.

18

On the Importance of the Question: What Do You Hear?

F. Blair Simmons, M.D.
Professor of Otolaryngology, Stanford University School of Medicine
Richard F. Dixon, Ph.D.
Director, Division of Communication Disorders, University of North Carolina at Greensboro

The utilitarian ubiquitousness of the audiometer has advanced clinical otology more than any tool of recent times, nor does its promise for the future seem dim. Yet this very success breeds danger—failure to appreciate the audiometer's innate limitations. The audiometer is not a substitute for clinical acumen. It cannot, for example, ask the patient what he hears during a test. The situation demands only that the subject respond by raising a finger or pressing a button, etc.

Our concern for this rather obvious fact lies in the observation that there seems to be an increasing tendency toward substitution of the techniques of electronic audiometry for careful questioning of patients with hearing losses. (Observe, for example, the number of audiograms published without comment about the patient's subjective observations of sounds in general, or even comments relevant to the audiometric tones themselves.) Perhaps this trend is due to the authoritarian appeal of lines on a graph, or to the convenience of relegating hearing testing to an office technician, or perhaps to failure to appreciate the severity of the audiometer's limitations in certain cases. Whatever the cause, the trend definitely seems to exist and can lead to diagnostic error.

Through the medium of a particular case, this article attempts to underscore one type of error that can occur. During this man's audiometric evaluation, he dutifully "raised his finger," through virtually every common clinical test. Yet, after many hours of testing, the most significant characteristic of his hearing loss remained unknown because not one examiner asked the question: *What do you hear?*

A 61-year-old male amateur musician and hi-fi enthusiast was in good health and was aware of no particular hearing problem until 12:45 PM on August 5. Then while driving his car, he felt slightly lightheaded and noted a severe hearing loss in his right ear. Two hours later he was examined by a resident otolaryngologist who described the patient's complaints: ". . . a sudden onset of hearing loss, rushing tinnitus and unsteady sensation involving the right ear." Except for the hearing loss, the neurological examination was normal. There was, however, a past history of a mild bilateral hearing loss and a vague vestibular disturbance five years earlier.

Figure 18-1 shows the audiogram taken by the resident immediately prior to the patient's admission to the hospital with a working diagnosis of "vascular spasm." Intravenous histamine therapy was initiated after consultation with a member of the clinical staff. Approximately three hours after admission, a second audiogram was taken (unchanged), and the other measurements shown in Figure 18-1 were obtained. Speech discrimination was poor (as estimated by running speech and a few words of one syllable). Vestibular examination by electronystagmography showed a type II (Nylen) left-beating positional nystagmus, most marked in the left lateral head position.

At this time, the presence of nearly complete recruitment and minimal tone decay seemed to confirm the admitting diagnosis, a cochlear lesion producing moderately severe damage between 125 and 2,000 cps. However, we felt that the supposed etiology of the loss was doubtful because the audiometric evidence strongly suggested a good deal of residual function in the involved apical half of the cochlea. Consequently, causes other than vascular spasm were considered including acute labyrinthine hydrops (edema), intracochlear hemorrhage, and

Reprinted by permission of the authors from *Arch. Otolaryng.*, **80**, 167–169 (1964). Copyright 1964, American Medical Association.

detachment, or rupture, of a scala media structure, cause unknown. (It was assumed that the bilateral high-frequency loss did not directly relate to the acute right-sided loss.)

This diagnostic uncertainty led, in the following 36 hours, to further audiological evaluation during which two more examiners were involved. Additional information thus obtained is shown in Figure 18–2. The Békésy audiogram and more recruitment studies still suggested an intracochlear lesion. Note that the speech discrimination score was 0 percent.

Not shown in Figure 18–2 are results of at least six pure-tone audiograms, which remained unchanged during three days of hospitalization. Four persons had been involved actively in conducting these hearing studies, and several others had reviewed the results. Yet at no time during the tests had any one actually asked the patient, who was considered an excellent listener, *What do you hear?*

By this time, the patient had made some rather astute observations of his own: All sounds had a high-pitched metalic quality—a ringing sensation.

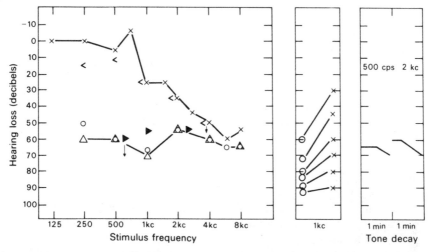

FIGURE 18-1. Pure tone audiogram, 1 kc binaural alternate loudness balance, 500 cps and 2 kc tone decay measurements obtained shortly after right-sided hearing loss.

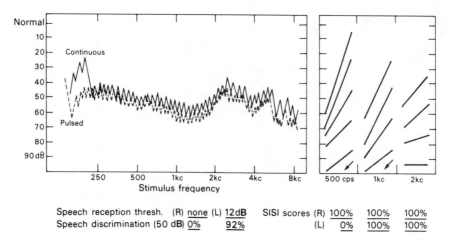

	(R)	(L)				
Speech reception thresh.	none	12dB	SISI scores (R)	100%	100%	100%
Speech discrimination (50 dB)	0%	92%	(L)	0%	100%	100%

FIGURE 18-2. Continuous and interrupted-stimulus Békésy audiogram of right ear and other test results obtained 24 to 48 hours after hearing loss.

Paper being crumpled sounded like broken glass being stirred in a metal bowl. Rubbing the skin of the ear sounded like rubbing the rim of a wine glass. Speech and other sounds seemed to reverberate in the ear.

These observations seemed a little bizarre, compared to the usual type of subjective dysacousic complaint. It occurred to us that both the patient's observations and the lack of speech discrimination might be explained by an abnormally prolonged damping of sound waves within the cochlea. Subsequently, on the fourth day, some special tests were administered to examine this hypothesis. The results were inconclusive after two hours of testing. Then as a final task the patient was asked to make some differential pitch judgments and *was* asked, What do you hear? The pitch studies proved to be most revealing and added significant information to the understanding of the hearing problem. They suggested, in fact, a lesion completely destroying the apical half of the cochlea.

The patient was completely unable to assign any pitch sensation whatsoever to frequencies in the lower portion of the hearing range tested, 200–730 cps; he noted only a "buzzing" sensation which varied somewhat in loudness. He was first able to assign a pitch to 750 cps but was unable to differentiate it from 1,000 cps, except for a slight increase in loudness. At still higher frequencies his difference limen for frequency was also poor, requiring an approximate 10 percent change in frequency.

The point in this story is a simple one. If the question, What do you hear? had been asked during any one of the pure-tone audiograms, a good deal of confused thinking could have been avoided. In retrospect the patient's audiograms were not, in fact, true *pure-tone* measurements at all below 1,000 cps. Rather, they signified the sound level at which he first heard an atonal buzz. This percept was also present for the Békésy tracings, for tone decay, and for SISI tests. Perhaps the most remarkable feat of all was his binaural alternate loudness balance at 500 cps, which was actually a balance between a buzz and a tone. Thus, these scores had one meaning from the audiometric reports, and perhaps quite a different meaning when interpreted in the light of the patient's sensations.

This case is unusual but far from unique. There are at least two other situations involving pure-tone acuity measurements where the patient's sensations have little or no relationship to the intended stimulus. Most clinicians are familiar with instances where patients with sharply falling audiograms hear clicks or noise when high-frequency tones are presented with the interrupter switch. Also an article by Carhart reports an instance where the patient apparently was responding to aural harmonics of the stimulus tones; this was determined only after the clinician investigated the nature of the patient's experience during the test.

The numbers on the frequency dial of an audiometer describe only generally the stimulus presented to the patient. The numbers themselves provide no information concerning harmonics of the stimulus frequency nor existence of possible unwanted transients.

Thus in some instances, the patient's report of the subjective sensation may bear little or no resemblance to the stimulus, the pure-tone audiogram being completed without the patient or the examiner being aware of anything unusual. To record the listener's "yes" response on an audiogram below a specific frequency heading may be misleading. The gap between audiometry and an adequate evaluation of hearing still exists. Perhaps a more persistent use of the question, *What do you hear?* will help to bridge it.

REFERENCE

Carhart, R. Atypical Audiometric Configurations Associated With Otosclerosis, *Ann Otol* **71**: 744–758 (Sept.) 1962.

19

Intertest Variability and the Air-Bone Gap

GERALD A. STUDEBAKER, Ph.D
*Professor of Speech and Hearing Science,
Memphis State University*

Among those concerned with the measurement of hearing loss there is a widespread belief that bone-conduction thresholds cannot be worse than air-conduction thresholds. Although an unqualified statement to this effect is rarely seen in the literature it is often heard in beginning audiology classes and is very often heard in lectures on audiogram interpretation given by "experts" to various medical and paramedical groups.

The reasoning usually is as follows: the air-conduction threshold is a measure of the sensitivity of the entire auditory system while the bone-conduction threshold is a measure of the sensitivity of only that part of the system excluding the outer and middle ear. Since a loss of sensitivity in part of a system cannot exceed the loss in the whole system, bone-conduction thresholds cannot be worse than air-conduction thresholds.

This argument is accurate as far as it goes, but it does not go far enough. Concluding the discussion at this point fails to take into consideration the very real subject of measurement variability and implies an exactitude of measurement which cannot be achieved in practice. This failure to discuss the effect of measurement variability on the air-bone relationship may be an effort to simplify the presentation or it may represent a lack of basic understanding on the part of the lecturer. In either case, it does create in idea about the air-conduction, bone-conduction threshold relationship which is misleading and which can result in several unfortunate consequences.

For example, the failure of test results in actual practice always to conform to "the way it is supposed to turn out" may make the inexperienced and insecure clinician anxious about his test findings. The tendency is to tamper with the test results or, at least, to be biased as to what is accepted as threshold. Even

experienced clinicians modify bone-conduction calibration values if bone-conduction thresholds are as much as 10 dB worse than air-conduction thresholds in more than a very rare instance. Those who view these "modified" audiograms become even more convinced that "bone cannot be worse than air" and the circle is thus completed. Finally, those who hold this belief may reach the conclusion, when viewing audiograms based on accurate calibration, that the results are invalid or that the audiologist is incompetent.

The following discussion attempts to demonstrate that not only can bone-conduction thresholds be worse than air-conduction thesholds, but that, in a group of persons with normal middle ears, the bone-conduction thresholds should exceed air-conduction thresholds in a predictable percentage of cases as a result of the variability associated with procedures for finding the threshold.

The variability of pure tone air- and bone-conduction thresholds is a result of the influence of a number of factors. Some of these factors, such as sensory-neural sensitivity, subject fatigue, attention, and experience, affect both air- and bone-conduction thresholds in a similar way. Other factors such as the normal variability in the efficiency of the middle ear, length and shape of the external meatus, thickness of skin and subcutaneous tissue, and pressure of the vibrator on the head may affect the threshold obtained by either air or bone conduction without influencing the threshold by the other. These latter factors together with the changes which occur in the patient, equipment, or examiner between one test and another, affect air- and bone-conduction thresholds differentially even in the absence of middle ear malfunction. Either a positive or a negative air-bone relationship may result because of the way in which the bone conduction system is calibrated which is in turn dictated by the fact that both air- and bone-conduction hearing loss is expressed relative to a normal reference.

Reprinted by permission of the author from *J. Speech Hearing Dis.*, **32**, 82–86 (1967).

The most commonly used method of calibrating the bone-conduction apparatus is that proposed by Roach and Carhart (1956). In this procedure air- and bone-conduction thresholds are obtained on a number of subjects with normal middle ears. Calibration is achieved by calculating the means of the air- and bone-conduction threshold distributions at each frequency and correcting the bone-conduction thesholds by the amount of the difference between the means. This can be done by applying mathematical corrections to the obtained bone-conduction thresholds or by modifying the output of the audiometer. The use of an "artificial mastoid" for calibration of the bone-conduction system does not change this basic procedure. In either case the means of two distributions are made equal, that is, the mean difference is made to equal 0. With "artificial ears" and "artificial mastoids" the data were simply collected at a more remote place and/or time.

When both air- and bone-conduction thresholds are obtained on the same individuals, the difference between air- and bone-conduction thresholds for each subject may be plotted as a single distribution at each frequency. When each individual difference value is corrected by the amount of the difference between the means of the two distributions, as above, the mean of the distribution of differences is 0. Approximately one-half of the differences then are positive and one-half negative. The distribution of differences approximates the normal curve. This is true whether the group has completely normal hearing or consists of those with purely sensory-neural hearing losses. The distribution, in practice, may be slightly skewed in the direction of "bone better than air" because of the inadvertent inclusion of some people with slight conductive losses which resulted from a disease process too insignificant or too long ago to be remembered by the subject or detected on physical examination. The degree of skewness depends on the stringency of the selection standards set up for the group.

Assuming that the sample is truly representative of patients with no middle ear disease, the air-bone relationship obtained on patients should be distributed in approximately the same way as in the sample. In other words, approximately one-half of the air-bone relationships obtained on patients without middle ear disease should have bone-conduction thresholds worse than air-conduction thesholds. To the extent that the sample is representative of the population, the measures of dispersion calculated for the sample should also predict the dispersion in the population.

Table 19-1 shows the frequency with which various relationships between air- and bone-conduction thresholds can be expected, assuming a normal distribution of differences between air- and bone-conduction thresholds. The percentages are given for a standard deviation of the distribution of differences of 5 dB. This value seems a good estimate on the basis of unpublished data obtained on several separate samples collected at this Center. Interestingly, this is about the same as the variability associated with speech reception threshold-pure tone average comparisons as reported by Graham (1960).

Table 19-1 was developed by listing in the first column the measured air-conduction threshold, bone-conduction threshold differences which can be reasonably expected when testing a group of people without middle ear malfunction. The assumptions are that 5 dB steps are used and that the equipment has been calibrated to make the mean bone-conduction threshold equal to the mean air-conduction threshold. The second column shows the range of actual air-conduction and bone-conduction threshold relationships for each of the nominal relationships shown in the first column.

The intervals in the second column are set up as −2.5 to +2.5 dB and +2.5 to +7.5 dB, and so forth, on the assumption that the actual average threshold of a group of persons assigned a given nominal

TABLE 19-1. EXPECTED DISTRIBUTION OF THE AIR-CONDUCTION, BONE-CONDUCTION THRESHOLD RELATIONSHIP IN SUBJECTS WITH NORMAL MIDDLE EAR FUNCTION ASSUMING A STANDARD DEVIATION OF THE DISTRIBUTION OF DIFFERENCES OF 5 dB.

Measured AC-BC Relationship	Actual AC-BC Relationship	Percentage in Interval
−20 or more	−20 or greater	0.02
−15	−17.5 to −12.5	0.60
−10	−12.5 to −7.5	6.06
−5	−7.5 to −2.5	24.17
0	−2.5 to +2.5	38.29
+5	+2.5 to +7.5	24.17
+10	+7.5 to +12.5	6.06
+15	+12.5 to +17.5	0.60
+20 or more	+20 or greater	0.02

threshold is approximately 2.5 dB below the nominal value. Therefore, the bone-conduction threshold, in order to have the same nominal value as obtained by air-conduction (i.e., 0 dB "air-bone gap"), must fall within ±2.5 dB of the actual average air-conduction threshold.

The percentages in the ±2.5 dB interval were obtained by noting that ±2.5 dB is equal to ±0.5 standard deviations assuming a standard deviation of 5 dB. The area under a normal curve between ±0.5 standard deviation is equal to 38.29 percent of the total area under the curve. In other words, about 38 percent of all air-bone comparisons obtained on a group of persons with normal middle ears will have a nominal "air-bone gap" of 0 dB. Using the same reasoning, it is noted that about 24 percent of all comparisons would show bone-conduction thresholds 5 dB worse than air-conduction thresholds ($z = 0.5$ to 1.5) and another 24 percent with bone-conduction thresholds better than air-conduction thresholds by 5 dB etc. A total of about 87 percent of the measures would be expected to fall within the nominal limits of ±5 dB. However, fully 13 percent of all comparisons fall outside the ±5 dB limits. Of particular interest is the number of instances in which bone-conduction thresholds are worse than air-conduction thresholds by 10 dB or more. Between 6 and 7 percent fall in this category.

In actual clinical testing, the percentage of instances in which bone-conduction thresholds are worse than air-conduction thresholds will be somewhat smaller since the total patient load of any clinic includes large numbers of patients with conductive hearing losses. Nevertheless, the appearance of bone-conduction thresholds worse than air-conduction thresholds by 10 to 15 dB at any given frequency should be expected with some regularity. Their appearance should be considered cause for a change in the bone-conduction calibration only when the number of instances in which bone-conduction thresholds are worse than air-conduction thresholds by any given amount exceeds the expected percentage of measurements for that relationship.

The purpose of this presentation has been to show that bone-conduction thresholds can be worse than air-conduction thresholds on the basis of intertest variability. This, however, should not be construed to mean that bone-conduction thresholds worse than air-conduction thresholds by 15 or 20 dB can be simply ignored. It is possible that bone-conduction thresholds can be worse than air-conduction thresholds by 20 dB on the basis of normal variability. However, a statement to the effect that this difference is due to expected intertest variability will be correct only once out of every 5,000 times the statement is made. An observation of this type in any individual instance should be viewed with great skepticism and cannot be accepted until all controllable sources of error have been eliminated.

One other aspect of this discussion concerns the situation when the bone-conduction threshold is better than the air-conduction threshold by 5 to 15 dB. Although probability favors that a difference of this size represents a pathologic loss of middle ear efficiency, it must not be forgotten that on a number of occasions such a difference may represent only intertest variability.

ACKNOWLEDGMENT

This discussion is, in part, based on research supported by Vocational Rehabilitation Administration Project No. RD-1717-S.

REFERENCES

Graham, J. T. Evaluation of methods for predicting speech reception threshold. *Arch. Otolaryng., 72,* 347–350 (1960).

Roach, R. E., and Carhart, R. A clinical method for calibrating the bone-conduction audiometer. *Arch. Otolaryng, 63,* 270–278 (1956).

20

The Variability of Occluded and Unoccluded Bone-Conduction Thresholds

DONALD D. DIRKS, Ph.D.
Professor, Head and Neck Surgery (Audiology)
UCLA School of Medicine, Los Angeles,
California
JOHN G. SWINDEMAN, M.A.
at UCLA School of Medicine when this article
was prepared

It is well known that partial or complete closure of the external auditory meatus results in an increase in sensitivity for bone-conducted signals. Although the magnitude of the effect had been studied under various conditions of occlusion (Pohlman and Kranz, 1926; Kelly and Reger, 1937; Watson and Gales, 1943; Sullivan et al., 1947; Naunton, 1957; Huizing, 1960), it was only recently that the stability and the intersubject variability of the effect was investigated by Elpern and Naunton (1963). These investigators, employing five occluding devices, obtained three estimates of the occlusion effect at each test frequency on normal hearing individuals. Two important conclusions emerged from their data. First, the occlusion effect was relatively unstable from test to retest; and second, the intersubject variability, as estimated by the standard error of estimate, was somewhat large. Since the standard deviations of the occlusion effect tended to vary inversely with frequency and the volume under the enclosure, the authors suggested that the occluding device itself was another source of variability—over and above that normally associated with bone conduction measurements. Thus, they reasoned that occluded thresholds might actually show a larger standard deviation than unoccluded thresholds.

More recent evidence, reported by Malmquist and Jerger (1966) indicated that the variability of occluded thresholds as exhibited by the intersubject standard deviations was smaller than the comparable variability of unoccluded thresholds. These investigators employed a TDH-39 earphone encased in a CZW-6 cushion as their occluding device, and covered the ears with Pederson earphones in the "unoccluded state." The latter condition was considered unoccluded, since the Pederson earphones cause no occlusion effect in the test frequency range from 500 to 4,000 Hz (Elpern and Naunton, 1963; Weston, 1965). The results of Malmquist and Jerger (1966) data led to the conclusion that the variability associated with occluded thresholds is no larger and is possibly smaller than the variability observed during the unoccluded state. This conclusion somewhat contradicts the conclusions reached by Elpern and Naunton (1963). Thus, it was decided to investigate in further detail the test-retest and intersubject variability of the occlusion effect.

This investigation is a report of three experiments to determine the variability of the occlusion effect and of occluded and unoccluded thresholds on normal listeners, using both supra-aural and circumaural cushions as the occluding devices. Repeated measurements were made with a MX41/AR cushion employed as the occluder in the first investigation and a Grason-Stadler 001 cushion in the second. In the final experiment, an attempt was made to substantially reduce the error of measurement by replicating each threshold 12 times on a group of highly sophisticated subjects with normal hearing. The latter procedure allowed us to determine whether the variability of the occlusion effect was due mainly to differences between individuals or between trials and if the variability could be reduced by employing a more compactly fitting circumaural cushion rather than the customary supra-aural cushion.

Reprinted by permission of the authors from *J. Speech Hearing Res., 10*, 232–249 (1967).

EXPERIMENT I: METHOD

Subjects

Eleven young adults with normal hearing served as subjects for the experiment. Eight female and three male subjects were included in the group. For this investigation and in the remaining experiments, normal hearing was defined as 15 dB re ISO norms at 250, 500, 1,000 and 2,000 Hz. Each subject was screened at the 15 dB level prior to his inclusion in the investigation. The subjects were paid for their services.

Apparatus

Subjects were tested in a double-walled IAC booth, Model 1200A. The ambient noise level was 30 dB SPL in the frequency range from 60 to 120 Hz. In the range above these frequencies, the noise level dropped to 22 dB.

The pure-tone stimuli were generated from an audio oscillator (Hewlett Packard, Model 200AB) and then passed through an elecronic switch (Grason-Stadler, Model 829D) and associated interval timer (Grason-Stadler, Model 471). The switch and timer were set to pass tones at the rate of 200 msec with a rise-decay time of 25 msec and a duty cycle of 50 percent. The signals were routed through a graphic attenuator of a Bekesy audiometer (Grason-Stadler, Type E800-4) at an attenuation rate of 2.5 dB per second. The signal was terminated in a TDH-39 earphone or in a Radioear B-70A bone-conduction vibrator. The TDH-39 earphones were encased in MX41/AR cushions.

Narrow bands of white noise, for conditions which required masking of the nontest ear, originated from a narrow-band masking unit (Beltone, Model NB 102). The noise was delivered to a second TDH-39 receiver mounted in an MX41/AR cushion. The masking noise was presented to the nontest ear at an effective level of 35 dB above the subject's air-conduction threshold at each test frequency.

The acoustic outputs of the pure-tone and noise channels were measured at intervals before, during, and after the experimental period. In the case of the pure-tone air conduction and noise stimuli, the signals were measured acoustically through a 6 cc coupler (Bruel and Kjaer, Type DB 0160) and associated Bruel and Kjaer microphone system. The output levels were read on the meter of an audio frequency spectrometer (Bruel and Kjaer, Type 2112).

The vibratory energy produced by the bone-conduction vibrator was measured on an artificial mastoid (Beltone, Model 5A). The output of the artificial mastoid was passed through an associated amplifier and the subsequent voltage was read on the audio frequency spectrometer (Bruel and Kjaer, Type 2112). The meter switch was set to read on the RMS scale. Appropriate corrections for the particular artificial mastoid, along with corrections for frontal bone measurements, were supplied by the manufacturer. These corrections were included in the computation of output levels in dB re I dyne RMS. The variations in output from both the air- and bone-conduction systems averaged less than 1.5 dB at any test frequency throughout the test period and, thus, were considered acceptable for the current investigations.

The bone-conduction vibrator was held in place on the frontal bone by a metal holder attached to an adjustable rubber strap. The headband was adjusted on each subject to approximate a relative application force on the forehead of 750 grams, as measured with a calibrated tension testing force gauge (Pelonze, Model 57).

Procedure

Experimental subjects were tested under three basic conditions:

A. Air conduction
   1. Air-conduction thresholds on the test ear.
B. Bone conduction, Quiet
   1. Bone-conduction thresholds with both ears open.
   2. Bone-conduction thresholds with both ears occluded.
C. Bone conduction, Masked
   1. Bone-conduction thresholds with the test ear open and the nontest ear masked.
   2. Bone-conduction thresholds with the test ear occluded and the nontest ear masked.

Each subject was tested under all experimental conditions at 250, 500, 1,000, and 2,000 Hz. Three estimates of threshold were obtained at each condition for every test frequency. The frequency of the test tone was presented in random order, and the order of presentation for the conditions was counterbalanced for subjects and for test sessions. The right ear was used with five subjects and the left ear with the remaining six.

The testing period involved five one-hour sessions for each subject. At the start of each subject's first testing session, four one-minute practice tracings were obtained on each ear. Additional practice periods were included at the beginning of subsequent sessions. The subjects were instructed in a manner similar to that described in detail by Jerger (1960). Each subject traced an individual threshold for a one-minute period. The threshold was determined by averaging the midpoints of the excursions at the 15-, 30-, and 45-second points during the tracing.

EXPERIMENT I: RESULTS

In the Elpern and Naunton (1963) study, the standard error of estimate and the correlation between trials of the occlusion effect were used primarily to determine the absolute and relative stability of the effect. For the present study, the results were analyzed not only in terms of the occlusion effect, but also from data of the occluded and unoccluded thresholds per se. The results of the average occluded and unoccluded thresholds from the Bekesy chart readings were converted into dB re 1 dyne RMS as determined on the Beltone artificial mastoid. All artificial mastoid outputs were read on the RMS volt meter of an audio spectrometer (Bruel and Kjaer, Type 2112).

Table 20-1 shows the average air-conduction and occluded and unoccluded bone-conduction thresholds for the 11 subjects, together with the average occlusion effect. The average results are based on three estimates of threshold for each subject in each condition. The occlusion effect was determined in the customary manner by subtracting the occluded bone-conduction threshold from the unoccluded bone-conduction threshold. The average occluded and unoccluded bone-conduction thresholds are reported graphically in Figure 20-1.

Table 20-1 and Figure 20-1 show that the occlusion effect decreased as a function of frequency. By 2,000 Hz, the occlusion effect was essentially negligible. Observe also that the bone-conduction thresholds obtained with noise in the contralateral ear mirror closely the threshold pattern found during the nonmasking condition. The two curves are separated by approximately 5 dB, indicating that greater intensity was required to reach threshold when masking was present in the nontest ear than during comparable nonmasking conditions. Similar observations were reported and explained in a previous investigation by Dirks and Malmquist (1964). Finally, it

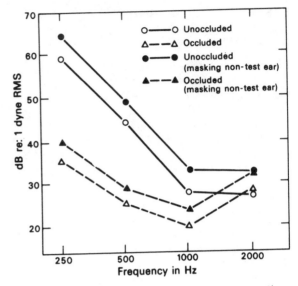

FIGURE 20-1. Mean absolute thresholds among three trials for 11 subjects with MX41/AR cushions (Experiment 1).

TABLE 20-1. MEAN ABSOLUTE THRESHOLDS AND OCCLUSION EFFECTS IN dB AMONG THREE TRIALS FOR 11 SUBJECTS WITH MX41/AR CUSHIONS (EXPERIMENT I).

Condition	Hz			
	250	500	1,000	2,000
Air Conduction	24.0*	7.2	1.2	4.5
Bone Conduction-Quiet				
Unoccluded	59.5†	45.6	28.8	28.7
Occluded	35.8	26.3	21.3	29.3
Bone Conduction-Masked				
Unoccluded	63.2†	49.6	34.0	34.4
Occluded	40.3	29.4	25.2	33.9
Occlusion Effect				
Quiet	23.7‡	19.3	7.5	−0.6
Masked	22.9	20.2	8.8	0.5

*In dB re SPL.
†In dB re 1 dyne RMS (measured on Beltone, Model 5A, artificial mastoid).
‡In dB re occlusion effect (unoccluded thresholds—occluded thresholds).

should be noted that the mean occlusion effect was similar for both masking and nonmasking conditions.

Intersubject variability as estimated from the standard deviations of the group over three trials is reported in Table 20–2 for each experimental condition. Standard deviations for test-retest stability over the three trials were so small that these have not been reported in the current paper. The test-retest standard deviations were all between 1.5 to 2.0 dB.

Some general results can be readily observed from Table 20–2. First, and possibly most important in this study, is the relatively small difference in the standard deviations between the occluded and unoccluded thresholds at any frequency. The results are, of course, in general agreement with the findings

TABLE 20–2. STANDARD DEVIATIONS IN dB FOR GROUPED THRESHOLDS AND OCCLUSION EFFECTS OBTAINED WITH MX41/AR CUSHIONS (EXPERIMENT I).

Condition	Hz			
	250	500	1,000	2,000
Air Conduction	3.6	3.5	3.9	5.9
Bone Conduction-Quiet				
Unoccluded	3.3	4.9	5.1	7.1
Occluded	3.5	5.4	5.4	6.6
Bone Conduction-Masked				
Unoccluded	3.0	6.5	6.4	7.9
Occluded	3.6	5.2	6.5	6.6
Occlusion Effect				
Quiet	4.1	3.7	4.0	2.7
Masked	4.4	5.1	4.5	2.9

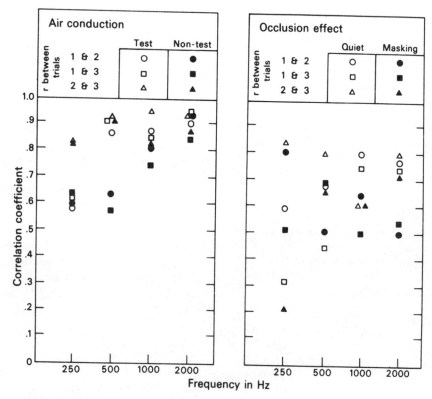

FIGURE 20-2. Correlations between trials for experimental conditions in Experiment I (air conduction and occlusion effect).

of Malmquist and Jerger (1966), although no significant reduction in variability was observed during the occluded state of the present investigation. The results do not agree with those of Elpern and Naunton (1963), who suggested that the variability of occluded thresholds might be larger than those expected in the unoccluded state. Second, the standard deviations for the occlusion effect itself are similar to those observed for either occluded or unoccluded bone-conduction thresholds, and are only slightly larger than those found for air-conduction measurements. An exception should be observed at 2,000 Hz, where a relatively small standard deviation for the occlusion effect probably suggests the reduction in range in the occlusion effect itself at this frequency. In other words, the fact that there is practically no occlusion effect at 2,000 Hz no doubt accounts for the considerable reduction in variability at this particular frequency, even though the standard deviations for the occluded and unoccluded thresholds themselves are as large at 2,000 Hz as at any other test frequency.

Analysis of variance was also applied to the data under all conditions and at each test frequency in order to determine whether the differences between individuals and/or between trials were the sources of variability. It would be much too lengthy to present the details of each analysis here, but the conclusions derived from the results patterned themselves in a clear-cut manner. As suggested from the data on standard deviations, the variability stems largely from variations between individuals rather than from test-retest variability, or from the trial factor. No greater test-retest variability was found for the occlusion effect than for bone-conduction thresholds themselves.

Pearson Product-Moment Correlations were also computed to determine the relative stability of air-conduction and occluded and unoccluded bone-conduction thresholds from trial to trial. These results are graphically displayed in Figures 20-2 and 20-3.

Observe that the test-retest air-conduction correlations are all high, ranging from 0.54 to 0.98. Correlations for bone-conduction thresholds (Figure 20-3) are generally high except for an occasional deviation. This result was found for the bone-conduction thresholds in both the occluded and unoccluded states. The test-retest correlations obtained for the occlusion effect itself are not quite as high as those

for either air- or bone-conduction thresholds. The latter result indicates that there are slightly more changes in rank order from trial to trial for the occlusion effect than for air- or bone-conduction thresholds. However, the correlations from trial to trial in the present study are substantially higher than those reported by Elpern and Naunton (1963) and are in closer agreement with those obtained by Malmquist and Jerger (1966).

In summary, the correlation data indicate that air-conduction thresholds are highly reliable from test to retest. A similar result was observed for bone-conduction thresholds, whether occluded or unoccluded, although a few deviations from this pattern did occur. Considering the fact that all the subjects in these experiments are normal listeners, so that the range in thresholds is somewhat restricted, the correlations were surprisingly high.

EXPERIMENT II

In the Malmquist and Jerger (1966) data, the investigators reported that intersubject variability was slightly smaller for occluded bone conduction thresholds than for unoccluded thresholds. In Experiment I of the present investigation, the standard deviations were essentially the same regardless of whether the test ear or ears were occluded or unoccluded. Malmquist and Jerger (1966) employed a TDH-39 earphone encased in a circumaural cushion as the occluder, whereas in the first investigation of the present series, the occluding device was a supra-aural cushion. The results from both investigations suggested that the variability in the occluded condition might be reduced further if a cushion were employed which fitted more effectively over the entire external ear than was possible with the supra-aural cushion. Thus, a second experiment was designed, similar to the first, except that a Grason-Stadler 001 circumaural cushion replaced the MX41/AR cushion used in the first study.

METHOD

Procedure

The procedure for the second experiment was essentially the same as that employed in Experiment I. Eleven young adult subjects with normal hearing were

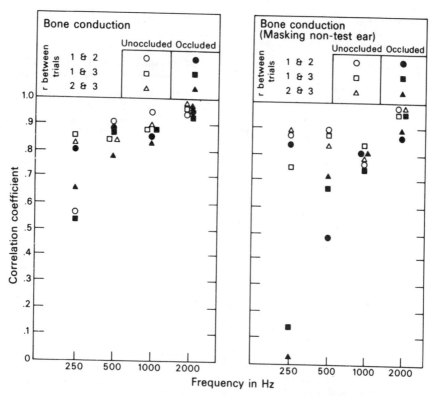

FIGURE 20-3. Correlations between trials for experimental conditions in Experiment I (bone conduction).

tested under the same experimental conditions as used in Experiment I. The order of presentation of the conditions was counterbalanced for subjects and for test sessions. During the occluded conditions, both ears were covered with the Grason-Stadler 001 cushions. In the occluded masking conditions, the narrow bands of noise were presented at effective levels of 35 dB. Actually, the level of the noise could not be determined as precisely for this experiment as in Experiment I, since there was no standard coupler available for the Grason-Stadler 001 cushions. The comparative difference in subjective pure-tone threshold between the 001 and the MX41/AR cushions was determined for several normal-hearing subjects prior to the experimental sessions. The results indicated that it took more intensity (approximately 1.5 dB at 250 Hz, 3.0 dB at 500 Hz, 6 dB at 1,000 Hz, and 3.0 dB at 2,000 Hz) to reach threshold with the Grason-Stadler 001 cushion than with the MX41/AR

cushion. These results became our guideline in determining the noise levels necessary to obtain an effective level of 35 dB. Thus, when masking was to be introduced to the nontest ear, the tester merely added the above differences to the masker dial reading used with an MX41/AR cushion.

EXPERIMENT II: RESULTS

The results for Experiment II were analyzed in a manner similar to that in Experiment I. Table 20-3 shows the average thresholds for the various experimental conditions while Figure 20-4 contains a graphic description of the average results for bone-conduction thresholds. The bone-conduction thresholds are reported in dB re 1 dyne RMS as measured through the Beltone artificial mastoid, while the air-

TABLE 20–3. MEAN ABSOLUTE THRESHOLDS AND OCCLUSION EFFECTS IN dB AMONG THREE TRIALS FOR ELEVEN SUBJECTS WITH GRASON-STADLER 001 CUSHIONS (EXPERIMENT II).

Condition	Hz			
	250	500	1,000	2,000
Air Conduction	25.8*	11.7	9.4	7.9
Bone Conduction-Quiet				
Unoccluded	59.8†	46.2	24.8	28.6
Occluded	37.3	26.7	17.4	28.2
Bone Conduction-Masked				
Unoccluded	64.4†	51.0	30.7	34.6
Occluded	44.6	32.5	21.1	32.8
Occlusion Effect				
Quiet	22.5‡	19.5	7.4	0.4
Masked	19.8	18.5	9.6	1.8

*In dB re SPL.
†In dB re 1 dyne RMS (measured on Beltone, Model 5 artificial mastoid).
‡In dB re occlusion effect (unoccluded thresholds—occluded thresholds).

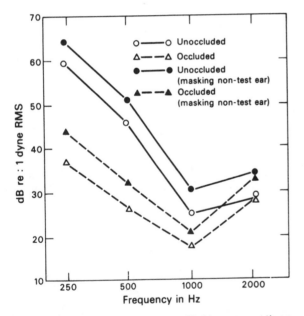

FIGURE 20–4. Mean absolute thresholds among three trials for 11 subjects with Grason-Stadler 001 cushions (Experiment II).

conduction thresholds are reported in dB re 0.0002 microbar as measured in a 6 cc coupler with the earphone encased in an MX41/AR cushion. Here the MX41/AR cushion was used only for calibration purposes, while the earphone was covered with the

Grason-Stadler 001 cushion during the experimental sessions.

The mean occluded and unoccluded bone-conduction thresholds are similar to those obtained in the first study. As in the first experiment, the bone-conduction thresholds obtained during the masking condition mirror those observed in the nonmasking condition, but again the curves are separated by approximately 5 dB. The occlusion effect is similar for both conditions.

The standard deviations for the group at each condition are reported in Table 20–4. Observe the small reduction in intersubject variability during the occluded state as compared to the standard deviations obtained with the test ear open. This result was obtained in both the nonmasking and masking conditions. The only exception was found at 250 Hz where the variability is substantially the same in both the occluded and unoccluded states. It should be noted that the test-retest standard deviations were again very small and hence are not reported separately.

Analysis of variance was applied to the data for each condition at every test frequency. As in the first experiment, the variability stems mainly from differences between individuals while the difference from test to retest is statistically insignificant.

The results of correlations on test-retest data are shown graphically in Figures 20–5 and 20–6 for all experimental conditions and for the occlusion effect. The results lead to substantially the same conclusion as in Experiment I. The test-retest correlations were high for air-conduction measurements and slightly reduced for bone-conduction thresholds, both oc-

TABLE 20–4. STANDARD DEVIATIONS IN dB FOR GROUPED THRESHOLDS AND OCCLUSION EFFECTS OBTAINED WITH GRASON-STADLER 001 CUSHIONS (EXPERIMENT II).

Condition	Hz			
	250	500	1,000	2,000
Air Conduction	3.8	2.9	4.8	2.8
Bone Conduction-Quiet				
Unoccluded	3.9	6.4	6.3	5.8
Occluded	4.2	4.7	5.7	5.4
Bone Conduction-Masked				
Unoccluded	3.4	6.8	7.3	8.1
Occluded	3.6	5.9	4.7	6.5
Occlusion Effect				
Quiet	6.0	4.2	3.1	1.9
Masked	5.2	4.8	4.8	4.4

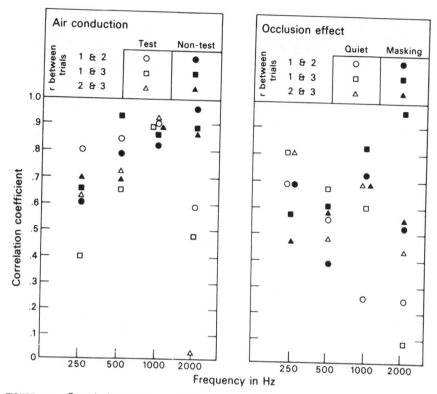

FIGURE 20-5. Correlations between trials for experimental conditions in Experiment II (air conduction and occlusion effect).

cluded and unoccluded. The test-retest correlations for the occlusion effect were not as high as for comparable air- and bone-conduction measurements.

EXPERIMENT III

The results of Experiments I and II suggested that the variability of occluded bone-conduction thresholds might be related to the type of occluder. In Experiment I, standard deviations were similar for both occluded and unoccluded thresholds, whereas in Experiment II, in which a circumaural cushion was used, standard deviations tended to be smaller for the occluded condition. Since the variability due to differences among persons was generally large in both sets of data, it was decided to reduce this source of variability as far as possible by using a more highly sophisticated group of subjects than in the previous

investigations. Further attempts to obtain the best estimate of a subject's threshold were accomplished by testing each individual a total of 12 times at each test frequency.

METHOD

Procedure

Nine subjects with previous experience in the Bekesy tracing task served as the experimental group in Experiment III. They were tested 12 times at each of 5 conditions with individual thresholds obtained at 500 and 1,000 Hz for each condition. These two frequencies were considered most desirable, since the occlusion effect is almost absent in the higher frequencies and since the lower frequencies present other problems, namely, harmonic distortion in the

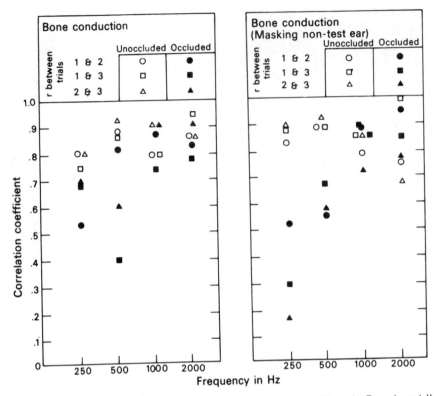

FIGURE 20-6. Correlations between trials for experimental conditions in Experiment II (bone conduction).

bone vibrator (Wilber and Goodhill, 1966) and difficulties in achieving appropriate masking levels which could interfere with the testing procedures.

The experimental conditions were as follows:

A. Air Conduction
    1. With an MX41/AR cushion
    2. With a Grason-Stadler 001 cushion
B. Bone Conduction (with masking in the nontest ear)
    1. Unoccluded
    2. Occluded with MX41/AR cushion
    3. Occluded with Grason-Stadler 001 cushion

Each of the above conditions was presented twice during a one-hour test session. Six one-hour test sessions per subject were necessary to trace 12 one-minute thresholds at both frequencies in each of the five conditions.

The conditions were presented in random order within each of the six sessions. The order of the frequency presentation was alternated from condition to condition and over trials. The noise levels necessary for an effective masking level of 35 dB, the instructions to the subjects, the practice for the subjects, and the method of scoring the tracings were comparable to procedures used in Experiments I and II.

Apparatus

The equipment used in this experiment was similar to that employed in the previous two, with one principal exception. A special apparatus was developed in order to couple the bone vibrator to the subject's forehead at a controlled and known force. The bone vibrator assembly is shown in Figure 20-7. It incorporates some of the features of a similar vibrator

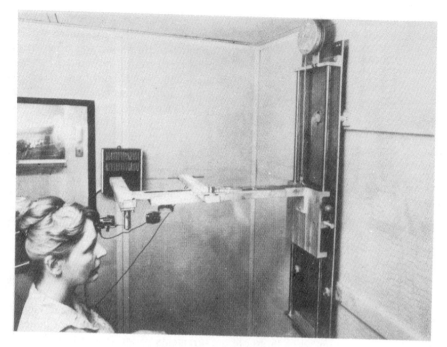

FIGURE 20-7. Bone vibrator assembly.

assembly described earlier by Jerger and Jerger (1965). The apparatus permits application of the vibrator to the forehead or the mastoid process without the use of headbands or other elastic straps. The relative tension of a calibrated spring was employed to control the amount of vibrator application force at each subject's head. The device was calibrated so that forces of 250, 500, 600, 750, and 1,000 grams could be used. The subject's head was fixed in place with the aid of a specially modified headrest. A gauge was located on an arm, parallel and in synchrony with the spring, which monitored any movements of the subject's head or changes in the desired force. Thus, if the subject's head moved slightly during the testing period, it could be immediately observed by the tester. If any movement took place, the force was readjusted and the test readministered.

RESULTS

The results of Experiment III are shown in Tables 20-5 and 20-6. Table 20-5 contains the mean thresholds at 500 and 1,000 Hz for the various experimental

TABLE 20-5. MEAN ABSOLUTE THRESHOLDS IN dB AMONG 12 TRIALS FOR NINE SOPHISTICATED SUBJECTS WITH NORMAL HEARING (EXPERIMENT III).

Condition	Hz 500	1,000
Air Conduction		
MX41/AR cushion	9.0*	2.4
Grason-Stadler cushion 001	11.7	7.4
Bone Conduction		
Unoccluded	48.3†	34.7
MX41/AR cushion	35.9	32.0
Grason-Stadler cushion 001	36.0	29.1

*In dB re SPL.

†In dB re 1 dyne RMS (measured on Beltone, Model 5A artificial mastoid).

conditions, while the standard deviations for the corresponding conditions are presented in Table 20-6.

Several results are noteworthy in Table 20-5. First, the air-conduction and unoccluded bone-conduction thresholds are in close agreement with those observed in the earlier studies. Second, the occluded bone-conduction thresholds are all slightly higher than those obtained during the first and second

TABLE 20-6. STANDARD DEVIATIONS IN dB FOR GROUPED
THRESHOLDS AND OCCLUSION EFFECTS OBTAINED FOR
NINE SOPHISTICATED SUBJECTS WITH NORMAL HEARING
(EXPERIMENT III).

	Hz	
Condition	500	1,000
Air Conduction		
MX41/AR cushion	2.2	2.8
Grason-Stadler cushion 001	3.2	4.1
Bone Conduction		
Unoccluded	4.9	4.5
Occluded with MX41/AR cushion	4.8	5.6
Occluded with Grason-Stadler		
001 cushion	4.7	4.9
Occlusion Effect		
MX41/AR cushion	5.8	2.3
Grason-Stadler 001 cushion	5.9	3.7

experiments. Thus, the occlusion effects are somewhat reduced from comparable results in the other
studies. Whether the reduction in the magnitude of
the occlusion effect is due to the sophistication of the
subjects, together with the large number of threshold
estimates obtained, is difficult to evaluate.

The standard deviations reported in Table 20-6
lead us to two major conclusions. First, the intersubject variability as estimated by the standard deviation
is essentially the same for occluded and unoccluded
bone-conduction thresholds. Second, the variability
of the occlusion effect itself is similar or smaller than
the variability estimates observed for occluded and
unoccluded bone-conduction thresholds. Since the
standard deviations at 1,000 Hz decrease substantially from those observed at 500 Hz, it appears that
the restricted range of the occlusion effect in the
higher frequencies probably accounts for the decreased standard deviations of the occlusion effect as
frequency rises.

The results from Experiment III essentially supported the conclusions reached in Experiments I and
II. Thus, no further statistical analysis was performed on the data than is reported in Tables 20-5
and 20-6.

DISCUSSION

In the present experiments, data were obtained on the
comparative variability between unoccluded and
occluded bone-conduction thresholds. One conclusion emerged consistently from the results, namely,
that the variability associated with occluded bone-
conduction thresholds was no greater than the variability observed for unoccluded bone conduction measurements. In general, these results lend support to
similar conclusions reached by Malmquist and Jerger
(1966). However, in the present studies, it was not
possible to substantiate their conclusion that occluded thresholds resulted in smaller intersubject variability than unoccluded thresholds, although there is a
definite tendency toward this result in Experiment II.
Thus, under controlled conditions, one should not
anticipate greater variability from occluded than
from unoccluded bone-conduction thresholds.

The source of the variability in all bone-conduction measurements, whether occluded or unoccluded, appears to stem primarily from differences between individuals rather than from variations from
test to retest. This result might have been anticipated
since numerous investigators (Carhart and Hayes,
1949; Dirks, 1964; Wilber and Goodhill, 1966) have
suggested that the stability of bone-conduction measurements from trial to trial may be acceptable
under controlled conditions. Fortunately, the intersubject variability for air conduction is substantially
smaller than that for comparable occluded or unoccluded bone-conduction measurements and, therefore, does not constitute as great a problem for the
clinician.

The variability of the occlusion effect itself was
generally no larger than the associated variability for
the occluded or unoccluded thresholds. As frequency
increased, the standard deviations for the occlusion
effect tended to decrease. Elpern and Naunton (1963)
have reported a similar result. It seems reasonable to
assume that the decrease in the variability of the
occlusion effect at higher frequencies is related directly to the decreased range in the occlusion effect as
frequency increases.

ACKNOWLEDGMENT

This investigation was supported by Public Health Service
Research Grant No. NB 05883 from the National Institute
of Neurological Diseases and Blindness and by the Hope
for Hearing Research Foundation. The authors are indebted to the Health Sciences Computing Facility, UCLA,
for statistical assistance.

REFERENCES

Carhart, R., and Hayes, C. The clinical reliability of bone conduction audiometry. *Laryngoscope,* 59, 1084–1101 (1949).

Dirks, D. Factors related to bone conduction reliability. *Arch. Otolaryng.,* 79, 551–558 (1964).

Dirks, D., and Malmquist, C. Changes in bone-conduction thresholds produced by masking in the non-test ear. *J. Speech Hearing Res.,* 7, 271–278 (1964).

Elpern, B. S., and Naunton, R. F. The stability of the occlusion effect. *Arch. Otolaryng,* 77, 376–384 (1963).

Huizing, E. H. Bone conduction—the influence of the middle ear. *Arch. Otolaryng.,* Suppl. 155 (1960).

Jerger, J. Bekesy audiometry in analysis of auditory disorders. *J. Speech Hearing Res.,* 3, 275–287 (1960).

Jerger, J., and Jerger, S. Critical evaluation of SAL audiometry. *J. Speech Hearing Res.,* 8, 103–128 (1965).

Kelley, N. H., and Reger, S. N. The effect of binaural occlusion of the external auditory meati on the sensitivity of the normal ear for bone conducted sound. *J. Exp. Psychol.,* 21, 211–217 (1937).

Malmquist, C. W., and Jerger, J. F. Some aspects of the normal occlusion effect. Paper presented at the Annual Convention of the American Speech and Hearing Association, Washington, D.C. (1966).

Naunton, R. F. Clinical bone-conduction audiometry: The use of a frontally applied bone-conduction receiver and the importance of the occlusion effect in clinical bone-conduction audiometry. *Arch. Otolaryng.,* 66, 281–298 (1957).

Pohlman, A. G., and Kranz, F. W. The influence of partial and complete occlusion of the external auditory canals on air and bone transmitted sound. *Ann. Oto. Rhino, Laryng.,* 35, 113–121 (1926).

Sullivan, J. A., Gotleib, C. C., and Hodges, W. E. Shift of bone conduction thresholds on occlusion of the external ear canal. *Laryngoscope,* 57, 690–703 (1947).

Watson, N. A., and Gales, R. S. Bone conduction threshold measurements: effects of occlusion, enclosures, and masking devices. *J. Acoust. Soc. Amer.,* 14, 207–215 (1943).

Wilber, L. A., and Goodhill, V. Real ear versus artificial mastoid methods of calibration. *J. Speech Hearing Res.* (in press).

Weston, P. Bone conduction and noise masking. *Acta Otolaryng.,* Suppl. 204 (1965).

21

Comparison of Frontal and Mastoid Bone-Conduction Thresholds in Various Conductive Lesions

DONALD D. DIRKS, Ph.D.
Professor, Head and Neck Surgery (Audiology), UCLA School of Medicine, Los Angeles, California
CAROLYN W. MALMQUIST
Research Audiologist, UCLA School of Medicine when this article was prepared

Unoccluded and occluded bone conduction (BC) and Sensorineural Acuity Level (SAL) thresholds at the frontal bone and the mastoid process were compared on 60 subjects with conductive hearing loss. The results were based on calibrated norms obtained on 32 subjects with normal hearing and validated on 10 cases with sensorineural hearing loss. The mastoid BC thresholds for the entire conductive group were more depressed than comparable frontal measurements, but the average difference was only five dB. The threshold data for subjects with surgically confirmed middle-ear lesions (N = 38) were analysed in greater detail by dividing the group by frontal-mastoid differences and observed physical changes within the middle ear. Approximately 20 percent of the group showed frontal-mastoid differences that exceeded the normal range, and these cases had either malleus fixation or an ossicular discontinuity due to incus necrosis or absence of the incus. Average results for 17 cases with stapes fixation suggested that there were no frontal-mastoid differences and that both BC curves were somewhat similarly influenced by the middle-ear impairment. The SAL and occluded BC thresholds at the frontal bone were always in close agreement and differed from the unoccluded frontal-bone measurements for the conductive cases by the amount of the average occlusion effect observed for normals. The advantages of unoccluded bone conduction at the frontal bone are stressed, and the possible use of a comparison of BC thresholds at the two sites for diagnostic purposes is suggested.

Traditionally, clinical bone-conduction measurements have been performed with the vibrator located on the mastoid process. However, it was suggested by Békésy (1932) and Barany (1938) that this position on the skull may be one of the least favorable for clinical testing. Of other possible sites on the skull, the frontal bone has received the most attention. Principally three arguments have been advanced in favor of placement of the vibrator on the frontal bone rather than on the mastoid process.

It is suggested that there is an increase in the test-retest reliability of bone-conduction measurements favoring forehead placement. Second, intersubject variability may be reduced when measurements are obtained at the frontal bone. Third, theory indicates that measurements performed at the frontal bone reduced the influence of the middle ear on the bone-conduction threshold.

There are a few other practical motives for testing at the frontal bone rather than at the mastoid process, such as the ease of performing the Weber and Bing tests without altering the vibrator position, avoiding replacement of the vibrator to the opposite side when testing the second ear, and reducing the

Reprinted by permission of the authors from *J. Speech Hearing Res.*, **12**, 725–746 (1969).

suggestion on the part of the patient and the tester that the ear being tested is the one closest to the vibrator. These latter reasons are of interest; however, they are not as significant as the initial three arguments.

First Argument. The hypothesis that the test-retest reliability of bone-conduction measurements on the forehead is more reliable than those on the mastoid process was based originally on observations by Bekesy (1932). He noted that the tip of the bone vibrator can be moved greater distances on the frontal bone than on the mastoid process without changing bone-conduction thresholds. Results by Hart and Naunton (1961) indicated there was less variation from the average of five repeated measurements when tests were performed at the frontal bone as compared to tests at the mastoid. However, the comparative results of other investigators on larger groups of individuals and using hearing-aid-type vibrators have not always been as impressive. Studebaker (1962) could find no statistical difference in test-retest reliability when comparisons were made between bone-conduction thresholds at the mastoid and the frontal bone on normal listeners. One of the current authors (Dirks, 1964) made similar test-retest comparisons on a group of 24 normal listeners. The results showed that test-retest scores at the frontal bone were not appreciably different from the measurements at the mastoid. When various sets of data were reviewed by the author, test-retest variability from measurements obtained at the frontal bone were more often smaller than for corresponding scores obtained at the mastoid process. However, the differences did not appear to be of great practical advantage. It may be noteworthy that these investigations (Studebaker, 1962, and Dirks, 1964) were performed with hearing-aid-type bone vibrators while the tests by Hart and Naunton (1961) were conducted with a vibrator containing a small vibrating tip excited by a driving system. The original observations may not apply as well when a large vibrating surface, such as found in the hearing-aid-type vibrator, is employed.

Second Argument. The second argument favoring frontal-bone placement has been concerned with intersubject variability, or the variations in thresholds among a group of normal listeners. It has been suggested that differences in bone-conduction thresholds among individuals would be reduced if they were obtained at the forehead rather than at the mastoid process. The results of Studebaker (1962) and one of the current authors (Dirks, 1964) seem to verify this argument. However, while intersubject variability was reduced at the forehead in both experiments, the difference in variability at the two positions was rather small.

Third Argument. The final argument for forehead placement evolved primarily from the classical investigation by Barany in 1938. He suggested that the participation of the middle ear in the bone-conduction threshold was greater for measurements made at the mastoid process than at positions along the median sagittal plane of the skull. Experimental results by Link and Zwislocki (1951) for cases with otitis media demonstrated less hearing loss from measurements at the frontal bone than at the mastoid process. Studebaker (1962) compared bone-conduction hearing loss measured at the forehead with similar measurements at the mastoid process on 39 individuals with middle-ear disease. Of these subjects, 22 were diagnosed as having otosclerosis, 7 had residuals of radical mastoid surgery, 6 had inactive otitis media, 3 had suppurative otitis media, and 1 had a retracted ear drum. There was less hearing loss by bone conduction for the group when measurements were carried out at the frontal bone rather than at the mastoid process. However, the average threshold difference over the test frequencies was approximately 4 dB.

It appeared to us that this final argument for measurements at the frontal bone was potentially the most powerful of the three and deserved more attention. Thus, our study was designed to explore the differences in hearing loss by bone conduction at the frontal bone and mastoid process on persons with conductive hearing loss for whom specific surgical findings were available following the measurements. A group of normal listeners was used in calibrating the bone-conduction and SAL systems, and subjects with sensorineural hearing loss were tested to validate the normative data. Because of the recent development of a reliable artificial mastoid, it was possible to calibrate the bone-vibrator system physically and report the results in force values. Finally, since recent emphasis (Jerger and Tillman, 1960; Herer, 1964; Jerger et al., 1965) has been placed on the SAL test and on occluded bone-conduction measurements as estimates of sensorineural acuity, these tests were included for comparison in the experimental battery.

METHOD

Subjects

Thirty-two subjects with normal hearing were our control group. Negative otologic histories and passage of a screening test at 15 dB re ISO-64 norms were required for inclusion in the normal group. The mean age for these subjects was 21.8 years, and the age range was 18–32 years.

The experimental group of subjects consisted of 70 individuals with hearing loss, 60 with conductive loss and 10 with sensorineural loss. The conductive group was divided on the basis of surgical information obtained after the preoperative audiological examination. Twenty-two cases were excluded from this subgrouping process because of incomplete medical or surgical information. The medical classification of the remaining 38 subjects with conductive loss was as follows:

1. Seventeen cases with stapes fixation due to otosclerosis.
2. Two cases with malleus fixation, one in which the malleus was fixed by a bony growth and the other in which the malleus and incus were fixed by granulation tissue. Both had intact ossicular chains and mobile stapes foot-plates.
3. Ten cases with ossicular discontinuity due to chronic otitis media. Three of these had a perforation of the tympanic membrane and cholesteatoma; one had a cholesteatoma with an intact tympanic membrane. Of the remaining six, three cases had a perforation of the tympanic membrane and three had no impairment other than the ossicular discontinuity.
4. One case with a perforated tympanic membrane only. The middle-ear cavity was clear and the ossicular chain intact and mobile.
5. Two cases with middle-ear fluid.
6. Six postoperative mastoidectomy cases on whom a second surgical procedure was later performed. Of these six cases, two had no ossicles or tympanic membrane, three had no ossicles with intact tympanic membranes, and one had an intact stapes and a small remnant of the incus which was attached to an intact tympanic membrane because of previous reconstruction.

Notice in the above classification that the emphasis had been placed on the physical change that had taken place in the middle ear rather than on the disease process. Although it is typical to divide conductive lesions on the basis of the disease process (such as otosclerosis, otitis media, etc.), the audiometric results are more closely related to the physical alterations of the system caused by the disease—not to the disease itself.

Apparatus

We used a Beltone 15C audiometer for the air- and bone-conduction signals. The pure tone was fed to a fixed attenuator which provided additional attenuation of the signal when necessary. The test signal was terminated either in an earphone (TDH-39 encased in MX41/AR cushion) or in a hearing-aid-type bone vibrator (Radioear B70-A).

We used a narrow-band masking unit (Beltone, Model NB 102) as our noise source for the SAL and for masking the nontest ear during bone-conduction measurements. The output of the masker went directly to an insert receiver (Beyer DT 507) during bone-conduction measurements; during the SAL test, the noise passed through an amplifier (McIntosh, Model 162K) and terminated in a second hearing-aid-type vibrator (Radioear B70-A). A volt meter monitored the output of the SAL noise across the terminal of the bone vibrator. When masking was required for air-conduction testing, the second channel of the Beltone 15C audiometer provided white noise. The air- and bone-conduction signals were calibrated, acoustically, prior to, and periodically throughout, the experiment. We used a 6 cc coupler and associated microphone (Bruel and Kjaer, Type 4132) and assembly (Bruel and Kjaer audio frequency spectrometer, Type 2112) to calibrate the air-conduction system. We calibrated the bone-conduction signals on an artificial mastoid (Beltone, Model 5A) with accompanying amplifier and volt meter. We made daily calibrations by monitoring the voltage at the receivers' terminals.

Procedure

Normal Listeners. Four tests were administered to each subject:

1. Sensorineural Acuity Level (SAL).
   a. Air conduction in quiet (ACq).
   b. Air conduction in the presence of bone-conduction noise (ACn).

2. Unoccluded bone conduction with mastoid placement (BCM).
3. Unoccluded bone conduction with frontal placement (BCFu).
4. Occluded bone conduction with frontal placement (BCFo).

The SAL test was always administered first, the ACq test to each ear and the ACn portion to the test ear only. The right or left ear was chosen alternately as the test ear. The subject's ACq thresholds in the nontest ear were collected only to determine appropriate masking levels for succeeding bone-conduction conditions. The order of presentation for the bone-conduction tests was counterbalanced according to site of vibrator placement (mastoid or frontal) and occlusion state (unoccluded or occluded). The frontal bone-conduction tests, however, were always presented consecutively so that it was not necessary to remove the vibrator from the forehead between tests.

Pure-tone thresholds were obtained at 250, 500, 1,000, 2,000, and 4,000 Hz for each of the test conditions. The ascending technique, described by Carhart and Jerger (1959), was used. The order of frequency presentation was 1,000, 2,000, 4,000, 1,000, 500, and 250 Hz.

With two modifications the SAL test was administered in the manner originally described by Jerger and Tillman (1960). First, we used narrow bands of noise and set the noise level for each band at 0.5 volts by monitoring the voltage at the terminals of the bone vibrator. Second, the resultant SAL norm was based on the difference between 0 dB HL re ISO-64 norms and the masked threshold (ACn).

For SAL and frontal-bone conduction, a commercially available holder and strap held the vibrator to the forehead. In both conditions force was kept constant at approximately 600 grams. For bone-conduction measurements at the mastoid process we used a standard bone-vibrator holder. No measurements of the vibrator's application force were performed during the experimental session. However, earlier measurements (Dirks, 1964) under very similar conditions suggested that the vibrator was affixed to the mastoid process of adults with an average pressure of 350 grams.

All threshold measurements were monaural. The test ear was unoccluded for BCM and BCFu and covered by an earphone (TDH-39 with an MX41/AR cushion) for the BCFo. The nontest ear always was masked for bone-conduction conditions at an effective level of 30 dB. Narrow bands of noise from a commercially available noise generator (Beltone, Model NB 102) were presented to the nontest ear via an insert receiver. The acoustic output of noise was calibrated with a 2 cc coupler and accompanying microphone and calibration assembly (Bruel and Kjaer, Type 2112).

Subjects with Hearing Loss. We used a method similar to that used for our normal group for our subjects with hearing loss, except for the masking procedure and the way we selected the experimental ear. The ear with the greatest loss of hearing, or the ear already selected for surgery, was routinely chosen as the experimental test ear. In most instances, the ear with the greatest loss was also the ear selected for surgery. We used the masking technique described by Hood (1957) for masking the nontest ear during the bone-conduction conditions and during the ACq condition when masking was required. If the nontest ear was masked during the ACq condition, the same level of contralateral masking was used to obtain the ACn portion of the SAL procedure. From a practical point of view, the plateau, determined by the Hood procedure, was usually found with the noise in the nontest ear at an effective level of 30 dB.

RESULTS

Normal Group

Figure 21–1 shows the results of the bone-conduction thresholds for the 32 listeners with normal hearing. Each datum point represents the mean threshold for the 32 subjects for the reported condition and frequency. The thresholds were reported in force values (dB re 1.0 dyne RMS) determined from measurements on the artificial mastoid. As previous investigators have observed (Studebaker, 1962; Dirks, 1964; Whittle, 1965; and Weston, Gengel and Hirsh, 1967), greater energy is required to reach threshold at the frontal bone than at the mastoid process. The differences in threshold between the two locations vary from 11.6 dB at 250 Hz to 1.7 dB at 4,000 Hz. The thresholds at the mastoid process that we obtained in this study are in good agreement with the values suggested for an interim norm by the standards committee of the Hearing Aid Industry Conference (HAIC) and reported by Lybarger (1966). The bone-conduction thresholds at the frontal bone are very similar to those recently published by Weston et al. (1967).

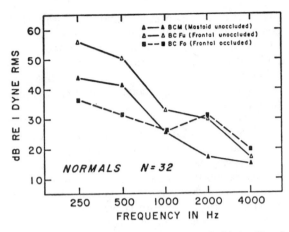

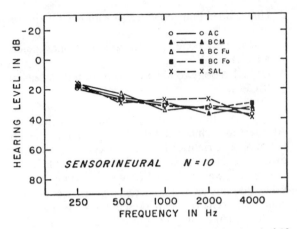

FIGURE 21-1. Mean bone-conduction thresholds in dB re 1 dyne RMS for 32 subjects on 3 conditions at 5 test frequencies.

FIGURE 21-2. Mean thresholds in dB re hearing level of 10 sensorineural cases for 5 test frequencies and conditions.

Figure 21–1 also contains the threshold measurements obtained at the frontal bone with the test ear occluded. The magnitude of the occlusion effect can be determined by comparing the BCFu and BCFo curves. The occlusion effect was 19.3 dB at 250 Hz, 19.0 dB at 500 Hz, and 7 dB at 1,000 Hz. At 2,000 and 4,000 Hz the occlusion effect was virtually absent. These results are in general agreement with previously published data on the magnitude of the occlusion effect obtained with similar earphones and cushions (Elpern and Naunton, 1963; Hodgson and Tillman, 1966; Dirks and Swindeman, 1967). The thresholds in Figure 21–1 were values we used for the calibrated bone-conduction norms in this investigation.

Sensorineural Group

We tested a group of 10 medically diagnosed cases of sensorineural hearing loss, using the SAL procedure and the three experimental bone-conduction conditions. We used only one ear from each of the cases to obtain the average thresholds in Figure 21–2. The primary purpose of including a group of individuals with sensorineural hearing loss in this study was to validate the normative data used for calibration purposes. We reasoned that the individuals with sensorineural hearing loss should demonstrate bone-conduction and SAL thresholds that were reduced from those obtained in the normal group by an amount equivalent to their air-conduction loss.

The results (Figure 21–2) suggests that our calibration values are appropriate for the normal listeners. Observe that the audiometric curves for SAL and bone-conduction thresholds interweave with the air-conduction thresholds at test frequencies. There is one minor exception. The spread of the test results at 2,000 Hz is somewhat larger than that observed at other frequencies. SAL and BCM differ from the air-conduction threshold by approximately 5 dB, the SAL tending to underestimate the degree of loss and the BCM to overestimate it. Except for these deviations, sensorineural group results emphasize the validity of the calibration values obtained from the normal group.

One other observation should be emphasized from the sensorineural group results. It concerns the good agreement of SAL and the three types of bone-conduction measurements with the air-conduction thresholds. Regardless of whether unoccluded (BCM, BCFu) or occluded (BCFo, SAL) measurements were performed, all the test results indicated equivalent thresholds for patients with sensorineural loss as long as the appropriate norm was applied. The results suggested that either relative (open ear) or absolute (occluded ear) bone-conduction and SAL measurements give equivalent estimates of sensorineural acuity on patients with sensorineural hearing loss.

Conductive Group

Studebaker (1962) reported the differences of calibrated frontal and mastoid bone-conduction thresholds on a group of 39 subjects with varied middle-ear lesions. Although the types of otologic impairments were listed, the comparison between results at the mastoid and frontal bone was based on threshold responses from the total group. We present the mean results for the total conductive group of this study to compare them with Studebaker's results (1962) and to illustrate the relationship of occluded and unoccluded test measurements on middle-ear lesion cases. The later division of patients into subgroups, however, provided the most informative and clinically useful "frontal-mastoid" results.

Figure 21–3 shows the mean threshold responses at the five test frequencies and conditions for the entire conductive group. Observe that the two unoccluded bone-conduction measurements (BCM and BCFu) differ slightly at most test frequencies. BCM is consistently poorer than BCFu, but the average difference is only 5 dB. Another interesting result (Figure 21–3) is the close agreement between the two occluded bone-conduction tests (BCFo and SAL). Tillman (1963) and Jerger and Jerger (1965) have cautioned against comparison of "occluded" SAL with unoccluded bone-conduction measurements. Our current findings again demonstrate the inappropriateness of such a comparison. Notice that SAL thresholds interweave with the occluded frontal-bone thresholds and that both differ from the unoccluded thresholds, the difference approximately equaling the average occlusion effect (BCFu − BCFo) found in the normal group.

Table 21–1 presents the average differences between the unoccluded bone-conduction thresholds at the mastoid process and frontal bone for the conductive group and the comparable differences reported

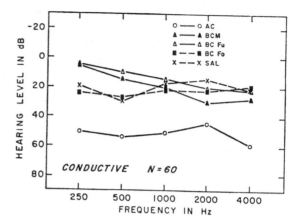

FIGURE 21-3. Mean thresholds in dB re hearing level of 60 cases with conductive hearing loss for 5 frequencies and conditions.

by Studebaker (1962). The results of both studies indicate a similar trend. The frontal bone-conduction thresholds show less hearing loss than those at the mastoid process, but the average differences are small.

Conductive Subgroups

It was our intent in this study to examine the relationship of various bone-conduction tests on individuals for whom rather precise medical and surgical information was available. Twenty-two cases were excluded from the final analysis because no surgery was performed. The remaining cases with conductive loss (N = 38) were divided initially into two groups: stapes fixation and no stapes fixation. It would have been desirable to divide the entire group into a larger number of categories specially related to the physical changes in the middle ear. However, the diversity of

TABLE 21-1. MEAN DIFFERENCE IN dB RE HEARING LEVEL BETWEEN FRONTAL AND MASTOID BONE-CONDUCTION THRESHOLDS (BCFu − BCM) FOR CONDUCTIVE LOSS GROUPS WITH DIVERSE MIDDLE-EAR IMPAIRMENTS. N = 60 FOR CURRENT DATA; N = 39 FOR STUDEBAKER'S DATA (1962).

| Data | \multicolumn{5}{c}{Frequency in Hz} | |
	250	500	1,000	2,000	4,000	Average Difference
Ours	−1.8	−4.7	−4.9	−8.1	−5.8	−5.1
Studebaker's	−1.4	−4.6	−4.1	−4.0	−5.2	−3.8

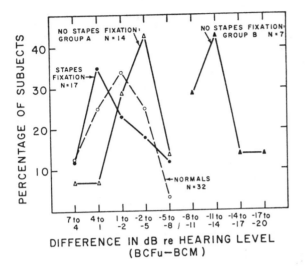

FIGURE   21-4. Frequency   distribution   of   average
BCFu – BCM difference scores for subjects with normal
hearing and for three conductive subgroups.

middle-ear lesions was large, as is true in most groups
of conductive hearing loss cases, and with an N of 38
it was impractical to subdivide the cases further by
precise physical changes.

Observation of the frontal-mastoid difference
scores for the two groups suggested reasonable
homogeneity for the stapes-fixation group but a wide
dispersion of scores for the no stapes-fixation subjects. Therefore, the no stapes-fixation group was
divided on the basis of the average BCFu – BCM
differences (5 test frequency scores were combined to
obtain average differences). Because the normal and
the stapes-fixation groups revealed frontal-mastoid
difference scores ranging from ±7 dB (in dB recalibrated norms), the arbitrary point for delineating a
significant BCFu – BCM difference was 8 dB. Thus,
individuals with a BCFu – BCM difference of ±7
dB fell into a no stapes-fixation group labeled *group
A*. Those with a difference of 8 dB or greater were
placed in the no stapes-fixation group, *group B*.

Figure 21-4 presents the frequency distributions
of the BCFu – BCM difference scores in dB re HL
for the normal and the three conductive subgroups.
Since the number of subjects in each group varied,
the ordinate in the figure designates the percentage of
subjects within each subgroup that demonstrated
various difference scores. The frequency distribution
of the difference scores (BCFu – BCM) for three of

the groups (normal, stapes fixation, and no stapes-
fixation group A) are relatively similar. Group B,
however, differs from the other three by definition,
for it includes the subjects who demonstrated BCFu
– BCM differences of 8 dB or greater. The average
difference between the mastoid and frontal bone-
conduction thresholds for group B was 12 dB. This
group, however, represents only 18 percent of the
conductive cases (N = 38).

Table 21-2 provides the mean and median difference scores for the subjects with normal hearing and
the three conductive subgroups. Note that these
scores for group A are negative and differ by 2 to 3
dB from the comparable difference scores for the
normal and the stapes-fixation group. Some individuals in group A had relatively large difference scores
at one or more of the test frequencies or consistent
but small differences over the frequency range. However, the limited number of cases and the use of a discrete frequency-testing technique did not permit a
more subtle analysis of the BCFu – BCM differences. The frontal-mastoid relationships for group B
are obviously different from the other groups. These
large differences are of significance and, unlike the
differences found in group A, should be easily differentiated from the normal group. Thus, the division
of the no stapes-fixation cases into only two groups
on the basis of BCFu – BCM difference scores is
considered to be a conservative approach.

Figure 21-5 includes the mean results for each
condition at the five test frequencies for the subjects
with stapes fixation. Although the stapes-fixation
group in Figure 21-5 was composed of 17 cases, the
number of responses varied slightly in the higher frequencies because the maximum shift for the SAL test
was not measurable in a few cases with severe air-
conduction losses. If the SAL threshold could not be

TABLE 21-2. MEAN AND MEDIAN BCFu – BCM DIFFERENCE
SCORES IN dB RE HEARING LEVEL FOR NORMAL LISTENERS
AND THREE CONDUCTIVE SUBGROUPS.

Test Groups	BCFu – BCM Difference Scores in dB Re Hearing Level		
	N	Mean	Median
Normal	32	0	0.5
Stapes Fixation	17	0.5	0.5
No Stapes Fixation			
Group A	14	−2.1	−2.8
Group B	7	−12.1	−12.0

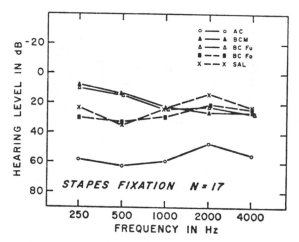

FIGURE 21-5. Mean thresholds in dB re hearing level of 17 cases with stapes fixation for 5 frequencies and conditions.

exactly determined for an individual at a particular frequency, the threshold values at that frequency for the SAL and the other experimental conditions were excluded in obtaining the mean results. The exclusion of these thresholds permitted a more accurate comparison of SAL with the BC thresholds and resulted in only minimal changes in the mean results. The group had approximately a 60-dB air-conduction loss, and the configuration of the curve demonstrated the characteristic stiffness tilt. The results for the two unoccluded bone-conduction tests (BCM and BCFu) were similar. This finding suggested that among cases with stapes fixation the frontal-mastoid differences were similar to those obtained on individuals with normal hearing.

The close agreement of the two occluded "bone conduction" tests (SAL and BCFo) in Figure 21-5 is also obvious. It appears that the only real difference among the battery of bone-conduction tests is related to the presence or absence of the occlusion effect in the normals. Although the SAL test is based on air-conduction shifts in the presence of bone-conducted noise, rather than actual bone-conduction thresholds, the SAL thresholds are equivalent to the BCFo thresholds.

In Figure 21-6, SAL was plotted with BCFu and BCM as an unoccluded-test result. The SAL was corrected at each frequency by the amount of the average occlusion effect for the normal group. The pur-

pose of this article is not to discuss all the merits of relative (unoccluded) or absolute (occluded) bone conduction. However, it is obvious that if one expects agreement between SAL and unoccluded frontal bone-conduction thresholds on conductive cases, such a correction must be made unless the earphone employed produces no occlusion effect for normals. Even after this correction, however, SAL can not always be expected to agree with unoccluded BCM, although the curves interweave for this particular group.

Figure 21-7 shows the mean thresholds for the experimental conditions at the five test frequencies for patients with no stapes-fixation group A. The average air-conduction loss for the group in the frequency range from 500 to 2,000 Hz was 46 dB. The configurations of the BCM, BCFu, and the corrected SAL thresholds interweave and indicate a substantial conductive loss. Each of the three estimates of sensorineural acuity is reduced in the high frequencies. The curve for BCM exhibits a small notch with the greatest reduction occurring at 2,000 Hz, but the results from the entire battery suggest that the threshold values at 2,000 and 4,000 Hz are practically equal. It is likely that this reduction in bone-conduction thresholds is primarily due to factors other than sensorineural loss. Notice that the air-conduction curve revealed a stiffness tilt, characteristic of conductive lesions, with only a mild drop between 2,000

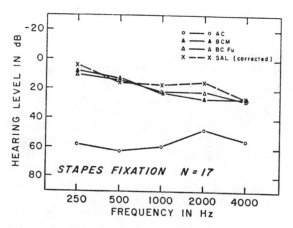

FIGURE 21-6. Comparison in dB re hearing level between "unoccluded," or corrected, SAL and unoccluded mastoid and frontal BC thresholds for 17 cases with stapes fixation.

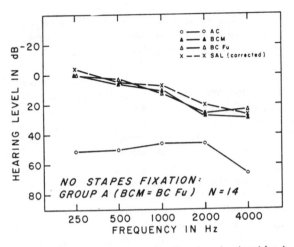

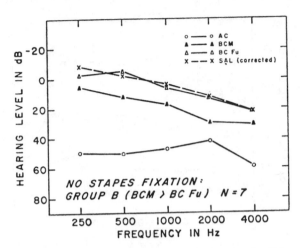

FIGURE 21-7. Mean thresholds in dB re hearing level for 4 test conditions for 14 subjects with no stapes fixation and in which BCM = BCFu.

FIGURE 21-8. Mean thresholds in dB re hearing level for four test conditions for seven subjects with no stapes fixation and BCM > BCFu by 8 dB or more.

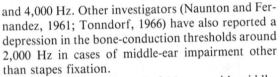

and 4,000 Hz. Other investigators (Naunton and Fernandez, 1961; Tonndorf, 1966) have also reported a depression in the bone-conduction thresholds around 2,000 Hz in cases of middle-ear impairment other than stapes fixation.

Group A was composed of 14 cases with middle-ear impairments. Four of the cases had no ossicles due to previous radical mastoidectomies, and two of these has perforations of the tympanic membrane. One case had a previous mastoidectomy and tympanoplasty. The surgery report from the day following the testing procedure indicated that the stapes was intact and a fragment of the incus was resting on the tympanic membrane. Two of the cases had fluid in the middle ear but an intact ossicular chain. Six of the cases had ossicular discontinuity and perforations of the tympanic membrane. In most of the cases with ossicular discontinuity there was either fibrous tissue or cholesteatoma present. It is possible that the fibrous connections or cholesteatoma may have substituted as a secondary ossicular chain for the transmission of sound. The final case had only a perforation of the tympanic membrane. To summarize, four cases had no ossicles, three patients had intact ossicular chains, and the remaining seven cases had an ossicular discontinuity with a cholesteatoma. Nine of the 14 cases had perforations of the tympanic membrane.

Figure 21-8 shows the results of the experimental conditions for the seven pathological subjects who formed group B. This group contains cases in which there was a difference between frontal and mastoid bone-conduction thresholds which exceeded the differences observed for the normal listeners. The air-conduction thresholds show an average deficit of approximately 47 dB in the range from 500 to 2,000 Hz. A stiffness tilt characterizes the configuration of the curve. The frontal-mastoid differences in this group averaged 12 dB. While the greatest difference between thresholds at the mastoid and frontal bone was 17 dB at 500 Hz, the smallest difference was 8 dB at 250 Hz. Observe again that the SAL results, corrected by the normal occlusion effect, agree extremely well with the BCFu results.

In comparing groups A and B (Figures 21-7 and 21-8), it is interesting to note that the average air-conduction losses for the two groups are practically identical. The frontal-bone thresholds are also quite similar. The marked difference between the two groups is found in the thresholds taken at the mastoid process. Although the configurations of the BCM curves are similar, the thresholds for group B are considerably more reduced than those for group A.

Four of the cases in group B had an ossicular discontinuity due to incus necrosis or absence of the incus. Two of the four cases had a perforation of the tympanic membrane and one of these had a cholesteatoma which filled the entire attic, antrum, and adicus. The fifth case had had a radical mastoidectomy and at the time of testing the attic was filled with cholesteatoma. The remaining two cases had malleus fixation: in one the malleus was fixed by bony growth to the lateral attic, and in the other thick granulation tissue enveloped the malleus and incus. As far as it can be determined, the interesting commonality of these cases is the presence of a mobile and intact stapes with a fixed malleus or a discontinuity due to necrosis or absence of the incus.

DISCUSSION

Theoretical Implications

The results of this study require some comment about the theory of bone conduction and the implications for the clinical testing of bone conduction. Recently Tonndorf (1966) presented a revised theory of bone conduction based in part on numerous experiments with laboratory animals. It is impossible to present all of the ramifications of Tonndorf's theory of bone conduction here, but some definite relationships appear to exist between our current results and the findings he derived from his laboratory investigations.

Tonndorf compared the changes in response to bone-conduction stimuli in four animal species following immobilization of the tympanic membrane or "amputation of the middle ear." The frequency of maximal loss by bone conduction correlated with the resonant point of the ossicular chain in each species. A similar result was found when the stapes of the cat was fixated with dental cement. The maximal loss in the bone-conduction response was found in the frequency area around 500–600 Hz, which corresponds to the resonant point of the ossicular chain in the cat. The explanation that the "Carhart notch" is due to the loss of the middle-ear inertial component generally has not been advanced, for it has often been suggested that this contribution to bone conduction is greatest in the low frequencies. Therefore, the accepted theory concerning inertia bone conduction and the presence of a BC notch at 2,000 Hz in man

did not appear to be related. Tonndorf suggests the earlier explanation of inertia bone conduction is too simple and overlooks the fact that the ossicular-chain vibrating system also has a resonant point which varies in different animals. Since the ossicular chain has a resonant point near 2,000 Hz (Groen, 1962) in man, the maximal loss should be found in this frequency area when the chain is fixated.

Tonndorf's evidence suggests that it is essentially the missing ossicular inertial component that determines the frequency value of the point of maximal bone-conduction loss when the middle ear is amputated. He reported reductions in bone conduction around 500–600 Hz due to amputation of the middle ear in the cats. However, a greater loss was observed when the middle-ear was amputated than when the stapes was fixed. Tonndorf suggested that somewhat similar results should occur in man after radical mastoidectomy and presented the audiogram of one such case.

Figure 21–9 shows the average air- and bone-conduction thresholds at the mastoid and frontal bone and the SAL results for seven patients who had radical mastoidectomies but no reconstructive surgery. Five of these cases are included in the Results section of this article, and we evaluated two patients recently, using similar experimental procedures. Our

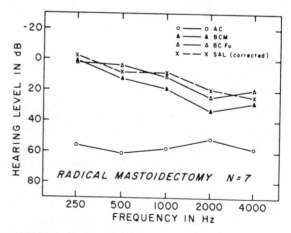

FIGURE 21-9. Mean thresholds in dB re hearing level for four test conditions for seven postoperative radical mastoidectomy cases who have had no reconstruction surgery.

results in Figure 21–9 agree on two major points with the conclusions reached by Tonndorf: (1) Bone-conduction thresholds are depressed from normal. (2) The frequency area of maximal loss corresponds to the resonance point of the ossicular chain in man.

The depression of the bone-conduction curves probably was not due to a sensorineural component, for the bone-conduction thresholds improved at 4,000 Hz, compared to those at 2,000 Hz, and speech discrimination scores were above 90 percent. Of further interest for this study is the general agreement between BCFu and corrected SAL thresholds. The results of tests conducted at the frontal bone indicated less hearing loss than the results obtained at the mastoid process. The average difference between the frontal and mastoid-process measurements is approximately 7 dB. As in earlier results, there is little difference at 250 Hz between frontal and mastoid measurements.

Compare the audiometric configuration of these seven patients who have had radical mastoidectomy (Figure 21–9) with the results observed on patients with surgically confirmed stapes fixation (Figure 21–6). Notice that in both groups the greatest reduction in bone conduction is observed in the higher frequencies, especially around 2,000 Hz. In the cases with stapes fixation the notch is not complete since the thresholds at 4,000 Hz remain equal to those at 2,000 Hz. This may be because some of the cases with stapes fixation also had sensorineural components or other secondary ossicular lesions. In general, our results for cases with stapes fixation and radical mastoidectomy support Tonndorf's theory that the maximal loss in bone conduction due to impairment or elimination of the ossicular inertial component will be found within frequencies of the resonance of the ossicular chain.

The purpose of our investigation was to test the hypothesis that cases with middle-ear lesions show less hearing loss for bone conduction at the frontal bone than at the mastoid process. While this may be true for some middle-ear problems, it does not necessarily hold true for all middle-ear impairments; results on the patients with stapes fixation (Figure 21–5) suggest that this concept is too elementary. In unpublished data, Herer (1964) also compared bone-conduction thresholds at the mastoid process with SAL thresholds on cases with stapes fixation. The two measurements showed equivalent reductions in

the higher frequency region. Thus, it would appear that some alterations in the middle ear similarly affect mastoid and frontal bone-conduction thresholds. It comes as no surprise that thresholds at the frontal bone can also be significantly affected by impairments in the middle ear. Studebaker's (1962) results showed only a small difference between thresholds at the frontal bone and the mastoid process on a group of various conductive lesions, and both sets of thresholds were depressed compared with normals. Naunton and Fernandez (1961) reported considerable changes in thresholds at the frontal bone in three cases of otitis media. They observed an improvement in bone-conduction thresholds in the low frequencies but a reduction around 2,000 Hz. In each of these studies, the contribution of middle-ear inertia was partially or completely eliminated and the largest reduction in bone-conduction or SAL threshold at the frontal bone was observed around 2,000 Hz.

Kirikae's (1959) evidence regarding oscillations of the skull from bone-conducted signals may be of interest here. Kirikae observed that in higher frequencies (above 1,500 Hz) the oscillations of the skull became extremely varied and complicated. He concluded that the location of the vibrator on the skull made relatively little difference for skull oscillations in high frequencies. Thus, the contribution from the middle-ear inertial effect would be similar regardless of vibrator placement in the higher frequency region. If middle-ear impairment eliminates this contribution to the total bone-conduction response, somewhat similar threshold changes could occur from measurements at the mastoid process and the frontal bone for frequencies around 2,000 Hz in man.

Among the individuals who demonstrated a substantial frontal-mastoid difference, one patient had surgically confirmed malleus fixation with an absence of other middle-ear changes. Results for this case are in Figure 21–10 and must be reviewed rather carefully since there was also a sensorineural component. Thresholds at the frontal bone indicated considerably less sensorineural involvement than mastoid process measurements did. The largest difference between measurements at the two sites was 21 dB at 2,000 Hz. A large difference was present also at 4,000 Hz. This difference gradually reduced as the test frequency was lowered and became nonexistent at 250 Hz. Results from the SAL test are not recorded in the figure; however, they were in good

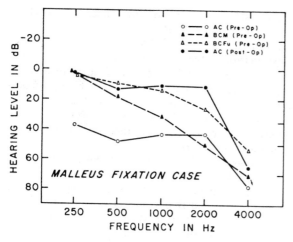

FIGURE 21-10. Preoperative AC, BCM, and BCFu thresholds and postoperative AC thresholds in dB re hearing level for an individual with malleus fixation.

It is obvious from our results that middle-ear lesion cases cannot be considered as a homogeneous group in terms of frontal-mastoid differences. Current evidence suggests the following:

1. When the stapes is fixated, the bone-conduction responses at the frontal bone and mastoid process are altered in a very similar manner.
2. If the ossicular chain is partially eliminated by a radical mastoidectomy, the thresholds for bone conduction at both sites are reduced maximally around 2,000 Hz; however, the reduction is not as large for measurements at the frontal bone as for measurements at the mastoid process.
3. Bone-conduction thresholds at the mastoid process appear to be considerably more reduced than those at the frontal bone—for cases in which the stapes is intact and mobile but the malleus and incus are fixated, or for some cases of discontinuity at or involving the incudo-stapedial joint.

agreement with the frontal-bone thresholds. Since the ossicular chain was probably fixated in this instance, the frontal-mastoid difference in the high frequencies was not anticipated in light of the aforementioned results of Kirikae (1959).

Notice that the postoperative air-conduction responses coincide closely with the preoperative frontal-bone hearing curve. The area of deviation is at 2,000 Hz at which the air-conduction curve is approximately 6 dB better than the preoperative bone-conduction result. This may be because there was also some reduction in the frontal-bone threshold due to the partial or complete elimination of the inertial effect or to variability in measurment.

Malleus fixation has some similarity with experimental fixation of the tympanic membrane, as reported by Tonndorf. In cats he found that fixation of the tympanic membrane resulted in a reduction of the bone-conduction response similar to that observed in stapes fixation; however, the notch became a flat-bottomed trough extending over a wider frequency range than that observed with stapes fixation. The case described in the current paper also demonstrates a reduction in mastoid bone-conduction thresholds covering a wider frequency range than that observed in stapes fixation.

Clinical Implications

The use of bone-conduction or SAL measurements in clinical evaluations is generally based on the assumption that the bone-conduction threshold is not as dependent on the external and middle ear as is the air-conduction threshold. While clinically useful, it is obvious that this assumption requires considerable modification, precisely because the external and middle ear do contribute to the total bone-conduction threshold. If, however, it becomes possible to determine and predict the changes in bone-conduction thresholds that occur with various middle-ear impairments, the very modifications that limit the basic clinical assumption may become useful in the differential diagnosis of middle-ear lesions.

The extensiveness of the clinical testing procedure and the selection of appropriate diagnostic tests depend on questions asked by the diagnostician. If separation of cases with conductive and sensorineural loss is the only objective, the majority of patients with conductive hearing loss can be adequately classified with only one of the tests included in our experimental battery. However, at least two types of cases may be incorrectly diagnosed if only one test of sensorineural acuity is employed:

1. Conductive cases with very mild hearing loss may present little or no air-bone gap, especially if BCM is the test of choice. Because of individual variations in bone-conduction thresholds and vibrator placement effects, it is hazardous to classify these on the basis of one bone-conduction test.
2. Cases with mixed hearing loss may be misdiagnosed because the effects of middle-ear impairment depress bone-conduction thresholds. Our results indicate that BCM measurements would be the most severely depressed compared to bone-conduction tests at the frontal bone or SAL.

If clinical constraints (time, personnel, equipment, etc.) do not permit an extensive evaluation of each patient, the clinician must choose the test of sensorineural acuity that will differentiate the largest number of cases possible. The results of this experiment and other similar bone-conduction investigations (Studebaker, 1962; Link and Zwislocki, 1951) suggest that we seriously consider BCFu as the test of choice. Although the middle ear's condition may influence both frontal and mastoid bone-conduction thresholds, as illustrated in cases with stapes fixation (Figure 21-6) and radical mastoidectomies (Figure 21-9), BCFu generally was equal to, or better than, BCM in this study. However, in certain cases (Figure 21-8) the results of the frontal bone tests showed considerably less hearing loss than BCM. Thus, the use of frontal bone-conduction measurements may maximize the air-bone gap and result in the proper diagnosis of the largest number of hearing impairments.

There are other dividends from testing bone-conduction thresholds at the frontal bone. Although results from clinical studies have not been as impressive as some laboratory investigations, measurements at the frontal bone always indicate equal or greater inter- and intrasubject reliability than do comparative measurements at the mastoid process. A minor advantage of unoccluded bone-conduction measurements at the frontal bone (BCFu) is the ease of administering such tests (e.g., the audiometric Weber and Bing) because their test results can be obtained without disturbing the original placement of the bone vibrator at the frontal bone.

The only obvious disadvantage of BCFu is that, in general, more intensity is required to reach threshold than for comparable mastoid measurements. The SAL test has the same disadvantage, for the placement of the vibrator at the frontal bone reduces the maximum shift available. In cases of severe hearing loss, mastoid placement of the vibrator may be necessary in order to obtain threshold values. However, an additional evaluation with BCFu is highly recommended, since in some instances threshold measurements obtained at the mastoid process may be considerably depressed from their frontal bone-conduction counterparts.

A question also arises concerning the use of occluded, frontal bone-conduction measurements or SAL. Our experimental results have demonstrated that the SAL and BCFo tests provide similar information and differ from BCFu only in conductive cases. SAL and BCFo both involve vibratory placement at the frontal bone and occlusion of the test ear. The SAL is a particularly valuable test for evaluating cases who are difficult to mask properly for bone-conduction testing. If a relative or unoccluded threshold is desired, however, one must use either earphones that cause no occlusion effect or correct the SAL results for conductive loss cases by subtracting the average occlusion effect obtained from normal listeners fitted with the occluding earphone cushions. The correction procedure is recognizably a hazardous one on individual cases, but currently there are no "non-occluding" earphones that are practical for clinical use. We caution that before SAL results can be corrected, the clinician must rule out the presence of an occlusion effect by administering unoccluded and occluded BC tests.

Our preference for unoccluded testing procedures, rather than occluded frontal bone-conduction or occluded SAL, is based partially on the most recent investigations of the occlusion effect by Tonndorf (1966). Tonndorf's evidence gathered from experimental animals indicates the occlusion effect for bone-conducted signals is based primarily on two factors: (1) When vibrating, the walls of the external canal radiate acoustic energy that is partially transmitted to the receptor organ via the middle ear, the open ear canal acting as a high-pass filter and its occlusion producing a low-frequency emphasis. (2) The air in the external canal constitutes a load upon the tympanic membrane, and changes in the resonant properties of the canal because modifications in length and/or occlusion alter the load effect. Thus, middle-ear impairments reduce or eliminate the occlusion effect.

Jerger et al. (1965) have suggested that SAL or occluded bone-conduction techniques give the best estimates of sensorineural acuity in conductive hearing loss cases because patients with middle-ear impairment have a built-in occlusion effect. The recent studies by Tonndorf (1966) however, suggest that the opposite is, indeed, the case. His results indicate that a functional tympanic membrane and ossicular chain are necessary for the presence of the occlusion effect, and middle-ear impairments generally eliminate the effect. Until substantial evidence to the contrary is presented, the use of an unoccluded bone-conduction or SAL test would be more appropriate.

Obviously, if a researcher or adventurous clinician wishes to perform tests at the frontal bone, he will need to collect normative data at this site. Clinics with an artificial mastoid may choose to perform threshold measurements on a group of normal subjects and calibrate their bone-conduction system in physical terms. The published data on frontal-bone measurements reported by Weston et al. (1967) or by Dirks, Malmquist, and Bower (1968) may prove helpful for comparison. Clinics lacking equipment to calibrate their systems in physical terms must periodically obtain threshold measurements at the frontal bone, as well as at the mastoid process, from normal hearing individuals, to determine dial corrections for their bone-conduction systems. We wish to emphasize that until the International Standards Organization has established bone-conduction norms for testing at the frontal bone and the mastoid process, rigorous calibration procedures (including testing of normal listeners) must be employed.

Rather than suggesting the abandonment of bone-conduction testing at the mastoid process, the results of our current study indicate that the use of several diagnostic tests might be valuable in differentiating between various middle-ear impairments. Knowledge and technology in otology and audiology have reached a stage at which the description of conductive losses in the gross terms of loss should no longer be considered completely adequate. For cases in which the otologic examination and routine audiological evaluation fail to facilitate a precise differential diagnosis, additional audiological information can often be helpful. Along with other tests of middle-ear function (i.e., absolute and relative acoustic impedance), the difference between bone-conduction thresholds at the mastoid process and frontal bone should be considered a possible diagnostic tool.

ACKNOWLEDGMENTS

This investigation was supported by Public Health Service Research Grant No. NB 0588303 from the National Institute of Neurological Diseases and Blindness and by the Hope for Hearing Research Foundation. The authors are indebted to Victor Goodhill and the resident doctors of the Head and Neck Surgery Department at UCLA.

REFERENCES

Barany, E. A contribution to physiology of bone conduction. *Acta Otolaryng. (Stockholm)*, suppl. **26**, 1–223 (1938).

Bekesy, G. Zur theorie des horens bei der schallaufnahme durch knochenleitung. *Ann. Physik*, **13**, 111–136 (1932).

Carhart, R., and Jerger, J. Preferred method for clinical determination of pure tone thresholds. *J. Speech Hearing Dis.*, **24**, 330–345 (1959).

Dirks, D. Factors related to bone conduction reliability. *Arch. Otolaryng.*, **79**, 551–558 (1964).

Dirks, D., Malmquist, C., and Bower, D. Toward the specification of normal bone conduction threshold. *J. Acoust. Soc. Amer.*, **43**, 1237–1242 (1968).

Dirks, D., and Swindeman, J. The variability of occluded and unoccluded bone conduction thresholds. *J. Speech Hearing Res.*, **10**, 232–249 (1967).

Elpern, B., and Naunton, R. The stability of the occlusion effect. *Arch. Otolaryng.*, **77**, 376–384 (1963).

Groen, J. J. The value of the Weber Test. Ch. 14 in H. F. Schuknecht (Ed.), *International Symposium on Otosclerosis*. Boston: Little Brown and Co. (1962).

Hart, C., and Naunton, R. Frontal bone conduction tests in clinical audiometry. *Laryngoscope*, **71**, 24–29 (1961).

Herer, G. A study of the effects of various forms of stapes surgery upon estimates of cochlear reserve. Unpublished doctoral dissertation, Northwestern Univ. (1964).

Hodgson, W., and Tillman, T. Reliability of bone conduction occlusion effects in normals. *J. Auditory Res.*, **6**, 141–151 (1966).

Hood, J. The principles and practice of bone conduction audiometry; a review of the present position. *Proc. Royal Soc. Med.*, **50**, 689–697 (1957).

Jerger, J. and Jerger, S. Critical evaluation of SAL audiometry. *J. Speech Hearing Res.*, **8**, 103–125 (1965).

Jerger, J., and Tillman, T. A new method for the clinical determination of sensorineural acuity level (SAL). *Arch. Otolaryng., 71,* 948–953 (1960).

Jerger, J., Verville, J., Shea, J., and Kinchen, K. Comparison of SAL and bone conduction audiometry in the prediction of gain from stapes surgery. *Acta Otolaryng., 60,* 467–478 (1965).

Kirikae, I. An experimental study on the fundamental mechanism of bone conduction. *Acta Otolaryng.* (Stockholm), suppl. **145,** 1–111 (1959).

Link, R., and Zwislocki, J. Audiometrische knochenleitungsuntersuchungen. *Arch. Ohr Nas Kehlkopfheilk,* **160,** 347–357 (1951).

Lybarger, S. Special report-interim bone conduction thresholds for audiometry. *J. Speech Hearing Res., 9,* 483–487 (1966).

Naunton, R., and Fernandez, C. Prolonged bone conduction: observations on man and animals. *Laryngoscope,* **71,** 306–318 (1961).

Studebaker, G. Placement of vibrator in bone conduction testing. *J. Speech Hearing Res.,* **5,** 321–331 (1962).

Tillman, T. Clinical applicability of the SAL test. *Arch. Otolaryng.* **78,** 36–48 (1963).

Tonndorf, J. Bone conduction studies in experimental animals. *Acta Otolaryng.* (Stockholm), suppl. **213,** 1–132 (1966).

Weston, P., Gengel, R., and Hirsh, I. Effects of vibrator types and their placement on bone conduction threshold measurements. *J. Acoust. Soc. Amer.,* **41,** 788–792 (1967).

Whittle, L. A determination of the normal threshold of hearing by bone conduction. *J. Sound Vibr.,* **2,** 227–248 (1965).

part III

SPEECH AUDIOMETRY

The status of speech audiometry as an integral part of basic hearing measurement has not changed much since the first edition of this book. The two major components of speech audiometry—the measurement of speech thresholds and the measurement of speech discrimination*—are used to assess the validity of the pure-tone audiogram, to evaluate hearing aids, to assist in differential diagnosis, and to predict communicative function in natural settings. Out of the multitude of articles on speech audiometry, we have selected twelve that appear to us to illustrate some basic principles, procedures, and problems. For a thorough discussion of speech audiometry, the reader is referred to a recent review by Olsen and Matkin (1979).

The first two articles in this part appeared in our earlier edition. They are reprinted again because they describe some of the basic principles underlying all speech audiometry. The Miller, Heise, and Lichten article, for example, introduces the student to the concept of the articulation function (also known as the "performance-intensity" function) and demonstrates succinctly the effects of different types of stimuli on that function. The Hirsh et al. article, on the other hand, details the development of the most widely used speech stimuli in audi-

ometry, the W-1 spondee and W-22 monosyllabic word lists.

The next three selections deal with the measurement of spondee threshold and the relation between spondee and pure-tone thresholds. The Chaiklin and Ventry article is again reprinted here because it appears that their method has gained some acceptance among audiologists; the article describes empirical evidence in support of measuring spondee thresholds in 5-dB steps and presents an alternative method for 2-dB steps. Note, too, that the ascending modification of the procedure described by Chaiklin, Font, and Dixon (1967) can be substituted readily for the descending technique recommended by Chaiklin and Ventry.

Another procedure for measuring spondee thresholds that has gained acceptance is one described originally by Tillman and Olsen (1973) and represented here by an article by Wilson, Morgan, and Dirks. Their article details the procedure, describes its statistical precedent, and offers some empirical data attesting to the adequacy of the method. We have chosen not to include here the American Speech-Language and Hearing Association's recent (1979) guidelines for measuring spondee thresholds since, at this writing, there appear to be no data supporting either the reliability or validity of the method advocated in the guidelines.

Although the two previous articles describe the relationships between spondee thresholds (obtained with the particular method under study) and pure-tone thresholds, the most recent and extensive treatment of this subject appears in Carhart and Porter (1971) and Carhart (1971). We chose to include the latter article because it speaks directly to

---

*Although we continue to use the traditional term *speech discrimination,* we recognize that some speech discrimination tests are, in reality, word recognition tasks that do not require speech sound discrimination. This is especially true of such open-response-set tests as the W-22 and the NU-6 word tests. In this section, we will use *speech discrimination* and *word recognition* interchangeably when referring to open-response-set monosyllabic word tests.

the clinician and it offers empirical support for the formula

$$ST = \frac{T_{500} + T_{1000}}{2} - 2 \text{ dB}$$

for predicting spondee threshold from pure-tone data when the pure-tone configuration is relatively flat. It is widely recognized, however, that a sloping configuration can have a marked influence on the spondee threshold/pure-tone average relationship. Readers are urged to consult Carhart and Porter's (1971) detailed discussion of the effect of slope on spondee thresholds and Fletcher's (1950) classic article concerning the two- and three-frequency pure-tone averages as predictors of spondee thresholds.

The remaining articles in this part all deal with various methodological aspects of speech discrimination testing. This subsection leads off with Carhart's overview of problems in speech discrimination testing, an article that also appeared in our first edition. The articles that follow amplify Carhart's remarks about phonemic equivalence, test-retest variability, and test procedures. But Carhart's article, published more than fifteen years ago, addresses issues that are still at the forefront of speech discrimination testing and that are still largely unresolved.

The next article, by Tillman and Carhart, was selected for several reasons. First, Northwestern University Auditory Test No. 6 (NU-6) is a widely used monosyllabic open-response-set test and, as Olsen and Matkin (1979) observe, the lists "... seem to have gained some popularity recently in research and clinical use" (p. 160). Second, the article should be of interest to clinicians who use the lists because it describes the research underly-

ing the development of NU-6. Finally, the reading is reprinted here because it is not readily available from government sources. Additional information concerning NU-6 may be found in Wilson et al.'s (1976) investigation of recorded versions of the NU-6 lists.

The inclusion of articles describing the development of the W-22 and NU-6 word lists reflects our opinion that clinicians should be familiar with the research underlying these tests of word recognition. Singling out these selections is no reflection on the quality or value of other speech discrimination tests that have been described in the literature. Rather, space limitations prevented us from including articles describing the development of tests such as the California Consonant Test (Owens and Schubert, 1977), the Modified Rhyme Test (Kreul et al., 1968), the Synthetic Sentence Indentification Test (Jerger, Speaks, and Trammel, 1968), and the Speech Intelligibility in Noise Test (Kalikow, Stevens, and Elliot, 1977). Readers are encouraged to consult these sources to familiarize themselves with alternatives to the more conventional monosyllabic discrimination tests.

Two recent articles by Thornton and Raffin and by Raffin and Thornton are included next because they address an extremely important question in speech discrimination testing: When can a difference in test-retest scores be considered a true difference rather than a chance difference? To put it in more clinical terms, if a patient scores 48 percent without an aid and 60 percent with an aid, is the 12 percent difference a statistically significant difference or could the difference have occurred merely by chance? In the first of the two articles, Thornton and Raffin explain the statistical basis for applying the binomial model to speech discrimination scores. While not easy reading, careful perusal should pay off in greater understanding of the model and its implications for clinical application. Note, too, the relevance of the model to any speech discrimination test using stimuli that are scored as correct or incorrect. In the second article, Raffin and Thornton provide tables that allow the clinician or researcher to determine at what confidence level two scores are different from one another when using fifty-item tests, twenty-five-item tests, or when comparing a twenty-five-item score to a fifty-item score. In the previous example, if a twenty-five-item test was used for both tests, the 12 percent difference would *not* be a significant difference (i.e., a confidence level of .4065). Penrod's article, reprinted later in this section, contains an example of the use of the Thornton and Raffin data. Further independent validation of the binomial model is contained in Raffin and Schafer (1980).

The effect of four different variables on speech discrimination scores was examined by Kreul, Bell, and Nixon in their 1969 study. Most significant was their finding that talker effects had an important influence on scores on the Modified Rhyme Test and that even an apparently innocuous change in the carrier phrase produced small but significant differences in discrimination scores. The conclusion of Kreul et al. is as apt today as it was more than ten years ago: "Tests ought not to be thought of as the written lists of words but as recordings of these words."

The research by Penrod extends the results of Kreul et al. by examining talker effects on the scores of subjects with sensorineural hearing impairment who responded to the W-22 word lists, spoken by four different talkers. The most relevant finding was that the talker-listener interaction poses the greatest threat to test stability and, further, that the greatest variability in scores occurs in individuals whose scores lie somewhere in the middle of the range. Penrod's data, as well as the data of Kreul et al., attest to the need to reduce talker effects in the clinical measurement of speech discrimination.

The final selection in this part examines still another aspect of speech discrimination testing—the scoring bias introduced when using talkback responses during speech discrimination testing. Nelson and Chaiklin's data show rather conclusively that scorer bias can affect discrimination scores and that with inexperienced listeners, the bias is such that higher scores are assigned than would be obtained using write-down responses. Nelson and Chaiklin caution that their data also reveal that experienced listeners are not immune to response bias and that bias increases somewhat as the listening situation deteriorates. Their suggestions for reducing response bias are worthy of attention: ask the patient for clarification; reduce examiner distractions; place the patient's microphone in an advantageous position; use adequate monitoring levels; and watch the patient's face.

REFERENCES AND ADDITIONAL READINGS

American Speech-Language and Hearing Association. Committee on Audiometric Evaluation. Guidelines for determining the threshold level for speech. *Asha,* **21,** 353–356 (1979).

Carhart, R., and Porter, L. S. Audiometric configuration and prediction of threshold for spondees. *J. Speech Hearing Res.,* **14,** 486–495 (1971).

Chaiklin, J. B.; Font, J.; and Dixon, R. Spondee thresholds measured in ascending 5-dB steps. *J. Speech Hearing Res.,* **10,** 141–145 (1967).

Fletcher, H. A method of calculating hearing loss for speech from an audiogram. *J. Acoust. Soc. Amer.,* **22,** 1–5 (1950).

Jerger, J.; Speaks, C.; and Trammel, J. A new approach to speech audiometry. *J. Speech Hearing Dis.,* **33,** 318–328 (1968).

Kalikow, D.; Stevens, K.; and Elliot, L. Development of a test of speech intelligibility in noise using sentence materials with controlled word predictability. *J. Acoust. Soc. Amer.,* **61,** 1337–1351 (1977).

Kreul, E.; Nixon, J.; Kryter, K.; Bell, D.; Lang, J.; and Schubert, E. A proposed clinical test of speech discrimination. *J. Speech Hearing Res.,* **11,** 536–552 (1968).

Olsen, W., and Matkin, N. Speech audiometry. In *Hearing Assessment,* ed. W. Rintelmann. Baltimore: University Park Press (1979).

Owens, E., and Schubert, E. Development of the California Consonant Test. *J. Speech Hearing Res.,* **20,** 463–474 (1977).

Raffin, M., and Schafer, D. Application of a probability model based on the binomial distribution to speech-discrimination scores. *J. Speech Hearing Res.,* **23,** 570–575 (1980).

Tillman, T., and Olsen, W. Speech audiometry. In *Modern developments in audiology,* 2nd ed., ed. J. Jerger. N.Y.: Academic Press (1973).

Wilson, R. H.; Coley, K. E.; Haenel, J. L.; and Browning, K. M. Northwestern University Auditory Test No. 6: Normative and comparative intelligibility functions. *J. Amer. Aud. Soc.,* **1,** 221–228 (1976).

22

The Intelligibility of Speech as a Function of the Context of the Test Materials

GEORGE A. MILLER, Ph.D.
The Rockefeller University, New York City
GEORGE A. HEISE, Ph.D.
Indiana University
WILLIAM LICHTEN
Undergraduate student at Harvard University when this study was conducted

For many years communication engineers have used a psychophysical method called the "articulation test" (Egan, 1948; Fletcher and Steinberg, 1929). An announcer reads lists of syllables, words, or sentences to a group of listeners who report what they hear. The articulation score is the percentage of discrete test units reported correctly by the listeners. This method gives a quantitative evaluation of the performance of a speech communication system.

There are three classes of variables involved in an articulation test: the *personnel,* talkers and listeners; the *test materials,* syllables, words, sentences, or continuous discourse; and the communication *equipment,* rooms, microphones, amplifiers, radios, earphones, etc. The present paper is directed toward the second of these three classes of variables, the test materials. The central concern can be stated as follows: Why is a stimulus configuration, a word, heard correctly in one context and incorrectly in another?

Three kinds of contexts are explored: (1) context supplied by the knowledge that the test item is one of a small vocabulary of items, (2) context supplied by the items that precede or follow a given item in a word or sentence, and (3) context supplied by the knowledge that the item is a repetition of the immediately preceding item. All three kinds of context enable the listener to limit the range of alternatives from which he selects his response. A word selected from a small vocabulary must be one of the few words agreed upon in advance. A word in a sentence must be one of the relatively few words that make a reasonable continuation of the sentence according to grammatical rules agreed upon in advance. A repeated word must be one of the few words

Reprinted by permission of the authors from *J. Exp. Psychol.,* **41,** 329–335 (1951).

similar to the word just heard. Not anything can happen, and the listener can set himself to make the required discrimination. Context, in the sense the word assumes here, is the S's knowledge of the conditions of stimulation. The experimental problem is to vary the nature and amount of this contextual knowledge in order to study its influence upon perceptual accuracy.

EQUIPMENT AND PROCEDURE

The apparatus consisted of components from military communication equipment used during the recent war. The output voltage of a carbon microphone was amplified and delivered to the listener's dynamic earphones. The talker monitored his speaking level with a volume indicator (VU meter) that responded to the voltage generated at the output of the amplifier. A random noise voltage, with a spectrum that was relatively uniform from 100 to 7,000 cps, was introduced at the listener's earphones. The signal-to-noise ratio (S/N) was varied by holding the average voice level constant and changing the level of the noise. The S/N was measured by a vacuum tube voltmeter across the terminals of the earphones, and the measurements reported in the following pages represent the ratio in decibels of the average peak deflection of the meter for the words (in the absence of noise) to the level of the noise in the 7,000-cycle band. A S/N of zero dB means, therefore, that the electrical measurements indicated the two voltages, speech and noise, were equal in magnitude. Since the earphones transduce frequencies only up to about 4,500 cps, however, the acoustic level of the noise was about 2 dB lower than these electrical measurements indicate. The over-all acoustic level of the voice at the listener's ears was approximately 90 dB re .0002 dyne/cm.*

The speech channel was not a high quality system. Only the speech frequencies between 200 and 3,000 cps were passed along to the listener.*

Only two Ss were used throughout the experiments. Both had normal auditory acuity, and both were familiar with the design and theory of the experiments. The Ss were located in different rooms, connected only by the communication channel described above, and they alternated as talker and listener. Some particular S/N was set up in the channel, and the talker proceeded to read a list of test items. These items were pronounced after a carrier sentence, "You will write . . . ." During this carrier sentence the talker adjusted his voice level to give the proper deflection of the monitoring VU meter, and then the test item was delivered with the same degree of effort. This procedure preserves the inherent variability of English words—the word "peep" has much less acoustic energy than the word "raw" when both words are pronounced with equal emphasis by a normal talker. By monitoring the carrier sentence rather than the test item, the relative intensities of the speech sounds are preserved in a natural fashion. The listener then recorded the item on a test blank, and these test sheets were later graded and the scores converted to percentages.

IMPORTANCE OF TEST MATERIALS

The kind of speech materials used to test communication systems is an important variable determining the results of the tests. Figure 22–1 illustrates how much difference the test materials can make. These three functions were obtained for the communication channel and the personnel described above. The test materials used for these three functions were the following:

(1) The *digits* were pronounced *zero, wun, too, thuh-ree, four, f-i-i-v, six, seven, ate, niner.* (2) The *sentences* were those constructed at the Psycho-

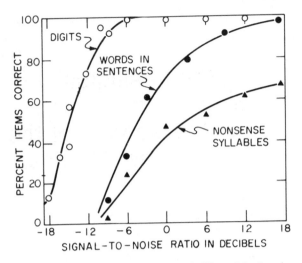

FIGURE 22-1. Relative intelligibility of different test materials.

Acoustic Laboratory (Egan, 1942). A sentence consists of five major words connected by auxiliary "of's," "the's," etc. The score shown in Figure 22–2 represents the percentage of these major words heard correctly. (3) The *nonsense syllables* used were also those published by Egan (1942). To standardize the pronunciation and recording of the nonsense syllables, an abbreviated phonetic symbolism was used.

The values of S/N necessary for 50 percent correct responses are approximately − 14 dB for digits, − 4 dB for the individual words in a sentence, and + 3 dB for nonsense syllables. At a S/N where practically no nonsense syllables were recorded correctly, nearly all the digits were correctly communicated. Differences of this magnitude require explanation. What differences among these spoken stimuli make some easy to hear and others quite difficult? A list of perceptual aspects—rhythm, accent, grouping, meaning, or phonetic composition—can be suggested. Our experiments indicate, however, that these various characteristics of the stimulus that *did* occur are less important than the characteristics of the stimuli that *could* have occurred but didn't. The most important variable producing the differences is the range of possible alternatives from which a test item is selected. A listener's expectation (or, more precisely, his freedom of choice) is determined by the context in which the particular phonetic pattern occurs. When

---

*For the convenience of those who may wish to apply one of the several schemes for predicting articulation scores, the frequency response of the system may be obtained by ordering Document 3250 from American Documentation Institute, 1719 N Street, N. W., Washington 6, D.C., for microfilm (images 1-inch high on standard 35 mm. motion picture film) or for photocopies (6 × 8 in.) readable without optical aid.

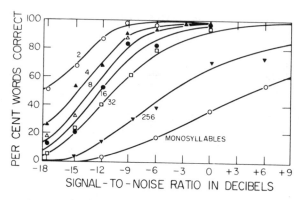

FIGURE 22-2. Intelligibility of monosyllables as a function of the size of the test vocabulary. (Data are not corrected for effects of chance.)

digits are used, the listener can respond correctly with a marginal impression of the relatively intense vowel sound alone, because all the digits, with the exception of *five* and *nine,* have different vowels. Since the alternatives are thus limited, the digit is interpreted correctly, although the same acoustic stimulus is quite ambiguous when the alternatives are not so limited. With nonsense syllables, however, this limitation of possibilities is far less helpful; the listener feels that anything can happen. To record the nonsense syllable correctly, a listener must perceive each phoneme correctly, and the perception of one phoneme in a syllable does not give a clue to the other phonemes in the same syllable. Not only must the listener hear the vowels correctly, but the less intense consonant sounds must also be distinguished.

SIZE OF TEST VOCABULARY

An articulation test is a rather unusual combination of the familiar psychophysical procedures. The experiment requires the listener to select, not one out of two or three, but one out of several thousand alternative responses. Thus the number of alternatives involved becomes an interesting variable.

Suppose we try to adapt spoken stimuli as closely as possible to the traditional method of constant stimuli. To this end we might use a single speech sound or a single syllable as the stimulus, present this speech unit at various intensities, and ask S to report whether or not he heard each presentation. This procedure determines a threshold of audibility for the

particular speech unit. The practical value of this isolated datum is negligible. The experiment must be repeated for all the forty or fifty different speech sounds or the thousands of different syllables of English. And then we know only about audibility, not intelligibility.

Consider this distinction between audible speech and intelligible speech. It is intuitively clear that the words *audible* and *intelligible* are not synonyms, and listeners give reliably higher thresholds when asked to make continuous discourse "just understandable" instead of "just audible" (Egan, 1948). The crux of the difference is that intelligibility involves a complex discrimination and identification, whereas audibility is simply a discrimination of presence or absence.

It seems reasonable, therefore, to call a speech unit intelligible when *it is possible for an average listener with normal hearing to distinguish it from a set of alternative units.* By a speech unit is meant any combination of vocal noises—phonemes, syllables, words, phrases, sentences. The act of distinguishing can take various forms—repeating the unit, writing it down, pointing to it, behaving in accordance with its content, etc. The critical part of this definition concerns the set of alternative speech units from which the particular unit is selected. This part of the definition reduces intelligibility to discriminability, and avoids the questions of semantic rules and meaning. Discriminability is a function of the number of alternatives and the similarities among them. The word "loot" is easily discriminated if all the alternatives are trisyllabic, but difficult to distinguish, other things being equal, in a set of alternatives that includes "boot," "loop," "jute," "lewd," "mute," "loose," etc.

An articulation test is analogous to a test of visual acuity where the percentage of correct judgments of a fixed set of test figures is plotted as a function of the level of illumination. A differential judgment is required under various favorable and unfavorable conditions. In such an experiment we determine the most unfavorable conditions under which the discrimination can be made, rather than the most unfavorable conditions under which the presence of the stimuli can be detected. These are clearly different thresholds and correspond to what we have called the thresholds of intelligibility and of audibility.

A difficult discrimination quickly becomes impossible as the conditions are made unfavorable, whereas an easy and obvious difference remains noticeable almost as long as the stimuli can be detected. The discrimination of a difference of 3 cycles in frequency, for example, is fairly accurate under favorable conditions—at 1,000 cps and 100 dB. If the intensity is progressively reduced, however, such a small difference becomes imperceptible. For a simpler discrimination, say 30 cycles difference in frequency, the listener can respond accurately at all intensities down to 5 or 10 dB above the threshold of audibility.

The situation is manageable so long as we have some index of the difficulty of the discrimination. Thus, in the tonal example, the difficulty can be gauged by the size of the difference in frequency. With the articulation test, however, such an index is not available. We could utilize known differences in the spectra of the sounds to construct an index of the distance between speech sounds, but this index is not yet available. For the present we must approach the problem in a simpler way.

Imagine a many-dimensional space with a separate coordinate for each one of the different frequencies involved in human speech sounds. Along each coordinate plot the relative amplitude of the component at that frequency. In this hyperspace each unique speech sound is represented by a single point. Each point in the hyperspace represents a single acoustic spectrum. The group of similar sounds comprising a phoneme is represented by a cluster of points in the hyperspace. If a language utilized only two different phonemes, the hyperspace could be split into two parts, one for each phoneme. The distance between the two phonemes could be made as large as the vocal mechanism permits, and discrimination would be relatively easy. But suppose the number of different phonemes in the language is increased from two to ten. With ten different phonemes the hyperspace must be divided into at least ten subspaces, and the average distance between phonemes must be smaller with ten phonemes that it is with two. The discriminations involved must be correspondingly more precise. If the number of alternative phonemes is increased to a thousand, then the listener is required to make even more precise discriminations.

In other words, the ease with which a discrimination of speech sounds can be made is limited according to the number of different speech sounds that must be discriminated. From this line of reasoning it follows that the number of alternatives can be used to gauge the difficulty of discrimination. This argument

TABLE 22–1. PERCENT WORDS CORRECT IN ARTICULATION TESTS WITH VOCABULARIES OF VARIOUS SIZES.

S/N in dB	Size of Vocabulary							Mono-syllables
	2	4	8	Digits	16	32	256	
−21	49							
−18	51	27	17	13	13	5		
−15	67	52	32	38	19	20	2	
−12	87	69	57	73	51	39	14	3
− 9	98	92	89	92	85	61	28	
− 6		94	95	99	82	81	39	17
− 3		96						
0				100	97	95	70	37
+ 6				100			76	53
+12				100			90	70
+18								82

has been developed by Shannon (1948) to give a measure of the amount of information in a message. The interesting aspect of this index of difficulty, or of amount of information, is that it does not depend upon the characteristics of the particular item, but upon the range of items that *could* occur.

The range of alternatives was used as the experimental variable in the following way. The listener was informed that each test word would be one of the items from a given restricted vocabulary. The size of the test vocabulary was alternatively 2, 4, 8, 16, 32, or 256 words. The talker always spoke one of the words from the prearranged list.

The words used in the restricted vocabularies were chosen at random from the list of phonetically balanced monosyllables published by Egan (1948). For the two-alternative vocabulary, different pairs of words were chosen and typed on the listener's answer sheet. The talker read one of the pair, and the listener checked the item he heard. A similar procedure was used for the four- and eight-word vocabularies. For the 16-, 32-, and 256-word vocabularies the listeners had a list of all the words before them, and studied this list until they made their choice. The choice was recorded and a signal given to the talker to proceed to the next item. The Ss studied carefully the particular list used in any test and arranged the words according to the vowel sounds before the tests began.

The results are summarized in Table 22–1 and in Figure 22–2. Included with the data for restricted vocabularies are data for words from the original list of 1,000 monosyllables, obtained with no list of choices available to the listener. When these data are corrected for chance, the two-word vocabulary gives a threshold (50 percent of the words correct) at − 14 dB, the 256-word vocabulary gives a threshold at −4 dB, and the unrestricted list of monosyllables gives a threshold at +4 dB. With the same test words the threshold is changed 18 dB by varying the number of alternatives. This result supports the argument that it is not so much the particular item as the context in which the item occurs that determines its intelligibility.

CONTEXT OF THE SENTENCE

A word is harder to understand if it is heard in isolation than if it is heard in a sentence. This fact is illustrated by Figure 22-3. Sentences containing five key words were read, and the listener's responses were scored as the percentage of these key words that were heard correctly. These data are shown by the filled circles in Figures 22-1 and 22-3. For comparison, the key words were extracted from the sentences, scrambled, and read in isolation. The scores obtained under these conditions are shown by the open circles of Figure 22-3. The removal of sentential context changes the threshold 6 dB.

The effect of the sentence is comparable to the effect of a restricted vocabulary, although the degree of restriction is harder to estimate. When the talker begins a sentence, "Apples grow on—," the range of possible continuations is sharply restricted. This restriction makes the discrimination easier and lowers the threshold of intelligibility. A detailed statistical discussion of the restrictions imposed by English sentence structure is given by Shannon (1948), and is used in a simple recall experiment by Miller and Selfridge (1950).

EFFECTS OF REPETITION

When an error occurs in vocal communication, the listener can ask for a repetition of the message. The repeated message is then heard in the context provided by the original message. If the original message enabled the listener to narrow the range of alternatives, his perception of the repeated message should be more accurate. A series of tests were run with various kinds of test materials to evaluate the importance of the context of repetition. These tests were run with automatic repetition of every item and, also, with repetitions only when the listener thought he had not received the test item correctly.

The improvement in the articulation scores obtained with automatic and with requested repetitions was found to be about the same. A slight but insignificant difference was found in favor of the requested repetition, and if we add to this the savings in time achieved by omitting the unnecessary repetitions, the requested repetition is clearly superior.

The advantage gained by repetition is small for all types of test materials. In Figure 22-4 data are given for the effects of repeating automatically the monosyllabic words. The difference in threshold between one presentation and three successive presentations is only 2.5 dB. Similar data for words heard in sentences show a shift of 2 dB, and for digits, 1.5 dB.

These results indicate that the improvement that can be achieved by the simple repetition of a message is slight. The repeated message contains approximately the same information, and the same omissions, that the original message contained. If the listener thinks he heard the word correctly, he persists in his original response, whether it is right or wrong. If he thinks he heard the word incorrectly, he does not use this presumably incorrect impression to narrow the range of possibilities when the item recurs. In any case, no strong factor is at work to improve the accuracy on repeated presentations, and so we obtain only the slight improvement indicated in Figure 22-4.

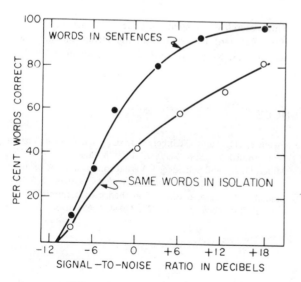

FIGURE 22-3. Effect of sentence context on the intelligibility of words.

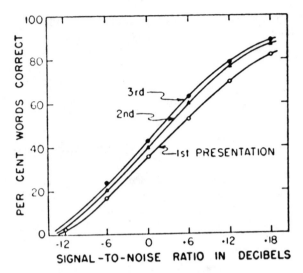

FIGURE 22-4. Effects of repetition of test words on the articulation score.

The results indicate that far more improvement in communication is possible by standardizing procedures and vocabulary than by merely repeating all messages one to two times.

In general, therefore, the results are in qualitative agreement with the mathematical theory of communication presented by Shannon (1948). A precise quantitative comparison of the data with the theory cannot be made in the absence of trustworthy information about the distributions of errors. Seemingly reasonable assumptions about the error distributions give results consistent with theoretical predictions, but a more thorough study would be rewarding. For a given signal-to-noise ratio the listener receives a given amount of information per second (according to Shannon's definition), and articulation scores can be predicted for different types of test materials on the basis of the average amount of information needed to receive each type of test item correctly.

SUMMARY

Articulation tests showed the effects of limiting the number of alternative test items upon the threshold of intelligibility for speech in noise. The number of alternative test items was limited by providing three kinds of context: (1) restricting the size of the test vocabulary, (2) using the words in sentences, and (3) repeating the test words. Differences among test materials with respect to their intelligibility are due principally to the fact that some materials require more information than others for their correct perception. The relative amount of information necessary for a given type of item is a function of the range of alternative possibilities. As the range of alternatives increases, the amount of information necessary per item also increases, and so the noise level must be decreased to permit more accurate discrimination.

ACKNOWLEDGMENT

This research was carried out under Contract N5ori-76 between Harvard University and the Office of Naval Research, U.S. Navy (Project NR147-201, Report PNR-74).

REFERENCES

Egan, J. P. *Articulation testing methods, II.* OSRD Report No. 3802, February, 1942. (Available through Office of Technical Services, U.S. Department of Commerce, Washington, D.C., as PB 22848.)

Egan, J. P. Articulation testing methods. *Laryngoscope,* 1948, 58, 955–991.

Fletcher, H., and Steinberg, J. C. Articulation testing methods. *Bell Syst. Tech. J.,* 1929, 8, 806–854.

Miller, G. A., and Selfridge, J. Verbal context and the recall of meaningful material. *Amer. J. Psychol.,* 1950, 63, 176–185.

Shannon, C. E. A mathematical theory of communication. *Bell Syst. Tech. J.,* 1948, 27, 379–423, 623–656.

23

Development of
Materials for
Speech Audiometry*

Ira J. Hirsh, Ph.D.

Professor of Psychology, Washington University, St. Louis, and Director of Research, Central Institute for the Deaf

Hallowell Davis, M.D.

Research Associate, Central Institute for the Deaf

S. Richard Silverman, Ph.D.

Director, Emeritus, Central Institute for the Deaf, Washington University

Elizabeth G. Reynolds

Research Assistant at Central Institute for the Deaf at the time this study was conducted

Elizabeth Eldert

Audiologist, Department of Otolaryngology, Washington University School of Medicine, at the time this study was conducted

Robert W. Benson, Ph.D.

Bonitron, Inc., Nashville, Tennessee

The sounds of speech have come to occupy an important place among the auditory stimuli that are used in clinical audiometry. By measuring a patient's ability to use his hearing in ways that are closer to everyday auditory experience, speech audiometry has not only added a kind of validity to pure-tone audiometry, but also certain speech tests have appeared to have diagnostic and prognostic value as well (Hirsh, 1952). The growth in the general acceptance and use of speech audiometry is accompanied by a need for standardization so that the test results in one clinic can be compared with those of another clinic. The present article deals with modifications of existing recorded auditory tests that yield new auditory tests, which appear to satisfy some clinical needs that were not fulfilled by older tests. In particular, tests will be described that permit the measurement of two clinical quantities: *hearing loss for speech* and *discrimination loss*.

*These materials were developed under contracts with the Veterans Administration (Contract V1001M-577) and the Office of Naval Research (Contract N60nr-272, Project No. NR142-170, Task Order III).

Reprinted by permission of the authors from *J. Speech Hearing Dis.*, **17**, 321–337 (1952).

BACKGROUND

During World War II, considerable effort was expended in the development of articulation testing methods for the evaluation of various types of military communications equipment. It turned out that certain of these tests, developed at the Psycho-Acoustic Laboratory, Harvard University, were applicable to the clinical evaluation of hearing.

Psycho-Acoustic Laboratory (PAL) Auditory Tests No. 9 and No. 12, for measuring the threshold of intelligibility for spondaic words and for sentences, respectively, were made available on phonograph records for clinical use—first for military rehabilitation centers and then for more general use. These two recorded tests permitted a quick and reliable measure of the threshold of intelligibility and its related clinical measure, the hearing loss for speech. They have been described by Hudgins et al. (1947), by Hirsh (1947), and others.

In a study of patients who were evaluated with respect to suitability for the fenestration operation, Davis (1948) and his co-workers have formulated a general estimate of a patient's ability to hear speech by coupling the results on the threshold of intelligibility (or the hearing loss for speech) with a measure of the ability to discriminate among speech sounds at levels considerably above the threshold. This latter ability was measured by using the Psycho-Acoustic Laboratory's PB-50 lists, which are the phonetically balanced lists described by Egan (1948). It appears that both types of tests are clinically useful and, indeed, that the latter measure of discrimination loss is the more useful clinical datum because the former, hearing loss for speech, can be predicted so reliably from the audiogram (Carhart, 1946; Fletcher, 1950; Harris, 1946).

Several years have passed during which many audiometrists have had a chance to try out the spondee words and the PB-lists both by live-voice techniques and by way of phonograph records. During these years, reports have accumulated of several deficiencies in the Harvard tests, deficiencies mostly with respect to clinical use. Specifically, it has been reported informally that certain of the records of Auditory Test No. 9 yield slightly different thresholds from other of these records. Further, the large vocabulary that was assembled for the 20 PB-lists [published in Egan (1948)] was too large for many clinical patients. The vocabulary appeared to need restriction in the dimension of familiarity. Finally, recorded versions of the PB-lists have not been available in suitably standard form.

This article does not purport to reveal any basically new concepts or techniques. It represents, rather, a report of modifications of these earlier tests in order to correct or eliminate some of these deficiencies that have been found as the tests have been used clinically.

Two basic improvements, from the clinical point of view, have been made. *First,* the vocabulary for the spondee lists and the PB-lists has been restricted so as to include only those words that meet certain criteria of familiarity. Furthermore, the vocabulary in each PB-list has been more rigidly phonetically balanced. The more rigid application of criteria of phonetic balance has resulted in a smaller test vocabulary, but one that appears to be sufficiently large for the small samples of lists that characterize clinical use. A *second* major improvement has been made possible by the use of recording on magnetic tape. With this recording technique it was possible to speak a given test word only once and then to copy it as many times as necessary to have it appear on different versions of a given test list. In the older tests, for example, the word *hothouse* appeared in each of

six scramblings (word orders) of one spondee list. Since the test was made from original disc recordings, the word had to be spoken six times, once within each scrambling. With tape, one would have to speak the word only once, copy it six times, and cut and resplice the actual tapes in order to produce the word in its proper place in each of the six word orders.

An improved version of the Auditory Test No. 9 for clinical use is C.I.D. Auditory Test W-2 (spondees at descending levels). The comparable modification of Auditory Test No. 14 is C.I.D. Auditory Test W-1 (spondees at constant level). Finally, recorded versions of the modified PB-lists appear as C.I.D. Auditory Test W-22. A general description, method of construction, and preliminary test results for each of these three tests follows.

DESCRIPTION AND DEVELOPMENT

C.I.D. Auditory Test W-1

Test W-1 consists of six scramblings of a single list of 36 spondaic words. These are recorded at a constant level, each word at a level 10 dB below the level of an introductory carrier phrase, "Say the word . . ." On the inside of each of the six record faces, a *1,000 cps tone has been recorded at the level of the carrier phrases, that is, 10 dB above the test words.* Since it was desirable that the carrier phrases be well above the level of the test words, especially for those playback levels at which the test words would be just barely intelligible, the tone could not be recorded at the level of the test words without endangering the monitoring meter of the test user. If, for example, the tone were recorded at the same level as the test words, and a playback were adjusted so that an ordinary VU meter read "0 VU," the carrier phrases would force the indicator to hit the pin at the right side of the scale.

Use of Test W-1. In general, Test W-1 permits the measurement of the threshold of intelligibility, the level at which a listener repeats correctly 50 percent of the words of a given list, by traditional methods of articulation testing. In clinical application, it may be used by the audiometrist who wishes to control manually (with an attenuator that is variable in decibel or some multiple of decibel steps) the intensity of the words presented to a listener.

Construction of Test W-1. The starting point for vocabulary was the group of 84 spondee words in PAL Test No. 9 (and No. 14). The most familiar spondees were obtained from ratings of judges who, working independently, rated the words in the Harvard tests on a three-point scale of familiarity. The words rated most familiar were spoken by an adult male and were recorded on a phonograph disc.

Two acetate discs were cut simultaneously, one for future rerecording and one for preliminary use. The talker monitored the carrier phrase "Say the word," carefully on a VU meter, and then spoke the following test word with "equal effort." When spoken in this manner the words varied from each other in intensity level by about ±2 dB. Some words were spoken several times until the talker felt that a satisfactory rendition had been obtained.

In a preliminary experiment, six listeners with normal pure-tone audiograms listened monaurally to the words through standard playback equipment (see Appendix A). The group included both experienced and inexperienced listeners. Instructions were as follows:

> You are going to hear a list of two-syllable words, like "baseball" and "armchair." A man's voice will say "Say the word" before each word. Listen for the word following. Some groups of words are louder, some are softer than others. Repeat through the microphone what you hear. If you hear only unintelligible sound after "Say the word," let me know by saying "Check."

Individual thresholds for speech (in dB re 0.0002 microbar) were obtained for the spondaic word lists in the PAL Test 9. The method of scoring was that described in Hudgins et al. (1947). Each listener then listened to the disc recording of the more familiar (CID) spondees at +4, +2, 0, −2, −4, and −6 dB relative to the threshold that had been obtained for PAL Test 9. The order in which the lists were presented was the same for each listener. The order in which the different levels appeared, however, was varied for each listener and each list according to a random Latin Square design. In this design, dependent variables, such as learning and fatigue, are presumably weighted equally at each level in the averaged data for six listeners. All data for each listener were obtained in one listening session.

Raw data were recorded in terms of the number of errors per word for each listener. One word, relatively much easier than the others, might be repeated

correctly even at levels 4 and 6 dB below the threshold. Consequently, there would be very few errors for that word. And conversely, a difficult word might not be heard correctly, even at levels 2 and 4 dB above the tnreshold, and would have many errors. In the analysis of this preliminary data an easy word was defined as one missed once or less by all six listeners. A difficult word was one missed five or more times by all six listeners. Words falling in both of these extreme categories were eliminated, and also the words that five of the six listeners found difficult or easy. In the 36 words left, a group of equally intelligible spondees was approximated.

The original disc reserve was then dubbed to tape. The 36 chosen words were cut out and spliced together with enough blank tape between words to facilitate the separate attenuation of individual words. This was called the *master tape* and all subsequent versions of the 36 words were recorded from this tape. One carrier phrase was recorded with good quality and even monitoring. This carrier was recorded separately from the words and therefore sounds qualitatively different from the words. This difference, however, in no way affects the results of the tests and is not very noticeable at levels around threshold where the test is given. This was called the *master carrier phrase.* It could be rerecorded any number of times by making a loop of it and running the tape around and around on the recording head of the tape recorder.

Six different word orders of the same 36 words were put together in the following manner. The master tape was dubbed to tape again six times. The order of the words in five dubbings was changed by cutting the words apart and resplicing them in different positions within each list. The master carrier phrase was then recorded once for each of the 216 words in the six lists at +10 dB relative to the words. A carrier phrase was spliced in front of each word and the timing made such that one carrier phrase plus the word following plus the pause for a listener's response took six seconds. The six word orders were designated as Lists A, B, C, D, E, and F of W-1 and an appropriate recorded introduction was spliced in front of each. A copy of these lists as just described was made for experimental purposes and the original spliced version was held in reserve.

An experiment similar to the preliminary testing was then run. One Latin Square was done with inexperienced listeners, however, and another with experienced listeners. The six word orders were given to all listeners in the same sequence, although the levels at which different listeners heard different word orders were determined by a random Latin Square. Tentative speech thresholds were determined this time by using one of the experimental word lists. The words were presented at this threshold (0 dB) and + 4, + 2, − 2, − 4, and − 6 dB. Raw data for each group of subjects were scored as errors for each word at each of the presentation levels.

Performance on the separate words varied little between the experienced and inexperienced listeners. For present purposes, therefore, their data were treated together. An inspection of the data showed that some words were still more difficult, some easier, than others in spite of the initial attempt to get a group of words homogeneous with respect to intelligibility. The degree of difficulty of a word was correlated with the intensity reading of the word on a VU meter. The easy words monitored at higher levels, the more difficult words at lower levels, relative to the average intensity reading for the 36 words. This correlation existed even though originally the words were spoken with "equal effort" and varied only ± 2 dB from an average intensity reading. It was therefore decided to push the more difficult words up 2 dB and the easier words down 2 dB.

A second set of the same six word orders was made from the master tape changing the levels of the more difficult or easier words by ± 2 dB in each rerecording of the master tape. The experiment described above was repeated. An analysis of the data showed that the words were now more homogeneous with respect to intelligibility and variations in the thresholds of individual words were, as adequately as could be measured by this method, chance variations. Since tape reproducers are not in general clinical use, and since there is no good way of copying large numbers of tape recordings, this last version of the six word lists was recorded on discs as Auditory Test W-1.

This final recording was done at the Technisonic Recording Studios. The word lists were recorded both at 78.26 rpm and 33⅓ rpm with the NARTB recording characteristic (*Recording and Listening Test Standards,* 1950). A half-minute of a 1,000 cps calibration tone, at the level of the carrier phrase, was put at the inner edge of each record so that individual operators can set their levels on a constant signal.

Preliminary Test Results for Test W-1. The articulation-vs.-gain function for Test W-1 as recorded on the final tapes is shown in Figure 23–1. The function

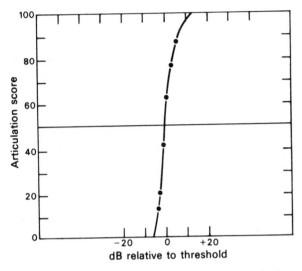

FIGURE 23-1. Articulation score as a function of level relative to individual threshold (Auditory Test W-1). Points represent average scores for 12 listeners.

represents the data of all listeners, six inexperienced and six experienced, and was drawn as the most representative curve for the series of individual curves superposed on each other at 0 dB, or threshold. Therefore the function is to be interpreted as showing slope relative to threshold with no indication of the absolute levels involved.

The articulation score rises from 0 to 100 percent within a range of about 20 dB. There is an increase from 20 to 80 percent within a range of 8 dB and throughout this range the slope or rate of rise in score is about 8 percent per dB. Since the threshold falls on the steepest part of the function, it is crossed very abruptly and, therefore, can be very sensitively determined with this test. There is a definite "tail" on the upper end of the curve. The rate of rise of the curve tapers off above 80 percent and does not reach the 100 percent point until about + 14 dB above threshold. Much of this tapering is due to the performance of the inexperienced listeners at levels above threshold. They were not familiar with the words or the listening situation and therefore continued to miss a few words even at levels above threshold where their scores should have been nearer 100 percent. Momentary inattention on the part of all listeners also contributed to the flattening of the function at the upper end. Below threshold the words drop out very quickly and there is little if any "tail" at this end of the curve.

The absolute thresholds for the experienced and inexperienced listeners were approximately the same, 20 dB and 21 dB re 0.0002 microbar, respectively. The difference between the two thresholds was not significant.

Preliminary checks were also made with the first disc recordings of Test W-1. Fourteen listeners (in groups of four or five) listened monaurally to all six scramblings at each of two levels, one below threshold and the other above. These levels were not the same for all listeners as each earphone used had a correction factor of its own which changed the output level. The two points obtained in each case were connected by a straight line, the slope of which was close to 8 percent per dB, and the approximate threshold was interpolated from this straight line function. The mean absolute threshold obtained in this way was 14.3 dB re 0.0002 microbar and the standard deviation of the individual mean thresholds around this mean was 2.2 dB.

It should be stressed here that the above results with the new W-1 disc recordings are tentative and await confirmation from those who use the test according to the instruction manual issued with the test.

C.I.D. Auditory Test W-2

Test W-2 employs the 36 words that were used in W-1 and also the same six word orders. Test W-2 differs from W-1, however, in that the intensity of the words is attenuated within each list at the rate of 3 dB every three words. In the older PAL Test 9 the rate of attenuation was 4 dB every six words. In the present test, it was attempted to employ a faster pace and also to avoid the necessity of a table for scoring by letting each word represent 1 dB of attenuation on the average.

Use of Test W-2. This test is designed specifically for a rapid estimate of the threshold of intelligibility. The six word orders, labelled lists A through F, are the same as those of Test W-1. Instead of presenting a whole list or a portion of a list at a fixed intensity or several intensities, this test sweeps through an intensity range of 33 dB by attenuating the level of the test words 3 dB every three words. The rationale for this procedure consists of sampling three-word portions

of the list at intensity levels that are 3 dB apart. Ideally the intensity level at which a listener repeats 50 percent of a group (i.e., 1.5 words) would be the threshold. Actually, the threshold is approximated by assuming that the words are attenuated at an average rate of 1 dB per word and that the threshold is the level at which the first group of three words is presented minus the number of words (or of decibels) that the listener repeats correctly.

Of course, a threshold calculated in this way will be in error because the 50 percent-criterion is not fully met unless 50 percent of the first group (i.e., the first 1.5 words) is first subtracted out of the total. The 1.5-dB error involved is a constant of small magnitude relative to ordinary test results and may be neglected in clinical use. The absolute thresholds to be given below have taken this correction into account and represent, therefore, the best approximation to a 50 percent-response level. In general, the clinical norms, if established without this correction, should be 1.5 dB lower.

Construction of Test W-2. When the master tape was dubbed again to tape for this test, the initial relative level of the same words was changed ±2 dB in each recording as they had been for the final version of Auditory Test W-1. In addition, in each rerecording every word was separately attenuated in such a way that when the words were spliced together in the same order as in W-1 the intensity within each list decreased 3 dB every three words.

Two hundred sixteen copies of the master carrier phrase were made, one for each word in W-2. The first nine carriers for each list were recorded at the level of the first three words. The intensity of the rest of the carrier phrases for each list was decreased 3 dB after every three carrier phrases. In the final spliced version of the test, therefore, the first nine carrier phrases are at the starting level of the test even though the intensity of the test words in these first three groups is already being attenuated. From the tenth item on, the carrier phrases are progressively attenuated, each carrier phrase remaining 6 dB above the word that follows it.

A carrier phrase at the correct relative level was then spliced in front of each word. The lists were designated as lists A, B, C, D, E, and F of W-2, corresponding to the same lists in W-1. Appropriate introductions were then spliced in front of the lists. Finally, copies of this original spliced version were made for experimental purposes.

The experimental problem was to find out if there were any differences in difficulty among the lists. A group of six experienced listeners were given the six word orders of Auditory Test W-2. The tests were started at 40 dB above 0.0002 microbar so that, assuming that the thresholds would be around 20 dB, a listener would repeat approximately half the list before reaching threshold. Instructions to the listener were the same as for the experiments with Auditory Test W-1. The order in which each listener heard the W-2 lists was determined by a random Latin Square design.

An analysis of variance showed that different thresholds obtained by using different word orders varied no more than would be expected by random error. There were differences, however, in the average thresholds for six listeners as obtained with the different lists. Differences were of the order of ±1 dB. It appears that the lists of words are not equal in difficulty unless each entire list is heard. When only part of the list is heard the difficulty of the list depends on which part is heard. For a given listener it cannot be said that all parts of the lists are equal in difficulty.

The six word lists were then recorded on discs at the Technisonic Recording Studios. These lists were also recorded at 78.26 rpm and at 33⅓ rpm with the NARTB recording characteristic (*Recording and Listening Test Standards,* 1950). Again, as for W-1, a 1,000 cps calibration tone was put at the inner edge of each record. This calibration tone is at the average level of the first nine carrier phrases and of the first three words.

Preliminary test results. The same 14 listeners who listened to the W-1 disc recordings also listened to the W-2 recordings. Each of the listeners heard all six scramblings of W-2 and individual thresholds were taken as the mean of the six scores for each listener. Lists were started at a level of 35 dB re 0.0002 microbar and, as described, the level of each successive three words decreased 3 dB. When the test is started at 35 dB for normal ears half or more of the test is heard before threshold is reached.

The mean absolute threshold for 14 listeners was 17.7 dB re 0.0002 microbar. (This includes the 1.5 dB correction mentioned earlier.) The standard deviation of the individual thresholds was 2.6 dB. The difference between the W-1 and the W-2 thresholds of about 3.5 dB in favor of W-1 may result from presenting all 36 words at a given level instead of only three. In actual clinical practice Test W-1 should be administered, as described in the manual, by "bracketing" the threshold using small samples of four or five words at levels around threshold. Thresholds obtained in this manner will undoubtedly be closer to those obtained with W-2.

An analysis of variance showed that there were no significant differences in difficulty between the W-2 lists as they were recorded on disc. Again, however, as with the tape versions, there were differences of the order of ±1 dB.

C.I.D. Auditory Test W-22

Test W-22 consists of a vocabulary of 200 monosyllabic words divided into four lists of 50 words each. Each list is phonetically balanced; that is, the speech sounds within the list occur with the same relative frequency as they do in a representative sample of English speech. Six scramblings of each list are available. The words have been spoken with the carrier phrase, "You will say," and the 1,000 cps calibration tone on the inner face of every record is at the average level of the carrier phrases.

Use of Test W-22. This test is used to determine a patient's discrimination loss for speech. The discrimination loss for speech is the difference between 100 percent and the percentage of given speech material that a listener repeats correctly at a level that is sufficiently high so that a further increase in intensity is not accompanied by a further increase in the amount of speech material repeated correctly. Low discrimination scores, i.e., large discriminations losses, have been found to yield important diagnostic distinctions (Davis, 1948).

Construction of Test W-22. The most important task was the selection of the vocabulary to make up the phonetically balanced word lists. The following criteria for the vocabulary were set up. First, all the words must be one-syllable words with no repetition of words in the different lists. Second, any word chosen should be a familiar word. This second criterion is to minimize the effect of differences in the educational background of subjects. Third, the phonetic composition of each word list should correspond to that of English as a whole as closely as possible.

This third criterion was the most difficult one to satisfy because there are no satisfactory studies of spoken English in the literature. The sources used were Dewey's study (1923) of the phonetic composition of newsprint and the Bell Telephone Laboratories' study (French et al., 1930) of business telephone calls in New York City. The two sources were given equal weight in the determination of the phonetic criteria for the word lists.

The sources were followed as closely as possible. First the distribution of syllable types (vowel-consonant, consonant-vowel-consonant, etc.) was determined. Then the distribution of vowels and consonants within each list was planned. Here the frequency of occurrence of consonants and consonant compounds in initial and final positions was considered. All distributions of phonetic elements were based on distributions of individual speech sounds rather than on groups of sounds.

The vocabulary of the 20 Psycho-Acoustic Laboratory PB-50 lists, a total of 1,000 words, was used as a pool from which words were drawn for Auditory Test W-22. From this pool 120 words were used. The remainder of the vocabulary (80 words) was not drawn from any specific source.

Five people independently rated the entire PAL vocabulary for familiarity. They were instructed to rate about half the words in each PB-50 list as 1 (most familiar), about 25 percent as 2 (fairly familiar), and approximately 25 percent as 3 (very unfamiliar). Agreement among the five raters was good. A final rating in familiarity, based on the rating given by the majority of the raters, was then assigned to each word. Of the 120 words from the PAL lists used in Auditory Test W-22, 112 were rated as 1, 7 as 2, and only one, "isle." as 3.

The entire W-22 vocabulary, a total of 200 words, was checked with the Thorndike list (1932). All words except "ace" appear on the Thorndike list. According to Thorndike, 190 are among the 4,000 most common English words; 171 are among the 2,000 most common words; and 144 are among the 1,000 most common words. The W-22 vocabulary was also checked with the Dewey list (1923). Of the 200 words, 128 appear on this list. All of these 128 words are among the first 2,000 most common words on the Thorndike list.

The only words of doubtful familiarity are "ace," "ale," and "pew." These words received a rating of 2 by the board of judges and are relatively unfamiliar according to the Thorndike lists. "Isle," which was given a rating of 3 by the judges, is among the 3,000 most common words according to Thorndike; as

TABLE 23-1. W-22 DISTRIBUTION OF SYLLABLE TYPES.

Type	Percentage of words
VC	20
CV	22
CVC	36
VCC	4
CCV	2
CVCC	10
CCVC	4
CCVCC	2

"aisle" it is in the first 5,000; and as "I'll" it is in the first 2,000. In general, the vocabulary consists of very common words.

The third criterion states that the phonetic composition of the lists shall correspond as closely as possible to that of English as it is generally spoken.

The first step in setting up a plan for phonetic balance was to decide on percentages for the various consonant-vowel arrangements found in monosyllabic words (Table 23-1). This decision was based on the analysis of syllable types in the study by French, Carter and Koenig (1930), with the following modifications. All vowel words were omitted. The high frequency of their occurrence depends on two words, "I" and "you." The percentage of consonant-vowel-consonant words was increased slightly and the percentage of words containing consonant compounds (two or more consonants in a row) was increased from 14.7 percent to 22 percent. The distribution of syllable types followed the French, Carter and Koenig study as closely as was practicable. In each W-22 list there were four initial consonant compounds and eight final compounds.

The next step was to decide on the distribution of vowels within each list (Table 23-2). The mean of the percentages given by Dewey (1923) and by French, Carter and Koenig (1930) for the frequency of occurrence of each vowel was followed as closely as possible. The following modifications were made. The neutral vowel was omitted from the distribution, since this vowel does not ordinarily appear in monosyllabic words. The percentages for the other vowels were increased, therefore, by an appropriate amount to make up for the absence of the neutral vowel from the distribution. Percentages for long vowels were also increased in order to fulfill requirements for syllable distribution. In general, a plan for the distribution of vowel sounds was worked out which was practicable, and it was followed exactly in each list.

TABLE 23-2. W-22 VOWEL DISTRIBUTION.

Vowel Sound	Percent occurrence in each W-22 list
I	12
æ	10
ε	10
ɑ	8
ʌ	8
i	10
e	10
o	6
u	6
ɑɪ	6
ɔ	4
ʊ	4
ɑʊ	2
ɪʊ	2
ɔɪ*	1
ɝ*	1

*The ɔɪ vowel occurs once in two lists and the ɝ sound in the other two lists.

Finally, the distribution of consonants was determined (Table 23-3). As for the vowel sounds, the mean of the percentages given by Dewey and by French, Carter and Koenig for the frequency of occurrence of each consonant sound was followed. The percentage for each consonant was divided into a quota for appearance of that consonant in initial and final positions. This was done by referring to both Dewey and the French, Carter and Koenig study and following their divisions roughly. The number of words in each PB-list (50 words) is too small to permit precise division of the consonants into quotas for initial and final positions.

Once the four PB-lists, each containing 50 different monosyllabic words, had been chosen they were recorded on magnetic tape. The talker used the carrier phrase "You will say." He monitored this phrase on a VU meter and then spoke the word as it would naturally follow in the phrase.

The four lists dubbed from live voice to magnetic tape were the master lists. Each list was then recorded six times and the words were cut and spliced in different orders to give six different word orders for each of the lists. There was no master carrier. Each phrase was kept intact as it had been spoken. The lists were designated Lists 1, 2, 3, and 4 and the word orders for each were lettered A through F. Appropriate introductions were then spliced into the recording. Copies on tape of the spliced version were made for experimental purposes and the original was kept for rerecording onto disc.

Trouble was encountered with signal transfer from one layer of tape to the layer directly under-neath on the reel both on the original recording and on the copies. This phenomenon is recognized by the tape manufacturer but usually the level of the transfer signal is very low and is not noticeable in a continuous recording. The transfer signal on the recordings was 45 to 50 dB below the signal and below threshold at lower playback levels. At the highest playback levels used in the experiment, however, particularly at 100 dB, the "echo" was above threshold in the pauses between phrases. In the following experiments, the words were presented at a level 20 dB above an intermixed white noise. The noise effectively masked the echo but did not interfere with the intelligibility of the words. When the lists were dubbed to disc the cutting head on the recording lathe was short-circuited between each phrase so that none of the echo was recorded.

An experimental check was made to determine whether the four lists were equal in difficulty. It was assumed that there would be no differences in difficulty among different word orders of the same list. Three groups of five listeners, a total of 15 in all, were used. They were screened at +10 dB relative to normal threshold for all test frequencies on the Maico pure-tone audiometer. Each group of five

TABLE 23-3. W-22 CONSONANT DISTRIBUTION.

Sound	Number of occurrences in each PB list Initial	Final
t	4	7
n	3	7
r	2	7
d	3	3
l	2	4
s	3	3
m	2	3
k	3	1
w	4	0
z	0	4
v	0	3
ð	2	1
h	3	0
f	1	1
p	1	1
b	2	0
j	2	0
ŋ	0	1
g	1	0
ʃ	1	0
θ	1	0
tʃ	1	0
dʒ	1	0
ʒ	0	0
	42	46

came on eight consecutive evenings (Saturdays and Sundays excluded) and listened each evening for 2½ hours including two or three rest periods.

Instructions were as follows:

> You are going to hear lists of one-syllable words. All the words you will hear are on the printed sheet I have just given you. At the beginning of each session you will be given the chance to look at this list. Some lists will be very loud and others will be very soft. Listen carefully and write down as many words as you can.

Group I first listened monaurally to all 24 lists (six word orders of each of four lists) at 100 dB re 0.0002 microbar. This procedure gave the listeners an indoctrination period in which the words were presented at a high level. Then they heard each of the 24 word lists at levels 10 dB apart from 20 to 70 dB re 0.0002 microbar. Lists and levels were randomized with the exception that no list was ever heard twice at the same level.

Group II listened under the same conditions. The lists and levels were in a different order, however, and an eighth level of 15 dB re 0.0002 microbar was also used when it was found that not enough low scores at 20 dB were being obtained to determine the bottom of the articulation curve. Group III first listened to all lists at 100 dB. Then they listened to each word order at 50, 40, 30, 20 and 15 dB re 0.0002 microbar. The scores from the first two groups were consistently near 100 percent correct above 50 dB and it was felt that the shape of the upper part of the curve was well determined without running Group III at 60 and 70 dB.

The articulation scores for each list are plotted as a function of sound pressure level in Figure 23-2. At higher levels there are no significant differences between the list scores. From 40 dB down, however, there are greater differences. The gain function for List 1 was consistently lower than for the other lists. A second articulation curve (the broken curve) drawn through the scores for List 1 alone is shifted over on the scale approximately 2 dB. A calculation of the average relative intensity of the words in each list as read from a VU meter showed that the words in List 1 were on the average 2.5 dB lower than the words in any other list. Therefore, in the final recordings from magnetic tape to disc the intensity of List 1 was increased 2 dB relative to the intensity at which the other three lists were recorded.

The threshold (50 percent-response) for these new PB-lists as determined from the experimental curve in Figure 23-2 is 24 dB re 0.0002 microbar.

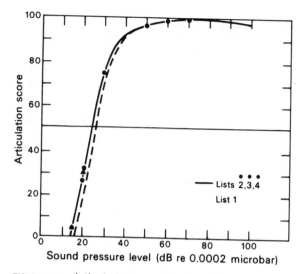

FIGURE 23-2. Articulation score (Auditory Test W-22) as a function of sound pressure level (experimental tape versions). Each point is the average of 15 listeners' scores on all six word orders of a list. The solid curve is drawn through points for Lists 2, 3, and 4. The broken curve is drawn through the points for List 1.

After inspection of the above data and the subsequent decision to raise the relative level of List 1 2-dB, the six word orders of each list were recorded onto disc from tape. The lists were recorded at 33⅓ rpm and 78.26 rpm. A calibration tone at the average level of the carrier phrase "You will say" was put on the inner band of every record.

Preliminary Test Results for Test W-22. The articulation function for Test W-22 has already been discussed under the construction of the test and is shown in Figure 23-2. This function was obtained using the experimental tapes. After the tapes were dubbed to disc for the final version of the test the articulation function was checked at two points using the disc recordings. The disc recordings were played to 15 listeners (in groups of 5) at 80 dB re 0.0002 microbar to check the maximum articulation score and at 25 dB to check scores close to threshold.

The average score at 80 dB using the disc recordings was 98 percent as compared to a score of approximately 99 percent at 80 dB read from the articulation function. At 25 dB scores were higher with the 78 rpm recordings than with the 33⅓ rpm recordings. The average score for the 78 rpm's was 63.4 percent, for the 33⅓ rpm's, 56.3 percent. The 33⅓ score agrees closely with the articulation score that would have been obtained at 25 dB with the experimental tapes (see Figure 23–2).

Although the same word orders of a list monitor alike on both the 78 and the 33⅓ rpm recordings, it is very possible that the high frequencies were given a boost of a few dB on the 78 rpm recordings. This boost does not show up in the monitoring as the VU meter is responding primarily to the energy around 250 cps which is the peak energy of the speaker's voice. Since the high frequencies are important in the discrimination of many consonants a high frequency boost in the recording might be accompanied by an increased articulation score for the recordings affected.

These data showed no consistent differences between scores on the four different lists. All listeners were given ample opportunity to study alphabetical lists of the words, however, and heard scramblings of each list at least three times. In a shorter clinical procedure where listeners may hear scramblings of two different lists once, some sort of differences between lists may appear from listener to listener. It can only be said that the averaged data of several listeners from several tests showed no consistent difference between lists.

As with the W-1 and W-2 results these results await verification from several clinics using a large number of listeners.

DISCUSSION

Although this report is intended to be only a description of some new auditory tests, it seems appropriate to discuss the relations among these tests and their predecessors. This discussion is supported by experimental data on a relatively few listeners. Most of the conclusions must remain tentative until a larger amount of clinical information is available.

Relations Among the New Tests

There are two outstanding relations that have been established with groups of normal listeners: one concerns the relation between W-1 and W-2 and the other between W-1 and W-22.

Descending-Level vs. Constant-Level Spondees. It has already been shown that the threshold for W-2 is about 4 dB above the threshold for W-1. That this difference is real is attested by some observations in which W-1 recordings were used as if they were W-2.

Otherwise said, the W-1 recording was begun at a certain sound pressure level and the experimenter attenuated the words by 3 dB every three words. The results of this procedure yielded thresholds of the order of 18 dB re 0.0002 microbar, the tentative standard threshold for W-2. It seems fair to conclude that the difference between the thresholds for W-1 and W-2 is attributable to the number of words that are presented at each level. From a restricted point of view, the W-1 threshold, at about 14 dB, represents the experimental ideal. When W-1 is put to clinical use, however, the tester ordinarily presents only four or five words at each level. Thus, in clinical use, when all 36 words are not presented at each test level, the expected threshold will be more nearly 18 dB, as for W-2.

Spondees vs. Monosyllables. Figure 23–3 shows the articulation-vs.-gain functions for all versions of W-1 and W-22. Two generalizations may be made: (1) The intelligibility of the spondee words (W-1) increases more rapidly with increase in intensity than does the intelligibility of the monosyllabic words of the PB-lists (W-22), and (2) the level at which a listener can repeat correctly 50 percent of a list of spondees is

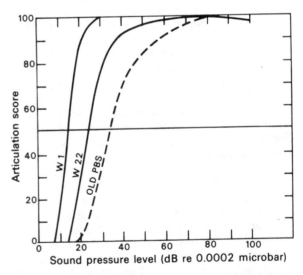

FIGURE 23-3. Relations between Auditory Test W-1, W-22, and the old PB-50 lists recorded at Technisonic Studios. The broken curve refers to the older version of the PB-lists. The solid curve labelled W-1 is the same curve found in Figure 23–1, but drawn relative to the average absolute threshold for 12 listeners. The curve labelled W-22 is the curve drawn for Lists 2, 3, and 4 in Figure 23–2.

lower than for one of the PB-lists of monosyllables. The reasons for the lower spondee threshold have been treated adequately elsewhere (Egan, 1948; Hudgins et al., 1947; Levin, 1952; Miller et al., 1951). It should be pointed out here, however, that the threshold for the present PB-lists (W-22) is much closer to the spondee threshold than have been the thresholds for previous PB-lists (see below).

Relations Between Present and Former Recorded Tests

It is clear that the results for normal listeners with these new recorded tests are not the same as the results for the older tests. Some of these differences need to be pointed out in detail.

Relation Between W-2 and PAL Auditory Test No. 9. The present W-2 threshold of 18 dB is somewhat lower than the threshold for Test No. 9 (22 dB). The reasons for this difference cannot be attributed entirely to the new recording procedure. First, the old threshold at 22 dB is a clinical threshold, somewhat higher than experimental ones. Furthermore, the total spondee vocabulary in W-2 is only 36 words while the total vocabulary for Auditory Test No. 9 is 84 words, or 42 words on either version. In view of the relation between the intelligibility of a given list of words and the size of the vocabulary for the list, which has been pointed out by Miller, Heise and Lichten (1951), it is not surprising that the threshold for the new tests with a smaller vocabulary should be lower. Again, it must be kept in mind that these thresholds are restricted to a psychophysical procedure in which only a few words are presented at each level. The low threshold that is obtained for W-1 indicates the order of difference that may be accounted for by these variations in the testing procedure.

Relation Between W-22 and the Older PB-lists. For some time a set of recordings of some of the PB-lists published by Egan has been available for distribution from the Technisonic Studios. These have enjoyed sufficient clinical use so that some tentative standards have become available. The articulation-vs.-gain function for these recordings is shown as a third curve in Figure 23–3. It is clear that the intelligibility of these older recordings at any given level is lower than for W-22 and that the function for the older recordings is not nearly so steep as that for W-22. Several reasons may be given for this difference. It has already been shown, in the above discussion of the development of Test W-1, that the intelligibility of a word is markedly dependent on its intensity relative to the other words in a list. The monitoring in W-22 is such that all of the words are much closer to each other in intensity than they were on the older recordings of the Egan lists. Furthermore, the vocabulary for W-22 consists of a total of 200 words while the total vocabulary in the Egan list was 1,000 words. Again, noting the relation between the intelligibility and vocabulary size (Miller et al., 1951), it is not surprising that the intelligibility of the smaller vocabulary should be higher at any given level than for the larger vocabulary.[1]

There are certain clinical questions that arise concerning the usefulness of W-22 in measuring discrimination loss. The smaller vocabulary makes W-22 an "easier" test than the older PB-lists. Both the vocabulary and the greater internal homogeneity contribute to a steeper gain function for W-22 than for the older PB-lists (Levin, 1952) (see Figure 23–3). There is not available as yet sufficient clinical information to predict whether this higher intelligibility and steeper gain function will make the use of W-22 more limited in the measurement of discrimination loss than the use of the older PB-lists.

SUMMARY

Three new recorded tests for the hearing of speech have been described. Tests W-1, W-2, and W-22 have been constructed to take the place of recorded versions of PAL Auditory Tests 14 and 9 and the PB-lists published by Egan respectively. Two novel techniques have been introduced: (1) The use of magnetic tape recording has permitted the construction of several versions or word orders of a given test list in which all occurrences of a test item in the several versions are physically identical; (2) The criterion of phonetic balance in W-22 and the criterion of familiarity of test items in both tests have been more rigidly followed, resulting in easier, more homogeneous lists, but with a more limited vocabulary.

Preliminary results have been presented in which the intelligibility for these new tests is shown as a function of intensity. Furthermore, a relation between intelligibility for these new tests and their analogous predecessors has been established. The authors' recommendation for the clinical adoption of these tests is tentative, pending the accumulation of results on larger groups of listeners in both clinical and laboratory situations.[2]

APPENDIX A

Equipment

The equipment necessary for reproducing the recordings of Auditory Tests W-1, W-2, and W-22 is represented by the American Standard Speech Audiometer[3] and includes the following elements:

1. A turntable and phonograph pickup with NARTB (National Association of Radio and Television Broadcasters) playback characteristic.
2. An amplifier.
3. A meter for monitoring the output of the amplifier.
4. An attenuator.
5. A calibrated earphone or loudspeaker.

The components are shown in the block diagram below:

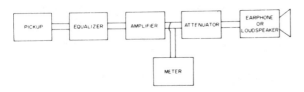

The turntable should be capable of playing recordings at a speed of 33⅓ rpm or of 78.26 rpm. The pickup should exert a force not greater than 10 grams. The pickup should be equalized so that it reproduces the frequencies in accordance with the NARTB characteristic.

Appropriate amplifiers should be used in order to obtain the power level necessary to drive either the earphone or the loudspeaker. The output noise of the amplifier should be at least 50 dB below the signal under all conditions. The meter should be provided to indicate the rms value of a 1,000 cps tone. A VU meter is very convenient but it is not essential.

An attenuator should be provided with a maximum insertion loss of at least 110 dB with indicated steps of 5 dB or less. If the indicated steps are 5 dB, an accessory vernier attenuator with steps of 2 dB or 1 dB is very desirable.

The earphone or loudspeaker should be of good quality in order to meet the following requirements. The over-all response characteristic including the pickup and equalizer, amplifier, attenuator and earphone or loudspeaker should not deviate more than plus or minus 5 dB from the NARTB characteristic over the frequency range from 200 to 5,000 cps. Furthermore, at no frequency from 50 cps to 10,000 cps should the pressure exceed the pressure at 1,000 cps by more than plus 5 dB.

APPENDIX B

The following lists of words constitute the vocabulary of the three Auditory Tests described in this report. Only an alphabetical order is given here. The ideal test lists used in the recorded versions are randomized orders of these words. The reader can make up equivalent test lists from these alphabetized orders by suitable scrambling.

Alphabetical List of the Spondaic Words Used in Auditory Tests W-1 and W-2

1. airplane	19. iceberg
2. armchair	20. inkwell
3. baseball	21. mousetrap
4. birthday	22. mushroom
5. cowboy	23. northwest
6. daybreak	24. oatmeal
7. doormat	25. padlock
8. drawbridge	26. pancake
9. duckpond	27. playground
10. eardrum	28. railroad
11. farewell	29. schoolboy
12. grandson	30. sidewalk
13. greyhound	31. stairway
14. hardware	32. sunset
15. headlight	33. toothbrush
16. horseshoe	34. whitewash
17. hotdog	35. woodwork
18. hothouse	36. workshop

Alphabetical Lists of the Words in Auditory Test W-22

List 1	List 2	List 3	List 4
1. ace	1. ail	1. add	1. aid
2. ache	2. air	2. aim	2. all
3. an	3. and	3. are	3. am
4. as	4. been	4. ate	4. arm
5. bathe	5. by	5. bill	5. art
6. bells	6. cap	6. book	6. at
7. carve	7. cars	7. camp	7. bee
8. chew	8. chest	8. chair	8. bread
9. could	9. die	9. cute	9. can
10. dad	10. does	10. do	10. chin
11. day	11. dumb	11. done	11. clothes
12. deaf	12. ease	12. dull	12. cook
13. earn	13. eat	13. ears	13. darn
14. east	14. else	14. end	14. dolls
15. felt	15. flat	15. farm	15. dust
16. give	16. gave	16. glove	16. ear
17. high	17. ham	17. hand	17. eyes
18. him	18. hit	18. have	18. few
19. hunt	19. hurt	19. he	19. go
20. isle	20. ice	20. if	20. hang
21. it	21. ill	21. is	21. his
22. jam	22. jaw	22. jar	22. in
23. knees	23. key	23. king	23. jump
24. law	24. knee	24. knit	24. leave
25. low	25. live	25. lie	25. men
26. me	26. move	26. may	26. my
27. mew	27. new	27. nest	27. near
28. none	28. now	28. no	28. net
29. not	29. oak	29. oil	29. nuts
30. or	30. odd	30. on	30. of
31. owl	31. off	31. out	31. ought
32. poor	32. one	32. owes	32. our
33. ran	33. own	33. pie	33. pale
34. see	34. pew	34. raw	34. save
35. she	35. rooms	35. say	35. shoe
36. skin	36. send	36. shove	36. so
37. stove	37. show	37. smooth	37. stiff
38. them	38. smart	38. start	38. tea
39. there	39. star	39. tan	39. tin
40. thing	40. tear	40. ten	40. than
41. toe	41. that	41. this	41. they
42. true	42. then	42. three	42. through
43. twins	43. thin	43. though	43. toy
44. up	44. too	44. tie	44. where
45. us	45. tree	45. use	45. who
46. wet	46. way	46. we	46. why
47. what	47. well	47. west	47. will
48. wire	48. with	48. when	48. wood
49. yard	49. young	49. wool	49. yes
50. you	50. your	50. year	50. yet

ENDNOTES

1. Comparison between the described speech-discrimination test and an older discrimination test based upon an earlier recording of the Harvard PB-Lists will be found in Silverman, S. R., and Hirsh, I. J., Problems related to the use of speech in clinical audiometry. *Ann. Otol. Rhinol. Laryngol.*, **64**, pp. 1234–1244 (1955): IJH, et al.

2. While this paper was in preparation clinical trials of W-2 and W-22 were conducted in the Hofheimer Audiology Laboratory (Washington University) and in the Hearing Clinic of Central Institute for the Deaf. Experience to date indicates (1) that W-2 is very satisfactory for determining the threshold for speech, but (2) that W-22 does *not* satisfactorily separate patients with mixed deafness from patients with pure conductive deafness. The older recordings of the Egan lists are more effective in this respect. The reasons for this difference are now being sought.

3. *American Standard Specification for Speech Audiometers.* New York: American Standards Association (in preparation).

REFERENCES

Carhart, R. Speech reception in relation to pattern of pure tone loss. *JSD,* **11**, 1946, 97–108.

Davis, H. The articulation area and the social adequacy index for hearing. *Laryngoscope,* **58**, 1948, 761–778.

Davis, H., Morrical, K. C. and Harrison, C. E. Memorandum on response characteristics and monitoring of word and sentence tests distributed by CID. *J. Acoust. Soc. Amer.,* **21**, 1949, 552–553.

Dewey, G. *Relative Frequency of English Speech Sounds.* Cambridge, Mass.: Harvard Univ. Press, 1923.

Egan, J. P. Articulation testing methods. *Laryngoscope,* **58**, 1948, 955–991.

Fletcher, H. A method of calculating hearing loss for speech from an audiogram. *J. Acoust. Soc. Amer.,* **22**, 1950, 1–5.

French, N. R., Carter, C. W. and Koenig, W. The words and sounds of telephone conversations. *Bell Syst. tech. J.,* **9**, 1930, 290–324.

Harris, J. D. Free voice and pure-tone audiometry for testing of auditory acuity. *Arch. Otolaryng., Chicago,* **44**, 1946, 452–467.

Hirsh, I. J. Clincial application of two Harvard auditory tests. *JSD,* **12**, 1947, 151–158.

—. *The Measurement of Hearing.* New York: McGraw-Hill, 1952.

Hudgins, C. V., Hawkins, J. E., Karlin, J. E. and Stevens, S. S. The development of recorded auditory tests for measuring hearing loss for speech. *Laryngoscope,* **57**, 1947, 57–89.

Levin, R. The intelligibility of different kinds of test material used in speech audiometry. M.A. Thesis, Washington Univ., 1952.

Miller, G. A., Heise, G. A. and Lichten, W. The intelligibility of speech as a function of the context of the test materials. *J. Exp. Psychol.,* **41**, 1951, 329–335.

Recording and Listening Test Standards. Washington, D.C.: Nat. Ass. Radio Telev. Broadcast., 1950.

Thorndike, E. L. *A Teacher's Word Book Of The Twenty Thousand Words Found Most Frequently and Widely In General Reading For Children and Young People.* New York: Teachers Coll., Columbia Univ., 1932.

24

Spondee Threshold Measurement: A Comparison of 2- and 5-dB Methods*

Joseph B. Chaiklin, Ph.D.
Supervisor, Audiology Section, Veterans Administration Medical Center, New Orleans
Ira M. Ventry, Ph.D.
Professor of Audiology, Teachers College, Columbia University

The general impression one gains from recent literature (Chaiklin, 1959; Jerger et al., 1959; Newby, 1958; Ruhm and Carhart, 1958; Tillman and Jerger, 1959) is that a 2-dB measurement interval is typically used in measuring spondee threshold.† Probably many clinicians use a 2-dB (or 1-dB) measurement interval because they believe a small interval provides spondee threshold estimates that are more precise and more reliable than could be obtained with a larger measurement interval. On theoretical grounds this rationale seems weak. If a variable is continuously distributed, a relatively small increase (2- or 3-dB) in size of measurement interval should have a negligible effect on precision, and no effect on reliability. A practical consideration that makes the use of small intervals questionable is that the intensity variations among currently used spondaic stimuli are larger than the small measurement intervals used by most clinicians. Finally, there is no apparent reason why spondee thresholds should be measured in steps smaller than the 5-dB step ordinarily used to measure pure-tone thresholds.

It should be noted that small measurement intervals have not always been used for spondee threshold sampling. Some of the early spondee threshold methodologies (Fletcher, 1950; Watson, 1949; Watson and Tolan, 1949, p. 449) employed a 5-dB measurement interval probably on the basis of equipment limitations rather than on theoretical bases. As far as we can determine, the most recent report of the use of a 5-dB spondee threshold measurement interval is contained in an article by Whipple and Kodman (1960). The primary purpose of this article is to report experimental evidence supporting the use of 5-dB steps in the measurement of spondee thresholds.

A secondary focus of the article is measurement method. Most descriptions of spondee threshold measurement methods have been imprecise or lacking in detail. A major portion of the present article is devoted to detailed descriptions of measurement methods that we believe will meet current needs in this area.

PROCEDURE

Subjects

Subjects were 100 adult male veterans selected from the clinic population of the Veterans Administration Audiology and Speech Pathology Clinic, San Francisco. They ranged in age from 23 to 62 years with a mean age of 42.2 years. The etiologies and types of hearing loss for the subjects are listed in Table 24–1. Seventy-one of the subjects were being seen at the clinic for routine audiometric testing related to otologic treatment, hearing aid evaluations, and diagnostic testing for the otolaryngology department. The remaining 29 subjects were being evaluated for compensation purposes and were part of a control

*The study was supported by U.S. Public Health Grant B-2741 (C2RI) and by the Veterans Administration.

†The term "spondee threshold" (Tillman and Jerger, 1959) is used here in place of the more traditional "speech reception threshold" (SRT). The term "spondee threshold" is a more direct statement of what is being measured.

This article has been revised from the original and is reprinted by permission of the authors from *J. Speech Hearing Dis.*, **29**, 47–59 (1964).

TABLE 24–1. DISTRIBUTION OF ETIOLOGIES AND TYPES OF HEARING LOSS FOR TOTAL SAMPLE; $N = 100$.

Category	N
Etiology	
Otosclerosis	49
Otitis Media (inactive)	19
Undetermined	15
Acoustic Trauma	13
Presbycusis	1
Normal*	3
Type	
Mixed	60
Sensory-neural	31
Conductive	6
Normal*	3

*Right ear was normal for three cases with unilateral loss.

group in a study of functional hearing loss (News Note, *JSHR*, 1962; Ventry, 1962).*

Subjects were selected using the following criteria: (1) absence of ear, nose, or throat conditions that might cause abnormal threshold fluctuations; (2) speech discrimination score not lower than 60 percent for the ear used in the study; (3) not more than 62 years of age; and (4) absence of functional hearing loss (Chaiklin and Ventry, 1963; Ventry and Chaiklin, 1962).

General Design

The general plan of the study was simple. First, pure-tone air-conduction thresholds were obtained for one or both ears. Next, spondee thresholds were measured using the 2-dB and 5-dB methods. To control order effects, 50 subjects had the 2-dB threshold measured first, followed by the 5-dB threshold. This order was reversed for the other 50 subjects. Eighty-five subjects has spondee threshold measurements on the right ear, and the remaining 15 had spondee threshold measurements on the left ear. An important feature of the general design was the control of bias that might result from the tester's knowledge of the results of a previous threshold measurement. The control of bias was accomplished either by having the

*For more complete details, see Chaiklin, J. B., and Ventry, I. M., Chapter I: Introduction and Research Plan. In I. M. Ventry and J. B. Chaiklin (Eds.), Multidiscipline study of functional hearing loss. *J. Aud. Res.*, **5**, 219–230 (1965). JBC, IMV.

second test conducted by a different tester who had no knowledge of the results of the first set ($N = 43$), or by means of an accessory "Random Variable Attenuator" ($N = 57$). The Random Variable Attenuator (RVA) permitted the tester to introduce an unknown amount of attenuation into the earphone line so that he could repeat a threshold measurement relatively free from the biasing effect of his knowledge of the first threshold obtained.[1] After making a threshold measurement the tester needed only to determine the amount of added attenuation in the line and then correct the audiometer dial reading by that amount. Following the measurement of spondee thresholds, the clinician proceeded with the remainder of the audiologic evaluation. All tests were administered by the authors or by the clinic's audiologists working under the close supervision of the authors. All tests were administered during a single test session except for the reliability substudy which required two sessions.

The test-retest reliability of the 2-dB and 5-dB methods was evaluated by retesting the 29 subjects referred to earlier. All reliability retests were conducted by the authors with the use of the RVA. The order of the retests was varied systematically to control order effects.

EQUIPMENT

Data were gathered in three test suites, two of which contained Industrial Acoustics Company audiometric testing rooms (Models 402 and 1201). The third two-room suite was of permanent construction. Two of the suites had Allison 21 series audiometers equipped with Telephonics Corporation TDH-39 earphones set in MX-41/AR cushions and Ampex 351 tape recorders as input sources for taped spondee stimuli. The third suite had an Allison 20A audiometer with provision for delivering only disc-recorded stimuli; the input source was a Garrard 301 turntable with a Garrard TPA 12 transcription arm and a General Electric variable reluctance cartridge (Model 4G-053). The calibration of both the pure-tone and speech circuits was checked periodically with an Allison Laboratories Audiometer Calibration Unit (Model 300). The pure-tone circuits were calibrated to the ASA standard (1951), but the speech circuits were calibrated to a zero hearing level of 29 dB re 0.0002 dyne/cm^2 rather than the 22-dB zero hearing level recommended by ASA (1953).*

Pure-Tone Threshold Measurement

Pure-tone air-conduction thresholds were measured with an ascending "on-effect" procedure similar to the procedure recommended by Carhart and Jerger (1959). Ascending series of short (approximately one sec.) tones were presented with successive stimuli separated by toneless intervals. The only important deviation from the procedure recommended by Carhart and Jerger was that each ascent was continued five dB above the level at which a subject first responded. Threshold was usually defined as the lowest hearing level at which at least a 60 percent response criterion was met. Of course, the criterion percentage was dependent on the number of stimuli presented at each level. Occasionally a 50 percent response criterion was applied. However, the 5-dB interval used in standard pure-tone audiometry is too large to allow routine application of the 50 percent response criterion frequently used with the classical psychophysical methods (Carhart and Jerger, 1959).

Spondee Threshold Measurement

The speech stimuli used in the measurement of thresholds were the 36 spondaic words of CID Auditory Test W-1 (Hirsh et al., 1952). All stimuli were presented either by means of the CID disc recordings

of Auditory Test W-1 (lists A through F) or by taped dubs of CID recordings with the identifying introduction to lists B through F omitted. Two further considerations should be noted: (1) the stimulus mode (tape or record) remained the same for a particular subject; that is, if the first spondee threshold was measured with taped stimuli, succeeding measurements employed taped stimuli; and (2) at no time was live-voice testing used in the measurement of spondee thresholds.

The procedure for instructing subjects before spondee threshold measurement was the same regardless of which of the two threshold measurement techniques was employed first. The following instructions, appropriate for both methods, were read to the subject before the first threshold measurement.

1. You're going to hear a recording of a man reading a list of two-syllable words such as "blackboard" and "earthquake." Before each word the man will say, "Say the word. . . ." For example, "Say the word 'earthquake.' "

2. Your job is to repeat each two-syllable word after you hear it, no matter how faint the word may be. You don't have to say, "Say the word." For example, if you hear "Say the word 'blackboard,' " you should say "blackboard." The words may become very faint, but please continue repeating them as well as you can until I tell you the test is over. It's important that you guess if you are uncertain of a word. Are there any questions?

3. The words you will hear are typed on cards lying on the table beside you. Please pick up the cards and read the words to me so that you can become familiar with them.

The subject then read aloud the 36 W-1 spondees which were typed on 3″ × 5″ cards. If a subject could not read the words the tester read them to him and asked him to repeat them aloud. The familiarization process served to reduce learning effects (Tillman and Jerger, 1959) and was consistent with the instructions provided with CID Auditory Test W-1 (undated). After the subject had been familiarized with the stimuli, he was told, "Remember, it's very important that you guess, no matter how faint the word may be, or if you only hear part of a word." Then the measurement of spondee threshold began.

---

*The ASA standard for pure-tone audiometers (1951) produces test results that underestimate loss of auditory sensitivity for pure tones (Davis, 1959; Jerger et al., 1959). The 22-dB (re 0.0002 dyne/cm^2) sound pressure output recommended by ASA (1953) for calibrating zero hearing level in speech audiometers is a good estimate of the SPL required to reach average normal threshold for spondaic words (Chaiklin, 1959; Hirsh et al., 1952; Jerger et al., 1959). Therefore, the ASA standard for speech audiometers produces spondee thresholds that tend to be higher than pure-tone averages (Jerger et al., 1959). Several years ago, the VA adopted a 29-dB (re 0.0002 dyne/cm^2) calibration level for speech audiometers. This was done to bring the results of pure-tone and speech audiometry into better agreement with each other. The result is that the VA calibration for speech audiometers yields results that underestimate spondee thresholds in the same way that the ASA standard for pure-tone audiometers results in under-estimates of loss of acuity for pure tones. It is important to recognize that some manufacturers of speech audiometers use the 22-dB ASA standard and some use other calibration values.

Procedure for 2-dB Method Spondee Threshold

A descending approach to threshold was used for both 2-dB and 5-dB methods. The initial descending approach to threshold for the 2-dB method was in 5-dB steps with one spondee per step presented at succeedingly lower levels until the subject failed to repeat a word correctly. The intensity of the signal was increased five or six dB to an even number on the hearing level dial. Sampling then proceeded in descending 2-dB steps with a minimum of three or a maximum of six stimuli presented at each step. The intensity was decreased by 2 dB each time it became apparent that a subject met or could not meet a 50 percent correct response criterion. It is obvious that six stimuli were not needed at each level. When a subject had made four errors (before getting three correct) it was impossible for him to meet the 50 percent criterion. Similarly, when three correct responses had been obtained, nothing would have been gained by presenting the maximum of six stimuli.

Sampling was discontinued when (1) four words were responded to incorrectly at each of three consecutive levels, or (2) four words were missed at each of two consecutive levels with no correct response at either level, that is, eight consecutive errors with none correct. Threshold was defined as the lowest hearing level at which three words were repeated correctly out of a theoretical maximum of six stimulus presentations. It should be noted that the criteria for determining the sampling end-point were designed to prevent premature designation of threshold when three correct responses were obtained at several levels.

Procedure for 5-dB Method Spondee Threshold

For the 5-dB method the initial descending approach to threshold was accomplished in 5-dB steps for 71 subjects and in 10-dB steps for the 29 reliability subjects. The remaining procedure was the same for all subjects. One word per step was presented until the subject failed to respond correctly. The signal was then raised five dB above the last level at which there was a correct response. Stimuli were presented in descending 5-dB steps, following at each level the same criteria for minimum and maximum sampling described above for the 2-dB method. The criterion for completion of threshold sampling with the 5-dB method was four incorrect responses at two consecutive levels (a total of eight errors). As with the 2-dB method, spondee threshold was defined as the lowest hearing level at which three words were repeated correctly out of a theoretical maximum of six stimulus presentations.

RESULTS

Order Effects

The first question considered was whether order of presentation resulted in a difference between spondee thresholds measured in 2-dB and 5-dB steps. Fifty subjects had the 2-dB threshold measured first; the order was reversed for the remaining 50 subjects. There was no significant difference ($t = .43$) between the mean difference scores for the 2-dB and 5-dB spondee thresholds as a function of order of presentation. All subjects, therefore, were considered as one group regardless of the order in which thresholds were measured.

Comparison of Measurement Methods

The mean spondee threshold obtained using the 2-dB method was 25.72 dB and the mean threshold for the 5-dB method was 27.55 dB. The difference (1.83 dB) between the means was significant ($t = 6.54$, $P < .001$).[2] The standard deviations were very similar for the two spondee thresholds ($SD_{2dB} = 20.26$ dB; $SD_{5dB} = 20.54$ dB); and there was little difference (.03 dB) between the standard errors of the means. As would be expected, there was high correlation[3] ($r = .99$) between the results of the 2-dB and 5-dB measurement methods. These results are summarized in Table 24–2.

TABLE 24–2. COMPARISON OF 2-dB AND 5-dB SPONDEE THRESHOLDS; $N = 100$.

Method	Mean	SD	t	r
2-dB	25.72	20.26		
			6.54*	.99
5-dB	27.55	20.54		

*Significant at < .001 level.

TABLE 24–3. MEAN PTAS (IN dB), CORRELATIONS BETWEEN SPONDEE THRESHOLDS AND PTAS, AND STANDARD ERROR OF ESTIMATES FOR PREDICTING SPONDEE THRESHOLDS FROM PTAS; $N = 100$.

Method	2-freq. PTA			3-freq. PTA		
	Mean	r	$SE_{est.}$	Mean	r	$SE_{est.}$
2-dB		.98	4.03		.97	4.90
	26.59			29.99		
5-dB		.97	4.97		.96	5.78

Table 24–3 shows the correlations between spondee thresholds obtained with the two measurement methods and the two- and three-frequency PTAs. The table also shows mean PTAs as well as the standard errors of estimate for predicting either the 2-dB or 5-dB spondee threshold from either the two- or three-frequency PTA. It is readily apparent that a 5-dB spondee threshold measurement method produces essentially the same degree of correlation with PTA as does the more commonly used 2-dB measurement interval. It is also apparent from the standard errors of estimate reported in Table 24–3 that little predictive power (approximately one dB) is lost when estimating a 5-dB threshold from the two- or three-frequency PTA. It is important to note that the correlation coefficients and standard errors of estimate reported in Table 24–3 are very similar to results reported by other investigators (Fletcher, 1950; Graham, 1960; Quiggle et al., 1957). The similarities are even more striking when one considers the important differences among these studies in terms of samples, measurement intervals, stimulus materials, and measurement methods.

One qualification should be made concerning the high spondee threshold-PTA correlations reported above. They are, in part, a function of our sample. No subject in our study had a sharply sloping pure-tone configuration, at least through the speech frequencies; and, further, no subject had a speech discrimination score less than 60 percent. It can be assumed that the presence of either of these problems might reduce the correlations between PTAs and spondee thresholds obtained with either a 2-dB or 5-dB method. This assumption is partially supported by Graham's (1960) data, at least for the 2-dB method. Nearly half of Graham's sample consisted of subjects with sensory-neural hearing loss, while only 31 percent of our sample had a similar loss. This difference could account for our finding a slightly higher correlation between spondee threshold and the three-frequency PTA than was found by Graham.

Measurement Method versus Pure-Tone Thresholds

Table 24–4 shows correlations between the spondee threshold measurement methods and each of the pure-tone thresholds from 500 cps through 2,000 cps including the interoctave frequencies of 750 cps and 1,500 cps. Also shown in Table 24–4 are the mean thresholds and standard deviations for each frequency tested. Once again the 5-dB method threshold compares favorably with the 2-dB method threshold. Both methods show similar high positive correlations (ranging from .79 to .96) with the speech-frequency pure-tone thresholds.

TABLE 24–4. MEANS AND STANDARD DEVIATIONS (IN dB) FOR PURE-TONE THRESHOLDS FROM 500 CPS TO 2,000 CPS AND CORRELATION COEFFICIENTS BETWEEN THE 2-dB AND THE 5-dB METHOD SPONDEE THRESHOLDS AND PURE-TONE THRESHOLDS; $N = 100$.

Frequencies	Mean	SD	$r_{2\text{-dB}}$	$r_{5\text{-dB}}$
500	26.30	21.80	.96	.95
750*	30.48	22.24	.96	.95
1,000	31.10	21.63	.96	.95
1,500†	33.52	21.16	.88	.87
2,000	33.60	21.05	.79	.79

*$N = 52$.
†$N = 61$.

Test-Retest Reliability

Twenty-nine subjects were used for the evaluation of test-retest reliability. For the 2-dB method 27 subjects (93 percent) had test-retest differences from 0 dB to ±6 dB; no subject had a test-retest difference greater than eight dB. For the 5-dB method all subjects had test-retest differences within ±5 dB; 59 percent had identical thresholds on both measurements with the 5-dB method. It is apparent that the small differences between the two methods are not significant.

DISCUSSION

The results of the data analyses indicate that spondee thresholds obtained with a 5-dB measurement interval agree well with spondee thresholds measured in 2-dB steps although the 5-dB method thresholds are slightly higher.

The 5-dB method is faster than the 2-dB method, agrees well with pure-tone audiometry, and is highly reliable. For clinics that have speech audiometers graduated in 2-dB steps, a 4-dB measurement interval is recommended. Spondee thresholds measured with a 4-dB measurement interval should have validity and reliability comparable to that demonstrated for a 5-dB measurement interval. The validity and reliability of any measure is dependent, to a large extent, on measurement method. If, on the basis of the results of this study, a 5-dB (or 4-dB) measurement interval is adopted for routine clinical use, the general method employed should conform to that described below or in the *Procedure* section.

The literature on measurement of spondee threshold is marked by meager descriptions of test methods. Sometimes the entire description of methodology consists of the instructions to present several words at successive levels until the patient misses about half of the words. Frequently, methodology is not described at all. Jerger and others (1959) have also commented on the prevalence of cursory descriptions of spondee threshold test methods. They reported that it was necessary to devise their own methodology to achieve some degree of objectivity in their study of pure-tone and speech thresholds. Their procedure was based on the method described by Newby (1958, p. 112), a method which, in our opinion, is too general and unsystematic. Newby's instructions are:

> . . . start the record (or the delivery of the words by live voice) at a level [unspecified] above the patient's presumed threshold. As the patient repeats two or three words successfully, decrease the intensity by a few dB. After two or three more words have been repeated correctly at this new level, decrease the intensity further. Continue in this way until the patient misses some words. By increasing or decreasing intensity in 1- or 2-dB steps, try to find the point at which the patient is correct about half the time. This is his SRT by spondees.

Jerger and others (1959) used the following adaptation of Newby's method.

> Two or three words were initially presented at a level 20 to 30 dB above the estimated threshold. Successive blocks of two or three words were then progressively attenuated in 10-dB steps until a level was reached at which two consecutive words were repeated incorrectly. At this point the tester simply "jumped around" in no set order, from level to level in 2-dB steps, presenting exactly four words per level. The spondee threshold was recorded as the lowest intensity at which a subject repeated two out of four words correctly.

This method is more explicitly described than Newby's method but still omits too many important procedural details.

The well-documented high correlation between spondee threshold and PTA may influence some clinicians to perform inappropriately casual spondee threshold measurements. Indeed, the measurement process and the resulting thresholds may be biased by the clinician's tendency to estimate spondee threshold from the PTA. Well-defined methods can serve as a protection against this kind of tester bias. The more specific the method, the fewer unique decisions the tester must make; by having most decisions predetermined for the tester the obtained spondee thresholds gain a degree of independence that does not exist with "flexible" clinical methods. In addition, the relative freedom from bias gained through precise methods makes the spondee threshold a much more meaningful independent check on the validity of pure-tone audiometry. The problems discussed above illustrate the need for a well-defined system for spondee threshold measurement. The following methodological proposals, which are based on the present research and several years of clinical trial, hopefully will meet this need.

The method we recommend for the measurement of spondee thresholds in 5-dB steps is similar to that described in the *Procedure* section. The method involves three major steps: (1) instructions, (2) familiarization, and (3) measurement. We suggest that the following instructions be read to the patient immediately before the measurement of spondee threshold.

The purpose of this test is to find the faintest level at which you hear words. You're going to hear some two-syllable words such as "baseball" and "mousetrap." Your job is to repeat each two-syllable word no matter how faint the word may be. For example, if you hear, "Say the word 'baseball,' " you should just repeat "baseball." The words may be very faint, but please continue repeating them as well as you can until I tell you the test is over. It's important that you guess at the word, even if you're not sure of it. Do you have any questions?

Now, I want you to pick up the stack of cards on the table and read the words aloud to me. These are the words that you'll hear during the test. I want you to become familiar with them. [The following final sentence of the instructions is to be read to the subject after he has been familiarized with the stimuli.] Remember, it's very importnt that you guess, no matter how faint a word may be or even if you only hear part of the word.

These instructions are similar to instructions used in previous research (Chaiklin, 1959; Jerger et al., 1959) and to the instructions provided with CID Auditory Test W-1. Deviations from the exact wording of the instructions may be far less critical than deviations involving essential ideas, such as the need for the patient to guess. We recognize that formal instructions may be inappropriate under certain circumstances, for example, in testing young children. However, we do believe it is important for clinics to adopt a specific set of instructions to be used whenever possible.

Familiarizing the patient with the spondee stimuli is the next important step. Familiarization serves to increase both the validity and reliability of spondee threshold results (Tillman and Jerger, 1959) and must, therefore, be incorporated into the measurement process. Familiarization can be accomplished by having the patient read the spondee words aloud, or by reading the words to the patient and having him repeat them back.

The 5-dB measurement method is as follows: (1) assuming that pure-tone thresholds have been measured,[4] begin the initial descent 25 dB above the two-frequency PTA (rounded to the nearest 5-dB step); (2) descend in 5-dB steps, presenting one spondee per level, until the patient misses a spondee; (3) increase the intensity 10 dB above the level arrived at in the previous step; (4) decrease the intensity in 5-dB steps,

presenting a minimum of three and a maximum of six spondees at each level; (5) continue to decrease the intensity in 5-dB steps until the patient fails to repeat correctly three spondees at two consecutive levels. Threshold is defined as the lowest level at which three spondees are repeated correctly out of a theoretical maximum of six stimuli. (See *Procedure* section for greater detail concerning sampling.) The entire measurement process for both ears, including instructions and familiarization, usually takes less than ten minutes.

We realize that some clinicians may be reluctant to change their measurement technique despite the evidence that a 5-dB method compares favorably to a 2-dB method and, in some respects, is superior. However, as was pointed out above, no detailed description of a 2-dB measurement method is currently available to these clinicians. To meet this need we suggest the following 2-dB measurement method (note that the instructions and familiarization process are the same for both the 2-dB and 5-dB methods): (1) begin initial descent 25 dB above the two-frequency PTA (rounded to the nearest 5-dB step); (2) descend in 5-dB steps, presenting one spondee per level, until the patient misses a spondee; (3) increase the intensity five dB or six dB above the level found in the previous step, the object being to start at an even number on the hearing loss dial; (4) decrease the intensity in 2-dB steps, presenting a minimum of two and a maximum of four spondees at each level*; (5) continue to decrease the intensity until three words are responded to incorrectly at each of three consecutive levels or until three words are missed at each of two consecutive levels with no correct responses at either level. Threshold is defined as the lowest level at which two spondees are repeated correctly out of a theoretical maximum of four stimuli.

The data sheet shown in Figure 24–1 has proved to be a useful aid in the measurement process. It provides a permanent record and is simple to use. Correct responses are indicated by a tally mark, and in-

approximat

---

*We should have explained that we determined empirically that essentially the same results are obtained with either a 2 out of 4 or a 3 out of 6 criterion for the 2-dB method. The 5-dB method, however, suffers when a 2 out of 4 criterion is used. JBC, IMV

SPONDEE RESPONSE DATA SHEET

Name: _N. K._   Date: _12/21/62_ Tester: _1. JFW 2. JGC_

HEARING LEVEL	RIGHT	ERROR 1	ERROR 2	ERROR 3	ERROR 4
TEST NO. 1			CIRCLE EAR Ⓡ L		
40	III				
38	III	shortstop			
36	II	baseball	N R	farewell	N R
(34)	III	N R	N R		
32	II	N R	sidewalk	N R	sandlot
30		N R	N R	sidewalk	N R
28		N R	N R	N R	N R
				ST = 34	
TEST NO. 2			CIRCLE EAR Ⓡ L		
40	III				
(35)	III	hotdog			
30	I	N R	N R	N R	N R
25		N R	N R	N R	N R
				ST = 35	

FIGURE 24-1. Spondee threshold data sheet showing examples of the sampling process used with the 5-dB and 2-dB measurement methods. Correct responses are indicated by tally marks; errors are written out (NR = no response). Note: Test No. 1 shows a 3 out of 6 threshold criterion rather than the 2 out of 4 criterion advocated in the discussion section.

correct responses are written to provide a means of examining error response patterns—some of which appear to have diagnostic significance.[5] The use of the data sheet is illustrated in Figure 24-1.

Our experience during another study suggested that an ascending method may be an even more rapid method of measuring spondee threshold than a descending method. Unfortunately, we did not evaluate an ascending 5-dB method and cannot, at this time, recommend such a procedure. It is not unreasonable to expect good agreement between thresholds obtained with either an ascending or descending measurement procedure.[6]

There are several observations we would like to make concerning spondee stimuli. The intensity and intelligibility differences among currently used spondee stimuli suggests that there may be value in research designed to select spondee stimuli that are more comparable on these two dimensions, as well as being equated for familiarity. These stimuli would be easier to record and easier to monitor in clinical situations where live-voice testing is necessary. It would also seem advisable, in any new set of stimuli, to avoid pairs of stimuli with identical syllables. Combinations such as "hotdog"—"hothouse" and "inkwell"—"farewell" in the W-1 list introduce a discrimination task, particularly at weak signal levels, that is peripheral to the threshold being measured. A smaller population of stimuli would also seem desirable to produce greater homogeneity and to facilitate the related task of familiarizing the subject with the stimuli. Reducing the number of stimuli would also make it easier to select spondees having equal intensity.

We found it convenient to use tape recorded stimuli in the measurement of spondee threshold. The use of taped stimuli provides obvious advantages such as preservation of fidelity and ease of handling. In any event, live-voice testing is the least desirable method because it introduces an unnecessary source (the speaker) of intra- and inter-test variability.

SUMMARY

The monaural spondee thresholds of 100 hard-of-hearing adult males were measured with two different measurement intervals—a 5-dB interval and a 2-dB interval. Measurements with both methods were repeated for 29 of the 100 subjects. All tests were controlled for tester bias to insure independent measures. Recordings of CID Auditory Test W-1 served as test stimuli. Carefully specified methods were used for all threshold measurements. The 5-dB measurement method resulted in spondee thresholds that (1) agreed well with 2-dB method thresholds, (2) had high correlations with pure-tone thresholds, and (3) had high reliability.

On the basis of the results of this study it is recommended that spondee thresholds be measured in 5-dB steps rather than in 2-dB steps. The 5-dB method is faster than the 2-dB method and provides more than adequate accuracy for clinical needs. The change to a 5-dB measurement interval should be accompanied by standard measurement techniques. Measurement techniques for both the 5-dB and 2-dB methods were described.

ACKNOWLEDGMENT

We wish to acknowledge the cooperation and assistance of the staff of the Audiology and Speech Pathology Clinic, Veterans Administration Hospital, San Francisco.

ENDNOTES

1. The auxiliary RVAs were designed and constructed by Mr. L. Glen Pew, Electro-Acoustic Company, San Carlos, California. The prototype for the RVA was designed for use in a study of simulated hearing loss conducted by Barrett (1959).

2. The journal version of this article reported an incorrect nonsignificant t ratio. In a letter to the editor (*J. Speech Hearing Dis.*, 30, pp. 99–100, 1965), Gaeth called attention to the error. Our reply to Gaeth (*J. Speech Hearing Dis.*, 30, pp. 100–101, 1965) acknowledged the mistake, which was caused by an arithmetical error, and presented supplementary data comparing the two methods. The following excerpt from our letter provides data that allow a fuller comparison of the two methods: "Of the 100 subjects used in the study, 49 had 5-dB method STs that were within ±2 dB of their 2-dB method STs, 32 differed by ±3 to ±5 dB, and the remaining 19 had STs from ±6 dB to ±9 dB of each other (one subject was +9 dB). Twenty-three of the 5-dB method STs were lower than the 2-dB STs, 59 were higher and 18 were identical. The larger differences constituted less than 20 percent of the cases and were often associated with sloping pure-tone configurations which seem to produce slightly more ST measurement error. In this connection, it should be noted that 20 percent of the test-retest differences for the 2-dB method were from +5 to +8 dB, which suggests that size of interval is not the sole factor operating in extreme cases. It is possible that some of these differences are related to stimulus differences rather than to measurement method." JBC, IMV

3. All correlations reported are Pearson product-moment correlation coefficients.

4. At least two methods can be used to establish a starting point for the initial descent if pure-tone thresholds have not been measured prior to the measurement of spondee threshold. The first method is one recommended by Carhart and Jerger (1959) for pure-tone audiometry. They suggest starting ". . . at a hearing level of 30 to 40 dB if the subject appears to have approximately normal acuity, and at a hearing [*sic*] of 70 dB if only a moderate impairment seems to be present. Provided these levels are inadequate, subsequent presentations are increased in steps of 15 dB until the subject's response is positive." The other methods is to start at −10-dB hearing level and ascend in 10-dB steps until the patient repeats two spondees correctly at a given level.

5. See Chaiklin, J. B., and Ventry, I. M., Patient errors during spondee and pure-tone threshold measurement. In I. M. Ventry and J. B. Chaiklin (Eds.), Multidiscipline study of functional hearing loss. *J. aud. Res.,* **5,** pp. 219–230 (1965). JBC, IMV

6. A study of the validity and reliability of spondee thresholds measured in ascending 5-dB steps was reported by Chaiklin, J. B., Dixon, R. F., and Font J., Spondee thresholds measured in ascending 5-dB steps. *J. Speech Hearing Res.,* **10,** pp. 141–145 (1967). Validity and reliability for the ascending method were highly similar to results reported in the present study, but contrary to our earlier speculation, the ascending method was not significantly faster. JBC, IMV

REFERENCES

American Standards Association. *American Standard Specification for Audiometers for General Diagnostic Purposes,* Z24.5-1951. New York: Amer. Standards Assoc., 1951.

American Standards Association. *American Standard Specification for Speech Audiometers.* Z24.13-1953. New York: Amer. Standards Assoc., 1953.

Barrett, L. S. Threshold relationships in simulated hearing loss. Ph.D. dissertation, Stanford Univ., 1959.

Carhart, R., and Jerger, J. F. Preferred method for clinical determination of pure-tone thresholds. *J. Speech Hearing Dis.,* **24,** 1959, 330–345.

Central Institute for the Deaf. *Auditory Tests W-1 and W-2, Spondaic Word Lists: Description and Instructions for Use.* St. Louis: Central Institute for the Deaf, undated.

Chaiklin, J. B. The relation among three selected auditory speech thresholds. *J. Speech Hearing Res.,* **2,** 1959, 237–243.

Chaiklin, J. B., and Ventry, I. M. Functional hearing loss. In J. F. Jerger (Ed.), *Modern Developments in Audiology.* New York: Academic Press, 1963.

Chaiklin, J. B., and Ventry, I. M. Functional hearing loss: V. Patient errors during measurement of speech reception threshold and the spondee error index (SERI), (in preparation). [See endnote 5 for reference. JBC,IMV]

Davis, H. For an international audiometric zero. *Asha,* **1,** 1959, 47–49.

Fletcher, H. A method for calculating hearing for speech from an audiogram. *Acta Otolaryng.,* Suppl. **90,** 1950, 26–37.

Graham, J. T. Evaluation of methods for predicting speech reception threshold. *Arch. Otolaryng.,* **72,** 1960, 347–350.

Hirsh, I. J.; Davis H.; Silverman, S. R.; Reynolds, Elizabeth G.; Eldert, Elizabeth; and Benson, R. W. Development of materials for speech audiometry. *J. Speech Hearing Dis.,* **17,** 1952, 321–337.

Jerger, J. F.; Carhart, R.; Tillman, T. W.; and Peterson, J. L. Some relations between normal hearing for pure tones and for speech. *J. Speech Hearing Res.,* **2,** 1959, 126–140.

Newby, H. A., *Audiology: Principles and Practice.* New York: Appleton-Century-Crofts, 1958.

Quiggle, R. R.; Glorig, A.; Delk, J. H; and Summerfield, Anne B. Predicting hearing loss for speech from pure tone audiograms. *Laryngoscope,* **67,** 1957, 1–15.

Research News Note. Multidisciplinary Investigation of Functional Hearing Loss Enters Fourth (Final) Year. *J. Speech Hearing Res.,* **5,** 1962, 291.

Ruhm, H. B., and Carhart, R. Objective speech audiometry: A new method based on electrodermal response. *J. Speech Hearing Res.,* **1,** 1958, 169–178.

Tillman, T. W., and Jerger, J. F. Some factors affecting the spondee threshold in normal hearing subjects. *J. Speech Hearing Res.,* **2,** 1959, 141–146.

Ventry, I. M. Relative efficiency of tests used to detect functional hearing loss. *International Audiol.,* **1,** 1962, 145–150.

Ventry, I. M., and Chaiklin, J. B. Functional hearing loss: A problem in terminology. *Asha,* **4,** 1962, 251–254.

Watson, L. A. *A Manual for Advanced Audiometry.* Minneapolis: Maico Company, 1949.

Watson, L. A., and Tolan, T. *Hearing Tests and Hearing Instruments.* Baltimore: Williams and Wilkins, 1949.

Whipple, C. I., and Kodman, F., Jr. The validity of objective speech audiometry. *J. Laryng. Oto.,* **74,** 1960, 84–89.

25

A Proposed SRT Procedure and Its Statistical Precedent

Richard H. Wilson, Ph.D.
Chief, Audiology Section VA Medical Center, Long Beach, California
Donald E. Morgan, Ph.D.
Associate Professor, Head and Neck Surgery, UCLA School of Medicine
Donald D. Dirks, Ph.D.
Professor, Head and Neck Surgery, UCLA School of Medicine

The procedure for establishing speech reception thresholds (SRTs) with spondee words as proposed by Tillman and Olsen is described, with a suggested modification of that protocol. These systemized techniques incorporate 2- and 5-dB intensity decrements with two and five words being presented at the respective intervals. Threshold derivations from these two procedures are discussed in terms of a long-standing statistical precedent, the Spearman-Kärber method. Our data from 100 ears tested validate the procedures. We conclude that these techniques are clinically practical and suggest that the procedures be considered for adoption as standardized clinical methods, if additional data support their validity and reliability.

Tillman and Olsen (1973) have proposed a method for establishment of speech reception thresholds (SRTs) for spondee words based on the principles set forth by Hudgins et al. (1947) and Hirsh et al. (1952). As Tillman and Olsen pointed out, a systemized procedure "confines all clinicians to the same operational definition of threshold, and thus reduces variability in estimates of the speech reception threshold produced by variations in this definition." Many audiologists acquainted with this SRT protocol are already employing it in their clinics. During the past year, we have incorporated this SRT procedure in our audiology clinic and have found it to be most useful because it is a defined technique, it is easily administered, and it provides SRTs that are in good agreement with the pure-tone thresholds. Details concerning the procedure, together with clinical results as reported in this paper, should encourage consideration of this method for general clinical use.

Reprinted by permission of the authors from *J. Speech Hearing Dis.*, **38**, 184–191 (1973).

TEST PROCEDURE

The SRT method proposed by Tillman and Olsen involves, basically, four steps: (1) Familiarization with test materials. Test words presented at a comfortable listening level are repeated by the patient. (2) Determination of initial test intensity. Starting 30–40 dB above the estimated SRT, one word is presented at each 10-dB decrement until two incorrect responses are elicited at a given intensity. When one word is missed, a second word is presented at the same intensity. Threshold determination is initiated 10 dB above the intensity at which two words are missed. (3) Determination of threshold. The systematic search for threshold involves the presentation of two words in 2-dB decrements. Two conditions govern the course of the testing. First, five of the initial six words must be repeated correctly; second, the test terminates when five of six words are missed. (4) Derivation of threshold. Threshold[1] is determined by subtracting the number of correct responses from the initial intensity, that is, the intensity at which

INTENSITY		INTENSITY		
0		40	✓	✓
8		8	✓	✓
6		6	✓	X
4		4	✓	✓
2		2	X	✓
0		30	✓	X
8		8	X	X
6		6	X	X
4		4		
2		2		
0		0		
8		8		
6		6		

INTENSITY				
0				
5				
0				
5				
0				
5				

0				
85	✓	✓	✓	✓ ✓
0	✓	X	✓	X ✓
75	X	X	X	X X
0				
5				

FIGURE 25-1. Part of the spondee-threshold worksheet used in the clinical application of the SRT procedure. Examples (see text) demonstrating the use of the proposed two words/2-dB decrement (left) and five words/5-dB decrement (right) methods are illustrated, with incorrect responses indicated by X. The tens column is filled in by the clinician in accordance with the initial intensity level.

Step 3 is begun. To this difference, a correction factor[2] of one (1) is added. The intensity derived is the SRT.

Figure 25–1 (left) illustrates a portion of the worksheet we have found useful in the clinical application of this SRT procedure. (For convenience, each clinical worksheet includes 24 copies of this form.) The initial intensity (Step 2) can be specified in the column headed "Intensity" with the correct/incorrect responses being recorded at each intensity level. With such a method, it is immediately apparent when the criterion for test termination (Step 3) has been met, and threshold derivation (Step 4) can be completed by subtracting the number of correct responses from the initial intensity recorded, plus the correction factor. This protocol of threshold derivation and its validity are the focus of this discussion.

STATISTICAL PROCEDURE

It is clear to us that the data generated by the proposed SRT procedure are amenable to a long-standing statistical precedent (Spearman, 1908), now termed the Spearman-Kärber method (Finney, 1952). This statistical protocol, in common use in the biological and medical fields, was developed independently in England by Spearman and in Germany by Kärber (1931). The following formula represents a refinement of the Spearman-Kärber method as it applies to the SRT procedure previously outlined (readers concerned with the mathematical derivation of this formula are referred to the aforementioned three references):

$$T_{50\%} = i + 1/2\,(d) - \frac{d\,(r),}{n}$$

where $T_{50\%}$ = threshold, i = the initial test intensity, d = the dB decrement, r = the total number of correct responses, and n = the number of words presented per decibel decrement. The worksheet exemplified in Figure 25–1 (left) should clarify applications of the formula. Given: $i = 40$ dB HL, $d = 2$-dB decrements, $r = 9$ correct responses, and $n =$ two words/decrement, then substituting we have

$$T_{50\%} = 40 + 1/2\,(2) - \frac{2\,(9)}{2}$$

$$T_{50\%} = 40 + 1 - 9$$
$$T_{50\%} = 32 \text{ dB HL.}$$

From this example, it is apparent that if $d = n$, then d and n cancel and the formula can be reduced to

$$T_{50\%} = i + 1/2\,(d) - r$$

This formula is directly applicable to the data generated by the proposed SRT method. Recall that two words are presented per 2-dB decrement, hence $d = n$. The threshold derivation described in Step 4 was accomplished using this formula and test procedure.

Variations in the proposed SRT method are appropriate, especially when consideration is given the clinical audiometers in use today. That is, the two words/2-dB decrement protocol is well suited for instruments with a 2-dB attenuator; however, individuals whose audiometers have 5-dB step attenuators may find their efforts to attain 2-dB decrements demanding and tedious. For these clinicians, we recommend that the following changes be incorporated into the procedure previously outlined: (1) 5-dB decrements, (2) five words/decrement, (3) termination of the test when all words at a single intensity are incorrect, and (4) threshold determination based on a correction factor of two instead of one. (The rationale for this choice is given later.) An example involving this five word/5-dB decrement technique is given in the lower right portion of Figure 25-1. Given: $i = 85$ dB HL, $d = 5$ dB, $r = 8$, and $n = 5$, then substituting we have

$$T_{50\%} = 85 + 1/2 (5) - 8$$
$$T_{50\%} = 79.5 \text{ dB HL.}$$

With the correction factor of two, the threshold would be 79 dB HL.

Finally, for those wishing to utilize combinations in which the words and decrements are not equal, the following serves as an example. Given: $i = 75$ dB SPL, $d = 3$ dB, $r = 12$, and $n = 5$, then substituting we have

$$T_{50\%} = 72 + 1/2 (3) - \frac{3 (12)}{5}$$

$$T_{50\%} = 72 + 1.5 - 7.2$$
$$T_{50\%} = 66.3 \text{ dB SPL.}$$

These three examples demonstrate (1) the procedure for applying the Spearman-Kärber method to data generated by the proposed SRT method, that is, two words/2-dB decrement; (2) the adaptation of the statistical procedure for other d and n values; and (3) the revisions necessary to utilize the method when unequal parameters of d and n are desired.

One comment about the use of this test procedure in research is in order. A dividend of this systematic data-collection process is the generation of intelligibility functions accomplished through the accumulation of the recorded responses at the respective intensity levels. Examples of this usage include the works of Wilson and Carhart (1969); Dirks, Wilson, and Bower (1969); and Dirks, Stream, and Wilson (1972).

VALIDATION

To substantiate the validity of the SRT method suggested by Tillman and Olsen and the modification of that procedure we have offered, data composed of pure-tone thresholds and two SRT estimates (two words/2-dB and five words/5-dB, counterbalanced) were gathered over several months from patients seen in the UCLA Audiology Clinic. The data are based on 100 ears from 76 adult patients undergoing

routine audiologic examination because of suspected hearing impairment. Except for eight ears with normal threshold sensitivity, these patients represent an unselected sample of conductive, mixed, and sensorineural hearing losses. The sample was composed of 25 individuals whose audiometric curves dropped off in the higher frequencies, of 57 individuals with flat configurations, and of 18 patients with impairments greater in the low than in the high frequencies. (The criterion for classifying the audiometric configurations was based on the 500-, 1,000-, and 2,000-Hz relationships. If the differences were no greater than 10 dB, then the audiogram was considered flat. When differences of 15 dB or more occurred, then the slope was categorized.)

Thirty-six spondee words were recorded on magnetic tape with the words peaking (± 2 dB) at the level of the 1,000-Hz calibration tone. The speech channels were calibrated to 20 dB SPL[3] and the pure-tone audiometers conformed to the ANSI 1969 norms. The mean data are presented in Table 25-1 in decibels re hearing level.

Several pertinent relationships and conclusions based on the data gathered in this study (Table 25-1) warrant discussion. First, the difference between the 2-dB (27.2 dB) and 5-dB (28.4 dB) SRTs was 1.2 dB, a significant difference, $F (1,99) = 8.12$. $p < 0.01$. This 1.2-dB difference is practically identical to the 1.8-dB difference, also significant ($t = 6.54$, $p < 0.001$), reported by Chaiklin and Ventry (1964, 1965; see also Gaeth, 1965) under conditions involving 2- and 5-dB decrements with three to six spondees per interval. We, like Chaiklin and Ventry (1965),

TABLE 25-1. THE MEAN THRESHOLDS AND STANDARD DEVIATIONS FOR THE DATA COLLECTED FROM 100 EARS (MEAN AGE, 50 YEARS) INCLUDED IN THIS STUDY.

Condition	Threshold dB HL*	SD
250 Hz	28.7	20.4
500 Hz	28.8	20.8
1,000 Hz	27.8	20.9
2,000 Hz	29.7	22.4
4,000 Hz	43.6	25.6
8,000 Hz	48.5	27.3
3 PT $\bar{\times}$	28.7	20.2
Fletcher $\bar{\times}$	25.3	20.0
Carhart $\times$	26.3	20.4
2-dB SRT	27.2	20.6
5-dB SRT	28.4	20.8

*re ANSI 1969 Standard (TDH-39).

attribute the 1.2-dB difference to the decrement size; that is, the 5-dB steps provide a less precise determination of the patients' perception of the words at or near threshold than do the 2-dB steps. Hence, slightly lower thresholds are found with the 2-dB intervals. Although the threshold difference derived from the two decrement sizes reached a level of statistical significance in both the current study and that of Chaiklin and Ventry, we conclude that for clinical purposes the difference is minimal and the comparative threshold can be considered essentially equivalent. Based on the small difference between the thresholds for the two methods, we suggest, for ease and convenience, that the correction factor for the 5-dB decrement procedure be two instead of the 2.5 called for in the Spearman-Kärber formula [½(d)].

Secondly, Chaiklin and Ventry concluded that 5-dB intervals were preferable to 2-dB decrements since under their protocol fewer words were required with the larger steps. This is not true with the procedures we employed since both decrement sizes involved one word per decibel; thus, essentially the same number of stimuli were required regardless of the interval. From the standpoint of test time needed to obtain threshold, the two decrement sizes are identical.

Third, the relationship between the threshold for 1,000 Hz and spondee words described by Jerger et al. (1959) has direct application to our data. In general, they found the difference in sound pressure level (SPL) between the two thresholds to be 12–13 dB and not the 6 dB as had been suggested in the ASA 1953 Standard (p. 9). Furthermore, a difference between the speech SPL (20 dB) and the 1,000 Hz SPL (7 dB) of 13 dB has been incorporated in the current specification for audiometers (ANSI, 1969). In contrast, we computed this difference from the Chaiklin and Ventry (1964) data to be only 7.5 dB, a result which may be attributable to the gradual slope in the pure-tone configuration of their data; that is, hearing loss increased with frequency (Chaiklin and Ventry, 1964, Table 4, p. 53). In our data, conversion of the 1,000-Hz pure-tone threshold and the two SRTs in Table 25–1 to SPL reveals differences between the pure-tone and speech threshold of 12.4 dB (2-dB decrement) and 13.6 dB (5-dB decrement). The remarkably close agreement between the current data, that reported by Jerger et al., and the relationship suggested in the 1969 ANSI Standard adds validity to the SRT procedures we are supporting.

The data in Table 25–1 permit observation of the relationships between the "pure-tone average" and the SRTs. This relationship has always been of interest to audiologists and has received recent detailed evaluation by Carhart (1971). For each ear included in the study, we derived the following pure-tone averages based on thresholds at 500, 1,000, and/or 2,000 Hz: (1) 3 PT $\bar{\times}$ average loss at the three frequencies (Fletcher, 1929); (2) Fletcher $\bar{\times}$, average loss at the two frequencies of least loss (Fletcher, 1950); and (3) Carhart $\bar{\times}$, average loss at 500 and 1,000 Hz minus 2 dB (Carhart, 1971). The data in the table demonstrate only a 3.4-dB spread among the three pure-tone averages used. The differences between the thresholds for spondee words and the pure-tone averages are minimal (0.3–3.1 dB). Correlation coefficients among these five variables (three averages and two SRTs) were extremely high (0.95–0.98). The similarity between the mean thresholds for speech and the pure-tone averages, together with the high correlations, attest to the validity of the proposed SRT methods on a clinic population.

Finally, during the preparation of this article, data on the 2-dB-step SRT procedure and pure tones were continually gathered in our audiology clinic. Since we now use only the 2-dB step method clinically, no further data were gathered with the 5-dB-step technique. Thus, data on 208 additional ears were gathered and are reported in Table 25–2 along with the 92 ears with hearing loss reported in Table 25–1. All ears in Table 25–2 (192 patients) had a hearing loss of at least 20 dB at one of the test frequencies. When these 300 ears were classified by general audiometric configuration, 82 dropped off in the higher frequencies, 154 were flat, and 64 demonstrated more loss in the low than the high frequencies. Com-

TABLE 25–2. THE MEAN THRESHOLDS AND STANDARD DEVIATIONS FOR THE DATA COLLECTED FROM 300 EARS (MEAN AGE, 52 YEARS).

Condition	Threshold dB HL*	SD
250 Hz	31.7	20.1
500 Hz	32.7	19.1
1,000 Hz	31.8	19.4
2,000 Hz	34.4	21.0
4,000 Hz	46.8	22.6
3 PT $\bar{\times}$	32.9	—
Carhart $\times$	30.1	—
2-dB SRT	31.2	18.9

*re ANSI 1969 Standard (TDH-39).

parison of the corresponding data in Table 25–1 and 25–2 reveals the only differences to be the degree of hearing loss, which amounted to ≈ 4 dB, with the larger group showing the greater loss. Specifically, the 1,000-Hz SRT differences are identical (0.6 dB), the 3 PT $\bar{x}$ /SRT differences are essentially the same (1.5–1.7 dB), and the Carhart $\bar{x}$ /SRT differences are approximately equal (0.9–1.1 dB). These additional findings confirm that the data in Table 25–1 from 100 ears are a valid representation of a population with hearing loss.

Based on the findings of this report, we suggest that these procedures be considered for adoption as standardized clinical methods if additional data from other audiology clinics support the validity and demonstrate the acceptable reliability of these SRT protocols.

ACKNOWLEDGMENT

The authors wish to thank Anne Betsworth and Joy Morros for their assistance with the data collection. Computing assistance was obtained from the Health Sciences Computing Facility, UCLA, sponsored by NIH Special Research Resources Grant RR-3.

ENDNOTES

1. Threshold is defined throughout this article as the intensity level at which 50 percent correct responses are achieved.

2. This correction factor is necessary to compensate for the extra word included in the initial intensity level.

3. A preliminary group of 24 normal ears yielded SRTs of 19.4 dB SPL. This indicates that the words and procedure used give speech thresholds for spondees that conform to the ANSI 1969 Standard.

REFERENCES

American National Standards Institute. *American National Standard Specification for Audiometers.* ANSI S3.6-1969. New York (1969).

American Standard Associations. *American Standard Specification for Speech Audiometers,* Z24.13-1953. New York (1953).

Carhart, R. Observations on relations between threshold for pure tones and for speech. *J. Speech Hearing Dis,* **36,** 476-483 (1971).

Chaiklin, J. B., and Ventry, I. M. Spondee threshold measurement: A comparison of 2- and 5-dB methods. *J. Speech Hearing Dis.,* **29,** 47-59 (1964).

Chaiklin, J. B., and Ventry, I. M. A reply to John Gaeth. *J. Speech Hearing Dis.,* **30,** 100-101 (1965).

Dirks, D. D.; Stream, R. W., and Wilson, R. H. Speech audiometry: Earphone and sound field. *J. Speech Hearing Dis.,* **37,** 162-176 (1972).

Dirks, D. D.; Wilson, R. H., and Bower, D. R. Effect of pulsed masking on selected speech materials. *J. Acoust. Soc. Amer.,* **46,** 898-906 (1969).

Finney, D. J. *Statistical Method in Biological Assay.* London: C. Griffen (1952).

Fletcher, H. *Speech and Hearing.* New York: Van Nostrand (1929).

Fletcher, H. A method of calculating hearing loss for speech from an audiogram. *Acta Otolaryng. Supp.,* **90,** 26-37 (1950).

Gaeth, J. Some comments for Chaiklin and Ventry. *J. Speech Hearing Dis.,* **30,** 99-100 (1965).

Hirsh, I. J.; Davis, H.; Silverman, S. R.; Reynolds, E. G.; Eldert, E.; and Benson, R. W. Development of materials for speech audiometry. *J. Speech Hearing Dis.,* **17,** 321-337 (1952).

Hudgins, C. V.; Hawkins, J. E.; Karlin, J. E.; and Stevens, S. S. The development of recorded auditory tests for measuring hearing loss for speech. *Laryngoscope,* **57,** 57-89 (1947).

Jerger, J. F.; Carhart, R.; Tillman, T. W.; and Peterson, J. L. Some relations between normal hearing for pure tones and for speech. *J. Speech Hearing Res.,* **2,** 126-140 (1959).

Karber, G. Beitrag zur kollektiven behandlung pharmakologischer reihenversuche. *Arch. Exp. Path um Pharm.,* **4,** 480-483 (1931).

Spearman, C. The method of "right and wrong cases" ("constant stimuli") without Gauss's formulae. *Brit. J. Psychol.,* **2,** 227-242 (1908).

Tillman, T. W., and Olsen, W. O. Speech audiometry. In J. Jerger (Ed.), *Modern Developments in Audiology.* (2nd ed.) New York: Academic Press (1973).

Wilson, R. H., and Carhart, R. Influence of pulsed masking on the threshold for spondees. *J. Acoust. Soc. Amer.,* **46,** 998-1,010 (1969).

26

Observations on Relations Between Thresholds for Pure Tones and for Speech

RAYMOND CARHART, Ph.D.
*Professor of Audiology, Northwestern University
when this article was prepared*

The prediction of SRT for spondees from pure-tone thresholds is considered in two ways. First, review of statistical studies on the relationship between sensitivity for pure tones and SRT for spondees shows their results to be inconclusive and confusing for the clinician except to demonstrate that frequencies outside the 500–2,000 Hz range are of minimal importance in estimating SRT. Second, regression equations derived from two new, audiometrically heterogeneous groups reveal that 500 and 1,000 Hz carry primary and nearly equal importance as predictors of SRT when audiometric contour is not taken into account. The clinician must bear in mind that any prediction he makes must incorporate a correction constant, which will vary with the calibration of his audiometers and other variables. A reasonable general formula for predicting clinical SRTs for spondees from pure-tone thresholds when audiometric contour is not taken into account and when the testing equipment is calibrated to the new ANSI threshold reference levels is:

$$SRT \ spondees = \frac{T_{500} + T_{1000}}{2} - 2 \ dB.$$

Various efforts have been made during the past five decades to quantify the relationships between impairment in sensitivity for speech and deficits in sensitivity for pure tones. Fletcher (1929) proposed that the average audiogram through the 500–2,000 Hz range be taken as the best prediction of hearing for speech. Sabine (1942) developed a system of weightings for pure-tone thresholds based on the normal hearer's capacity to make loudness and pitch discriminations. Concurrently, Fowler (1941, 1942) proposed a series of weightings for pure-tone thresholds which emerged from his copious clinical experience. The views of these two men exerted heavy influence on the system for estimating percentage of hearing loss which the American Medical Association adopted in 1942 and revised in 1947.

The first study to measure directly the SRTs of hearing-impaired patients was conducted by Hughson and Thompson (1942). They demonstrated interdependence between the threshold for sentences and sensitivity for pure tones in the midfrequencies. Carhart (1946a) extended empirical observations on clinical populations in several directions. He showed that SRTs determined with Harvard spondees and with connected sentences are relatively equivalent, and he explored the comparative efficiencies of several systems for predicting SRTs. These systems ranged from prediction from a single pure-tone threshold to prediction from either the 1942 AMA method for computing percentage loss or from one of several regression equations derived from averaging the data at his disposal. He found several of the predictive procedures to be relatively comparable and suggested the simple averaging of octave thresholds from 512 through 2,048 Hz as both an adequate and a clinically expedient method for estimating a patient's sensitivity for either spondees or connected speech.

Reprinted by permission of the American Speech-Language-Hearing Association from *J. Speech Hearing Dis.*, 36, 476–483 (1971).

Fletcher (1950) presented a formula for weighting audiometric frequencies and applied it to several sets of data. He wrote, "The formula yields a calculated value which generally is in closer agreement with the observation than is the value calculated by the familiar rule of averaging the losses at 500, 1,000 and 2,000 cps." He then suggested a simplified computational rule which he found to be almost as reliable as his formula: "This simplified rule is to examine the hearing losses measured by means of the audiometer at the three frequencies 500, 1,000 and 2,000 cps and to take the average of the two smallest values of loss" (1950, p. 35). Fletcher refined his weighting system in 1953, but he proposed this refinement as a means of computing percentage impairments for speech rather than for predicting decibels of impairment in the speech threshold.

The medicolegal aspects of estimating loss for speech from the audiogram have received much attention since World War II. This work has culminated in several systems for computing percentage of disability from pure-tone audiometry. One example is the current AMA system (1961) which represents the outcome of the work by the Committee on Conservation of Hearing of the American Academy of Ophthalmology and Otolaryngology. Such methods are tangential to our discussion because their goal is to yield a legally acceptable expression of disability rather than to supply a clinical estimate of the amount of impairment, but their influence has crept into the clinical world.

Another major trend which has impinged on the clinical thinking has been the evolution of the concept of the Articulation Index (French and Steinberg, 1947; Beranek, 1947; Kryter, 1962; and others). Of course, this concept is applicable to the estimation of the threshold for speech in quiet. However, use of the method in its original form requires knowledge of thresholds at more frequencies than ordinarily tested clinically, and the primary use of the Articulation Index has been estimating efficiencies of speech reproducing systems or of reception against background noise. However, several attempts to adapt the underlying premises of the Articulation Index to clinical use by weighting the clinical audiogram have been made (Lightfoot, Carhart, and Jerger, 1953; Kryter, Williams, and Green, 1962). The resulting methods have not received wide clinical acceptance as predictors of SRT because they are cumbersome when the task at hand is merely estimating the threshold in quiet, whether for spondees or for analogous test material.

The foregoing resume, though brief and incomplete, illustrates the confusion which has beset the clinician. He must answer the question, Which system from among the several available for estimating the SRT in quiet from the pure-tone audiogram should I employ? This uncertainty has prompted a number of studies. Harris, Haines, and Myers (1956), Graham (1960), and Siegenthaler and Strand (1964) have evaluated already existing methods by determining the efficiencies these methods achieved when applied to clinical data. The generalization which emerges from such studies is that differences among methods are demonstrable and that some of these differences are substantial. However, other differences are small. Moreover, complicated predictive formulas appear to be only slightly superior to several of the simple averages that can be more easily abstracted from the audiogram.

One technique of searching for interdependencies between thresholds for pure tones and thresholds for speech is to derive regression equations from empirical data gathered from clinical populations. Among earlier investigators using this technique are Harris, Haines, and Myers (1956), Quiggle et al. (1957), and Hirsh and Bilger (1956). Harris, Haines, and Myers used measures obtained on 197 partially defective ears. Their criterion for the speech threshold was the level where 50 percent intelligibility for PB-50 words was achieved. Quiggle et al. analyzed data on the right ears of 319 men aged 20–29 examined during the Wisconsin State Fair Survey. Spondee thresholds were obtained with W-1 recordings. Hirsh and Bilger, also using spondee thresholds as the criterion of impairment for speech, studied data on 179 ears drawn from clinical files.

Both Harris, Haines, and Myers and Quiggle et al. confirmed the often-observed fact that in heterogeneous populations frequencies above 2,000 Hz play such minimal statistical roles in prediction of SRT in quiet that these frequencies can be ignored. Hence, the present discussion will limit itself to comparison of regression equations incorporating frequencies in the 500–2,000 Hz range. Table 26–1 presents a series of such equations (and the corresponding coefficients of correlation) derived from two clinical populations whose SRTs were measured with spondees: a series of 341 better ears derived from a consecutive series of audiological patients seen in one of Northwestern University's Hearing Clinics during a single six-month period and a second series of better ears from another group of audiometrically heterogeneous patients. The only other provisos for inclusion in

TABLE 26–1. ILLUSTRATIVE REGRESSION EQUATIONS FOR PREDICTION OF SPONDEE THRESHOLDS IN QUIET FROM PURE-TONE THRESHOLDS FOR FREQUENCIES IN THE 500–2,000-Hz RANGE. EQUATIONS DERIVED FROM TWO SETS OF UNSELECTED CLINICAL DATA OBTAINED AT NORTHWESTERN UNIVERSITY AFTER ADJUSTMENT OF THRESHOLD LEVELS TO CONFORM TO THE NEW ANSI REFERENCE LEVELS. ONLY BETTER EAR OF EACH SUBJECT USED.

Subjects	Correlation Coefficient	Predicted SRT
Group 1	$r = 0.90$	$3.6 \text{ dB} + 0.85T_{500}$
$N = 341$ Ears	$r = 0.92$	$2.6 \text{ dB} + 0.77T_{1000}$
	$r = 0.78$	$9.5 \text{ dB} + 0.56T_{2000}$
	$R = 0.95$	$-3.8 \text{ dB} + 0.45T_{500} + 0.54T_{1000}$
	$R = 0.95$	$-5.3 \text{ dB} + 0.46T_{500} + 0.41T_{1000} + 0.15T_{2000}$
Group 2	$r = 0.89$	$3.1 \text{ dB} + 0.94T_{500}$
$N = 200$ Ears	$r = 0.91$	$4.3 \text{ dB} + 0.81T_{1000}$
	$r = 0.76$	$6.3 \text{ dB} + 0.65T_{2000}$
	$R = 0.95$	$0.8 \text{ dB} + 0.46T_{500} + 0.49T_{1000}$
	$R = 0.96$	$-1.1 \text{ dB} + 0.47T_{500} + 0.37T_{1000} + 0.14T_{2000}$

either population were that each patient must have been between 10 and 80 years old and he must have yielded measurable thresholds for spondees and for all frequencies of importance in the study. Incidentally, both sets of data have been brought into conformity with the new American National Standards Institute's (1969) reference threshold levels for spondees and for pure tones, and the equations should be read accordingly.

Note first that all coefficients of correlation are highly positive. The Pearson rs for interdependence between SRT and a single frequency range from 0.76 to 0.92, with all correlations involving either 500 or 1,000 Hz being at least 0.89. These coefficients definitely improved when a second frequency was brought into the predictive formula. By contrast, bringing in the third frequency (2,000 Hz) caused almost no further change. (Computations of higher order regressions were also carried out, but they failed to produce any appreciable increase in R.) Thus, there does not seem to be any reason for favoring the use of regression equations employing more than two pure tones.

Note next that the regression equations vary substantially in both the constants they require and in the weightings (beta coefficients) by which pure-tone thresholds are multiplied. Such variation is to be expected among the several equations for a single clinical population because each equation was derived from a different array of thresholds. It is also

attributable to the transition from one set of data to the other because two patient populations will not be identical. Bearing the latter consideration in mind, one is impressed by the reasonable parallelism which usually characterizes the corresponding beta coefficients for the two groups in any pair of equivalent equations. However, in the face of the foregoing variables it is well to remember that no one regression equation can be designated as most applicable for general clinical use. Harris (1965) pointed this up when he said, "The multiple R's in the literature. . . . are statistically justified, but they may apply with reasonable precision only to the population from which they were derived" (p. 828).

Despite this observation, clinical guidelines can be abstracted from the materials just reviewed. The two frequencies which emerge as particularly intimately related to the spondee threshold in quiet are 500 and 1,000 Hz. One may reason from the material in Table 26–1 that the threshold for either frequency is, after appropriate weighting, a good predictor. However, precision improves when the two are combined and reweighted in a multiple regression equation. Moreover, we note that in these two instances the beta coefficients that emerged in a single formula received nearly equal weightings (0.45 and 0.54 for the first group, and 0.46 and 0.49 for the second group). Furthermore, these beta coefficients are close enough to 0.5 so that a reasonable clinical approximation would be to consider these two frequencies as contributing equally. Doing so reduces the clinician's task when predicting SRT for spondees to one of averaging the thresholds at these two frequencies.

In this regard, however, it is imperative that the clinician remember two other facts as he proceeds.

The first of these is that the various studies which have examined relations between SRT and pure-tone thresholds have all employed audiometrically heterogeneous populations. It does not follow that weighing 500 and 1,000 Hz equally is applicable to all patterns of pure-tone loss. In fact, Fletcher's (1950) findings that the two best thresholds in the 500–2,000 Hz range have good predictive value suggests that relations do vary with audiogram shape, but neither Fletcher's work nor any other published study clarifies how relations change with audiometric configuration. Thus, the present suggestion (as well as any other predictive system now advocated) offers an approximation which will probably be modified when we learn more about the role which pattern of hearing loss plays in the clinical population.

Secondly, the clinician must realize that whatever predictive formula he employs will probably require use of a constant to be added to or subtracted from the value he derives from weighting the pure-tone thresholds as called for by his formula. Such constants appear as the first terms in the several regression equations reported in this paper. Their magnitude differs substantially from formula to formula, and most are large enough so that one cannot justify ignoring them. Note, for example, that the use of the regression equations using 500 and 1,000 Hz require a −3.8 dB correction in the regression equations generated from the data on 341 ears. There are several reasons why the correction constant varies. It shifts as the number of frequencies in the regression equation vary. It is also influenced by the reference levels to which one's audiometers are calibrated and by the precision with which these instruments actually conform to these levels. An appreciable variation in the size of the correction constant will occur even when audiometers are within the tolerance limits allowed by current calibrational standards, and miscalibration increases its range greatly.

Clinicians have largely ignored the need to employ a correction constant when estimating the SRT from the pure-tone audiogram. Those who have realized the need to do so have often felt baffled by the disparities in correction constant to be found in formulas reported in the literature. Some of these constants have been so large they seemed clinically incredible. Others have been smaller and have been disregarded as having only second order clinical significance. Finally, some proponents of averaging techniques (Carhart, 1946b, for example) have implied that no correction is necessary.

The foregoing discussion makes clear that clinicians can develop an improved frame of reference for estimating SRT from the pure-tone audiogram. For one thing, the data in the literature which bear on prediction of SRT from pure-tone thresholds supply only an approximate foundation for modern clinical practice. These data were obtained with pure-tone and speech audiometers calibrated to antiquated reference levels. We have reached the era where the ISO 1964 reference levels for pure-tone audiometers are in general use and the ANSI reference threshold levels for spondees as well as pure tones have been adopted. Sophisticated clinicians are insightfully monitoring the calibration of their equipment. We need to have our predictive formulas expressed in relation to our new audiometric standards and our improved calibrational competence, so that we can employ the proper correction constants in using these formulas.

As to the choice of what predictive formula to use, the unanswered question is whether or not the clinician should employ the same formula irrespective of the patient's audiometric pattern. We already have indirect evidence that the correction constant cannot be assumed to be the same irrespective of configuration (Carhart, 1946b). It may well be that the frequencies that are critical and the beta-weights they embody also vary importantly with audiometric configuration. Today, as he faces this question, the clinician can only employ tenuously based rules of thumb derived from his workaday clinical experience. Such a state of affairs is historically understandable, but it should be rectified by further research as rapidly as possible.

Meanwhile there are two steps the clinician can take. One of these is to reassess the appropriateness of the formula he is using for prediction of SRT from pure-tone audiogram. On the basis of the results shown in Table 26–1, plus an evaluation of the evidence in the literature, the writer now suggests that the estimate of the SRT be based on the average of 500 and 1,000 Hz; but the important thing is for the clinician to make his choice after weighing the several alternatives insightfully. The other step is for the clinician to examine his own cumulating data to ascertain what correction constant is applicable in his situation for the formula he has chosen. Doing so takes into account local variables, such as the specifics of audiometer output, which will affect his results.

As a final comment, and pending confirmation from further statistical studies, it seems, on the basis of the data reported in this paper, that the following equation offers a reasonable general formula for predicting clinical SRTs for spondees from pure-tone thresholds when one's audiometric equipment is calibrated to ANSI reference levels:

$$\text{SRT spondee} = -2 \text{ dB} + 0.5 \; T_{500} + 0.5 \; T_{1,000}$$

$$\text{or } \frac{T_{500} + T_{1,000}}{2} - 2 \text{ dB}.$$

This formula takes cognizance of the prime importance of 500 and 1,000 Hz as predictor frequencies when audiometric pattern is not taken into account.

It also embodies the reasonable simplification of giving equal weight to these two frequencies. In addition, it includes the minor correction constant (rounded to the nearest 2-dB step) which the data for the two groups reported above require when the formula is applied to these data. In view of these considerations, this formula seems to offer a good starting point from which the clinician can proceed until he has ascertained more accurately on the basis of his own experience what correction constant best applies to his situation and until the role of audiometric configuration in prediction of spondee threshold is clarified.

ACKNOWLEDGMENT

The study reported in this paper was supported by Grant NS-01310, National Institute of Neurological Diseases and Stroke, and preparation of the paper was supported by Grant K6 NS 16,224, NINDB.

REFERENCES

American Medical Association. Guides to the evaluation of permanent impairment: Ear, nose, throat and related structures. *J. Amer. Med. Ass.,* **177,** 489–501 (1961).

American Medical Association. Tentative standard procedure for evaluating the percentage of useful hearing loss in medicolegal cases. *J. Amer. Med. Ass.,* **119,** 1,108–1,109 (1942).

American Medical Association. Tentative standard procedure for evaluating the percentage of useful hearing loss in medicolegal cases. *J. Amer. Med. Ass.,* **133,** 396–397 (1947).

American National Standard Specifications for Audiometers, ANSI S3.6-1969. New York: American National Standards Institute (1969).

American Standard Specification for Audiometers for General Diagnostic Purposes, Z24.5-1951. New York: American Standards Association (1951).

Beranek, L. L. The design of speech communication systems. *Proc. Inst. Radio Engin.,* **35,** 880–890 (1947).

Carhart, R. Monitored live-voice as a test for auditory acuity. *J. Acoust. Soc. Amer.,* **17,** 339–349 (1946*a*).

Carthart, R. Speech reception in relation to pattern of pure tone loss. *J. Speech Dis.,* **11,** 97–108 (1946*b*).

Fletcher, H. *Speech and Hearing.* New York: Van Nostrand (1929).

Fletcher, H. A method of calculating hearing loss for speech from an audiogram. *Acta Otolaryng. Supp.,* **90,** 26–37 (1950). See also *J. Acoust. Soc. Amer.,* **22,** 1–5 (1950).

Fletcher, H., *Speech and Hearing in Communication.* New York: Van Nostrand (1953).

Fowler, E. P., Hearing standards for acceptance, disability rating and discharge in the military services and in industry. *Trans. Amer. Otol. Soc.,* **45,** 243–263 (1941).

Fowler, E. P., A simple method of measuring percentage of capacity for hearing speech. *Arch. Otolaryng.,* **36,** 874–890 (1942).

French, N. R., and Steinberg, J. C., Factors governing the intelligibility of speech sounds. *J. Acoust. Soc. Amer.,* **19,** 90–119 (1947).

Graham, J. T., Evaluation of methods for predicting speech reception threshold. *Arch. Otolaryng.,* **72,** 347–350 (1960).

Harris, J. D., Pure-tone acuity and the intelligibility of everyday speech. *J. Acoust. Soc. Amer.,* **37,** 824–830 (1965).

Harris, J. D.; Haines, H. L.; and Myers, C. K. A new formula for using the audiogram to predict speech hearing loss. *Arch. Otolaryng.,* **63,** 158–176 (1956) (and correction, **64,** 477, 1956).

Hirsh, I. J., and Bilger, R. C., Prediction of speech threshold from the pure tone audiogram by multiple-regression technique. Paper presented at the Annual Convention of the American Speech and Hearing Association, Chicago, Illinois (1956).

Hughson, W., and Thompson, E., Correlation of hearing acuity for speech with discrete frequency audiograms. *Arch. Otolaryng.,* **36,** 526–540 (1942).

Kryter, K. D., Methods for the calculation and use of the articulation index. *J. Acoust. Soc. Amer.,* **34,** 1689–1697 (1962).

Kryter, K. D.; Williams, C.; and Green, D. M. Auditory acuity and the perception of speech. *J. Acoust. Soc. Amer.,* **34,** 1217–1223 (1962).

Lightfoot, C., Carhart, R.; and Jerger, J. F. Efficiency of impaired ears in noise: C. Perception of speech at suprathreshold levels. Project No. 21-1203-0001, Report No. 6, USAF School of Aviation Medicine, Randolph Field, Texas (1953).

Quiggle, R. R.; Glorig, A.; Delk, J. H.; and Summerfield, A. B. Predicting hearing loss for speech from pure tone audiograms. *Laryngoscope,* **67,** 1–15 (1957).

Sabine, P. E., On estimating the percentage loss of useful hearing. *Trans. Amer. Acad ophthal. Otolaryng.,* **46,** 179–196 (1942).

Siegenthaler, B. M., and Strand, R., Audiogram-average methods and SRT scores. *J. Acoust. Soc. Amer.,* **36,** 589–593 (1964).

Standard Reference Zero Calibration for Pure-Tone Audiometers, ISO/R 389-1964. International Organization for Standardization (1964).

27

Problems in the Measurement of Speech Discrimination

Raymond Carhart, Ph.D.

Professor of Audiology, Northwestern University when this article was prepared

I. INTRODUCTION

Traditionally, a speech discrimination score is the percentage of test items a person can identify correctly by ear. Two decades ago lists of monosyllabic words, the PB-50 tests, were adapted to the measurement of the speech discrimination of the hearing impaired. These materials have since become thoroughly entrenched in otological and audiological practice. Unfortunately, a number of confusions regarding their use has persisted to the present. Our purpose is to review some of the factors that contribute to these confusions. The goal is to examine problems which, when kept in mind, can help otologists stabilize measurement of speech discrimination and unify their interpretation of its results.

II. TEST MATERIALS

The first problem is, "Which test materials shall one use?"

A test of discrimination for speech, as opposed to a threshold test, must consist of relatively nonredundant items. Otherwise, the multiplicity of clues available to the patient will obscure many of his inabilities to differentiate consonants and vowels accurately. It is for this reason that monosyllabic words have been chosen instead of conversational sentences or multisyllabic words, such as spondees. Monosyllabic words are sufficiently unpredictable for clinical subjects so that individual speech elements must be perceived relatively independently. On the other hand,

they are not as confusing as nonsense syllables, which are so abstract that they baffle many subjects.

The traditional discrimination test in this country consists of 50 PB monosyllables. The original materials of this kind were the 20 PB-50-word lists developed at Harvard (1948) during World War II. These lists are still used in some clinics and laboratories, but they contain enough unfamiliar words so that they can somewhat confound linguistically naive subjects. Consequently, several workers have since composed lists which are more familiar. For example, Haskins (1949) developed four PB-50-word lists restricted to monosyllables taken from the speaking vocabularies of young children. Again, Hirsh et al. (1952) constructed the well-known W-22 test from words that (with one exception) appear in Thorndike's tabulation of 20,000 familiar words.

The foregoing lists were all patterned so that they yielded only rough approximations of the phonetic balance found in everyday spoken English. Lehiste and Peterson (1959), therefore, devised ten 50-word lists that conform very closely in balance to monosyllabic words as a class. These CNC lists, as they were called, were later improved by giving they more uniform distributions of word familiarity (Peterson and Lehiste, 1962). Still more recently, Tillman et al. (1963) assembled other versions of the CNC test pattern, and other tests may be expected in the future.

Probably the most important consideration in choosing a particular discrimination test for clinical use is the linguistic background of the patient. Unfamiliar material tends to make the test more difficult (Owens, 1961). This fact does not mean that highly familiar words must always be used, since there are times when a relatively difficult test is preferable. However, the clinician must be on the lookout for instances where some words become nonsense

Reprinted by permission of the American Medical Association from *Arch. Otolaryng.*, **82**, 253-260 (1965). Copyright 1965, American Medical Association.

items for his patient, as can occur particularly often with a young child.

Conversely, differences in phonetic balance among lists seem to be of only secondary influence as long as these are only moderate differences. This fact became apparent with the original PB-50-word lists. These 20 lists have proved to be reasonably equivalent forms, in spite of some deviation in phonetic balance. Likewise, we have found in our laboratory that discrimination scores are not changed importantly by shift from the PB-50 to the Lehiste-Peterson criterion of phonetic balance. In general as long as the test items are meaningful monosyllables for the patient and their phonetic distribution is appropriately diversified, one 50-word compilation is relatively equivalent to another.

III. TEST PRESENTATION

This generalization does not imply that major differences in discrimination scores do not occur. The contrary is true, but these large differences are brought about by other factors, such as changes in talker, in method of reproducing the test, in characteristics of the test equipment, and the like.

This circumstance brings us to the second problem facing the clinician: namely, the problem of determining the details of test presentation which he shall specify.

A major point of past controversy has been whether material should be administered by monitored live-voice, i.e., spoken by the tester at the time of the test, or from a prerecording. Critics of the live-voice procedure argue correctly that results obtained by different speakers cannot be compared unless the talkers have been demonstrated to be equivalent. Lacking this information, the best one can do is to make comparisons only among the results obtained by a single talker and to remember that the significance of any particular score varies from one talker to the next.

A point often ignored in use of prerecorded material is that each talker's unique characteristics are permanently built into the test he has recorded. There may be as much difference between one recording and another as between two live-voice talkers.

An excellent example of this fact is the well-known dissimilarity between the Rush-Hughes recordings and the W-22 recordings of PB-50 mate-

rials. The former, it will be recalled, constitute the version with which data were gathered in the late 1940s by Davis (1948) and others. The latter are the later and widely used version prepared by Hirsh et al. (1952). The difference between the two versions is illustrated in Figure 27-1, which plots normal articulation functions for both versions. Notice that discrimination for W-22 improves rapidly as the presentation level is raised, and that scores become nearly perfect relatively close to the speech reception threshold. The Rush-Hughes version is much more exacting, as evidenced by the more gradual improvement in discrimination as the presentation level is increased. It is not until extremely high levels are used that the Rush-Hughes scores are as good as the W-22 scores.

A somewhat comparable dissimilarity between these versions appears for clinical subjects, although the details of the relationship vary from person to person. Figure 27-2 presents an illustrative set of results. Notice first that performance on both tests is poorer than that obtained by normal listeners. This is apparent in two ways: namely each articulation function rises more gently, and it reaches a plateau before 100 percent scores are achieved. However, the most dramatic feature is that the deterioration in performance is proportionately much greater with Rush-Hughes than with W-22. For example, the plateau level is 94 percent for W-22 but it drops to 71 percent for Rush-Hughes.

As these examples emphasize, the clinician must remember that recorded tests are inflexible. Each ver-

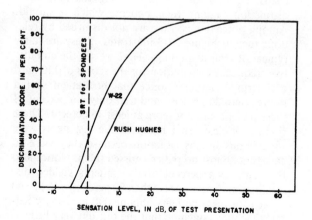

FIGURE 27-1. Articulation curves for normal hearers showing relation between two recorded tests.

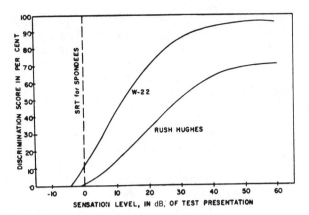

FIGURE 27-2. Articulation curves for an illustrative sensorineural loss showing relation between two recorded tests.

sion possesses a degree of difficulty which he must accept and to which he must adapt as best he can. Moreover, he has at his disposal only a very few recorded versions that are easily available. One or the other of these may serve his clinical need, or neither may be very applicable.

Let us illustrate the clinician's dilemma by a further consideration of W-22. This version has become extremely popular for several reasons, one of which is that the Veterans Administration arbitrarily made it the basis for adjudicating service-connected hearing losses. Many clinicians now use the test without seriously questioning its appropriateness to their own needs. They do not ask whether it reveals the critical distinctions among their patients which it should. Among other things, they are not disturbed by relations such as Figure 27-3 illustrates. These are fairly typical of clinical findings. Here we see the cumulative frequency distribution for the scores of 170 hard of hearing veterans. Notice that no patient scored poorer than 26 percent, and that only 3.6 percent of these patients did not score at least 46 percent. These findings indicate that many of the test items were superfluous in this situation because they were so easy that almost no patient missed them. Notice also that only 39.4 percent of the patients yielded discrimination scores poorer than 90 percent. That is, 60 percent of these patients obtained 90 percent or better. One may conclude that the test did very little to separate the performances of six out of every ten of these patients.

Please do not misunderstand the intent of these remarks. They are not a criticism of W-22 per se. They are a criticism of the clinician, be he audiologist or otolaryngologist, who uses a test without concern for its characteristics and for how these characteristics affect the test's usefulness to him. The Rush-Hughes version can be used just as uninsightfully, as can any other existing test. The simple fact is that no one has ever laid out the clinical criteria he felt a test should satisfy and then developed a set of recordings meeting those criteria.

Of course, variables other than the recording itself affect a test's characteristics.

One such variable is the equipment used. The American Standards Association (1953) has decreed the specifications which a speech audiometer should meet. Since discrimination tests are particularly susceptible to variations in reproduction, one is not justified in comparing discrimination scores from two clinics where the same materials are presented in the same way unless the clinics also use comparable equipment.

Another variable that is critically important is the presentation level at which testing is done. Here we get into very complex problems even though the issue

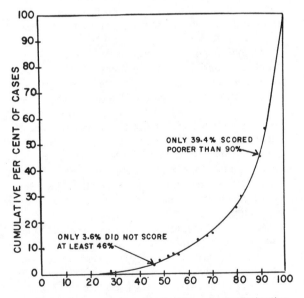

FIGURE 27-3. Cumulative distribution of discrimination scores obtained from 170 patients tested with W-22 recordings in a VA Audiology Center.

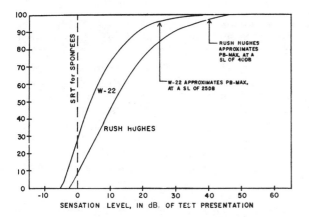

FIGURE 27-4. Articulation curves for normal hearers illustrating that the lowest presentation level yielding the maximum discrimination score varies with the test used.

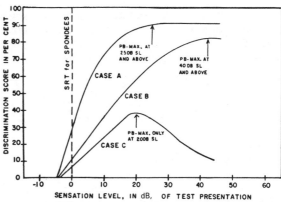

FIGURE 27-5. Three types of abnormal articulation curves illustrating that sensation levels at which maximum discrimination scores occur vary with the individual case.

as it sometimes is stated by clinicians appears very simple. To explain: clinicians often argue as to whether a discrimination test should be given 25 dB above the patient's speech reception threshold, at 40 dB above, or at some other level (such as the 110 dB SPL advocated by Davis [1948]). Here the underlying assumption has been that one should be measuring the best discriminations the patient can achieve on the test material. This maximum discrimination has sometimes been called the PB-Max score (Carhart, 1952). The question is, "At what level is the PB-Max score achieved?"

The difficulties in selecting a presentation level which will guarantee measuring the PB-Max score can be illustrated by considering Figures 27-4 and 27-5.

Figure 27-4 compares normal articulation scores for W-22 and Rush-Hughes recordings when plotted against the sensation level of presentation. Note that W-22 yields scores good enough at a sensation level of 25 dB to approximate maximum. It is necessary to rise to a 40 dB sensation level before the same outcome is obtained with Rush-Hughes. Thus, one can be fairly certain of a score at 25 dB approaching PB-Max if he is using W-22 on a patient with normal discrimination for speech, but he has no chance of this outcome if he is using Rush-Hughes. Incidentally, most talkers when using live voice obtain results close to those shown here for W-22.

Figure 27-5 expands the illustration by showing three types of abnormal articulation function. These

curves demonstrate that the presentation levels at which maximum discrimination scores are obtainable vary with individual clinical patients. Note that any level from 25 dB up will yield PB-Max with patient A, but that this same situation is true for patient B only from 40 dB up. Moreover, only a small range of levels around 20 dB SL will allow patient C to achieve his best discrimination score. If, in these instances, the clinician were to test only at a sensation level of 25 dB he would fail to obtain a reasonable estimate of the maximum discrimination score achievable by patient B, while using the 40 dB SL would yield results far short of PB-Max for patient C.

The foregoing examples make eminently clear the fact that the clinician who tests only at one presentation level can be sure that he has a valid estimate of a person's maximum discrimination score only if the score approximates 100 percent. If the score is lower than this there is no way of knowing whether it represents the patient's best performance, i.e., whether it is a score on the plateau of his articulation curve, or whether the test condition precludes his responding at his best capacity. The only way to resolve this dilemma is to administer enough lists at enough levels to allow the upper part of the patient's articulation function to be plotted. Admittedly, there are many circumstances wherein time limitations and other restrictions make it necessary to test discrimination for speech at only one level. Here the clinician has no choice but to use a level that is practical and likely to evoke maximum discrimination scores from most patients. But the clinician must recollect the uncertainty attending a single test score whenever he compares different patients or compares the same person under different circumstances of listening.

IV. MARGIN OF UNCERTAINTY

Another question of importance is, "What allowance must one make for the margin of uncertainty of the test he is using?"

Of course, precision of a patient's score depends on many factors. Some of these are related to the considerations which we have already mentioned. Obviously, failure to control key factors may increase the margin of error substantially. It is possible for a clinician to carry on such sloppy testing that his results have little meaning. We can discard such eventualities from further discussion with the comment that here we are discussing the uncertainty in test scores which remains after proper precautions are observed. The important point is that there is an irreducible minimum in the repeatability of test results. The problem before us is one of estimating this minimum so that allowance can be made for it.

Reliability varies from one test version to another, but an approximate picture of the precision possible with tests consisting of 50 monosyllables emerges from the following data obtained in our laboratory. Two versions of NU Auditory Test 4 were administered twice at each of five sensation levels to three groups of 16 subjects each. One group consisted of normal hearers, the second of patients with conductive losses, and the third of patients with sensorineural impairments.

A meaningful way to examine the results is to consider averages of the individual differences between test and retest scores, since these averages represent the means of the absolute discrepancies in scores. The Table presents these averages after the results have been corrected to compensate for the learning effect introduced by the experimental design.

The table highlights two relationships. As long as sensation levels were low, which meant that performance on the rising slope of the articulation function was being measured (notably at 0 and +8 dB SL), averages of discrepancies tended to be a little less than 6 percent. Here, then, the margin of uncertainty as gauged by averages of discrepancies was about three test words. As soon as scores became high enough to evoke response on the plateau of the articulation function (at 32 dB for sensorineurals but from 16 dB up for conductives and normals) the averages of discrepancies dropped to 2 percent or less. This represents a margin of error of one test word.

To the degree that one may generalize from these data, two conclusions seem justified. First, precision varies with presentation level, being sharpest when the test is given so that the patient is able to do his best in discriminating speech. Second, the precision of a 50 monosyllable test, as gauged by the average discrepancy between test and retest scores, can be relatively good. There is little to be gained clinically by using a 100-item test so as to enhance the representativeness of the score.

Some authors, notably Elpern (1961), have contended that the converse also is true: namely, that there is no point in using a 50-item test because adequate precision can be maintained with 25 words, i.e., a so-called half-list. Elpern bases his argument on an analysis of W-22 scores. What he fails to re-

AVERAGES OF DIFFERENCES IN PERCENT BETWEEN DISCRIMINATION SCORES FOR TEST
AND RETEST WITH NU AUDITORY TEST 4*

Sensation Level of Presentation	Normal Hearers†	Conductive Loss Group†	Sensorineural Loss Group†	All Groups Combined‡
0 dB	7.2	5.5	3.6	5.3
8 dB	3.5	5.1	5.3	4.6
16 dB	2.3	2.5	5.6	3.5
24 dB	0.3	1.8	4.9	2.3
32 dB	0.6	1.2	1.8	1.2

*Results shown are combined data for lists 1 and 2 after correction to compensate for the learning effect introduced by experimental design.

†16 subjects, 32 test-retest comparisons.

‡48 subjects, 96 test-retest comparisons.

member is that about four tenths of the W-22 words are too easy to help differentiate among scores except very rarely. Consequently, when a half-list is used only about 15 of its 25 words function as effective test items under ordinary circumstances. This number cannot be considered adequate when W-22 is used.

V. MEASUREMENT OF DISCRIMINATION

We come now to the question as to how measurement of discrimination for speech may serve the otologist in his diagnoses of auditory maladies.

First, we must recall Walsh's early emphasis on the idea that discrimination tests can help classify the amount of sensorineural involvement attending clinical otosclerosis. In an article that he wrote with Thurlow et al. (1949) we find the statement, "The maximum PB score varies with clinical diagnosis. It is highest in conductive deafness, slightly lower in conductive deafness with some nerve involvement causing high-tone hearing loss, and still lower if nerve involvement predominates." However, in accepting this conclusion, one must remember that discrimination must be measured with a difficult test like the Rush-Hughes version. The same degree of delineation will not occur with an easy test like W-22. Instead, as Walsh (1964) has put it recently in speaking of responses of otosclerotic patients to W-22, " . . . everybody either gets 100 percent or 30 percent."

Second, we must remember that measurement of speech discrimination has in recent years become a helpful aid in differential diagnosis of relatively diverse conditions. For example, presbycusis may be classified in terms of whether patients have suffered a breakdown in clarity of speech perception which is out of proportion to the pattern of their pure tone loss. Schuknecht (1955) has expressed the view that such a breakdown characterizes presbycusis due to neural rather than epithelial atrophy.

Another illustration is found when there is need to distinguish unilateral Meniere's disease from eighth nerve tumor. Moderate deterioration in speech discrimination is a frequent symptom in Meniere's disease. Thus Shambaugh (1959), in describing the symptomatology of Meniere's, has said, " . . . impaired discrimination beyond the degree of pure tone loss is very characteristic . . . ." However, fair ca-

pacity in discrimination remains in this instance. By contrast, as is well known, acoustic neurinoma very often produces radical disruption of discrimination for speech. Here, the patient's score is likely to be near zero even with a very easy test. Hence, when the differentiation must be made between unilateral Meniere's disease and an eighth nerve tumor there are advantages in using an easy test, such as W-22 or NU Test 4, because scores on a harder test, like Rush-Hughes are likely also to be so poor for Meniere's disease that one malady will give results akin to the other.

Finally, we turn to use of speech discrimination in diagnosis of lesions within the central auditory system. Here the situation becomes very complex. Jerger (1960) states, "Brain stem lesions may produce severe discrimination problems with no depression in the audiogram whatsoever." By contrast, lesions at higher levels in the auditory system do not disrupt speech discrimination to a noteworthy degree unless the material is distorted in some way to reduce its redundancies. Several kinds of material and various systems of distortion have been used. For example, Bocca (1965) pioneered the use of filtered lists of phonetically balanced words. Such material can be presented via only one ear, in which event the score is appreciably poorer when hearing is done through the ear contralateral to a unilateral lesion of the higher auditory system. Or the same material can be administered binaurally with dissimilar distortions to the two ears, in which case the integrative mechanisms of the central auditory system are subjected to test. It is worth noting that the Rush-Hughes test is difficult enough so that it can serve as a distorted speech test when presented unilaterally (Goldstein, Goodman, and King, 1956), but it is of little value in binaural presentation because the same sound patterns are reaching both ears. It would appear that for the latter purpose one must have differential stimulation such as Matzger's (1962) system for filtering a single signal so that each ear gets a distinctive band of frequencies, although Linden (1964) has failed to confirm Matzger's findings on the usefulness of this procedure.

One may epitomize the present situation by noting that, although speech audiometry has come to be recognized as an important tool in otoneurology, its present status in this area confuses the clinician. A plethora of special procedures has been suggested, but their significance and validity await confirmation. Already, however, the general principles are clear enough to suggest some of the ways that measurement with speech audiometry can assist in otoneurological diagnosis. Its contributions here are in addition to those it makes to differential diagnosis among more peripheral disorders.

VI. DIAGNOSING SOCIAL EFFICIENCY

An entirely different purpose for measuring speech discrimination is to evaluate a patient's everyday difficulties in hearing and to assess the practical significance of therapeutic and rehabilitative procedures for him. Here, the goal is to diagnose the social efficiency of his audition.

At present, one can perform such a diagnosis only in general and qualitative terms. We have very little positive information regarding the work-a-day meaning of discrimination scores. True, it is sometimes assumed that PB-word lists are representative of spoken English because of their parallelisms in phonetic composition. Every sophisticated person recognizes immediately that this cannot be the case. Monosyllables are more difficult to understand than are either longer words or connected utterances. Moreover, clinical measurement of discrimination for monosyllables is usually performed in quiet, whereas most everyday listening situations are characterized by fluctuating background noise of one degree or another. Finally, no one has done the extensive validational study that would be needed to estimate confidently a person's practical handicap from his discrimination score. Probably the closest approximation to such validation is the system for computing the Social Adequacy Index detailed by Davis (1948), but this system merely ranks patients along a scale whose practical significance has not been clarified throughout its entire range. Consequently, every clinician must recognize that regardless of the monosyllabic word list he uses he is obtaining information which he cannot relate directly to everyday auditory efficiency.

Nonetheless, discrimination tests stand as the primary method by which we can ascertain whether or not a person has a multiple problem in receiving speech. That is, we can learn whether or not the patient combines loss of acuity, which is shown by pure tone audiometry and requires that signals be made more intense, with loss in precision of perceiving speech elements, which is shown by a discrimination test and is not improved by amplifying the signal. With this information at hand the insightful clinician can reach a qualitative judgment both about the circumstances in which his patient will have difficulty and about the magnitude of the trouble his patient will face. Of course, in reaching this judgment the clinician must consider both the life patterns of his patient and the characteristics of the test with which speech discrimination was measured.

As one example of how speech audiometry may be used in assessing therapeutic and rehabilitative procedures we have the question as to whether, after stapes surgery, a patient has maintained the clarity of perception he knew preoperatively. A good decibel gain can be at least partially nullified by a loss in discrimination. A relatively exacting test, like Rush-Hughes, is preferable in exploring such a question, because an easy test can fail to reveal moderate shifts which affect everyday efficiency.

Another important question is whether discrimination is affected adversely when a hearing aid is used. Again, a good decibel gain can be nullified by a loss in discrimination. Two issues arise in this instance. One is whether the patient suffers breakdown in discrimination with hearing aids as a class of amplifier. Many an elderly person, for example, is a poor hearing aid user because his phonemic regression interacts adversely with the limitations inherent in the good hearing aids of today. The second issue is whether the patient's discrimination changes importantly from one instrument to the next. We should assure ourselves that the particular hearing aid he procures is one with which he performs satisfactorily. Here a discrimination test serves as the basis for discarding undesirable instruments.

Today clinicians feel particularly frustrated when faced with the need to assess hearing aid performance. Negativistic attitudes have predominated ever since the Harvard research was reported in 1946 (Davis, 1946). It is often argued that differences in aided discrimination score are happenstance and are clinically meaningless.

Without attempting full consideration of the arguments involved, one comment must nonetheless be made. Almost without exception the tests used in the past to evaluate hearing aids have been inadequate in one of two ways. Sometimes, as in the study by Shore, Bilger, and Hirsh (1960), tests have been too short to assure reliability. More often, as when W-22 is used, the test has been so easy that it lacks resolving power. This criticism applies to tests administered in noise as well as in quiet.

The present need, if we are to assess practical efficiency in speech discrimination relatively directly, is for new tests which pit their test items against backgrounds that simulate the competition encountered in everyday situations. Laboratory versions of such tests have been developed, but they are neither fully standardized nor available as yet to the clinician.

Meanwhile the clinician can recognize the limitations of contemporary tests and avoid attempting more precision of interpretation than they justify. Accepting this precaution, measurement of speech discrimination is useful in reaching the qualitative estimate of the outcome of surgery, of potential for hearing aid use, of relative efficiency with different instruments, and of phonemic perception in everyday life.

VII. SUMMARY AND CONCLUSIONS

A number of monosyllabic word tests designed to measure discrimination for speech are available today. The clinician must be clear as to the purpose for which he is measuring discrimination. He must choose both the test to use and the method for administering it so as to satisfy his purpose. Different criteria apply when a test is used in the diagnosis of auditory pathology and in determination of site of lesion than when it is used in estimating either the efficiency of hearing in everyday life or the potential value of a rehabilitative procedure such as a hearing aid. Finally, the clinician must remember that existing tests for speech discrimination are imperfectly standardized and lack validation. They have qualitative usefulness today, but with appropriate revision they can become much more definitive clinical tools.

ACKNOWLEDGMENT

This work was supported by grant K6 NB 16,244-02 from the National Institute of Neurological Diseases and Blindness, the Public Health Service, and by contract AF 41 (657)-418, School of Aerospace Medicine, U.S. Air Force, Brooks Air Force Base, Tex.

REFERENCES

American Standard Specifications for Speech Audiometers. New York: American Standards Association, 1953.

Bocca, E. Binaural Hearing: Another Approach, *Laryngoscope* 65: 1164–1171, 1965.

Carhart, R. Speech Audiometry in Clinical Evaluation, *Acta Otolaryng* 41: 18–42, 1952.

Davis, H. The Articulation Area and the Social Adequecy Index for Hearing, *Laryngoscope* 58: 761–778, 1948.

Davis, H., et al. The Selection of Hearing Aids, *Laryngoscope* 56: 85–115 and 135–163, 1946.

Egan, J. P. Articulation Testing Methods, *Laryngoscope* 58: 955–991, 1948.

Elpern, B. S. The Relative Stability of Half-List and Full-List Discrimination Tests, *Laryngoscope* 71: 30–35, 1961.

Goldstein, R.; Goodman, A. C.; and King, R. B. Hearing and Speech in Infantile Hemiplegia Before and After Left Hemispherectomy, *Neurology* 6: 869–875, 1956.

Haskins, H. *A Phonetically Balanced Test of Speech Discrimination for Children,* thesis, Northwestern University, Chicago, 1949.

Hirsh, I. J., et al. Development of Materials for Speech Audiometry, *J. Speech Hearing Dis.,* 17: 321–337, 1952.

Jerger, J. Audiological Manifestations of Lesions in the Auditory Nervous System, *Laryngoscope* 70: 417–425, 1960.

Lehiste, I., and Peterson, G. E. Linguistic Considerations in the Study of Speech Intelligibility, *J. Acoust. Soc. Amer.* 31: 280–286, 1959.

Linden, A. Distorted Speech and Binaural Speech Resynthesis Tests, *Acta Otolaryng* 58: 32–48, 1964.

Matzker, J. The Sound Localization Test, *Int. Audiol.* 1: 248–249, 1962.

Owens, E. Intelligibility of Words Varying in Familiarity, *J. Speech Hearing Res.* 4: 113–129, 1961.

Peterson, G. E., and Lehiste, I. Revised CNC Lists for Auditory Tests, *J. Speech Hearing Dis.* 27: 62–70, 1962.

Schuknecht, H. F. Presbycusis, *Laryngoscope* 65: 402–419, 1955.

Shambaugh, G. E., Jr. *Surgery of the Ear,* Philadelphia: W. B. Saunders and Co., 1959.

Shore, I.; Bilger, R. C.; and Hirsh, I. J. Hearing Aid Evaluation: Reliability of Repeated Measurements, *J. Speech Hearing Dis.* 25: 152–170, 1960.

Tillman, T. W.; Carhart, R.; and Wilber, L. "A Test for Speech Discrimination Composed of CNC Monosyllabic Words," technical documentary report No. SAM-TDR-62-135, USAF School of Aerospace Medicine, Brooks Air Force Base, Tex, 1963.

Thurlow, W. R., et al. Further Statistical Study of Auditory Tests in Relation to the Fenestration Operation, *Laryngoscope* 59: 113–129, 1949.

Walsh, T. Informal comment, *Trans Amer. Otol. Soc.* 52: 79, 1964.

28

An Expanded Test for Speech Discrimination Utilizing CNC Monosyllabic Words: Northwestern University Auditory Test No. 6

Tom W. Tillman, Ph.D.
Professor of Audiology and Associate Dean,
School of Speech, Northwestern University
Raymond Carhart, Ph.D.
Professor of Audiology, Northwestern University,
when this report was prepared

I. INTRODUCTION

In 1963, a new test for speech discrimination was described by Tillman et al. (1963). It consisted of six randomizations of each of two 50-word lists and was designated Northwestern University Auditory Test No. 4. The monosyllabic words used in constructing the test were of the consonant-nucleus-consonant (CNC) variety and were selected from a pool of such words compiled by Lehiste and Peterson (1959). The scheme of phonemic balance followed in constructing the two parent lists was described in detail earlier (Tillman et al., 1963).

This new tool, N.U. Test No. 4, was utilized extensively in the Auditory Research Laboratories at Northwestern for a two-year period. It proved to be a valuable addition to the array of materials available for the measurement of phonemic discrimination. In both its original form and under conditions of differential filtering it has been shown to possess high interlist equivalence and good reliability. The major

shortcoming of the test has evolved from the fact that the pool of test materials which it makes available is too restricted. Even with six equivalent forms of each list, the exploration of a large number of listening conditions cannot be accomplished without several repetitions of the various forms and lists. Such repetition, of course, adds variables such as learning factors which may exert differential effects over subjects.

Because of the limitation just described, it became desirable to revise and expand N.U. Auditory Test No. 4. The foremost consideration was to produce a larger repertoire of test lists which retained the worthwhile features of the original pair. That is, we wished to achieve a new tool with maximum interlist equivalence and high reliability, and one which would yield articulation functions with approximately the same slopes as those associated with the original test.

The difficulties which Peterson and Lehiste (1962) encountered in constructing ten lists of 50 CNC words so that all lists incorporated the same phonemic balance, led us to set a goal of only four such lists. A new speech discrimination test comprising four phonemically equivalent lists has now been developed and evaluated. The test, Northwestern University Auditory Test No. 6, is described in this report.

Prepared in the Auditory Research Laboratory of Northwestern University under Contract No. AF 41 (609)–2643 and task No. 775508, USAF School of Aerospace Medicine and promulgated as report No. SAM–TR–66–55, June, 1966. Reprinted by permission of the senior author and Department of the Air Force.

II. NATURE OF N.U. AUDITORY TEST NO. 6

Characteristics of the Word Lists

In developing the two lists of words which comprise N.U. Auditory Test No. 4, Tillman et al. (1963) were careful to conform as rigorously as possible to the scheme of phonemic balance advocated by Lehiste and Peterson (1959). This pattern was developed by selecting all the 1,263 monosyllables of the consonant-vowel-consonant type which Thorndike and Lorge (1944) listed as occurring at least once per million words. Lehiste and Peterson then determined the frequency with which each initial, medial, and final phoneme occurred in this pool of 1,263 words. They specified that each such phoneme should appear in a single list of 50 words with the same relative incidence as it exhibited in the total pool of words.

The first step in the construction of the four CNC lists which were to comprise N.U. Auditory Test No. 6 was to make the tabulation shown in Table 28-1. The table indicates the number of times each phoneme must be used in a given list if one is to preserve the phonemic distribution which characterizes the pool of 1,263 words selected initially by Lehiste and Peterson (1959).

The second step was to select four mutually exclusive groups of 50 words that conformed as exactly as possible to the distributions of phonemes shown in Table 28-1. These four groupings of words appear in Table 28-2. They have been designated as lists I, II, III, and IV of N.U. Auditory Test No. 6. All but 15 of the 200 words were selected from the 500-word pool comprising the revised CNC lists published by Peterson and Lehiste (1962). The remaining 15 words all appear in the larger pool of 1,263 words. More-

TABLE 28-1. THE PROPORTIONS (p) OF INCIDENCE OF PHONEMES WHICH CONSTITUTE THE LEHISTE-PETERSON PATTERN OF PHONEMIC BALANCE FOR CNC WORDS AND THE NUMBER (N) OF INCLUSIONS OF EACH PHONEME IN EACH OF THE FOUR LISTS OF N.U. AUDITORY TEST NO. 6.

Initial consonant				Vowel nucleus			Final consonant		
		N				N			N
Sound	p	List I	List* II, III, IV	Sound	p	All lists*	Sound	p	All lists*
p	.0642	3	3	i	.0832	4	p	.0564	3
b	.0658	3	3	I	.1116	5	b	.0264	1
t	.0578	3	3	e^I	.0942	5	t	.1102	6
d	.0594	3	3	ε	.0744	4	d	.0778	4
k	.0658	3	3	æ	.1038	5	k	.0818	4
g	.0420	2	2	ə	.0864	4	g	.0392	2
m	.0584	3	3	a	.0592	3	m	.0542	3
n	.0460	2	2	ɔ	.0626	3	n	.1054	5
f	.0452	2	2	o^U	.0736	4	ŋ	.0208	1
v	.0182	1	1	U	.0222	1	f	.0310	2
θ	.0118	1	1	u	.0586	3	v	.0288	1
ð	.0080	0	0	a^U	.0278	1	θ	.0240	1
s	.0680	3	3	a^I	.0736	4	ð	.0090	0
z	.0032	0	0	$ɔ^I$	.0126	1	s	.0564	3
ʃ	.0354	2	2	ɚ	.0562	3	z	.0390	2
r	.0736	4	4				ʃ	.0200	1
l	.0736	4	4				ʒ	.0018	0
tʃ	.0316	2	2				r	.0628	3
dʒ	.0332	2	2				l	.1032	5
h	.0606	3	3				tʃ	.0318	2
w	.0476	1	2				dʒ	.0200	1
wh	.0156	2	1						
j	.0150	1	1						

$N = \dfrac{100_p}{2}$ rounded to nearest integer.

*Identical to configuration associated with two lists of N.U. Auditory Test No. 4.

TABLE 28-2. ALPHABETICAL ARRANGEMENT OF CNC MONOSYLLABIC WORDS COMPRISING
THE FOUR LISTS OF N.U. AUDITORY TEST NO. 6.

List I		List II		List III		List IV	
bean*	met	bite	merge*	bar*	mouse	back*	mob
boat	mode*	book*	mill	base*	name	bath*	mood*
burn	moon	bought*	nice*	beg	note*	bone	near
chalk	nag*	calm	numb	cab*	pain	came	neat*
choice	page	chair	pad*	cause	pearl*	chain*	pass*
death*	pool	chief	pick*	chat*	phone	check*	peg*
dime*	puff*	dab*	pike	cheek	pole	dip*	perch*
door	rag*	dead*	rain	cool	rat*	dog*	red*
fall*	raid*	deep*	read*	date	ring	doll	ripe*
fat*	raise*	fail	room	ditch*	road*	fit*	rose*
gap	reach*	far*	rot*	dodge*	rush*	food	rough*
goose	sell*	gaze	said	five*	search	gas*	sail
hash*	shout*	gin*	shack*	germ	seize	get*	shirt
home	size*	goal	shawl	good*	shall	hall	should
hurl*	sub	hate*	soap*	gun*	sheep*	have*	sour*
jail	sure	haze	south*	half	soup	hole*	such*
jar	take	hush*	thought*	hire*	talk	join	tape
keen	third	juice	ton*	hit*	team	judge*	thumb*
king	tip*	keep	tool	jug*	tell*	kick*	time*
kite*	tough*	keg	turn*	late	thin*	kill*	tire*
knock	vine*	learn	voice	lid*	void*	lean	vote*
laud	week*	live	wag*	life*	walk*	lease	wash*
limb	which	loaf	white*	luck	when	long	wheat*
lot	whip	lore	witch	mess	wire*	lose	wife*
love*	yes*	match	young	mop*	youth*	make	yearn

*Also in original PB-50 lists.

over, list I in Table 28-2 is identical in content to list I of N.U. Test No. 4. In addition, list II in Table 28-2 differs by only 4 words from the original list II (N.U. Test No. 4). Lists III and IV in the table represent two entirely new compilations.

The third step in the development of N.U. Test No. 6 was to randomize each of the four parent lists four times. This procedure yielded four forms (A, B, C, D) of each of the four lists. These randomizations were subsequently recorded on magnetic tape.

Since the relative familiarity of test items is a significant variable in intelligibility testing, it is important to describe N.U. Test No. 6 in terms of this characteristic before recounting the procedure followed in recording the new test. Table 28-3 reports the number of words in each test list which fall into each of seven categories of word familiarity. Also shown in the table is analogous information based on the average of the ten Peterson-Lehiste (1962) revised CNC lists. Note that the average list of N.U. Test No. 6 is quite similar to the average Peterson-Lehiste list so far as the relative distribution of test words among these seven classes is concerned. Furthermore, as was the case with the previous test (N.U.

Test No. 4), the four lists of N.U. Test No. 6 include a sizeable proportion of very common words and at the same time cover a wide range of familiarity.

Recording Procedures

The apparatus and technical procedure employed in storing the four lists of N.U. Test No. 6 on magnetic tape were essentially the same as those described in relation to N.U. Test No. 4 (Tillman et al., 1963). However, in order to achieve a better signal-to-noise ratio on the new test, the record gain of the tape recorder was adjusted so as to achieve a VU level of 0 dB rather than the −20-dB level used previously.

In the recording of N.U. Test No. 6, a 32-year-old male spoke the test items. In connected discourse his dialect may be described as General American, Southern Fringe (southwest Oklahoma region). Prior to this activity, he had extensive experience in the monitored live voice technic of speech audiometry. Nevertheless, he practiced extensively with the materials to be recorded prior to the final recording session.

TABLE 28-3. DISTRIBUTION ACCORDING TO FREQUENCY OF USAGE OF THE CNC MONOSYLLABLES IN N.U. AUDITORY TEST NO. 6 AND IN THE REVISED PETERSON-LEHISTE TEST.

Familiarity rating	List I	List II	List III	List IV	Average of four lists	Average per list for Peterson-Lehiste test
Among most common 500 words	11	13	14	14	13	10.8
Among next most common 500 words	11	9	6	12	9.5	8.4
More than 100 occurrences per million words	2	0	2	3	1.8	0.8
50 through 99 occurrences per million words	3	6	12	5	6.5	7.7
25 through 49 occurrences per million words	10	6	6	9	7.8	8.3
10 through 24 occurrences per million words	9	5	8	5	6.8	7.8
1 through 9 occurrences per million words	4	11	2	2	4.8	6.2

As stated earlier, each of the four lists of N.U. Test No. 6 was prepared in four alternate forms. In order to insure equivalence from form to form in the recorded tapes, only form A of each of the four lists was actually spoken by the talker. This tape was then copied four times and through a process of cutting and splicing, master copies of each list in its four forms (randomizations) were prepared in the manner detailed in an earlier report (Tillman et al., 1963).

III. METHOD OF EVALUATION

Administration of Lists at Selected Presentation Levels

Interlist equivalence, test-retest reliabilities and other characteristics of N.U. Auditory Test No. 6 were evaluated using two groups of subjects. One of these groups contained 24 normal hearing individuals while the remaining group was composed of 12 persons with sensorineural-type hearing impairments.

Each of the 36 subjects involved was examined twice. During each session, all four lists of the test were administered to the subjects six times beginning at a presentation level 4 dB *below* the subject's spondee threshold (SRT). Succeeding presentations were at progressively higher intensity levels. The rationale for this procedure was discussed in an earlier report (Tillman et al., 1963).

A modified Latin-square design was utilized so as to counterbalance as completely as possible both list and form order of presentation. Since only four forms of each of the four lists were available and it was necessary to present each list a total of six times, two forms of a given list were repeated once in each test session. Care was taken to insure that a given form never recurred until three other forms of the list had intervened.

Subjects

The 24 normal hearing subjects used in the experiment were drawn from the student population at Northwestern University. The group consisted of 7 males and 17 females ranging in age from 19 to 28 years with a mean age of 21.1 years. In 12 subjects the left ear served as the test ear, while in the remaining 12 the right ear was selected for test. No subject was included who failed to respond in a screening test to pure tones from 125 through 8,000 cps at a 10-dB hearing level (re ASA 1951 norm) in his test ear. The nontest ear was not held to this criterion because all measurements were conducted monaurally.

The 12 hypoacousic subjects used in evaluating Test No. 6 were drawn from the files of the Northwestern University Hearing Clinics. They were individuals who had experienced progressive hearing loss during adulthood, and they were selected primarily from the diagnostic categories of sensorineural loss and labyrinthine otosclerosis. No person was chosen as a potential subject unless his audiometric data on file in the hearing clinic indicated that his spondee threshold hearing level fell within the range of 20 to 60 dB and his discrimination score exceeded 70 percent. The final decision to include a subject in this group was made on the basis of audiometric tests conducted at the time of his initial visit. If the results of this examination indicated significant change in the individual's hearing since his last examination in the hearing clinic, he was not included in the experimental group.

The 11 females and 1 male finally selected ranged in age from 41 to 67 years showing an average age of 52.3 years. In all cases, the hearing loss had first been noted prior to age 50. As a group, these individuals were characterized by a mild to moderate gradually sloping, bilaterally symmetrical audiometric configuration. In those persons who showed a difference in acuity between ears, the better ear served as the test ear. Otherwise the test ear was selected arbitrarily.

Test Procedures

As stated earlier, each of the 36 subjects examined in this study participated in two test sessions. Considering both groups, the interval between the test and retest sessions ranged from 6 to 17 days with a mean interval of 8.8 days. The two sessions differed from each other in only one respect—namely, the pure tone audiometry necessary for subject selection was carried out only in the initial session.

Prior to presentation of any CNC materials in either test session, the SRT for the test ear was measured after the subject had been familiarized with the spondee test vocabulary in the manner described previously (Tillman et al., 1963). These materials were delivered to the subject via a speech audiometer (Grason-Stadler, model 162), calibrated to conform to the ASA norm which specifies 22 dB re: 0.0002 microbar as the strength of the signal at 0-dB hearing level. The taped test materials were reproduced by a tape recorder (Ampex, model 351–2) whose output drove the external input to one of the channels of the speech audiometer. In all instances, the level of the 1,000 cps calibration tone, recorded on the tapes at the level of the test materials, was set so that the VU meter of the speech audiometer registered 0 dB. Actual determination of the SRT followed the procedure described below.

An initial presentation level, 10 to 20 dB above the estimated SRT, was selected and two test words were presented at this level. The initial presentation level was selected so that the subject correctly repeated a minimum of five of the first six test items. In the event that this criterion was not met with the initial selection of a starting level, a higher presentation level was chosen and the test run was begun anew. The intensity of the signal was then attenuated by 2 dB and two more words were presented. This procedure was continued until the subject either failed to respond or responded incorrectly to six consecutive test words. Threshold was then computed by subtracting the number of words correctly repeated from the intensity of the signal at the starting level and then adding 1 dB to compensate for the fact that the 50 percent-criterion is not fully met via this procedure.

In each test session, the spondee threshold was established in two consecutive runs and the lower (better) of the two values was accepted as the reference level from which to present the CNC words. Since the attenuator of the speech audiometer was calibrated in 2-dB steps, in the case of an odd-integer spondee threshold, the reference intensity used was the level 1-dB higher than the actual SRT.

The next step in the procedure involved the measurement of discrimination scores for each of the four test lists. As stated earlier, the sensation levels of presentation were expressed relative to the SRT measured in the particular session. That is, in the event of a change in the SRT from test to retest, the new level, regardless of whether it was higher or lower than the initial SRT, served as 0-dB sensation level in the retest session. The six sensation levels at which the CNC materials were presented were: −4, 0, 8, 16, 24, and 32 dB. As stated previously, so far as possible, the order of presentation of lists and forms was rotated over subjects to guard against systematic order effects. However, for a given subject, the same sequence of presentation was followed in the two test sessions.

IV. RESULTS

Articulation Functions for Normal Hearing Subjects

Table 28–4 displays the data obtained with normal hearing subjects during the first test run, while Table 28–5 summarizes the like information obtained in the retest session. In these two tables, means, medians, and standard deviations of discrimination scores are reported separately for each of the four lists at each presentation level. The mean values reported in these two tables are displayed in graphic form in Figure 28–1. Since the data points clustered within a relatively narrow range of discrimination scores, a single articulation function was utilized to describe them (see Figure 28–1).

The data in Tables 28–4 and 28–5 and in Figure 28–1 reveal that the four lists yielded articulation functions of essentially equivalent slope. Further, it is apparent that for a given list, the slope of the function changed little from test to retest.

As was the case with N.U. Auditory Test No. 4 (Tillman et al., 1963), the characteristic feature of the curve in Figure 28–1 is that it represents a linear func-

TABLE 28-4. MEDIAN (MED), MEAN (M), AND STANDARD DEVIATIONS (SD) OF DISCRIMINATION SCORES OBTAINED WITH N.U. AUDITORY TEST NO. 6 FOR SUBJECTS WITH NORMAL HEARING DURING THE FIRST TEST SESSION (SCORES REPRESENT PERCENT OF ITEMS CORRECTLY REPEATED).

Sensation level of presentation*	List I			List II			List III			List IV		
	Med	M	SD	Med	M	SD	Med	M	SD	Med	M	SD
−4	6	8.2	8.2	8	9.4	9.8	6	6.7	5.9	6	8.8	7.7
0	29	30.9	14.1	24	28.1	16.1	25	25.7	10.8	32	31.1	15.3
8	74	70.8	14.3	72	72.3	12.1	74	73.8	9.4	77	74.1	10.6
16	89	88.6	10.6	93	91.3	7.2	94	92.3	5.3	94	92.5	6.1
24	98	96.0	5.2	98	97.8	2.8	99	96.6	8.1	98	97.7	2.8
32	100	98.6	3.8	100	99.3	1.5	100	99.6	1.0	100	99.5	2.4

*Mean SRT = 21.9 dB SPL re: 0.0002 microbar.

TABLE 28-5. MEDIAN (MED), MEAN (M), AND STANDARD DEVIATIONS (SD) OF DISCRIMINATION SCORES OBTAINED WITH N.U. AUDITORY TEST NO. 6 FOR SUBJECTS WITH NORMAL HEARING DURING RETEST SESSION (SCORES REPRESENT PERCENT OF ITEMS CORRECTLY REPEATED).

Sensation level of presentation*	List I			List II			List III			List IV		
	Med	M	SD	Med	M	SD	Med	M	SD	Med	M	SD
−4	6	8.2	7.7	7	8.7	9.0	3	5.8	5.9	6	8.1	7.4
0	32	31.5	13.0	38	37.4	13.1	30	29.6	12.9	33	34.1	13.0
8	76	75.8	10.0	81	79.8	6.8	84	79.6	11.1	77	77.8	9.8
16	94	92.0	5.4	94	94.4	3.6	94	94.2	3.5	96	94.0	6.8
24	98	97.5	2.4	100	98.9	2.0	98	98.3	2.0	100	97.8	4.4
32	100	99.7	1.0	100	99.8	0.7	100	99.3	2.2	100	99.2	3.3

*Mean SRT = 21.2 dB SPL re: 0.0002 microbar.

tion which undergoes saturation. The lower segment of the curve is linear and rises at the rate of approximately 5.6 percent per decibel increase in signal presentation level. The linear segment appears to terminate at a sensation level of about 9 dB where the average discrimination score approaches 80 percent. These characteristics are almost identical to those of the earlier test (N.U. Test No. 4). As was also the case with this latter test, the upper portion of the function in Figure 28-1 describes a curvilinear progression in which scores increase less and less with progressive elevation in signal strength, finally reaching an asymptote, characterized by almost perfect discrimination. This asymptote is not reached until a presentation level of 32 dB is achieved. With the previous test (N.U. Test No. 4) the asymptotic level was reached at the 24-dB sensation level.

Another way of considering the features just discussed is to examine the variability of scores at the different presentation levels (see Tables 28-4 and 28-5). In this consideration the values at the −4-dB sensation level are excluded, since at this level the range of scores was restricted by the fact that negative scores cannot occur and the standard deviation is, therefore, not an adequate measure of the variability. Note, however, that at the 0-dB and 8-dB sensation levels, both of which fall within the linear portion of the articulation functions, the variability of the discrimination scores was great. Observe further that as the stimulus intensity became high enough to saturate the curve with correct responses, variability decreased markedly and systematically. In fact, as the asymptote of the function is approached—i.e., at 32-dB sensation level—the standard deviations approach zero, ranging from 0.7 percent to 3.8 percent. At this level, variation in response among normal hearing subjects is probably due predominantly to occasional errors arising from lack of attention, masking produced by head movement or vocal productions and other secondary factors.

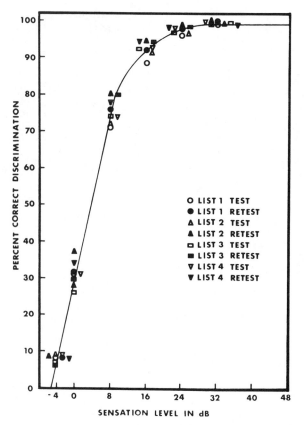

Articulation Functions for
Subjects with Sensorineural Loss

Our previous experience with N.U. Test No. 4 had revealed that the basic pattern of the articulation function for subjects with conductive hearing losses was essentially the same as that for normal subjects. Thus, in the evaluation of N.U. Test No. 6 a sample of subjects with conductive losses was not included. However, since subjects with sensorineural hearing impairment had differed markedly from those of normal subjects when exposed to Test No. 4, the various lists of Test No. 6 were administered to a group of subjects with sensorineural impairment. The data yielded by these subjects in the test and retest sessions are summarized in Tables 28–6 and 28–7. The mean data from these two tables are displayed graphically in Figure 28–2. In two respects, these data closely approximate those reported earlier for the normal hearing subjects. However, one also notes three major discrepancies.

As was the case with the normal hearing group, the articulation functions yielded by the hypoacousic subjects for the four lists are highly equivalent to one another in configuration. In fact, a single function describes the entire array of data points rather well (see Figure 28–2). As was true with the normal group, the pattern of the articulation functions for the sensorineural group also bespeaks a saturation curve with the point of nonlinearity occurring at a score of approximately 74 percent (16-dB SL). Recall that this point occurred at about 80 percent (SL = 9-dB) for the normal group.

The first discrepancy between the results for the normal group and the sensorineural group concerns the slope of the articulation functions for the various lists. While the linear portions of the functions yielded by the normal hearing subjects rose at the rate of about 5.6 percent per decibel increase in signal intensity, the functions for the hearing impaired group sloped more gradually, approximately 3.4 percent per decibel in the linear segment. As a concomitant, the nonlinear upper segments of the functions for the sensorineural group do not reach full saturation within the range of presentation levels employed in this experiment. At the maximum level, 32-dB SL, the average score was approximately 91 percent. If one extrapolates the functions as has been done in Figure 28–2, it appears that the average

FIGURE 28-1. Mean discrimination scores yielded by normal hearing group for lists I, II, III, and IV during both test and retest sessions. A single articulation function fits all sets of data.

As emphasized above, the important features of the articulation functions for N.U. Test No. 6 were essentially invariant from list to list and from test to retest. It is true that careful examination of the data presented so far reveals that minor changes in performance did occur as a consequence of both these variables. However, it may be stated that the characteristics of N.U. Test No. 6, as these reveal themselves through data collected from normal hearing subjects, are almost identical to those of N.U. Test No. 4 (Tillman et al., 1963). In fact, the articulation function for these latter materials is not shown in Figure 28–1 because it would be essentially indistinguishable from the curve displayed there.

TABLE 28-6. MEDIAN (MED), MEAN (M), AND STANDARD DEVIATIONS (SD) OF DISCRIMINATION SCORES OBTAINED WITH N.U. AUDITORY TEST NO. 6 FOR SUBJECTS WITH SENSORINEURAL HEARING LOSS DURING THE FIRST TEST SESSION (SCORES REPRESENT PERCENT OF ITEMS CORRECTLY REPEATED).

Sensation level of presentation*	List I			List II			List III			List IV		
	Med	M	SD	Med	M	SD	Med	M	SD	Med	M	SD
−4	7	7.5	6.3	4	8.8	9.8	3	6.0	7.1	8	8.2	7.2
0	16	16.8	10.7	18	20.7	14.7	11	16.7	13.1	18	17.3	12.5
8	55	49.0	17.5	49	47.3	19.6	41	41.0	17.3	49	46.2	16.1
16	75	71.0	16.2	74	71.3	18.2	74	67.2	24.1	78	70.8	17.3
24	87	85.8	9.2	91	87.3	10.2	84	81.8	13.9	93	89.2	9.3
32	91	90.7	5.3	96	93.2	6.5	92	89.3	8.5	96	93.3	5.1

*Mean SRT = 57.5 dB SPL re: 0.0002 microbar.

TABLE 28-7. MEDIAN (MED), MEAN (M), AND STANDARD DEVIATIONS (SD) OF DISCRIMINATION SCORES OBTAINED WITH N.U. AUDITORY TEST NO. 6 FOR SUBJECTS WITH SENSORINEURAL HEARING LOSS DURING THE RETEST SESSION (SCORES REPRESENT PERCENT OF ITEMS CORRECTLY REPEATED).

Sensation level of presentation*	List I			List II			List III			List IV		
	Med	M	SD	Med	M	SD	Med	M	SD	Med	M	SD
−4	5	7.0	7.2	7	9.7	10.2	1	4.7	9.6	8	8.8	7.7
0	21	19.8	11.3	17	21.0	10.7	10	14.5	10.5	16	17.3	10.4
8	57	53.5	20.5	61	54.8	17.7	38	42.2	21.2	47	48.0	18.4
16	82	74.5	16.4	82	77.5	15.1	76	67.7	21.4	80	73.7	17.9
24	90	85.7	12.8	94	91.0	6.7	87	81.5	17.5	94	87.5	12.3
32	93	90.7	10.4	95	93.0	5.7	92	86.0	18.5	97	92.8	8.2

*Mean SRT = 56.5 dB SPL re: 0.0002 microbar.

saturation asymptote would occur at a mean discrimination score of approximately 93 percent and that this mean score would have occurred at a sensation level of about 40 dB.

A second feature which distinguishes the results for the sensorineural group from those for the normal group concerns the variability of the discrimination scores about the mean values at the various presentation levels. At the 8-dB sensation level and above, the intersubject variability in performance, as estimated by the standard deviation of the responses, was much greater for the hypoacoustic group than for the normal group. This fact merely emphasizes that, as a group, the hearing impaired subjects were much less homogeneous in discriminatory capacity than were the normal hearers.

The third and perhaps the most significant difference between the results of these tests for the two groups studied concerns the group performance from list to list. Recall that, for the normal listeners, only minor differences in group performance occurred in

this regard. However, in the sensorineural group, although the functions for the various lists rose with approximately the same slope, they seemed to be slightly displaced from one another on the sensation level scale. For example, the function for list II would appear to be shifted somewhat further to the left than the other three while that for list III seems to be displaced to the right of the other functions. These circumstances suggest, of course, that the close interlist equivalence, apparent from a study of the data from the normal hearing group, is not completely preserved when the tests are administered to subjects with sensorineural hearing impairment. This discovery is hardly surprising when one considers the effects which variations in the audiometric configuration and other features of hearing loss may exert. The important point to make is that the N.U. Auditory Test No. 6 possesses good interlist equivalence as judged from the performance of the present hypoacousic sample, and this picture is not likely to change significantly as other samples are evaluated.

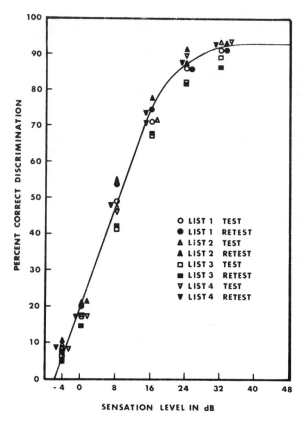

FIGURE 28-2. Mean discrimination scores yielded by subjects with sensorineural hearing loss for lists I, II, III, and IV during both test and retest sessions. A single articulation function fits all sets of data.

Test-Retest Relationships

Two important relationships emerge from a study of the test-retest data yielded by the two subject groups. First, there was a highly systematic tendency for discrimination scores to improve slightly from test to retest. This trend was particularly apparent within the range of sensation levels where the articulation functions were linear. Second, test-retest reliability was good.

Table 28-8 allows one to evaluate the absolute differences between mean performance from test to retest. Note that for both subject groups, the maximum test-retest difference is less than 10 percent and only 4 out of 48 times did it exceed 6 percent. Furthermore, for the normal group only 4 of the 24 test-retest differences were found to be statistically significant.

Similarly, only 3 of the differences between test-retest performance proved to be statistically significant for the sensorineural group. It is interesting to note that 6 of these 7 significant outcomes are associated with list II which, for the sensorineural group at least, appeared to be the easiest of the four lists.

On the basis of the data from this experiment, it is impossible to say whether the improvement in performance from test to retest occurred in consequence of practice in the task involved or of increase in familiarity with the test vocabulary. Be that as it may, the data in Table 28-8 allow one to conclude that with this test the differences in performance from test to retest are not sufficiently large to cause major concern. Recall that, within the linear segment, the articulation functions for the normal and sensorineural subjects rose at rates of 5.6 percent and 3.4 percent per decibel, respectively. Thus, the mean changes in performance from test to retest were of the order of magnitude which would have been produced by a 1- to 2-dB increase in signal presentation level (see Table 28-8). With N.U. Test No. 6, as with its predecessor (N.U. Test No. 4), one can thus have confidence in the discrimination score that is obtained when a particular form of any of the four lists must be used a second time. This conclusion, of course, implies that the experimenter will take care to insure that a given list is not repeated over and over in the same form or without other lists intervening between successive presentations of a given list.

The test-retest reliability of the four lists of N.U. Test No. 6 can be judged by a study of the correlation coefficients shown in Table 28-9. If one disregards the data for the −4-dB sensation level, where the distribution of scores was obviously truncated, and confines attention to the data obtained in the remainder of the region where the articulation function rose with a linear slope, the following facts emerge. First, in the normal hearing group the correlations are all positive and they range from a low of .27 to a high of .59. Secondly, in the sensorineural group, the correlations are again all positive and generally much higher, ranging from .36 to .93. This difference between the two groups is undoubtedly related to the fact that the range of discriminatory capacities in the normal group was quite restricted relative to that of the sensorineural group. Other things being equal, such a restriction in the range of the characteristic under study tends to reduce the magnitude of the Pearson r.

TABLE 28-8. DIFFERENCE BETWEEN MEAN DISCRIMINATION SCORES FROM TEST TO RETEST AT THE SEVERAL PRESENTATION LEVELS FOR THE TWO GROUPS ON N.U. AUDITORY TEST NO. 6 (NEGATIVE DIFFERENCE INDICATES HIGHER SCORE IN RETEST THAN IN TEST SESSION).

Sensation level of presentation	Normal hearing group				Sensorineural loss group			
	List I	List II	List III	List IV	List I	List II	List III	List IV
−4	−0.1	0.8	0.8	0.8	0.5	−0.8	1.3	−0.7
0	−0.6	−9.3*	−3.9	−3.0	−3.0	−0.3	2.2	0.0
8	−4.9	−7.5†	−5.8*	−3.7	−4.5	−7.5†	−1.2	−1.8
16	−3.4	−3.1*	−1.9	−1.5	−3.5	−6.2*	−0.5	−2.8
24	−1.5	−1.2	−1.8	−0.2	0.2	−3.7*	0.3	1.7
32	−1.1	−0.4	0.2	0.3	0.0	0.2	3.3	0.5

*t statistic associated with difference equals or exceeds that required for significance at 5 percent confidence level.
†t statistic associated with difference equals or exceeds that required for significance at 1 percent confidence level.

TABLE 28-9. COEFFICIENTS OF CORRELATION* (PEARSON) BETWEEN TEST AND RETEST FOR N.U. AUDITORY TEST NO. 6 ADMINISTERED TO SUBJECTS WITH NORMAL HEARING AND SUBJECTS WITH SENSORINEURAL HEARING LOSS.

Sensation level	Normal hearing group				Sensorineural loss group			
	List I	List II	List III	List IV	List I	List II	List III	List IV
−4	.30	.29	.34	.15	.59	.84	.74	.48
0	.41	.35	.41	.36	.47	.72	.62	.50
8	.54	.27	.43	.59	.93	.92	.83	.79
16					.92	.86	.93	.91

*For each group, analysis is restricted to the range of sensation levels within which the slopes of the articulation functions were judged to be linear.

The array of test-retest correlations shown in Table 28-9 compares favorably with that associated with N.U. Auditory Test No. 4 (Tillman et al., 1963). Moreover, the various values reported in the table are of the general order of magnitude usually considered to indicate acceptable test-retest reliability.

V. CONCLUSIONS

On the basis of the material presented here, we conclude that we have achieved the goal that we are seeking. It seems clear that N.U. Auditory Test No. 6 compares favorably with its predecessor (N.U. Test No. 4) in interlist equivalence and test-retest reliability. In addition, the new tool yields articulation functions which rise with approximately the same slope as those associated with the original test. As stated earlier, N.U. Test No. 4 has proved to be a highly useful tool for the measurement of phonemic discrimination in the laboratory as well as in the clinical setting. We thus expect N.U. Test No. 6, which possesses twice the vocabulary of the original test, to be a valuable addition to the armanentarium of the audiologist.

REFERENCES

Lehiste, I., and G. E. Peterson. Linguistic considerations in the study of speech intelligibility. *J. Acoust. Soc. Amer.* **31:** 280–286 (1959).

Peterson, G. E., and I. Lehiste. Revised CNC lists for auditory tests. *J. Speech Hearing Dis.* **27:** 62–70 (1962).

Thorndike, E. L., and I. Lorge. The teacher's word book of 30,000 words. New York: Columbia University Teachers College, 1944.

Tillman, T. W., R. Carhart, and L. Wilber. A test for speech discrimination composed of CNC monosyllabic words (N.U. auditory test No. 4). SAM-TDR-62-135, Jan. 1963.

29

Speech-Discrimination Scores Modeled as a Binomial Variable

Aaron R. Thornton, Ph.D.
Assistant Professor of Otolaryngology (Audiology), Harvard University, and Clinical Audiologist, Massachusetts Eye and Ear Infirmary, Boston, Massachusetts
Michael J. M. Raffin, Ph.D.
Professor of Audiology, University of Montana, Missoula, Montana

Many studies have reported variability data for tests of speech discrimination, and the disparate results of these studies have not been given a simple explanation. Arguments over the relative merits of 25- vs 50-word tests have ignored the basic mathematical properties inherent in the use of percentage scores. The present study models performance on clinical tests of speech discrimination as a binomial variable. A binomial model was developed, and some of its characteristics were tested against data from 4,120 scores obtained on the CID Auditory Test W–22. A table for determining significant deviations between scores was generated and compared to observed differences in half-list scores for the W–22 tests. Good agreement was found between predicted and observed values. Implications of the binomial characteristics of speech-discrimination scores are discussed.

Speech-discrimination tests are used in clinical audiometry for several purposes, including diagnosis of ear disease, assessment of communicative impairment, and evaluation of hearing aid performance. To serve a useful purpose, a test must be able to place a subject in an appropriate category of subjects or differentiate his performance in a variety of listening situations. In the first of these cases, the clinician must be concerned with two sources of error (1) the relation between test performance and the parameter of interest (diagnostic category or extent of communicative impairment), and (2) consistency across alternate forms of the test. When different forms of a test are used to compare performance across listening conditions (for example, quiet vs noise), the variations in test-form difficulty are a limiting factor in the ability to measure differences among conditions, and the clinician cannot always determine whether dif-

ferences in scores are a result of differences in test conditions or differences in test forms. Although test forms are constructed to be equally difficult, this equivalence is usually determined by mean performance on each of the test forms by a group of subjects. For an individual subject, however, the tests are seldom equally difficult, and performance can be expected to vary across forms. In clinical practice the differences in test-form difficulty must be considered when scores are evaluated.

Many previous studies have addressed the question of test-retest reliability, particularly with the 25- and 50-word tests. In most cases the within-subject variability was confounded with between-subject differences by the comparisons of mean data across subjects or the use of correlation coefficients that are greatly dependent on the spread of scores in the sample of subjects being studied. An additional problem has been probable failure to recognize the special characteristics inherent in percentage scores. Egan (1948) suggested that variability of a test score

Reprinted by permission of the authors from *J. Speech Hearing Res.*, **21**: 507–518 (1978).

is a function of the test score itself. He pointed out that variability is at a minimum near the extremes of the articulation scale (0 and 100 percent) and at a maximum in the middle of the range. He also recognized that variability is dependent on the length of a test list and that error is distributed normally only for mid-range scores. He did not, however, provide a theoretical framework for these observations.

The present paper proposes a simple model to describe variability (across forms) of speech-discrimination tests. Although the model is not original or new, it has largely been ignored in the past.

Examination of the construction of the majority of clinical speech-discrimination tests shows that variance among test forms can be estimated using probabilistic models. Test administration typically requires a subject to respond to each of a series of stimuli, and each response is categorized as correct or incorrect. The test score is reported as the percentage (proportion) of correct responses. Alternate forms of the test are composed of an equal number of similar stimuli. The most frequently used tests are 50-item lists of monosyllabic words. These will be used to discuss the prediction of variability across test forms —however, the discussion is applicable to any stimulus (for example, syllable, word, sentence) that is scored as having only two possible outcomes (such as, correct, incorrect).

If the responses to test stimuli are assumed to be independent of each other, then test results can be treated as binomial distributions and the statistics of proportions can be used to describe their characteristics. Hagerman (1976) reached this conclusion by examining individual word difficulties. He noted that scores on theoretical lists of words having uniform difficulty could be described as a binomial variable. However, for lists of words having variable difficulty, he reported data to show that these lists could be equated to slightly longer lists of words having uniform difficulty, and variability then could be described by the binomial distribution corresponding to the longer list.

Hagerman's data also are consistent with a simpler binomial model based on sampling theory. Let us define a pool of stimuli to be used in a test of speech discrimination. For example, we can specify a pool of all common, monosyllabic English words selected to achieve phonetically balanced proportions, and spoken by a single person. For a given subject on a particular occasion each word of the original pool can be assigned to one of two categories—words that will be responded to correctly and words that will be responded to incorrectly. The proportion of words in the original pool to which the subject would respond correctly can be considered the subject's true score $\tilde{p}$ for the test. It is also the expected score for any randomly selected sample from the pool. The distribution of scores obtained by repeated testing using random samples of equal length drawn from the original pool is described by a binomial distribution with $\tilde{p}$ = proportion of correct responses in the original pool and n = number of items in the (sample) test. This situation is not unlike that encountered with most speech-discrimination tests; each of the alternative test forms can be modeled as a random sample of stimuli drawn from a larger pool defined by the characteristics of the stimuli in all forms of the test combined.

To the extent that speech-discrimination test scores can be described by a binomial distribution, the clinician and researcher should be familiar with the unique characteristics of proportions, particularly with their variability, confidence intervals, and statistical tests of significance. A binomial distribution is completely specified when we know $\tilde{p}$, the proportion of successes in a population (in this case true score or proportion of correct responses in the pool of stimuli), and n, the number of cases drawn from the population (in this case number of words in a list). All other characteristics of the population are irrelevant with respect to variability across test forms. Confidence intervals for estimating a subject's true score and critical differences for determining when two test scores deviate significantly may be computed from the obtained test scores without regard to type of stimulus, subject, or listening conditions as long as these remain constant across test administrations.

METHOD AND RESULTS

Characteristics of the binomial model were compared to the performance of hearing-impaired listeners on a widely used clinical test of speech discrimination. Records of 4120 administrations of the Central Institute for the Deaf (CID) Auditory Test W-22 (Hirsh et al., 1952) were drawn from patient files in the Department of Speech Pathology and Audiology at the Veterans Administration Hospital in Iowa City. The clinic case load typically consisted of patients in their late 50s to early 60s, but they ranged in age from approximately 20 to 80 years. The recorded, 50-item, monosyllabic word lists were presented at 40 dB re SRT whenever possible. Each of the four alternate forms of the test (Lists 1–4) were used with 1030 ears, and six standard randomizations (A–F) of word order for each list were represented as shown in Table 29–1. Table 29–2 shows the distribution of scores for each of the lists. Table 29–3 shows the distribution of item difficulty within each list.

The standard deviation of a binomial distribution depends on both the probability of a success and the number of cases drawn. In percentage,

$$SD = 100 \sqrt{\left[\frac{(\tilde{p})(1 - \tilde{p})}{n}\right]}. \qquad (1)$$

A comparison was made between standard deviations computed for binomial variables and standard deviations of scores on subsets of the 50-word tests. Each 50-word list (1–4) was divided into two 25-word lists and five 10-word lists by a sequential division of randomization A. Scores on these shorter lists were then computed from each of the 4120 50-word tests. Tests were grouped by 50-word scores, which were used as the best estimate of $\tilde{p}$ (true score), and an analysis of variance was used to compute variability at 25 levels of $\tilde{p}$ (50-word scores of 50–96 percent) for the 25-word scores, and 17 levels of $\tilde{p}$ (50-word scores of 44–98 percent) for the 10-word scores. The 44–56, 58–64, and 66–70 percentage levels were pooled as three broader groupings in the 10-word analysis.

TABLE 29–1. NUMBER OF CASES SAMPLED FOR EACH RANDOMIZATION OF THE FOUR 50-WORD LISTS OF THE CID AUDITORY TEST W-22.

Randomization	List 1	2	3	4
A	131	126	175	181
B	63	57	177	182
C	174	182	197	178
D	248	248	174	174
E	158	156	62	65
F	256	261	245	250
Total	1030	1030	1030	1030

TABLE 29–2. DISTRIBUTION OF SCORES FOR EACH OF THE FOUR 50-WORD LISTS OF THE CID AUDITORY TEST W-22.

Score	List 1	2	3	4	Total
0	2	6	5	10	23
2	0	1	1	2	4
4	0	1	0	2	3
6	0	2	1	2	5
8	0	0	2	2	4
10	2	1	3	5	11
12	2	4	3	3	12
14	0	2	2	2	6
16	0	2	2	5	9
18	2	0	1	3	6
20	2	4	3	2	11
22	0	3	0	2	5
24	1	4	4	2	11
26	2	4	2	5	13
28	4	2	4	5	15
30	2	3	2	5	12
32	1	4	4	3	12
34	1	6	4	4	15
36	1	6	5	4	16
38	3	0	3	7	13
40	5	5	6	6	22
42	7	5	3	5	20
44	3	4	10	4	21
46	2	5	2	4	13
48	1	4	5	6	16
50	1	8	4	7	20
52	6	5	2	6	19
54	9	4	9	8	30
56	6	4	8	10	28
58	5	8	11	16	40
60	6	6	6	13	31
62	7	10	10	19	46
64	7	13	12	9	41
66	11	13	10	17	51
68	13	9	4	9	35
70	10	12	19	20	61
72	19	16	19	26	80
74	25	19	23	21	88
76	19	23	22	29	93
78	25	27	29	25	106
80	36	41	41	45	163
82	56	50	45	46	197
84	47	44	52	36	179
86	59	45	56	51	211
88	59	44	66	77	246
90	67	71	77	68	283
92	73	84	83	73	313
94	106	96	107	88	397
96	127	141	121	99	488
98	139	123	96	80	438
100	49	36	21	32	138
Total	1030	1030	1030	1030	4120

TABLE 29–3. PERCENTAGE OF INCORRECT RESPONSES MADE TO EACH WORD OF THE CID AUDITORY TEST W-22. EACH LIST WAS MEASURED ON AN INDEPENDENT SAMPLE OF 1,030 EARS.

	List 1		List 2		List 3		List 4	
Item	Word	% Incorrect	Word	% Incorrect	Word	% Incorrect	Word	% Incorrect
1	up	2.82	now	5.24	out	3.79	why	5.53
2	none	2.91	well	5.63	when	3.98	men	6.41
3	what	2.91	one	5.73	on	4.27	ought	8.06
4	yard	3.40	eat	5.83	book	4.56	in	8.64
5	him	3.59	that	6.31	no	5.24	jump	8.84
6	us	3.88	odd	6.80	are	6.02	cook	9.03
7	you	3.98	yore	6.89	oil	6.51	my	9.32
8	it	4.18	by	7.28	ate	7.28	wood	9.32
9	hunt	4.37	air	7.38	done	7.57	who	9.61
10	dad	4.76	tree	7.38	this	7.67	toy	9.81
11	there	4.76	star	8.25	he	8.45	pale	9.90
12	me	5.34	own	9.03	pie	8.74	aid	10.10
13	poor	5.53	die	9.13	jar	8.84	at	10.19
14	or	5.92	flat	9.42	add	10.00	bread	10.19
15	wet	6.60	young	9.42	may	10.00	our	10.97
16	low	6.70	hurt	9.52	glove	10.58	of	11.26
17	could	6.80	too	9.52	have	10.49	they	12.62
18	not	6.89	oak	9.71	if	10.58	shoe	13.01
19	as	7.57	and	9.81	raw	10.87	yet	13.88
20	isle	7.86	smart	10.29	shove	11.17	leave	13.98
21	give	8.06	live	10.58	bill	11.46	bee	15.24
22	day	8.25	off	11.07	cute	12.14	will	15.44
23	law	8.35	does	11.26	do	12.82	clothes	16.02
24	true	8.74	way	11.36	lie	13.20	through	16.21
25	felt	9.03	dumb	11.85	end	13.40	yes	16.70
26	toe	9.03	then	12.33	farm	13.40	am	16.89
27	ran	9.22	jaw	13.40	smooth	13.59	where	17.48
28	skin	9.61	bin	14.47	tie	13.59	his	18.16
29	wire	10.10	see	14.56	hand	13.69	so	20.78
30	earn	10.49	new	16.12	is	18.06	arm	20.87
31	she	11.07	hit	17.28	three	18.54	go	20.78
32	high	11.94	ham	17.77	ten	18.74	few	22.52
33	them	12.82	ill	18.35	chair	20.29	eyes	23.20
34	stove	15.34	show	18.35	though	20.49	all	23.30
35	twins	16.12	cars	20.49	we	22.04	hang	23.79
36	see	19.03	thin	20.49	use	23.50	ear	26.12
37	owl	20.10	tare	21.36	say	24.08	chin	26.60
38	carve	20.19	with	22.43	king	24.56	than	28.64
39	jam	20.29	chest	22.52	wool	25.15	save	28.93
40	thing	23.01	ease	23.20	camp	27.09	can	32.91
41	east	24.27	gave	23.98	year	28.64	near	33.11
42	an	25.56	move	24.37	aim	29.17	darn	34.27
43	bells	27.48	cap	25.24	start	30.78	tin	34.95
44	chew	28.84	else	25.73	dull	33.40	stiff	36.41
45	ace	33.79	ail	26.41	owes	36.89	art	38.84
46	bathe	35.44	key	34.76	ears	37.57	tea	39.42
47	ache	37.77	pew	33.98	tan	38.64	net	39.81
48	knees	38.35	rooms	46.99	west	39.90	nuts	48.64
49	deaf	52.23	send	48.74	knit	40.19	dust	48.74
50	mew	58.93	knee	74.85	nest	49.81	dolls	52.43
Mean		14.48		17.06		17.63		20.76
SD		12.86		12.85		11.38		12.07

Standard deviations were computed as

$$SD = \sqrt{\left(\frac{SS\,\text{total} - SS\,\text{subjects}}{df\,\text{total} - df\,\text{subjects}}\right)}$$

$$\text{or} \quad \sqrt{\left(\frac{SS\,\text{within-subjects}}{df\,\text{within-subjects}}\right)}. \tag{2}$$

For example, Table 29–2 shows that 80 subjects were estimated to have a true score p of 72 percent based on their 50-word test scores. The tests were rescored as 160 25-word tests and 400 10-word tests. The standard deviations of these part-list scores were 8.22 percent and 13.51 percent respectively. The correspondence between the empirically measured standard deviations at each level and theoretical binomial standard deviations is shown in Figure 29–1. Test variability appears to be dependent on a subject's true score and the number of words in the test.

When the form of a distribution is known, an inference about the population mean can be made from a sample mean. This frequently takes the form of a confidence interval, a range of scores about the sample mean that has a specified probability of encompassing the population mean. The range is usually positioned about the sample mean such that the probabilities of the population mean falling outside either end of the range are equal. Tables and charts of confidence intervals for proportions (for example, Steel and Torrie, 1960; Pearson and Hartley, 1966) may be supplemented by use of a Z-table and an equation explained by Hays and Winkler (1970). The size of the confidence interval and its symmetry about the sample score are dependent on both the sample score and the number of events in the sample. For example, when a subject scores 92 percent on a 50-word test, the 95 percent confidence interval of the true score is from 81 percent (92 − 11) to 98 percent (92 + 6). For a score of 68 percent it is 54 percent (68 − 14) to 80 percent (68 + 12). When the test is shortened to 25 words, scores of 92 percent and 68 percent have confidence intervals of 74 percent to 99 percent (92 − 18, 92 + 7) and 46 percent to 85 percent (68 − 22, 68 + 17). As can be seen, a simple rule cannot be generated to describe all cases.

Although the binomial confidence intervals may be useful in estimating a range of uncertainty about the location of a subject's true score, they cannot be used to solve the more common problem of determining when two scores are significantly different. To test an obtained difference in scores against a hypothesis of no difference, the theoretical distribution of difference scores must be defined, but the characteristics of the distribution of differences between binomial variables are not available.

An approximate solution to determining the significance of observed differences in scores may be made by first transforming the scores to a variable that has uniform variance, then calculating the variance of a difference between transformed scores and, finally, estimating the probability of an observed difference occurring by chance by using a Z-table. The Freeman and Tukey (1950) averaged angular transformation for stabilization of variance in binomial data was used as the basis for generating tables of critical differences. For a word list of a specific length, each possible score was transformed to an angle by

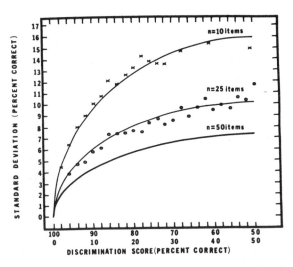

FIGURE 29-1. Within-subject standard deviations for 10- and 25-word tests grouped by estimated true scores (50-words). Solid lines show standard deviations of binomial distributions as a function of p (in percentage) for $n = 10$, $n = 25$, and $n = 50$. Measured standard deviations for $n = 10$ and $n = 25$ are shown by X and 0 respectively.

$$\theta = \sin^{-1}\sqrt{\left(\frac{x}{n+1}\right)} + \sin^{-1}\sqrt{\left(\frac{x+1}{n+1}\right)}, \tag{3}$$

where n = number of words in the list and x = number of correct responses. The estimated variance of

TABLE 29-4. LOWER AND UPPER LIMITS OF THE 95 PERCENT CRITICAL DIFFERENCES FOR PERCENTAGE SCORES. VALUES WITHIN THE RANGE SHOWN ARE NOT SIGNIFICANTLY DIFFERENT FROM THE VALUE SHOWN IN THE PERCENTAGE SCORE COLUMNS (P > 0.05).

% Score	$n = 50$	$n = 25$	$n = 10$	% Score	$n = 100*$
0	0–4	0–8	0–20	50	37–63
2	0–10			51	38–64
4	0–14	0–20		52	39–65
6	2–18			53	40–66
8	2–22	0–28		54	41–67
10	2–24		0–50	55	42–68
12	4–26	4–32		56	43–69
14	4–30			57	44–70
16	6–32	4–40		58	45–71
18	6–34			59	46–72
20	8–36	4–44	0–60	60	47–73
22	8–40			61	48–74
24	10–42	8–48		62	49–74
26	12–44			63	50–75
28	14–46	8–52		64	51–76
30	14–48		10–70	65	52–77
32	16–50	12–56		66	53–78
34	18–52			67	54–79
36	20–54	16–60		68	55–80
38	22–56			69	56–81
40	22–58	16–64	10–80	70	57–81
42	24–60			71	58–82
44	26–62	20–68		72	59–83
46	28–64			73	60–84
48	30–66	24–72		74	61–85
50	32–68		10–90	75	63–86
52	34–70	28–76		76	64–86
54	36–72			77	65–87
56	38–74	32–80		78	66–88
58	40–76			79	67–89
60	42–78	36–84	20–90	80	68–89
62	44–78			81	69–90
64	46–80	40–84		82	71–91
66	48–82			83	72–92
68	50–84	44–88		84	73–92
70	52–86		30–90	85	74–93
72	54–86	48–92		86	75–94
74	56–88			87	77–94
76	58–90	52–92		88	78–95
78	60–92			89	79–96
80	64–92	56–96	40–100	90	81–96
82	66–94			91	82–97
84	68–94	60–96		92	83–98
86	70–96			93	85–98
88	74–96	68–96		94	86–99
90	76–98		50–100	95	88–99
92	78–98	72–100		96	89–99
94	82–98			97	91–100
96	86–100	80–100		98	92–100
98	90–100			99	94–100
100	96–100	92–100	80–100	100	97–100

*If score is less than 50%, find % Score = 100-observed score and subtract each critical difference limit from 100.

this angle was adjusted for sample size as suggested by Mosteller and Youtz (1961):

$$\text{For } n > 50: \quad \sigma_\theta^2 = \frac{1}{n + \frac{1}{2}}, \tag{4}$$

$$\text{for } 10 \le n \le 50: \quad \sigma_\theta^2 = \frac{1}{n + 1}. \tag{5}$$

The estimated variance of a difference between two independent angles would simply be twice the above values when n's are equal. Using this variance and a Z-table, 95 percent confidence intervals about a hypothesized angular difference of zero were computed for $n = 10, 25, 50,$ and 100. For $n = 25$ a 90 percent confidence interval was also computed.

The angular confidence intervals were used to generate tables of critical differences that might be used clinically (see Table 29-4). The term critical difference is used to avoid confusion with the confidence interval for predicting a true score. With respect to any test score, the critical difference is specified by upper and lower limits, which are the largest and smallest test scores whose transformed θ-values fall within the angular confidence interval (for a hypothesized true difference of 0) (see Appendix). Because binomial test-score distributions change in steps, the critical differences will usually have a confidence level less than that specified for the angular confidence interval. Also, the angular transformation does not work well at the tails of the distribution, and this error is carried to the critical differences.

The critical differences (shown in Table 29-4) show an asymmetry and dependence on sample score and n similar to that described for the confidence intervals of the true scores. For example, if a subject scored 92 percent on one form of a 50-word test, there is a 95 percent probability that his score on another form of the test would fall within the range 78–98 percent (-14 percent, $+6$ percent). For a score of 68 percent the range is 50–84 percent (-18 percent, $+16$ percent), which is greater but also more symmetrical. For the 25-word tests the critical differences for scores of 92 percent and 68 percent increase to 72–100 percent and 44–88 percent respectively.

The 95 percent critical differences (shown in Table 29-4) and 90 percent critical differences (not shown) were compared to observed differences between

25-word scores for each of the 4120 50-word tests. Each of the four lists was divided into two 25-word tests by a random assignment of the 50 words different from randomizations A–F. The number of differences in half-list scores that exceeded the theoretical critical differences were tallied and are shown in Table 29-5. Good agreement is seen between predicted and obtained results. The total percentage of scores falling outside the suggested critical differences was 5.4 percent for the 95 percent limits and 7.9 percent for the 90 percent limits. The imbalance between upper and lower limit errors for high scores is consistent with the corresponding skewness of the binomial distribution at these points and with the discrete characteristics of the distribution. The total proportion of differences falling beyond the limits, however, is consistent with the specified confidence

TABLE 29-5. NUMBER OF SCORES ON SECOND 25-WORDS THAT ARE LESS THAN THE LOWER LIMIT (<LL) OR GREATER THAN THE UPPER LIMIT (>UL) OF THE 90 PERCENT AND 95 PERCENT CRITICAL DIFFERENCES SHOWN IN TABLE 29-4.

Score on First 25	n	90% <LL	90% >UL	95% <LL	95% >UL
0	23	0	0	0	0
4	12	0	3	0	0
8	17	0	1	0	1
12	12	1	1	1	1
16	15	1	0	1	0
20	19	2	0	0	0
24	19	1	0	1	0
28	22	0	1	0	0
32	28	3	1	0	0
36	26	0	0	0	0
40	35	3	3	0	0
44	38	1	2	0	1
48	31	3	2	1	2
52	64	2	2	1	2
56	58	4	1	3	1
60	81	7	6	4	1
64	93	1	8	0	8
68	102	2	9	1	6
72	147	5	10	3	1
76	221	1	9	1	9
80	290	4	25	3	5
84	383	6	16	4	16
88	455	14	35	8	35
92	537	11	0	5	0
96	687	35	0	12	0
100	705	85	0	85	0
Totals	4120	192	135	134	89
		327		223	
		7.9%		5.4%	

levels. A change in the upper limits would only result in greater discrepancies. For example, if the upper limit of the 95 percent critical difference for a score of 92 percent were lowered one step from 100 percent to 96 percent, then 19.7 percent (106) of the 537 observed differences would fall beyond the upper limit.

CONCLUSIONS

The binomial characteristics of speech-discrimination tests make variability among test forms dependent on both the number of items in the test and the subject's true score for the class of items used. The optimal number of items for a test must be determined from an estimate of the true scores of the subjects to be tested and a recognition of the trade-off between administration time and variability. For some clinical purposes, 25 words may be sufficient, whereas 100 may not be enough for others. In selecting the number of stimuli, the clinician needs to know how accurately he must estimate a true score or, alternatively, how small a difference between test scores that he must be able to measure with certainty. For example, if a clinician determines a subject's score to be 100 percent on 25 words, then he can estimate the true score of the subject to be within the range of 86 percent to 100 percent (95 percent confidence interval; see Steele and Torrie, 1960, p. 454). For some clinical screening purposes this may be sufficient precision. However, a 25-word score of 48 percent would place the range of uncertainty for the true score at 28–69 percent, which permits only a gross classification. If the person having the 100 percent score were retested at a later date and the 25-word score dropped to 88 percent, the 12 percent difference in scores would be strong evidence that the true score was different on the two occasions (see Table 29-4). However, a similar (12 percent) decrease of the 48 percent score to 36 percent would be only weak evidence of a change in true score because the second score lies well within the 95 percent critical difference. When judging and comparing the performance of hearing aids, it is important to use as many words as may be needed to measure changes in true scores associated with differences in the hearing aids. These shifts in true score cannot be determined when they do not exceed chance variation. Testing in the presence of noise often lowers the true scores and consequently increases the variability and error. Increased differences among the scores obtained with various hearing aids tested in noise may in many cases be explained by the increased variability of the measuring instrument as opposed to real differences in the true scores for the different hearing aids.

We recommend that clinicians always indicate the number of items used in a test, or report the confidence interval in addition to the obtained score. This would accurately reflect the uncertainty of the location of a subject's true score. For comparison of scores, the critical differences should be used to determine significance. The skewness of the critical differences and their dependency on the number of items and subject's score make it difficult to judge the significance of differences in scores without the help of a table. This is particularly true for the clinician in training.

We wish to emphasize that the binomial characteristics of speech-discrimination tests are relatively independent of subject characteristics, listening conditions, and type of stimulus. These factors will, however, influence the true score of a subject. Although it is tempting to try to devise a test with fewer items that will have the same variability across forms as a larger test, it is unlikely that this can be done without substantial changes in construction and scoring to eliminate the binomial characteristics. As shown by our sample, most subjects score high on currently used clinical tests. From Figure 29-1 we can see that the variance changes rapidly as 100 percent is approached, and this feature makes it imperative to use variance stabilization transformations on test scores before performing statistical tests that assume that variance is independent of the score. Finally, application of the binomial model might be extended to other tests used in the field of communicative disorders when these tests meet the basic assumptions required for the model. This application is particularly important when the test scores are used to classify subjects or measure progress during treatment.

ACKNOWLEDGMENT

Appreciation is extended to Herbert Jordan for making his clinical records available for this study. The majority of the work on this paper was completed while both authors were at the University of Iowa, and portions of the work have been presented at the 1976 Annual Convention of the American Speech and Hearing Association in Houston, Texas and the May 1977 Meeting of the Canadian Speech and Hearing Association in Victoria, British Columbia.

REFERENCES

Egan, J. P. Articulation testing methods. *Laryngoscope,* **58,** 955–991 (1948).

Freeman, M. F., and Tukey, J. W. Transformations related to the angular and the square root. *Ann. Math. Statist.,* **21,** 607–611 (1950).

Hagerman, B. Reliability in the determination of speech discrimination. *Scand. Audiol.,* **5,** 219–228 (1976).

Hays, W. L., and Winkler, R. L. *Statistics: Probability, Inference and Decision.* (Vol. 1) New York: Holt, Rinehart and Winston, 332 (1970).

Hirsh, I. J; Davis, H.; Silverman, S. R.; Reynolds, E. G.; Eldert, E.; and Benson, R. W. Development of materials for speech audiometry. *J. Speech Hearing Res.,* **17,** 321–337 (1952).

Mosteller, F., and Youtz, C. Tables of the Freeman-Tukey transformations for the binominal and Poisson distributions. *Biometrika,* **48,** 433–440 (1961).

Pearson, E. S., and Hartley, H. O. *Biometrika Tables for Statisticians.* (Vol. 1) Cambridge (Eng.): Cambridge Univ. Press (1966).

Steele, R. G. D., and Torrie, J. H. *Principles and Procedures of Statistics.* New York: McGraw-Hill (1960).

APPENDIX

The procedure for computing critical differences will be illustrated by the following example. Consider the problem of determining the 95 percent critical differences for a score of 90 percent on a 50-word test (45 correct).

By Equation (3) $\Theta_{90\%} = 2.473$ radians

By Equation (4) $\sigma_\Theta^2 = 0.0199$ radians

$2\sigma_\Theta^2 = 0.0398$ radians

For a difference between two angles $\Theta_1 - \Theta_2$:

$$\sigma_{\Theta_1 - \Theta_2} = 0.1996 \text{ radians } \sqrt{(2\sigma_\Theta^2)}$$

The 95 percent confidence interval for an angular difference will be bounded by upper (UL) and lower limits (LL).

$$\Theta_{LL} = \Theta - 1.96 \, \Theta_{\Theta_1 - \Theta_2} \quad \Theta_{UL} = \Theta + 1.96 \, \sigma_{\Theta_1 - \Theta_2}$$

For $\Theta_{90\%}$: $\Theta_{LL} = 2.082$ radians $\Theta_{UL} = 2.864$ radians .

By a process of iteration with Equation (3), one can determine minimum and maximum scores that have Θs within the computed limits.

$\Theta_{76\%} = 2.106$ radians

$\Theta_{98\%} = 2.697$ radians (within the limits)

$\Theta_{74\%} = 2.061$ radians

$\Theta_{100\%} = 3.001$ radians (exceed the limits)

Critical differences for a score of 90 percent are 76 percent and 98 percent.

30

Confidence Levels for Differences Between Speech-Discrimination Scores: A Research Note

MICHAEL J. M. RAFFIN, Ph.D.
Professor of Audiology, University of Montana, Missoula, Montana
AARON R. THORNTON, Ph.D.
Assistant Professor of Otolaryngology (Audiology), Harvard University, and Clinical Audiologist, Massachusetts Eye and Ear Infirmary

Tables of confidence levels for determining the probability of differences between speech-discrimination scores are presented. These tables were generated by a computer program developed for that purpose, and they are based on arc-sine transforms applied to a binomial distribution.

In a recent article (Thornton and Raffin, 1978), we proposed a model to describe variability in speech-discrimination scores. This model is applicable to open set tests in which each item is scored as correct or incorrect and the total score is expressed in percentage correct. To assist in the clinical application of this model, we provided a table of critical differences for 10-item, 25-item, 50-item, and 100-item tests at the 0.05 level of confidence. Although the 0.05 level of confidence may be appropriate for some applications, it may be too stringent or too lenient for other applications (Raffin and Schafer, 1980; Schafer, 1978). In addition, it would be useful to be able to determine the significance of differences in scores based on tests which do not contain the same number of items. For example, it may be necessary to compare a score obtained on a half-list (25 items) with a score obtained on a full-list (50 items). To meet these stated needs, a computer program was developed to generate more complete tables showing the probabilities of chance differences between any two scores for tests of any length and for tests based on a different number of items.*

*Tables generated by this program, for any number of test items and for comparisons of any test desired may be obtained by contacting the senior author.

Reprinted by permission of the authors from *J. Speech Hearing Res.,* **23,** 5–18 (1980).

Tables 30–1 and 30–2 show the probabilities of differences among performance scores based on 25 items and 50 items respectively. For example, if an individual scores 60 percent and 84 percent on two 25-item tests, the difference in performance indicated by these two scores is significant at the 0.06 level of confidence. That is, differences this great or greater will occur by chance alone six times out of 100. Alternatively, if an individual obtains a score of 60 percent on a 50-item test, then in order to show a significant improvement (at the 0.01 level of confidence), the individual must obtain a score of 84 percent, since a score of 82 percent is significant only at the 0.0151 level of confidence (from Table 30–2). Finally, from Table 30–3, it can be determined that if a subject obtains a score of 60 percent on a 25-item test, a significant improvement (at the 0.10 level of confidence) in performance based on a 50-item test would be indicated by a score of 80 percent or greater (*significance* = 0.0703); since a score of 78 percent is significant only at the 0.1096 level of confidence (greater than the desired significance level). These tables may be used to construct tables of critical differences at any confidence level for easy clinical reference. Discrepancies from our previous tables are due to differences in the number of significant digits carried by the two computers.

TABLE 30–1. CONFIDENCE LEVELS FOR DIFFERENCES BETWEEN PERCENT SCORES BASED ON A 25-ITEM TEST.

Second Score (Percent Correct)	First Score (Percent Correct)										
	0.00	4.00	8.00	12.00	16.00	20.00	24.00	28.00	32.00	36.00	40.00
—	1.0000	0.3077	0.1188	0.0455	0.0178	0.0069	0.0014	0.0014	0.0003	0.0001	0.0001
4.00	0.3077	1.0000	0.5961	0.3320	0.1707	0.0873	0.0404	0.0178	0.0093	0.0037	0.0014
8.00	0.1188	0.5961	1.0000	0.6599	0.4065	0.2340	0.1285	0.0673	0.0332	0.0160	0.0069
12.00	0.0455	0.3320	0.6599	1.0000	0.7039	0.4593	0.2801	0.1645	0.0910	0.0477	0.0238
16.00	0.0178	0.1707	0.4065	0.7039	1.0000	0.7188	0.4965	0.3173	0.1936	0.1141	0.0601
20.00	0.0069	0.0873	0.2340	0.4593	0.7188	1.0000	0.7339	0.5222	0.3421	0.2187	0.1285
24.00	0.0014	0.0404	0.1285	0.2801	0.4965	0.7339	1.0000	0.7490	0.5419	0.3628	0.2340
28.00	0.0014	0.0178	0.0673	0.1645	0.3173	0.5222	0.7490	1.0000	0.7642	0.5552	0.3843
32.00	0.0003	0.0093	0.0332	0.0910	0.1936	0.3421	0.5419	0.7642	1.0000	0.7718	0.5687
36.00	0.0001	0.0037	0.0160	0.0477	0.1141	0.2187	0.3628	0.5552	0.7718	1.0000	0.7718
40.00	0.0001	0.0014	0.0069	0.0238	0.0601	0.1285	0.2340	0.3843	0.5687	0.7718	1.0000
44.00	—	0.0003	0.0037	0.0111	0.0316	0.0703	0.1416	0.2501	0.3953	0.5687	0.7718
48.00	—	0.0003	0.0014	0.0037	0.0151	0.0366	0.0801	0.1527	0.2543	0.3953	0.5823
52.00	—	0.0001	0.0003	0.0014	0.0069	0.0188	0.0424	0.0873	0.1585	0.2627	0.4065
56.00	—	0.0001	0.0001	0.0014	0.0037	0.0093	0.0214	0.0455	0.0910	0.1585	0.2627
60.00	—	—	0.0001	0.0003	0.0014	0.0037	0.0099	0.0226	0.0477	0.0910	0.1645
64.00	—	—	0.0001	0.0001	0.0003	0.0014	0.0037	0.0105	0.0238	0.0500	0.0910
68.00	—	—	—	0.0001	0.0001	0.0003	0.0014	0.0037	0.0105	0.0238	0.0477
72.00	—	—	—	—	0.0001	0.0003	0.0003	0.0014	0.0037	0.0105	0.0226
76.00	—	—	—	—	0.0001	0.0001	0.0003	0.0003	0.0014	0.0037	0.0099
80.00	—	—	—	—	—	0.0001	0.0001	0.0003	0.0003	0.0014	0.0037
84.00	—	—	—	—	—	—	0.0001	0.0001	0.0001	0.0003	0.0014
88.00	—	—	—	—	—	—	—	—	0.0001	0.0001	0.0003
92.00	—	—	—	—	—	—	—	—	—	0.0001	0.0001
96.00	—	—	—	—	—	—	—	—	—	—	—
100.00	—	—	—	—	—	—	—	—	—	—	—

TABLE 30-1. (CONTINUED)

Second Score (Percent Correct)	First Score (Percent Correct)								
	44.00	48.00	52.00	56.00	60.00	64.00	68.00	72.00	76.00
—	—	—	—	—	—	—	—	—	—
4.00	0.0003	0.0003	0.0001	0.0001	—	—	—	—	—
8.00	0.0037	0.0014	0.0003	0.0001	0.0001	0.0001	—	—	—
12.00	0.0111	0.0037	0.0014	0.0014	0.0003	0.0001	0.0001	—	—
16.00	0.0316	0.0151	0.0069	0.0037	0.0014	0.0003	0.0001	0.0001	0.0001
20.00	0.0703	0.0366	0.0188	0.0093	0.0037	0.0014	0.0003	0.0003	0.0001
24.00	0.1416	0.0801	0.0424	0.0214	0.0099	0.0037	0.0014	0.0003	0.0003
28.00	0.2501	0.1527	0.0873	0.0455	0.0226	0.0105	0.0037	0.0014	0.0003
32.00	0.3953	0.2543	0.1585	0.0910	0.0477	0.0238	0.0105	0.0037	0.0014
36.00	0.5687	0.3953	0.2627	0.1585	0.0910	0.0500	0.0238	0.0105	0.0037
40.00	0.7718	0.5823	0.4065	0.2627	0.1645	0.0910	0.0477	0.0226	0.0099
44.00	1.0000	0.7872	0.5823	0.4065	0.2627	0.1585	0.0910	0.0455	0.0214
48.00	0.7872	1.0000	0.7872	0.5823	0.4065	0.2627	0.1585	0.0873	0.0424
52.00	0.5823	0.7872	1.0000	0.7872	0.5823	0.3953	0.2543	0.1527	0.0801
56.00	0.4065	0.5823	0.7872	1.0000	0.7718	0.5687	0.3953	0.2501	0.1416
60.00	0.2627	0.4065	0.5823	0.7718	1.0000	0.7718	0.5687	0.3843	0.2340
64.00	0.1585	0.2627	0.3953	0.5687	0.7718	1.0000	0.7718	0.5552	0.3628
68.00	0.0910	0.1585	0.2543	0.3953	0.5687	0.7718	1.0000	0.7642	0.5419
72.00	0.0455	0.0873	0.1527	0.2501	0.3843	0.5552	0.7642	1.0000	0.7490
76.00	0.0214	0.0424	0.0801	0.1416	0.2340	0.3628	0.5419	0.7490	1.0000
80.00	0.0093	0.0188	0.0366	0.0703	0.1285	0.2187	0.3421	0.5222	0.7339
84.00	0.0037	0.0069	0.0151	0.0316	0.0601	0.1141	0.1936	0.3173	0.4965
88.00	0.0014	0.0014	0.0037	0.0111	0.0238	0.0477	0.0910	0.1645	0.2801
92.00	0.0001	0.0003	0.0014	0.0037	0.0069	0.0160	0.0332	0.0673	0.1285
96.00	0.0001	0.0001	0.0003	0.0003	0.0014	0.0037	0.0093	0.0178	0.0404
100.00	—	—	—	—	0.0001	0.0001	0.0003	0.0014	0.0014

TABLE 30–1. (CONTINUED)

Second Score (Percent Correct)	First Score (Percent Correct)					
	80.00	84.00	88.00	92.00	96.00	100.00
4.00	—	—	—	—	—	—
8.00	—	—	—	—	—	—
12.00	—	—	—	—	—	—
16.00	—	—	—	—	—	—
20.00	0.0001	—	—	—	—	—
24.00	0.0001	0.0001	—	—	—	—
28.00	0.0003	0.0001	—	—	—	—
32.00	0.0003	0.0001	0.0001	—	—	—
36.00	0.0014	0.0003	0.0001	0.0001	—	—
40.00	0.0037	0.0014	0.0003	0.0001	—	—
44.00	0.0093	0.0037	0.0014	0.0001	0.0001	—
48.00	0.0188	0.0069	0.0014	0.0003	0.0001	—
52.00	0.0366	0.0151	0.0037	0.0014	0.0003	—
56.00	0.0703	0.0316	0.0111	0.0037	0.0003	—
60.00	0.1285	0.0601	0.0238	0.0069	0.0014	0.0001
64.00	0.2187	0.1141	0.0477	0.0160	0.0037	0.0001
68.00	0.3421	0.1936	0.0910	0.0332	0.0093	0.0003
72.00	0.5222	0.3173	0.1645	0.0673	0.0178	0.0014
76.00	0.7339	0.4965	0.2801	0.1285	0.0404	0.0014
80.00	1.0000	0.7188	0.4593	0.2340	0.0873	0.0069
84.00	0.7188	1.0000	0.7039	0.4065	0.1707	0.0178
88.00	0.4593	0.7039	1.0000	0.6599	0.3320	0.0455
92.00	0.2340	0.4065	0.6599	1.0000	0.5961	0.1188
96.00	0.0873	0.1707	0.3320	0.5961	1.0000	0.3077
100.00	0.0069	0.0178	0.0455	0.1188	0.3077	1.0000

TABLE 30–2. CONFIDENCE LEVELS FOR DIFFERENCES BETWEEN PERCENT SCORES BASED ON A 50-ITEM TEST.

Second Score (Percent Correct)	First Score (Percent Correct) 0.00	2.00	4.00	6.00	8.00	10.00	12.00	14.00	16.00
—	1.0000	0.3173	0.1236	0.0500	0.0193	0.0093	0.0037	0.0014	0.0003
2.00	0.3173	1.0000	0.5961	0.3421	0.1868	0.0969	0.0500	0.0238	0.0117
4.00	0.1236	0.5961	1.0000	0.6745	0.4237	0.2543	0.1471	0.0836	0.0455
6.00	0.0500	0.3421	0.6745	1.0000	0.7039	0.4839	0.3077	0.1936	0.1141
8.00	0.0193	0.1868	0.4237	0.7039	1.0000	0.7339	0.5222	0.3524	0.2263
10.00	0.0093	0.0969	0.2543	0.4839	0.7339	1.0000	0.7642	0.5552	0.3843
12.00	0.0037	0.0500	0.1471	0.3077	0.5222	0.7642	1.0000	0.7718	0.5687
14.00	0.0014	0.0238	0.0836	0.1936	0.3524	0.5552	0.7718	1.0000	0.7872
16.00	0.0003	0.0117	0.0455	0.1141	0.2263	0.3843	0.5687	0.7872	1.0000
18.00	0.0003	0.0069	0.0238	0.0673	0.1416	0.2627	0.4065	0.5961	0.7872
20.00	0.0001	0.0014	0.0121	0.0366	0.0873	0.1707	0.2801	0.4354	0.6101
22.00	0.0001	0.0014	0.0069	0.0203	0.0500	0.1052	0.1868	0.3077	0.4473
24.00	—	0.0003	0.0037	0.0105	0.0293	0.0629	0.1236	0.2077	0.3271
26.00	—	0.0003	0.0014	0.0069	0.0160	0.0366	0.0767	0.1362	0.2263
28.00	—	0.0001	0.0003	0.0014	0.0093	0.0214	0.0455	0.0873	0.1527
30.00	—	0.0001	0.0003	0.0014	0.0037	0.0117	0.0264	0.0549	0.0969
32.00	—	0.0001	0.0001	0.0003	0.0014	0.0069	0.0151	0.0332	0.0629
34.00	—	—	0.0001	0.0003	0.0014	0.0037	0.0093	0.0193	0.0385
36.00	—	—	0.0001	0.0001	0.0003	0.0014	0.0037	0.0105	0.0226
38.00	—	—	0.0001	0.0001	0.0003	0.0014	0.0014	0.0069	0.0128
40.00	—	—	—	0.0001	0.0001	0.0003	0.0014	0.0037	0.0093
42.00	—	—	—	0.0001	0.0001	0.0003	0.0003	0.0014	0.0093
44.00	—	—	—	—	0.0001	0.0001	0.0003	0.0014	0.0037
46.00	—	—	—	—	0.0001	0.0001	0.0001	0.0014	0.0014
48.00	—	—	—	—	—	0.0001	0.0001	0.0003	0.0014
50.00	—	—	—	—	—	—	0.0001	0.0003	0.0003
52.00	—	—	—	—	—	—	0.0001	0.0001	0.0003
54.00	—	—	—	—	—	—	0.0001	0.0001	0.0001
56.00	—	—	—	—	—	—	—	0.0001	0.0001
58.00	—	—	—	—	—	—	—	—	0.0001
60.00	—	—	—	—	—	—	—	—	0.0001
62.00	—	—	—	—	—	—	—	—	—
64.00	—	—	—	—	—	—	—	—	—
66.00	—	—	—	—	—	—	—	—	—
68.00	—	—	—	—	—	—	—	—	—
70.00	—	—	—	—	—	—	—	—	—
72.00	—	—	—	—	—	—	—	—	—
74.00	—	—	—	—	—	—	—	—	—
76.00	—	—	—	—	—	—	—	—	—
78.00	—	—	—	—	—	—	—	—	—
80.00	—	—	—	—	—	—	—	—	—
82.00	—	—	—	—	—	—	—	—	—
84.00	—	—	—	—	—	—	—	—	—
86.00	—	—	—	—	—	—	—	—	—
88.00	—	—	—	—	—	—	—	—	—
90.00	—	—	—	—	—	—	—	—	—
92.00	—	—	—	—	—	—	—	—	—
94.00	—	—	—	—	—	—	—	—	—
96.00	—	—	—	—	—	—	—	—	—
98.00	—	—	—	—	—	—	—	—	—
100.00	—	—	—	—	—	—	—	—	—

TABLE 30–2. (CONTINUED)

Second Score (Percent Correct)	First Score (Percent Correct) 18.00	20.00	22.00	24.00	26.00	28.00	30.00	32.00	34.00
—	0.0003	0.0001	0.0001	—	—	—	—	—	—
2.00	0.0069	0.0014	0.0014	0.0003	0.0003	0.0001	0.0001	0.0001	—
4.00	0.0238	0.0121	0.0069	0.0037	0.0014	0.0003	0.0003	0.0001	0.0001
6.00	0.0673	0.0366	0.0203	0.0105	0.0069	0.0014	0.0014	0.0003	0.0003
8.00	0.1416	0.0873	0.0500	0.0293	0.0160	0.0093	0.0037	0.0014	0.0014
10.00	0.2627	0.1707	0.1052	0.0629	0.0366	0.0214	0.0117	0.0069	0.0037
12.00	0.4065	0.2801	0.1868	0.1236	0.0767	0.0455	0.0264	0.0151	0.0093
14.00	0.5961	0.4354	0.3077	0.2077	0.1362	0.0873	0.0549	0.0332	0.0193
16.00	0.7872	0.6101	0.4473	0.3271	0.2263	0.1527	0.0969	0.0629	0.0385
18.00	1.0000	0.8026	0.6241	0.4715	0.3421	0.2420	0.1645	0.1096	0.0703
20.00	0.8026	1.0000	0.8026	0.6384	0.4839	0.3524	0.2543	0.1770	0.1188
22.00	0.6241	0.8026	1.0000	0.8181	0.6455	0.4965	0.3628	0.2627	0.1868
24.00	0.4715	0.6384	0.8181	1.0000	0.8181	0.6599	0.5093	0.3735	0.2713
26.00	0.3421	0.4839	0.6455	0.8181	1.0000	0.8181	0.6599	0.5093	0.3843
28.00	0.2420	0.3524	0.4965	0.6599	0.8181	1.0000	0.8337	0.6599	0.5222
30.00	0.1645	0.2543	0.3628	0.5093	0.6599	0.8337	1.0000	0.8337	0.6745
32.00	0.1096	0.1770	0.2627	0.3735	0.5093	0.6599	0.8337	1.0000	0.8337
34.00	0.0703	0.1188	0.1868	0.2713	0.3843	0.5222	0.6745	0.8337	1.0000
36.00	0.0424	0.0767	0.1236	0.1936	0.2801	0.3953	0.5287	0.6745	0.8337
38.00	0.0264	0.0477	0.0836	0.1336	0.2005	0.2891	0.4065	0.5287	0.6745
40.00	0.0151	0.0300	0.0524	0.0873	0.1416	0.2077	0.2983	0.4065	0.5419
42.00	0.0093	0.0168	0.0316	0.0574	0.0949	0.1471	0.2187	0.3077	0.4179
44.00	0.0037	0.0099	0.0193	0.0349	0.0601	0.0969	0.1527	0.2187	0.3077
46.00	0.0014	0.0069	0.0111	0.0214	0.0385	0.0629	0.1010	0.1527	0.2263
48.00	0.0014	0.0037	0.0069	0.0121	0.0226	0.0404	0.0673	0.1052	0.1585
50.00	0.0003	0.0014	0.0037	0.0069	0.0135	0.0238	0.0424	0.0673	0.1052
52.00	0.0003	0.0014	0.0014	0.0037	0.0093	0.0143	0.0251	0.0424	0.0703
54.00	0.0001	0.0003	0.0014	0.0014	0.0037	0.0093	0.0151	0.0264	0.0455
56.00	0.0001	0.0003	0.0003	0.0014	0.0014	0.0037	0.0093	0.0160	0.0278
58.00	0.0001	0.0001	0.0003	0.0003	0.0014	0.0014	0.0037	0.0093	0.0160
60.00	0.0001	0.0001	0.0001	0.0003	0.0003	0.0014	0.0014	0.0037	0.0093
62.00	—	0.0001	0.0001	0.0001	0.0003	0.0003	0.0014	0.0014	0.0037
64.00	—	—	0.0001	0.0001	0.0001	0.0003	0.0003	0.0014	0.0014
66.00	—	—	—	0.0001	0.0001	0.0001	0.0003	0.0003	0.0014
68.00	—	—	—	—	0.0001	0.0001	0.0001	0.0003	0.0003
70.00	—	—	—	—	—	0.0001	0.0001	0.0001	0.0003
72.00	—	—	—	—	—	—	0.0001	0.0001	0.0001
74.00	—	—	—	—	—	—	—	0.0001	0.0001
76.00	—	—	—	—	—	—	—	—	0.0001
78.00	—	—	—	—	—	—	—	—	—
80.00	—	—	—	—	—	—	—	—	—
82.00	—	—	—	—	—	—	—	—	—
84.00	—	—	—	—	—	—	—	—	—
86.00	—	—	—	—	—	—	—	—	—
88.00	—	—	—	—	—	—	—	—	—
90.00	—	—	—	—	—	—	—	—	—
92.00	—	—	—	—	—	—	—	—	—
94.00	—	—	—	—	—	—	—	—	—
96.00	—	—	—	—	—	—	—	—	—
98.00	—	—	—	—	—	—	—	—	—
100.00	—	—	—	—	—	—	—	—	—

TABLE 30–2. (CONTINUED)

	First Score (Percent Correct)								
	36.00	38.00	40.00	42.00	44.00	46.00	48.00	50.00	52.00
—	—	—	—	—	—	—	—	—	—
2.00	—	—	—	—	—	—	—	—	—
4.00	0.0001	0.0001	—	—	—	—	—	—	—
6.00	0.0001	0.0001	0.0001	0.0001	—	—	—	—	—
8.00	0.0003	0.0003	0.0001	0.0001	0.0001	0.0001	—	—	—
10.00	0.0014	0.0014	0.0003	0.0003	0.0001	0.0001	0.0001	—	—
12.00	0.0037	0.0014	0.0014	0.0003	0.0003	0.0001	0.0001	0.0001	0.0001
14.00	0.0105	0.0069	0.0037	0.0014	0.0014	0.0003	0.0003	0.0001	0.0001
16.00	0.0226	0.0128	0.0093	0.0037	0.0014	0.0014	0.0003	0.0003	0.0001
18.00	0.0424	0.0264	0.0151	0.0093	0.0037	0.0014	0.0014	0.0003	0.0003
20.00	0.0767	0.0477	0.0300	0.0168	0.0099	0.0069	0.0037	0.0014	0.0014
22.00	0.1236	0.0836	0.0524	0.0316	0.0193	0.0111	0.0069	0.0037	0.0014
24.00	0.1936	0.1336	0.0873	0.0574	0.0349	0.0214	0.0121	0.0069	0.0037
26.00	0.2801	0.2005	0.1416	0.0949	0.0601	0.0385	0.0226	0.0135	0.0093
28.00	0.3953	0.2891	0.2077	0.1471	0.0969	0.0629	0.0404	0.0238	0.0143
30.00	0.5287	0.4065	0.2983	0.2187	0.1527	0.1010	0.0673	0.0424	0.0251
32.00	0.6745	0.5287	0.4065	0.3077	0.2187	0.1527	0.1052	0.0673	0.0424
34.00	0.8337	0.6745	0.5419	0.4179	0.3077	0.2263	0.1585	0.1052	0.0703
36.00	1.0000	0.8337	0.6892	0.5419	0.4237	0.3173	0.2263	0.1585	0.1096
38.00	0.8337	1.0000	0.8337	0.6892	0.5419	0.4237	0.3173	0.2340	0.1645
40.00	0.6892	0.8337	1.0000	0.8337	0.6892	0.5419	0.4237	0.3173	0.2340
42.00	0.5419	0.6892	0.8337	1.0000	0.8493	0.6892	0.5552	0.4237	0.3173
44.00	0.4237	0.5419	0.6892	0.8493	1.0000	0.8493	0.6892	0.5552	0.4237
46.00	0.3173	0.4237	0.5419	0.6892	0.8493	1.0000	0.8493	0.6892	0.5552
48.00	0.2263	0.3173	0.4237	0.5552	0.6892	0.8493	1.0000	0.8493	0.6892
50.00	0.1585	0.2340	0.3173	0.4237	0.5552	0.6892	0.8493	1.0000	0.8493
52.00	0.1096	0.1645	0.2340	0.3173	0.4237	0.5552	0.6892	0.8493	1.0000
54.00	0.0703	0.1096	0.1645	0.2340	0.3173	0.4237	0.5552	0.6892	0.8493
56.00	0.0455	0.0735	0.1096	0.1645	0.2340	0.3173	0.4237	0.5552	0.6892
58.00	0.0278	0.0455	0.0735	0.1096	0.1645	0.2340	0.3173	0.4237	0.5552
60.00	0.0160	0.0278	0.0455	0.0735	0.1096	0.1645	0.2340	0.3173	0.4237
62.00	0.0093	0.0168	0.0278	0.0455	0.0735	0.1096	0.1645	0.2340	0.3173
64.00	0.0037	0.0093	0.0160	0.0278	0.0455	0.0703	0.1096	0.1585	0.2263
66.00	0.0014	0.0037	0.0093	0.0160	0.0278	0.0455	0.0703	0.1052	0.1585
68.00	0.0014	0.0014	0.0037	0.0093	0.0160	0.0264	0.0424	0.0673	0.1052
70.00	0.0003	0.0014	0.0014	0.0037	0.0093	0.0151	0.0251	0.0424	0.0673
72.00	0.0003	0.0003	0.0014	0.0014	0.0037	0.0093	0.0143	0.0238	0.0404
74.00	0.0001	0.0003	0.0003	0.0014	0.0014	0.0037	0.0093	0.0135	0.0226
76.00	0.0001	0.0001	0.0003	0.0003	0.0014	0.0014	0.0037	0.0069	0.0121
78.00	0.0001	0.0001	0.0001	0.0003	0.0003	0.0014	0.0014	0.0037	0.0069
80.00	—	0.0001	0.0001	0.0001	0.0003	0.0003	0.0014	0.0014	0.0037
82.00	—	—	0.0001	0.0001	0.0001	0.0001	0.0003	0.0003	0.0014
84.00	—	—	—	0.0001	0.0001	0.0001	0.0001	0.0003	0.0003
86.00	—	—	—	—	-	0.0001	0.0001	0.0001	0.0003
88.00	—	—	—	—	—	—	0.0001	0.0001	0.0001
90.00	—	—	—	—	—	—	—	—	0.0001
92.00	—	—	—	—	—	—	—	—	—
94.00	—	—	—	—	—	—	—	—	—
96.00	—	—	—	—	—	—	—	—	—
98.00	—	—	—	—	—	—	—	—	—
100.00	—	—	—	—	—	—	—	—	—

Second Score (Percent Correct)

TABLE 30–2. (CONTINUED)

	First Score (Percent Correct)								
	54.00	56.00	58.00	60.00	62.00	64.00	66.00	68.00	70.00
—	—	—	—	—	—	—	—	—	—
2.00	—	—	—	—	—	—	—	—	—
4.00	—	—	—	—	—	—	—	—	—
6.00	—	—	—	—	—	—	—	—	—
8.00	—	—	—	—	—	—	—	—	—
10.00	—	—	—	—	—	—	—	—	—
12.00	—	—	—	—	—	—	—	—	—
14.00	0.0001	—	—	—	—	—	—	—	—
16.00	0.0001	0.0001	0.0001	—	—	—	—	—	—
18.00	0.0001	0.0001	0.0001	0.0001	—	—	—	—	—
20.00	0.0003	0.0003	0.0001	0.0001	0.0001	—	—	—	—
22.00	0.0014	0.0003	0.0003	0.0001	0.0001	0.0001	—	—	—
24.00	0.0014	0.0014	0.0003	0.0003	0.0001	0.0001	0.0001	—	—
26.00	0.0037	0.0014	0.0014	0.0003	0.0003	0.0001	0.0001	0.0001	—
28.00	0.0093	0.0037	0.0014	0.0014	0.0003	0.0003	0.0001	0.0001	0.0001
30.00	0.0151	0.0093	0.0037	0.0014	0.0014	0.0003	0.0003	0.0001	0.0001
32.00	0.0264	0.0160	0.0093	0.0037	0.0014	0.0014	0.0003	0.0003	0.0001
34.00	0.0455	0.0278	0.0160	0.0093	0.0037	0.0014	0.0014	0.0003	0.0003
36.00	0.0703	0.0455	0.0278	0.0160	0.0093	0.0037	0.0014	0.0014	0.0003
38.00	0.1096	0.0735	0.0455	0.0278	0.0168	0.0093	0.0037	0.0014	0.0014
40.00	0.1645	0.1096	0.0735	0.0455	0.0278	0.0160	0.0093	0.0037	0.0014
42.00	0.2340	0.1645	0.1096	0.0735	0.0455	0.0278	0.0160	0.0093	0.0037
44.00	0.3173	0.2340	0.1645	0.1096	0.0735	0.0455	0.0278	0.0160	0.0093
46.00	0.4237	0.3173	0.2340	0.1645	0.1096	0.0703	0.0455	0.0264	0.0151
48.00	0.5552	0.4237	0.3173	0.2340	0.1645	0.1096	0.0703	0.0424	0.0251
50.00	0.6892	0.5552	0.4237	0.3173	0.2340	0.1585	0.1052	0.0673	0.0424
52.00	0.8493	0.6892	0.5552	0.4237	0.3173	0.2263	0.1585	0.1052	0.0673
54.00	1.0000	0.8493	0.6892	0.5419	0.4237	0.3173	0.2263	0.1527	0.1010
56.00	0.8493	1.0000	0.8493	0.6892	0.5419	0.4237	0.3077	0.2187	0.1527
58.00	0.6892	0.8493	1.0000	0.8337	0.6892	0.5419	0.4179	0.3077	0.2187
60.00	0.5419	0.6892	0.8337	1.0000	0.8337	0.6892	0.5419	0.4065	0.2983
62.00	0.4237	0.5419	0.6892	0.8337	1.0000	0.8337	0.6745	0.5287	0.4065
64.00	0.3173	0.4237	0.5419	0.6892	0.8337	1.0000	0.8337	0.6745	0.5287
66.00	0.2263	0.3077	0.4179	0.5419	0.6745	0.8337	1.0000	0.8337	0.6745
68.00	0.1527	0.2187	0.3077	0.4065	0.5287	0.6745	0.8337	1.0000	0.8337
70.00	0.1010	0.1527	0.2187	0.2983	0.4065	0.5287	0.6745	0.8337	1.0000
72.00	0.0629	0.0969	0.1471	0.2077	0.2891	0.3953	0.5222	0.6599	0.8337
74.00	0.0385	0.0601	0.0949	0.1416	0.2005	0.2801	0.3843	0.5093	0.6599
76.00	0.0214	0.0349	0.0574	0.0873	0.1336	0.1936	0.2713	0.3735	0.5093
78.00	0.0111	0.0193	0.0316	0.0524	0.0836	0.1236	0.1868	0.2627	0.3628
80.00	0.0069	0.0099	0.0168	0.0300	0.0477	0.0767	0.1188	0.1770	0.2543
82.00	0.0014	0.0037	0.0093	0.0151	0.0264	0.0424	0.0703	0.1096	0.1645
84.00	0.0014	0.0014	0.0037	0.0093	0.0128	0.0226	0.0385	0.0629	0.0969
86.00	0.0003	0.0014	0.0014	0.0037	0.0069	0.0105	0.0193	0.0332	0.0549
88.00	0.0001	0.0003	0.0003	0.0014	0.0014	0.0037	0.0093	0.0151	0.0264
90.00	0.0001	0.0001	0.0003	0.0003	0.0014	0.0014	0.0037	0.0069	0.0117
92.00	0.0001	0.0001	0.0001	0.0001	0.0003	0.0003	0.0014	0.0014	0.0037
94.00	—	—	0.0001	0.0001	0.0001	0.0001	0.0003	0.0003	0.0014
96.00	—	—	—	—	0.0001	0.0001	0.0001	0.0001	0.0003
98.00	—	—	—	—	—	—	—	0.0001	0.0001
100.00	—	—	—	—	—	—	—	—	—

Second Score (Percent Correct)

TABLE 30–2. (CONTINUED)

Second Score (Percent Correct)	First Score (Percent Correct)								
	72.00	74.00	76.00	78.00	80.00	82.00	84.00	86.00	88.00
—	—	—	—	—	—	—	—	—	—
2.00	—	—	—	—	—	—	—	—	—
4.00	—	—	—	—	—	—	—	—	—
6.00	—	—	—	—	—	—	—	—	—
8.00	—	—	—	—	—	—	—	—	—
10.00	—	—	—	—	—	—	—	—	—
12.00	—	—	—	—	—	—	—	—	—
14.00	—	—	—	—	—	—	—	—	—
16.00	—	—	—	—	—	—	—	—	—
18.00	—	—	—	—	—	—	—	—	—
20.00	—	—	—	—	—	—	—	—	—
22.00	—	—	—	—	—	—	—	—	—
24.00	—	—	—	—	—	—	—	—	—
26.00	—	—	—	—	—	—	—	—	—
28.00	—	—	—	—	—	—	—	—	—
30.00	0.0001	—	—	—	—	—	—	—	—
32.00	0.0001	0.0001	—	—	—	—	—	—	—
34.00	0.0001	0.0001	0.0001	—	—	—	—	—	—
36.00	0.0003	0.0001	0.0001	0.0001	—	—	—	—	—
38.00	0.0003	0.0003	0.0001	0.0001	0.0001	—	—	—	—
40.00	0.0014	0.0003	0.0003	0.0001	0.0001	0.0001	—	—	—
42.00	0.0014	0.0014	0.0003	0.0003	0.0001	0.0001	0.0001	—	—
44.00	0.0037	0.0014	0.0014	0.0003	0.0003	0.0001	0.0001	—	—
46.00	0.0093	0.0037	0.0014	0.0014	0.0003	0.0001	0.0001	0.0001	—
48.00	0.0143	0.0093	0.0037	0.0014	0.0014	0.0003	0.0001	0.0001	0.0001
50.00	0.0238	0.0135	0.0069	0.0037	0.0014	0.0003	0.0003	0.0001	0.0001
52.00	0.0404	0.0226	0.0121	0.0069	0.0037	0.0014	0.0003	0.0003	0.0001
54.00	0.0629	0.0385	0.0214	0.0111	0.0069	0.0014	0.0014	0.0003	0.0001
56.00	0.0969	0.0601	0.0349	0.0193	0.0099	0.0037	0.0014	0.0014	0.0003
58.00	0.1471	0.0949	0.0574	0.0316	0.0168	0.0093	0.0037	0.0014	0.0003
60.00	0.2077	0.1416	0.0873	0.0524	0.0300	0.0151	0.0093	0.0037	0.0014
62.00	0.2891	0.2005	0.1336	0.0836	0.0477	0.0264	0.0128	0.0069	0.0014
64.00	0.3953	0.2801	0.1936	0.1236	0.0767	0.0424	0.0226	0.0105	0.0037
66.00	0.5222	0.3843	0.2713	0.1868	0.1188	0.0703	0.0385	0.0193	0.0093
68.00	0.6599	0.5093	0.3735	0.2627	0.1770	0.1096	0.0629	0.0332	0.0151
70.00	0.8337	0.6599	0.5093	0.3628	0.2543	0.1645	0.0969	0.0549	0.0264
72.00	1.0000	0.8181	0.6599	0.4965	0.3524	0.2420	0.1527	0.0873	0.0455
74.00	0.8181	1.0000	0.8181	0.6455	0.4839	0.3421	0.2263	0.1362	0.0767
76.00	0.6599	0.8181	1.0000	0.8181	0.6384	0.4715	0.3271	0.2077	0.1236
78.00	0.4965	0.6455	0.8181	1.0000	0.8026	0.6241	0.4473	0.3077	0.1868
80.00	0.3524	0.4839	0.6384	0.8026	1.0000	0.8026	0.6101	0.4354	0.2801
82.00	0.2420	0.3421	0.4715	0.6241	0.8026	1.0000	0.7872	0.5961	0.4065
84.00	0.1527	0.2263	0.3271	0.4473	0.6101	0.7872	1.0000	0.7872	0.5687
86.00	0.0873	0.1362	0.2077	0.3077	0.4354	0.5961	0.7872	1.0000	0.7718
88.00	0.0455	0.0767	0.1236	0.1868	0.2801	0.4065	0.5687	0.7718	1.0000
90.00	0.0214	0.0366	0.0629	0.1052	0.1707	0.2627	0.3843	0.5552	0.7642
92.00	0.0093	0.0160	0.0293	0.0500	0.0873	0.1416	0.2263	0.3524	0.5222
94.00	0.0014	0.0069	0.0105	0.0203	0.0366	0.0673	0.1141	0.1936	0.3077
96.00	0.0003	0.0014	0.0037	0.0069	0.0121	0.0238	0.0455	0.0836	0.1471
98.00	0.0001	0.0003	0.0003	0.0014	0.0014	0.0069	0.0117	0.0238	0.0500
100.00	—	—	—	0.0001	0.0001	0.0003	0.0003	0.0014	0.0037

TABLE 30–2. (CONTINUED)

Second Score (Percent Correct)	First Score (Percent Correct)					
	90.00	92.00	94.00	96.00	98.00	100.00
—	—	—	—	—	—	—
2.00	—	—	—	—	—	—
4.00	—	—	—	—	—	—
6.00	—	—	—	—	—	—
8.00	—	—	—	—	—	—
10.00	—	—	—	—	—	—
12.00	—	—	—	—	—	—
14.00	—	—	—	—	—	—
16.00	—	—	—	—	—	—
18.00	—	—	—	—	—	—
20.00	—	—	—	—	—	—
22.00	—	—	—	—	—	—
24.00	—	—	—	—	—	—
26.00	—	—	—	—	—	—
28.00	—	—	—	—	—	—
30.00	—	—	—	—	—	—
32.00	—	—	—	—	—	—
34.00	—	—	—	—	—	—
36.00	—	—	—	—	—	—
38.00	—	—	—	—	—	—
40.00	—	—	—	—	—	—
42.00	—	—	—	—	—	—
44.00	—	—	—	—	—	—
46.00	—	—	—	—	—	—
48.00	—	—	—	—	—	—
50.00	—	—	—	—	—	—
52.00	0.0001	—	—	—	—	—
54.00	0.0001	0.0001	—	—	—	—
56.00	0.0001	0.0001	—	—	—	—
58.00	0.0003	0.0001	0.0001	—	—	—
60.00	0.0003	0.0001	0.0001	—	—	—
62.00	0.0014	0.0003	0.0001	0.0001	—	—
64.00	0.0014	0.0003	0.0001	0.0001	—	—
66.00	0.0037	0.0014	0.0003	0.0001	—	—
68.00	0.0069	0.0014	0.0003	0.0001	0.0001	—
70.00	0.0117	0.0037	0.0014	0.0003	0.0001	—
72.00	0.0214	0.0093	0.0014	0.0003	0.0001	—
74.00	0.0366	0.0160	0.0069	0.0014	0.0003	—
76.00	0.0629	0.0293	0.0105	0.0037	0.0003	—
78.00	0.1052	0.0500	0.0203	0.0069	0.0014	0.0001
80.00	0.1707	0.0873	0.0366	0.0121	0.0014	0.0001
82.00	0.2627	0.1416	0.0673	0.0238	0.0069	0.0003
84.00	0.3843	0.2263	0.1141	0.0455	0.0117	0.0003
86.00	0.5552	0.3524	0.1936	0.0836	0.0238	0.0014
88.00	0.7642	0.5222	0.3077	0.1471	0.0500	0.0037
90.00	1.0000	0.7339	0.4839	0.2543	0.0969	0.0093
92.00	0.7339	1.0000	0.7039	0.4237	0.1868	0.0193
94.00	0.4839	0.7039	1.0000	0.6745	0.3421	0.0500
96.00	0.2543	0.4237	0.6745	1.0000	0.5961	0.1236
98.00	0.0969	0.1868	0.3421	0.5961	1.0000	0.3173
100.00	0.0093	0.0193	0.0500	0.1236	0.3173	1.0000

TABLE 30-3. CONFIDENCE LEVELS FOR DIFFERENCES BETWEEN PERCENT SCORES; ONE OF WHICH IS BASED ON A 25-ITEM TEST, THE OTHER ON A 50-ITEM TEST.

Percent Correct (50-Item Test)	Percent Correct (25-Item Test)							
	0.00	4.00	8.00	12.00	16.00	20.00	24.00	28.00
—	0.8181	0.1585	0.0424	0.0117	0.0037	0.0014	0.0003	0.0001
2.00	0.5552	0.5687	0.2340	0.0873	0.0316	0.0105	0.0037	0.0014
4.00	0.3077	0.8808	0.4473	0.2077	0.0873	0.0349	0.0128	0.0037
6.00	0.1707	0.8337	0.6892	0.3628	0.1707	0.0767	0.0316	0.0121
8.00	0.0910	0.6101	0.9203	0.5419	0.2891	0.1416	0.0658	0.0278
10.00	0.0500	0.4354	0.8650	0.7339	0.4354	0.2340	0.1188	0.0549
12.00	0.0278	0.2983	0.6745	0.9362	0.5961	0.3524	0.1868	0.0949
14.00	0.0143	0.2005	0.5093	0.8808	0.7718	0.4839	0.2801	0.1527
16.00	0.0093	0.1336	0.3735	0.7039	0.9522	0.6384	0.3953	0.2263
18.00	0.0037	0.0873	0.2713	0.5552	0.8808	0.7872	0.5222	0.3173
20.00	0.0014	0.0549	0.1936	0.4237	0.7188	0.9522	0.6599	0.4237
22.00	0.0014	0.0332	0.1336	0.3173	0.5823	0.8808	0.8181	0.5552
24.00	0.0003	0.0203	0.0910	0.2340	0.4593	0.7339	0.9681	0.6892
26.00	0.0003	0.0128	0.0601	0.1707	0.3524	0.5961	0.8808	0.8337
28.00	0.0001	0.0093	0.0385	0.1188	0.2627	0.4839	0.7490	0.9681
30.00	0.0001	0.0037	0.0251	0.0836	0.2005	0.3735	0.6101	0.8808
32.00	0.0001	0.0014	0.0160	0.0549	0.1416	0.2891	0.4965	0.7490
34.00	0.0001	0.0014	0.0099	0.0366	0.1010	0.2187	0.3953	0.6241
36.00	—	0.0014	0.0069	0.0238	0.0703	0.1585	0.3077	0.5093
38.00	—	0.0003	0.0037	0.0151	0.0477	0.1188	0.2340	0.4065
40.00	—	0.0003	0.0014	0.0099	0.0316	0.0836	0.1770	0.3173
42.00	—	0.0001	0.0014	0.0069	0.0214	0.0574	0.1285	0.2420
44.00	—	0.0001	0.0003	0.0037	0.0135	0.0385	0.0910	0.1868
46.00	—	0.0001	0.0003	0.0014	0.0093	0.0264	0.0658	0.1362
48.00	—	0.0001	0.0003	0.0014	0.0069	0.0168	0.0444	0.0969
50.00	—	—	0.0001	0.0003	0.0037	0.0105	0.0300	0.0703
52.00	—	—	0.0001	0.0003	0.0014	0.0069	0.0193	0.0477
54.00	—	—	0.0001	0.0003	0.0014	0.0037	0.0121	0.0316
56.00	—	—	0.0001	0.0001	0.0003	0.0014	0.0093	0.0214
58.00	—	—	—	0.0001	0.0003	0.0014	0.0037	0.0135
60.00	—	—	—	0.0001	0.0003	0.0014	0.0037	0.0093
62.00	—	—	—	0.0001	0.0001	0.0003	0.0014	0.0037
64.00	—	—	—	—	0.0001	0.0003	0.0014	0.0037
66.00	—	—	—	—	0.0001	0.0001	0.0003	0.0014
68.00	—	—	—	—	0.0001	0.0001	0.0003	0.0014
70.00	—	—	—	—	—	0.0001	0.0001	0.0003
72.00	—	—	—	—	—	0.0001	0.0001	0.0003
74.00	—	—	—	—	—	—	0.0001	0.0001
76.00	—	—	—	—	—	—	0.0001	0.0001
78.00	—	—	—	—	—	—	—	0.0001
80.00	—	—	—	—	—	—	—	0.0001
82.00	—	—	—	—	—	—	—	—
84.00	—	—	—	—	—	—	—	—
86.00	—	—	—	—	—	—	—	—
88.00	—	—	—	—	—	—	—	—
90.00	—	—	—	—	—	—	—	—
92.00	—	—	—	—	—	—	—	—
94.00	—	—	—	—	—	—	—	—
96.00	—	—	—	—	—	—	—	—
98.00	—	—	—	—	—	—	—	—
100.00	—	—	—	—	—	—	—	—

TABLE 30-3. (CONTINUED)

Percent Correct (50-Item Test)

| | Percent Correct (25-Item Test) | | | | | | | | |
	32.00	36.00	40.00	44.00	48.00	52.00	56.00	60.00	64.00
—	0.0001	—	—	—	—	—	—	—	—
2.00	0.0003	0.0001	0.0001	—	—	—	—	—	—
4.00	0.0014	0.0003	0.0001	0.0001	—	—	—	—	—
6.00	0.0037	0.0014	0.0003	0.0001	0.0001	0.0001	—	—	—
8.00	0.0105	0.0037	0.0014	0.0003	0.0001	0.0001	0.0001	—	—
10.00	0.0226	0.0093	0.0037	0.0014	0.0003	0.0001	0.0001	—	—
12.00	0.0424	0.0188	0.0093	0.0014	0.0014	0.0003	0.0001	0.0001	—
14.00	0.0735	0.0332	0.0143	0.0069	0.0014	0.0003	0.0003	0.0001	0.0001
16.00	0.1188	0.0574	0.0264	0.0111	0.0037	0.0014	0.0003	0.0001	0.0001
18.00	0.1770	0.0910	0.0444	0.0193	0.0093	0.0037	0.0014	0.0003	0.0001
20.00	0.2543	0.1416	0.0703	0.0332	0.0143	0.0069	0.0014	0.0003	0.0003
22.00	0.3421	0.2005	0.1096	0.0524	0.0238	0.0099	0.0037	0.0014	0.0003
24.00	0.4473	0.2801	0.1585	0.0801	0.0385	0.0168	0.0069	0.0014	0.0014
26.00	0.5687	0.3628	0.2187	0.1188	0.0601	0.0278	0.0121	0.0037	0.0014
28.00	0.7039	0.4715	0.2983	0.1707	0.0910	0.0444	0.0193	0.0093	0.0037
30.00	0.8337	0.5823	0.3843	0.2340	0.1285	0.0673	0.0316	0.0135	0.0037
32.00	0.9840	0.7188	0.4839	0.3077	0.1835	0.0969	0.0477	0.0214	0.0093
34.00	0.8808	0.8493	0.5961	0.3953	0.2420	0.1362	0.0703	0.0332	0.0143
36.00	0.7490	0.9840	0.7188	0.4965	0.3173	0.1868	0.1010	0.0500	0.0226
38.00	0.6241	0.8808	0.8493	0.6101	0.4065	0.2543	0.1416	0.0735	0.0349
40.00	0.5222	0.7490	0.9840	0.7339	0.5093	0.3320	0.1936	0.1052	0.0500
42.00	0.4179	0.6384	0.8808	0.8650	0.6241	0.4179	0.2543	0.1471	0.0735
44.00	0.3320	0.5222	0.7490	1.0000	0.7490	0.5222	0.3320	0.1936	0.1052
46.00	0.2543	0.4237	0.6384	0.8808	0.8650	0.6241	0.4237	0.2627	0.1471
48.00	0.1936	0.3320	0.5222	0.7490	1.0000	0.7490	0.5222	0.3320	0.1936
50.00	0.1416	0.2543	0.4237	0.6241	0.8808	0.8808	0.6241	0.4237	0.2543
52.00	0.1010	0.1936	0.3320	0.5222	0.7490	1.0000	0.7490	0.5222	0.3320
54.00	0.0735	0.1471	0.2627	0.4237	0.6241	0.8650	0.8808	0.6384	0.4237
56.00	0.0500	0.1052	0.1936	0.3320	0.5222	0.7490	1.0000	0.7490	0.5222
58.00	0.0332	0.0735	0.1471	0.2543	0.4179	0.6241	0.8650	0.8808	0.6384
60.00	0.0226	0.0500	0.1052	0.1936	0.3320	0.5093	0.7339	0.9840	0.7490
62.00	0.0143	0.0349	0.0735	0.1416	0.2543	0.4065	0.6101	0.8493	0.8808
64.00	0.0093	0.0226	0.0500	0.1010	0.1868	0.3173	0.4965	0.7188	0.9840
66.00	0.0069	0.0143	0.0332	0.0703	0.1362	0.2420	0.3953	0.5961	0.8493
68.00	0.0037	0.0093	0.0214	0.0477	0.0969	0.1835	0.3077	0.4839	0.7188
70.00	0.0014	0.0037	0.0135	0.0316	0.0673	0.1285	0.2340	0.3843	0.5823
72.00	0.0014	0.0037	0.0093	0.0193	0.0444	0.0910	0.1707	0.2983	0.4715
74.00	0.0003	0.0014	0.0037	0.0121	0.0278	0.0601	0.1188	0.2187	0.3628
76.00	0.0003	0.0014	0.0014	0.0069	0.0168	0.0385	0.0801	0.1585	0.2801
78.00	0.0001	0.0003	0.0014	0.0037	0.0099	0.0238	0.0524	0.1096	0.2005
80.00	0.0001	0.0003	0.0003	0.0014	0.0069	0.0143	0.0332	0.0703	0.1416
82.00	0.0001	0.0001	0.0003	0.0014	0.0037	0.0093	0.0193	0.0444	0.0910
84.00	0.0001	0.0001	0.0001	0.0003	0.0014	0.0037	0.0111	0.0264	0.0574
86.00	—	0.0001	0.0001	0.0003	0.0003	0.0014	0.0069	0.0143	0.0332
88.00	—	—	0.0001	0.0001	0.0003	0.0014	0.0014	0.0093	0.0188
90.00	—	—	—	0.0001	0.0001	0.0003	0.0014	0.0037	0.0093
92.00	—	—	—	0.0001	0.0001	0.0001	0.0003	0.0014	0.0037
94.00	—	—	—	—	0.0001	0.0001	0.0001	0.0003	0.0014
96.00	—	—	—	—	—	—	0.0001	0.0001	0.0003
98.00	—	—	—	—	—	—	—	0.0001	0.0001
100.00	—	—	—	—	—	—	—	—	—

TABLE 30-3. (CONTINUED)

	Percent Correct (25-Item Test)								
	68.00	72.00	76.00	80.00	84.00	88.00	92.00	96.00	100.00
—	—	—	—	—	—	—	—	—	—
2.00	—	—	—	—	—	—	—	—	—
4.00	—	—	—	—	—	—	—	—	—
6.00	––	—	—	—	—	—	—	—	—
8.00	—	—	—	—	—	—	—	—	—
10.00	—	—	—	—	—	—	—	—	—
12.00	—	—	—	—	—	—	—	—	—
14.00	—	—	—	—	—	—	—	—	—
16.00	0.0001	—	—	—	—	—	—	—	—
18.00	0.0001	—	—	—	—	—	—	—	—
20.00	0.0001	0.0001	—	—	—	—	—	—	—
22.00	0.0001	0.0001	—	—	—	—	—	—	—
24.00	0.0003	0.0001	0.0001	—	—	—	—	—	—
26.00	0.0003	0.0001	0.0001	—	—	—	—	—	—
28.00	0.0014	0.0003	0.0001	0.0001	—	—	—	—	—
30.00	0.0014	0.0003	0.0001	0.0001	—	—	—	—	—
32.00	0.0037	0.0014	0.0003	0.0001	0.0001	—	—	—	—
34.00	0.0069	0.0014	0.0003	0.0001	0.0001	—	—	—	—
36.00	0.0093	0.0037	0.0014	0.0003	0.0001	—	—	—	—
38.00	0.0143	0.0037	0.0014	0.0003	0.0001	0.0001	—	—	—
40.00	0.0226	0.0093	0.0037	0.0014	0.0003	0.0001	—	—	—
42.00	0.0332	0.0135	0.0037	0.0014	0.0003	0.0001	—	—	—
44.00	0.0500	0.0214	0.0093	0.0014	0.0003	0.0001	0.0001	—	—
46.00	0.0735	0.0316	0.0121	0.0037	0.0014	0.0003	0.0001	—	—
48.00	0.1010	0.0477	0.0193	0.0069	0.0014	0.0003	0.0001	—	—
50.00	0.1416	0.0703	0.0300	0.0105	0.0037	0.0003	0.0001	—	—
52.00	0.1936	0.0969	0.0444	0.0168	0.0069	0.0014	0.0003	0.0001	—
54.00	0.2543	0.1362	0.0658	0.0264	0.0093	0.0014	0.0003	0.0001	—
56.00	0.3320	0.1868	0.0910	0.0385	0.0135	0.0037	0.0003	0.0001	—
58.00	0.4179	0.2420	0.1285	0.0574	0.0214	0.0069	0.0014	0.0001	––
60.00	0.5222	0.3173	0.1770	0.0836	0.0316	0.0099	0.0014	0.0003	—
62.00	0.6241	0.4065	0.2340	0.1188	0.0477	0.0151	0.0037	0.0003	—
64.00	0.7490	0.5093	0.3077	0.1585	0.0703	0.0238	0.0069	0.0014	
66.00	0.8808	0.6241	0.3953	0.2187	0.1010	0.0366	0.0099	0.0014	0.0001
68.00	0.9840	0.7490	0.4965	0.2891	0.1416	0.0549	0.0160	0.0014	0.0001
70.00	0.8337	0.8808	0.6101	0.3735	0.2005	0.0836	0.0251	0.0037	0.0001
72.00	0.7039	0.9681	0.7490	0.4839	0.2627	0.1188	0.0385	0.0093	0.0001
74.00	0.5687	0.8337	0.8808	0.5961	0.3524	0.1707	0.0601	0.0128	0.0003
76.00	0.4473	0.6892	0.9681	0.7339	0.4593	0.2340	0.0910	0.0203	0.0003
78.00	0.3421	0.5552	0.8181	0.8808	0.5823	0.3173	0.1336	0.0332	0.0014
80.00	0.2543	0.4237	0.6599	0.9522	0.7188	0.4237	0.1936	0.0549	0.0014
82.00	0.1770	0.3173	0.5222	0.7872	0.8808	0.5552	0.2713	0.0873	0.0037
84.00	0.1188	0.2263	0.3953	0.6384	0.9522	0.7039	0.3735	0.1336	0.0093
86.00	0.0735	0.1527	0.2801	0.4839	0.7718	0.8808	0.5093	0.2005	0.0143
88.00	0.0424	0.0949	0.1868	0.3524	0.5961	0.9362	0.6745	0.2983	0.0278
90.00	0.0226	0.0549	0.1188	0.2340	0.4354	0.7339	0.8650	0.4354	0.0500
92.00	0.0105	0.0278	0.0658	0.1416	0.2891	0.5419	0.9203	0.6101	0.0910
94.00	0.0037	0.0121	0.0316	0.0767	0.1707	0.3628	0.6892	0.8337	0.1707
96.00	0.0014	0.0037	0.0128	0.0349	0.0873	0.2077	0.4473	0.8808	0.3077
98.00	0.0003	0.0014	0.0037	0.0105	0.0316	0.0873	0.2340	0.5687	0.5552
100.00	0.0001	0.0001	0.0003	0.0014	0.0037	0.0117	0.0424	0.1585	0.8181

Percent Correct (50-Item Test)

REFERENCES

Raffin, M. J. M., and Schafer, D. Application of a probability model based on the binomial distribution to speech-discrimination scores. *J. Speech Hearing Res.,* to be published, (1980).

Schafer, D. *Application of a Probability Model Based on the Binomial Distribution to Speech Discrimination Scores.* M.A. Thesis, Northwestern University (1978).

Thornton, A. R., and Raffin, M. J. M. Speech-discrimination scores modeled as a binomial variable. *J. Speech Hearing Res.,* **21,** 507–518 (1978).

31

Factors Affecting Speech Discrimination Test Difficulty

E. JAMES KREUL, Ph.D
Professor of Audiology, California State University at Chico, Chico, California
DONALD W. BELL, Ph.D.
Senior Research Psychologist, SRI International, Menlo Park, California
JAMES C. NIXON, Ph.D.
Stanford Research Institute when this article was prepared

Changes in item and overall test difficulty of speech discrimination and intelligibility tests were examined as a function of: carrier phrase, talker, reutterances by a talker, and level of accompanying noise. The results indicate that all of these variables must be considered in test development. Only the actual recordings of the spoken lists of words can be considered to be the test material; the word lists, in and of themselves, should not be thought of as test material.

In spite of the early experiments of Egan (1944) and Hirsh et al. (1952), which reported test results for specific recordings, it has become practice to consider tests of speech discrimination as lists of printed words rather than sets of recorded utterances. It is common practice for audiologists to speak "standardized" lists of words to the patients they examine. Reviews of the literature such as that of Heath and Bartlett (1961) show that difficulty of speech discrimination and intelligibility tests varies for different talkers—both on individual item and overall test list. This was most recently demonstrated in the work of Kreul et al. (1968). Further, the work of Brandy (1966) shows that reutterances of given list of words even by the same talker result in significant differences in listener performance.

The goal of this experiment was to examine the influence of carrier phrase and accompanying levels of noise on speech discrimination for two talkers. Another purpose was to determine how reliable speech discrimination mean scores are when a list of words is reread.

METHOD

The level of speech discrimination difficulty was examined as two talkers spoke and respoke a list of test words* (1) within a single recording session; (2) between two recording sessions; (3) as the carrier phrase was changed; and (4) for talker EJK, as the noise level was changed.

Test Materials and Format

The Modified Rhyme Test (MRT), developed by House et al. (1963, 1965), was employed for this investigation. Briefly, the test consists of 300 common monosyllabic words arranged in six 50-word lists. As each stimulus item is presented the subject must select the correct response from an ensemble of six words. Only one of the six MRT lists was used, but it was rearranged in eight different random orders. The item selection for each order was accomplished by randomly selecting each of the 50 items as it appeared without replacement.

---

*Throughout this paper *test-retest* refers to a contrast of test results for the same recording of a list of words; *reutterance* refers to a contrast of test results for the same word list that has been reordered and rerecorded.

Reprinted by permission of the authors from *J. Speech Hearing Res.*, **12**, 281–287 (1969).

Talkers

Talkers were two of the experimenters, both of whom speak General American English.

Recording Procedure

Four orders of the test were spoken at each of two recording sessions by each of the talkers. The test words, as is common practice, were produced within a carrier phrase. The two carrier phrases employed were:

You will strike *through*-------*now.*   (TN)
You will *strike*-------*please.*   (SP)

One recording session was arranged for the morning and the second for the afternoon of the same day. At each recording session a talker produced two orders of the MRT list with the *Through-Now* (TN) carrier phrase, and two with the *Strike-Please* (SP) carrier phrase. During the second recording session, the same procedure was followed by each of the two talkers. The purpose of two recording sessions was to examine the reutterance reliability for orders of MRT lists spoken at a given recording session in contrast to reliability between orders of the MRT list produced at two recording sessions.

The recording order of the spoken test list with the two carrier phrases was:

Morning	Afternoon
TN-1	TN-3
TN-2	TN-4
SP-1	SP-3
SP-2	SP-4

The test recordings were made in a double-walled IAC test booth. A Breul and Kjaer 4131 microphone was placed approximately 12 in. from the talker's lips. The carrier phrase and stimulus item were uttered at a comfortable speaking level as in a simple declarative sentence. The recordings were made on an Ampex 351 tape recorder. A new test item was begun every six seconds with six seconds between homologous points of two adjacent test items. To accomplish the sequencing of the test items, the sweep frequency on a cathode ray oscilloscope was set to recycle every six seconds. Watching the trace, the talker began a new item each time the trace

crossed the middle of the oscilloscope face. This technique allowed the talker to pace his speaking time. The talker and two observers outside the test booth monitored the adequacy of articulation and the level of the carrier phrase on a volume level (VU) indicator. The test word was controlled by monitoring the level of the word *strike*, assuming equal effort for the test word. The level of the word *strike* in each of the two carrier phrases was achieved by peaking the VU indicator to the middle (−2) of the scale. The level was considered incorrect if the peak VU reading varied ± 1 dB on the word *strike*. Lists were rerecorded when errors of articulation or level were noted. A calibration tone and noise were recorded at the beginning of each test list so that the VU reading for the calibration signals was at the same level as the word *strike* in the carrier phrase.[1]

Listeners

Three listening crews of Foothill Junior College students were presented the eight recorded MRT list orders of each talker. Two crews were composed of eight listeners, the third of seven listeners. All listeners demonstrated normal hearing and spoke General American English.

Test Presentation Equipment

An Ampex 351 tape recorder was used to present the test lists. The speech signals were mixed with broadband white noise (100–7,000 Hz) from a Grason-Stadler noise generator. The tests were presented in right ears over eight matched sets of earphones. White noise (100–7,000 Hz) from a second Grason-Stadler noise generator was presented to the left ear at 70 dB SPL to prevent cross hearing.

Test Presentation

The listening crews were presented two TN and two SP orders of the test per day. The MRT lists were presented to the listening crews with other speech tests interposed between the lists to minimize learning effects that might occur if the test lists were presented too often and too close together. The first two listening crews were given only the recorded lists for EJK. One crew received all eight orders of the MRT list spoken by EJK at both 0 and −10 dB signal-to-noise ratio (S/N).[2] The other crew received all eight orders of the MRT list spoken by EJK at both −10 and −15 dB S/N. Thus, 15 listeners were presented the test materials at a −10 S/N; 15 listeners were presented all eight forms of the MRT list spoken by DWB at −10 dB S/N. The speech level was held constant at 75 dB equivalent SPL. The S/N was attained by adjusting the noise level while maintaining the same speech level for all forms of the MRT list. Test list presentation was counterbalanced to reduce order effects. All the subjects were given the same instructions prior to testing.

RESULTS

Means and standard deviations of the number of errors for EJK at three S/Ns (0, −10, and −15 dB) and at one S/N (−10 dB) for DWB are presented in Table 31-1. The means are plotted in Figure 31-1.

Test Difficulty and Reutterance

Data for both carrier phrases are independently analyzed at each S/N. A Friedman analysis of variance (Siegel, 1956) indicated scores obtained from repeat testing on different occasions at any S/N for either carrier phrase or for either talker were not significantly different. Thus, overall level of difficulty remained stable over several utterances and orders of the MRT list used. This result does not agree with the findings of Brandy (1966); however, there are major differences in procedure.

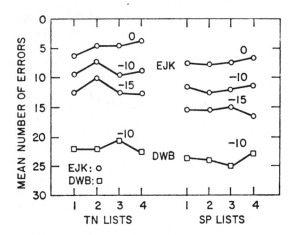

FIGURE 31-1. Mean number of errors for four reutterances of the same 50 words with two carrier phrases for two talkers. Modified Rhyme Test.

Test Difficulty with Carrier Phrase

The data in Table 31-1 reveal that, for both talkers, the mean number of errors with the TN carrier phrase is fewer than with the SP carrier phrase. For EJK, this difference occurs at all three S/Ns. The difference in number of errors between the two carrier phrases was more striking for EJK.

For the only condition in common for both talkers, the −10 dB S/N, the number of errors was notably fewer for EJK. Increased number of errors for listeners responding to lists spoken by DWB as compared with lists spoken by EJK cannot be explained

TABLE 31-1. MEANS AND STANDARD DEVIATIONS IN NUMBER OF LISTENER ERRORS ON THROUGH-NOW (TN) AND STRIKE-PLEASE (SP) CARRIER PHRASES FOR TWO TALKERS. MODIFIED RHYME TEST.

Talker	S/N		TN-1	TN-2	TN-3	TN-4	SP-1	SP-2	SP-3	SP-4	Number of Listeners
EJK	0	Mean	6.1	4.6	4.6	3.9	7.4	7.9	7.4	6.9	7
		σ	2.22	1.29	1.72	1.95	2.49	3.09	2.49	1.88	
EJK	−10	Mean	9.4	7.3	9.5	8.9	11.5	12.5	12.1	11.4	15
		σ	2.49	2.57	3.70	2.38	3.15	2.72	3.28	3.91	
EJK	−15	Mean	12.4	9.9	12.6	12.7	15.4	15.5	15.1	16.5	8
		σ	3.15	0.77	3.19	1.91	2.39	2.34	1.96	5.72	
DWB	−10	Mean	22.0	21.8	20.6	22.5	23.4	23.8	24.8	22.9	8
		σ	3.27	3.63	4.79	4.74	4.55	4.57	3.26	3.85	

by the measured S/N difference, but this difference in number of errors between talkers is not unusual (Heath and Bartlett, 1961).

As previously stated, when a Friedman analysis of variance was performed treating the data from the two carrier phrases separately, no significant differences between lists were found. But when the treatment included the variance due to carrier phrase by combining the two sets of data, significant differences were found at each S/N between the list orders with the TN carrier phrase and the list orders with the SP carrier phrase. Table 31–2 gives a summary of these analyses. Clearly, carrier phrase does affect speech discrimination, the words are more easily discriminated with the TN carrier phrase, and the effect is sufficiently striking to emerge through repeated presentations even though variance was added by rearranging and reuttering the test items for each presentation.

Differences between VU values for the test items in the TN and SP lists are approximately a decibel and do not explain the relatively large differences in listener performance with the two carrier phrases.

Confusion matrices were prepared for the data of talker EJK to examine the patterning of word confusions as a function of utterances versus carrier phrases (TN and SP) at three S/Ns. An evaluation of the matrices indicates that easily identified words tend to remain easily identified even though the carrier phrase has been changed. The rank order of item difficulty tends to persist over all S/Ns. The degree to which the level of word difficulty persisted was examined for talker EJK by tabulating the number of errors, across subjects, for each of the 50 words. Each of the 50 words had six total number of errors associated with it, one for each of the six carrier phrases and S/N combinations. The words were then ranked for each carrier phrase and S/N combination

according to number of errors, and the ranks correlated (Spearman rho). Table 31–3 presents the correlations. With either carrier phrase, the rank order of item difficulty persisted across noise levels. The strongest relationship, $r_s = 0.89$, were found between the two conditions presented at the least favorable S/N.

CONCLUSIONS

Test difficulty changes significantly with changes in talker and carrier phrase. Test difficulty does not change significantly with reutterances of the same test materials by a given speaker over two recording sessions. These results held over a 15 dB S/N. Finally, the rank order of test item difficulty tends to persist with a change in carrier phrase and as the level of the accompanying noise is increased.

In speech discrimination and intelligibility test development, selection of the talker, his specific set of utterances, the carrier phrase, and the deliberately in-

TABLE 31–3a. CORRELATION BETWEEN LEVELS WITHIN TN CARRIER PHRASE.

TN S/N	TN carrier phrase	
	−10	−15
0	0.64	0.64
−10	—	0.89

TABLE 31–3b. CORRELATION BETWEEN LEVELS WITHIN SP CARRIER PHRASE.

SP S/N	SP carrier phrase	
	−10	−15
0	0.76	0.70
−10	—	0.89

TABLE 31–2. SUMMARY OF ANALYSES OF THE EFFECT OF CARRIER PHRASE ON WORD INTELLIGIBILITY OF TWO TALKERS. MODIFIED RHYME TEST.

Talker	S/N	χ_r^2	df	P<
EJK	0	23.31	7	0.01
	−10	44.88	7	0.001
	−15	22.47	7	0.01
DWB	−10	12.16	7	0.10

TABLE 31–3c. CORRELATION BETWEEN CARRIER PHRASES WITHIN LEVELS.

TN carrier phrase S/N	SP carrier phrase		
	0	−10	−15
0	0.61		
−10		0.91	
−15			0.82

troduced distortion will all interact to determine level of test difficulty. Speech intelligibility and discrimination test development can and should be designed to meet the specific need of the user. Accomplishing the requirements of the test can only be determined empirically and requirements of the test are embodied only in the recorded form of the test.

Tests ought not be thought of as the written lists of words but as recordings of these words. In the development of equivalent lists for a test of speech discrimination or intelligibility, it is cautioned that the test standards be based on listener responses to the recorded lists. Further, the test standards are only applicable for the specific set of conditions and for the population of listeners represented in the standardization of the test.

ACKNOWLEDGMENT

This research was supported in part by Stanford Research Institute's Research and Development Program No. 188531-171 and in part by Public Health Service Grant No. NB-UI 07908–03CMS from the National Center for Urban and Industrial Health. Donald W. Bell was a National Institute of Mental Health Postdoctoral Fellow (5-F2-MH-32105-02) at Stanford University during the period of this research.

ENDNOTES

1. The level of the 1 kHz calibration tone and 100–7,000 Hz noise band were recorded to match the peak reading of the word *strike* as measured at the middle of a Davin VU meter. For the recorded speech samples, this match in levels is designated in equivalent SPL. Thus, the SPL of the 1 kHz tone defines the speech monitoring level. This level is approximately 7 dB above the long-term rms overall level of speech (Williams et al., 1967).

2. The S/N was determined by the relationship between the speech monitoring level (see first endnote) and the band pressure level of the white noise masker (100–7,000 Hz).

REFERENCES

Brandy, W. T. Reliability of voice tests of speech discrimination. *J. Speech Hearing Res.,* **9,** 461–465 (1966).

Egan, J. P. Articulation testing methods II. OSRD Rept. 3802, 92 pp. AD-20 504 (Nov. 1944).

Heath, R. W., and Bartlett, S. C. Speaking and listening variables in jammed communications. Tech. Rept. of Task No. 1, U.S. Army Electronic Proving Ground, Fort Huachuca, Ariz., Contract No. DA-36-039-SC-80492 (1961).

Hirsh, I. J.; Davis H.; Silverman, S. R.; Reynolds, E. G.; Eldert, E.; and Benson, R. W. Development of materials for speech audiometry. *J. Speech Hearing Dis.,* **17,** 321–337 (1952).

House, A. S.; Williams, C. E.; Hecker, M. H. L.; and Kryter, K. D. Articulation-testing methods: Consonantal differentiation with a closed response set. *J. Acoust. Soc. Amer.,* **37,** 158–166 (1965).

House, A. S.; Williams, C. E.; Hecker, M. H. L.; and Kryter, K. D. Psychoacoustic speech tests: A Modified Rhyme Test. U.S. Air Force Systems Command, Hanscom Field, Electronics Systems Division, Tech. Doc. Rept. ESD-TDR-63-403 (June 1963).

Kreul, E. J.; Nixon, J. C.; Kryter, K. D.; Bell, D. W.; Lang, J. S.; and Schubert, E. D. A proposed clinical test of speech discrimination. *J. Speech Hearing Res.,* **11,** 536–552 (1968).

Siegel, S. *Nonparametric Statistics for the Behavioral Sciences.* New York: McGraw-Hill (1956).

Williams, C. E.; Stevens, K. N.; Hecker, M. H. L.; and Pearsons, K. S. The speech interference effects of aircraft noise. Tech. Rept. Aircraft Development Service, Washington, D.C., Contract No. FA66WA-1566 (1967).

32

Talker Effects on Word-Discrimination Scores of Adults with Sensorineural Hearing Impairment

John P. Penrod, Ph.D.
Assistant Professor of Audiology, University of Georgia, Athens, Georgia

Speech discrimination testing was completed on 30 adults with varying degrees of sensorineural hearing impairment. Tape recordings of four talkers' utterances of CID W-22 word lists served as the stimulus materials. Listeners' responses were scored independently by three experienced judges. For 26 of the 30 subjects, the difference between the lowest and highest word-discrimination score was 8 percent or greater. Variations in scores could not be attributed to a single talker but were spread across all talkers. A moderate negative correlation was found between each listener's average word-discrimination score and amount of variability among his or her individual scores. The statistical analysis indicated that talker differences were responsible for only a small portion of the variability in scores and suggested that a factor of greater importance is the talker-listener interaction.

Speech audiometric tests may be administered by means of either recordings or by monitored live voice (MLV) presentation. A procedure for determining the speech reception threshold (SRT) using MLV was described by Hughson and Thompson (1942). The use of MLV has also been prevalent in word-discrimination testing because of its flexibility, rapidity, and ease of administration. The variation inherent in this procedure has not gone unnoticed by researchers and clinicians (Asher, 1958; Brandy, 1966; Carhart, 1965; Goetzinger, 1972; Kreul, Bell, and Nixon, 1969; Palmer, 1955; Silverman and Hirsh, 1955).

The variability in clinical word-discrimination scores (WDS) is probably of greater concern than variability that might occur for the SRT. It is a rather simple procedure to compare the SRT to the average pure-tone loss as a quick reliability check because there is a strong relationship between these two mea-

sures (Carhart, 1946; Fletcher, 1950; Harris, Haines, and Myers, 1956; Hughson and Thompson, 1942; Sieganthaler and Strand, 1964). Unfortunately, the relationship between the degree of loss and the WDS is not so clear.

Carhart (1965) and Goetzinger (1972) have stated that test results obtained by different talkers are not comparable unless their equivalency has been demonstrated. Where equivalency has not been shown, comparisons must be restricted to a single talker. Brandy (1966) later demonstrated that upon retesting, even a single talker will vary his presentations on the same words. Kreul et al. (1969) in a study of several variables affecting reliability of WDS, reported that scores for repeat testing for either of two talkers on different occasions were not significantly different. Major procedural differences exist between these two studies. Kreul et al. (1969) used the Modified Rhyme Test which employs a closed set response paradigm, while Brandy (1966) used 25 words selected from List 3 of CID W-22 and written re-

Reprinted by permission of the author from *J. Speech Hearing Dis.*, **44**, 340–349 (1979).

sponses. Tillman and Olsen (1973) indicate that a standardized test is not possible unless recordings are used. Despite the evidence, MLV testing continues to have widespread clinical use.

Campbell (1965) states: "Clinical practice would make it apparent that only differences in discrimination scores in excess of about 5 percent are commonly thought to be meaningful. This reflects the general impression that test-retest variability is about 5 percent" (p. 14). Resnick (1962) reported discrimination scores differing by no more than 6 percent for five subjects tested the same day with different lists but one tester. Scores differed within subjects by a maximum of 6 percent between the lowest and highest score (test-retest reliability) and averaged only 3.4 percent. Based on these findings, variations of 8 percent or more between listeners' scores on different talkers in this study shall be considered clinically significant.

This study examined the word discrimination scores of subjects with sensorineural hearing impairment obtained using MLV, and determined whether clinically significant variations occurred in their scores as a result of different talkers. The use of individualized MLV presentations by different talkers is questionable, in view of Brandy's (1966) findings of significant variability within a single talker upon repeated presentations. Campbell (1965) has also commented on the differences that exist between individual testers using MLV, saying that it is the most vulnerable area for criticism. To ensure that each listener received exactly the same stimuli, and that presentations were representative of each talker's clinical delivery of the stimulus words, tape recordings of each talker's clinical presentations of word discrimination materials were made and served as the stimuli for this study.

PROCEDURES

Preparation of Stimulus Materials

Eighteen audiologists who reported using MLV speech audiometry routinely, were available to serve as talkers. Four of the 18 were selected randomly to serve as talkers (three males and one female). Each had at least 2 years of professional experience before the experimental study. They ranged in age from 26 to 45 years with a mean age of 34 years.

It was desired that the recordings of each talker should represent his or her usual clinical monitored-live-voice presentation of speech discrimination material. Therefore, all recordings were made at the clinic of the respective talker during actual evaluations of listeners' word-discrimination ability. A cardioid microphone (Northern Electric 633A) was placed directly in front of the talker. Recordings of the stimulus lists were made using a tape recorder (Ampex AG440) operated at 15 ips. The same apparatus was used for all recordings. The calibration of the tape recorder was checked immediately before and after each recording session using the National Association of Broadcasters reproduce-aligment tape. The playback response of the tape recorder was found to be within ± 2 dB of the manufacturer's specifications during each of these calibration checks.

Tape recordings of scramblings A, B, C, and D of List 2 of CID Auditory Test W-22 served as the speech discrimination materials. All talkers used the carrier phrase *Say the word* before presenting each stimulus word. Talker 1 was recorded presenting List 2A, Talker 2 presenting List 2B, Talker 3 presenting List 2C, and Talker 4 presenting list 2D. During all presentations the complete 50-word list was recorded. A minimum of four recordings was made of each audiologist delivering the stimulus words. In all cases the first recording was discarded. It was thought that the presence of recording equipment might initially cause some talkers to alter their presentations. From the remaining presentations, one was selected randomly as representative of the MLV presentation under clinical conditions.

Any extraneous conversation such as directions to the patient, questions regarding responses, or answers to patients' questions, was cut from the tape leaving only the 50 stimulus words preceded by the carrier phrase. Each original recording was dubbed onto a separate master tape for use during this study. The interstimulus intervals ranged from 2.8 to 6 seconds for the four talkers. No attempt was made to alter the presentations in any manner.

Analysis of Intensity

Each of the four master tapes was analyzed for variations in intensity. Graphic level recordings were made using a Bruel and Kjaer 2305 graphic level recorder. The peak intensity of each stimulus word was measured, and the range and mean were computed for each talker. Talkers 1 and 4 showed a range of intensity variation of 8 dB while 2 and 3 showed a range of intensity variation of only 6 dB among the peak intensities of the stimulus words. The mean total range of intensity variation was 7 dB.

To determine whether the range of intensity variations discussed previously should be considered excessive, the identical procedure was carried out using a commercially available recorded version (Technisonic Studios) of List 2A of CID Auditory Test W-22. The test items on the recording were found to have intensity variations of 14 dB; this observation suggests a relatively high degree of homogeneity in level maintained by the talkers of this study.

Following the completion of measurements of the relative intensities of the stimulus words, a 1,000-Hz calibration tone of at least 30 seconds was placed at the beginning of each tape to permit accurate control of intensity by the experimenter. The calibration tone was recorded at the average level of the peaks of the carrier phrase for the 50 items on each tape recordings, as measured on the B & K graphic level recorder.

Subjects

Thirty adults having sensorineural hearing impairment were the subjects. There were 17 males and 13 females, who ranged in age from 27 to 79 years, with a mean age of 61.5 years. The criteria for subject selection were: (1) bilateral sensorineural hearing loss averaging at least 25 dB through the speech frequencies (500, 1,000, and 2,000 Hz) in the better ear; (2) word discrimination ability no greater than 90 percent in the ear to be tested as determined from previous MLV testing; (3) ability to tolerate speech at a sensation level of 25 dB; (4) no history of frequent or gross shifts in speech discrimination ability; and (5) native speaker of the English language.

Each subject was tested individually. The subject was seated in the test room of a two-room audiometric suite that met the American National Standards Institute (ANSI-S3.1-1960) specifications for ambient noise level.

Test Procedure and Instrumentation

An SRT was first established for the test ear using commercially available recordings of CID Auditory Test W-1 (Technisonic Studios) and the method described by Chaiklin, Font, and Dixon (1967), with the exception that 2-dB rather than 5-dB steps were used. In those individuals whose loss of sensitivity was equal in each ear and whose speech discrimination met the criterion stated previously, the stimuli were delivered to the ear for which the subject stated a preference. In no instance were the stimuli delivered to one ear if masking of the other ear would have been necessary. The record of the spondees was played at a speed of 33⅓ rpm on a turntable (Thorens, TD 124) and presented to the subject via TDH-39 headphones mounted in MX-41/AR cushions. Only one earphone was used. The stimuli were routed through a Maico MA-18 audiometer and calibrated for intensity by monitoring the prerecorded 1,000 Hz tone on the VU meter of the audiometer.

After the SRT was established, the headphones were removed and the subject was read the following instructions for the experimental task.

> You are going to hear some recordings of speakers saying a list of words. Each word will be preceded by the phrase *say the word*. You are to repeat the word you think the speaker said. If you are not sure of the word, it is all right to make a guess. Please give only one response to each word and say the words clearly into the microphone in front of you.

Each subject listened to all four talkers. A 2-minute rest period was interposed between each test. The presentation of the four different talkers was independently randomized for each listener.

The master tape of each talker was played on a tape recorder (Ampex AG440) at 15 ips. The same audiometer and earphone were used. Intensity was calibrated by monitoring the prerecorded 1,000 Hz tone on the audiometer's VU meter. Each subject listened to the stimulus tapes at a sensation level of 25 dB relative to his or her SRT.

Recording and Scoring of Responses

Listeners' oral responses to the four test lists were recorded on another tape recorder (Uher model 5500). The recorder was located in the control booth and operated by the examiner. A lavalier microphone (Shure 575SB) was placed on each subject for recording responses.

The responses of each subject were scored independently by three speech-language pathology graduate students. All scorers had thresholds of 15 dB or better through the frequency range 250–8,000 Hz, speech discrimination scores of 98 to 100 percent as measured by CID W-22, and all had at least one course in phonetics. Each scorer was provided with a typewritten score sheet containing the words on each list in the order that they were presented to each subject. The only scoring undertaken by the examiner was to indicate those items to which no response had occurred, so as to assist the scorers in maintaining position on the score sheets.

Tape recordings of subject responses were reproduced by the same Uher model 5500 tape recorder on which they had been originally recorded. The final score for each subject was determined by comparing results of the three independent judges and recording the majority response on a master score sheet. Any response scored as incorrect by at least two of the three judges was considered to be incorrect and was recorded as such.

RESULTS

The average word-discrimination scores for the 30 listeners across the four talkers ranged from 38 percent to 96.5 percent. The absolute range of scores

was from a low of 30 percent to a high of 100 percent. The score of 100 percent occurred even though one of the criteria for subject selection was a word-discrimination score of 90 percent or less on previous MLV testing. It should be noted, however, that of the 120 presentations, only a single listener made a perfect score on one of the presentations.

A total of 1,235 responses were scored as incorrect by either two or more of the judges. Only 46 of these were items to which there had been no response by subjects. Of the remaining 1,189 responses, 1,060 (89.2 percent) were judged as incorrect by all three judges and 129 (10.8 percent) were judged as incorrect by only two judges, indicating high agreement among the judges.

Table 32-1 displays the frequency of errors for each stimulus word as a function of talker. Included are all incorrect responses including nonresponses. Eleven words were incorrect on more than 40 of the 120 presentations (*else, cap, rooms, knee, bin, buy, off, thin, gave, does,* and *pew*). These 11 words accounted for 45.16 percent of the total errors. Although not a single word was recognized correctly by all listeners on every list, four to six words presented

TABLE 32-1. SUMMARY OF ERRORS MADE FOR EACH WORD OF LIST 2 OF CID W-22 FOR FOUR DIFFERENT TALKERS. WORDS PRESENTED IN ORDER OF MOST TO LEAST DIFFICULTY.

Stimulus Word	Talker 1	2	3	4	Total Errors	Stimulus Word	Talker 1	2	3	4	Total Errors
else	19	21	19	15	74	tare	5	6	3	7	21
cap	18	7	16	24	65	chest	5	4	7	4	20
rooms	15	14	16	8	53	ill	6	6	7	1	20
knee	4	12	17	16	49	own	2	7	4	6	19
bin	9	12	14	12	47	air	3	1	7	7	18
buy	5	2	29	11	47	dumb	3	5	4	6	18
off	12	9	14	12	47	oak	14	2	2	2	18
gave	13	5	14	14	46	star	4	3	5	3	15
does	6	13	13	12	44	and	1	4	7	4	16
pew	11	10	10	11	42	tree	2	1	3	7	13
thin	9	11	17	5	42	way	3	4	3	3	13
case	5	9	16	8	38	hit	2	1	8	1	12
ale	12	8	10	9	34	live	0	3	4	3	10
ham	6	7	8	10	31	new	6	1	2	1	10
with	6	8	14	3	31	show	3	3	4	0	10
ice	0	7	16	7	30	smart	2	3	2	3	10
send	4	10	5	11	30	your	4	0	0	6	10
then	2	7	7	11	27	young	0	0	4	3	7
key	3	6	6	11	26	hurt	2	1	0	3	6
cars	4	8	8	5	25	too	1	4	0	1	6
that	6	3	10	6	25	well	0	2	2	2	6
pie	8	3	7	6	24	one	3	1	0	1	5
move	8	2	9	5	24	now	0	0	1	3	4
jaw	10	1	6	5	22	eat	2	0	0	0	2
flat	5	0	13	3	21	odd	2	0	0	0	2

SPEECH AUDIOMETRY

by each talker were identified correctly by all listeners. Only 13 of the 50 stimulus words were missed a total of 10 times or less (*odd, eat, now, one, too, hurt, young, new, show, smart, well, your,* and *live*) and these accounted for only 7.4 percent of the total errors. The results substantiate those of Campbell (1965), who carried out a similar study using hearing-impaired listeners and the CID W-22 recorded auditory tests. He reported that the words were not all of equal difficulty and presented a listing of the words ranked in order of difficulty based on the number of errors that had been observed for each word. Even though the stimulus words in this study were spoken by four different talkers and were presented at a lower sensation level, many of the test items appear at the same general location with respect to degree of difficulty.

Statistical Analysis of the Data

A repeated measures analysis of variance (ANOVA) was done on the word-discrimination scores obtained across the four different talkers. The results of the ANOVA were not significant at the 0.05 level ($F = 2.23$, $df = 3/116$, $p < 0.08$). Although the means of the four conditions are not significantly different statistically, there are large variations present across individual subjects. Table 32–2 presents the

TABLE 32–2. SUMMARY OF DISCRIMINATION SCORES FOR EACH OF 30 LISTENERS ACROSS 4 DIFFERENT TALKERS. MEANS AND STANDARD DEVIATIONS FOR EACH LISTENER ACROSS ALL TALKERS AND FOR ALL LISTENERS ACROSS EACH TALKER. MAXIMUM VARIATION IS THE PERCENTAGE DIFFERENCE BETWEEN EACH LISTENER'S LOWEST AND HIGHEST DISCRIMINATION SCORE ON CID W-22 LIST 2 OBTAINED ACROSS THE 4 TALKERS.

Listener	Talker 1	Talker 2	Talker 3	Talker 4	$\overline{X}$	SD	Maximum Variation
1.*	74	90	92	98	88.5	10.24	24
2.*	80	70	66	42	64.5	16.11	38
3.	70	74	58	76	69.5	8.06	18
4.*	90	88	90	74	85.5	7.72	16
5.	76	88	78	78	80.0	5.42	12
6.	88	78	76	90	83.0	7.02	14
7.	80	86	72	74	78.0	6.32	14
8.	86	84	84	92	86.5	3.78	8
9.*	70	66	48	60	61.0	9.59	22
10.*	84	82	52	50	67.0	18.51	34
11.	90	98	96	96	95.0	3.46	8
12.*	74	86	60	70	72.5	10.75	26
13.	96	98	98	94	96.5	1.91	4
14.*	88	70	82	94	83.5	10.24	24
15.*	84	70	64	84	75.5	10.11	20
16.*	88	96	80	80	86.0	7.66	16
17.	78	86	70	82	79.0	6.83	16
18.	66	74	60	62	65.5	6.19	14
19.*	84	88	70	92	83.5	9.57	22
20.	82	86	80	90	84.5	4.43	8
21.	92	90	78	88	87.0	6.21	12
22.*	76	88	60	56	70.0	14.78	32
23.	94	94	92	88	92.0	2.82	6
24.	70	72	74	80	74.0	4.32	10
25.	90	92	88	90	90.0	1.63	4
26.*	76	84	60	78	74.5	10.25	24
27.*	94	100	86	94	93.5	5.74	14
28.	90	80	88	84	85.5	4.43	10
29.	48	40	30	34	38.0	7.83	18
30.	92	98	94	96	95.0	2.58	6
	$X = 81.67$ $SD = 10.47$	$X = 83.20$ $SD = 12.50$	$X = 74.20$ $SD = 16.09$	$X = 78.87$ $SD = 16.71$			

*Scores achieved between two or more talkers exceeded the upper or lower limits of the 95 percent critical differences for percentage scores as presented by Thornton and Raffin (1978).

listener by talker scores and means and standard deviations for individual listeners across all talkers and for all listeners across each talker.

Only four of the 30 listeners had variations between their lowest and highest word-discrimination scores of 6 percent or less. The range of variation for the remaining 26 listeners was from 8 percent to 38 percent and the average maximum variation was 18.23 percent. Such excessive differences in scores are clearly not within the range of acceptable clinical variation as defined earlier.

Additional strong support of excessive variation is apparent when the scores presented in Table 32–2 are compared to Thornton and Raffin's (1978) criteria for statistical differences between speech discrimination scores. In their study, the performance of subjects on CID Auditory Test W-22 was modeled as a binomial variable. Based on 4120 test administrations, a model was devised that provides confidence intervals for determining the presence of significant differences between scores. Application of their criteria to the scores of the subjects in this study reveals that 43 percent (13 of 30 subjects) of the subjects had scores falling outside the suggested confidence intervals (critical difference) for the 95 percent limits. Of 180 possible comparisons between pairs of scores, 29 or 16 percent were different beyond the 0.05 level.

It is clear that there is substantial variability among the word-discrimination abilities of the different subjects as evidenced by their wide range of scores. It is the amount of within-subject variability, however, that must be considered. If excessive within-subject variability exists, large differences could be present across the scores attained by each of the listeners but group means might be relatively unaffected. If the variability were spread across all four talkers, this pattern could account for nonsignificant differences in means for talkers. This pattern is apparently present and is an accurate description of the distribution of scores for the subjects of this study. Individual variability is clearly discernible in Table 32–2.

The data were reanalyzed using a two-way ANOVA without replication, and are reported in Table 32–3. When the sum of squares for listeners, which accounted for 73.8 percent of the total variance, was subtracted from the sum of squares for residual, there remained the more appropriate error term of talker-listener interaction. This accounts for 20.5 percent of the variance and resulted in an F ratio of 8.02, which is significant beyond the 0.01 level. Only 5.7 percent of the variance could be attributed to the talkers.

A Spearman rank-order correlation coefficient was calculated to determine if there was any relationship between variations in listeners' scores and each listener's average word-discrimination score. A coefficient of correlation of -0.63 was obtained. A correction factor was used because of the large number of tied ranks. A test of significance was completed on this correlation. The resultant t of -4.29 is significant beyond the 0.01 level of confidence ($df = 28$, $p < 0.01$). This observation indicates that there is a greater probability of observing larger variations in discrimination scores for patients with poor word discrimination. A similar finding was reported by Beattie, Svihovec, and Edgerton (1978) in a study comparing half- and full-list intelligibility scores. They reported that variability in scores was greatest for subjects in the 30–70 percent range and least for those near the extremes of 0 and 100 percent. Thornton and Raffin (1978) also reported a corresponding increase in variability for scores within the middle range and less variation at the extremes.

DISCUSSION

This study indicates that considerable variability exists in the word-discrimination scores of sensorineural-hearing-loss subjects on a single word list when it is presented by different talkers. Clinically significant variations (for this study taken to be ≥ 8 percent) occurred for 26 of the 30 subjects. Differ-

TABLE 32–3. ANALYSIS OF VARIANCE.

Source	ss	df	F	Significance of F	Proportion of Variation
Talker	1,406.233	3	2.33	NS	5.7%
Listener	18,226.967	29	10.76	<0.01	73.8%
Talker-Listener	5,082.767	87	8.02	<0.01	20.5%
Total	24,715.967	119	—	—	100%

ences in scores could not be attributed to a single talker but were apparent for all talkers. The observed tendency for variability to increase with lower word-discrimination scores indicates a greater probability of observing larger variations when testing individuals with generally reduced word-discrimination ability. This finding also suggests the need for sampling such individuals' word-discrimination ability on more than a single presentation. Also, it seems that greater test-retest reliability can be expected using MLV when word discrimination scores are near the maximum value of 100 percent.

Although large variation in word-discrimination scores is apparent for the majority of the subjects in this study, the primary factor responsible for the variability does not seem to be the talker but rather talker-listener interaction. If only one of the talkers were different, then it would be expected that errors could be consistently ascribed to that talker. The data in this study offer no support for this premise as the variability is spread across all talkers. Apparently there is some factor or factors that make the identifi-

cation of a particular word by a given talker very difficult for some listeners but not for others. At present, there is no evidence to suggest what factor or factors might be responsible for this variability.

Campbell (1965) believes that the greatest reliability of measurement is needed for those with discrimination scores in the 30 to 90 percent range. He commented on the effects that variations in scores might have on surgical decisions, recommendations for amplification, aural rehabilitation efforts, and the like. Such decisions could be inordinately difficult in the presence of extremely variable scores such as those seen in this study. The large differences in the scores across individual subjects clearly reflect the need for a standardized presentation.

ACKNOWLEDGMENT

This article is based on a doctoral dissertation completed under the direction of Lloyd L. Price.

REFERENCES

American National Standards Institute. Criteria for background noise in audiometer rooms. New York: ANSI S3.1–1960 (1960).

Asher, W. J. Intelligibility tests: A review of their standardization, some experiments, and a new test. *Speech Monographs, 25,* 14–28 (1958).

Beattie, R. C.; Svihovec, D. A.; and Edgerton, B. J. Comparison of speech detection and spondee thresholds and half-versus full-list intelligibility scores with MLV and taped presentations of NU-6. *J. Am. Aud. Soc., 3,* 267–272 (1978).

Brandy, William T. Reliability of voice tests of speech discrimination. *J. Speech Hearing Res., 9,* 461–465 (1966).

Campbell, R. A. Discrimination test word difficulty. *J. Speech Hearing Res., 8,* 13–22 (1965).

Carhart, R. A. Monitored live-voice as a test of auditory acuity. *J. Acoust. Soc. Am., 17,* 338–349 (1946).

Carhart, R. Problems in the measurement of speech discrimination. *Arch. Otolar., 82,* 253–260 (1965).

Chaiklin, J. B.; Font, J.; and Dixon, R. F. Spondee thresholds measured in ascending 5-dB steps. *J. Speech Hearing Res., 10,* 141–145 (1967).

Fletcher, H. A method of calculating hearing loss for speech from the audiogram. *Acta Otolaryng. Sup., 90,* 26–37 (1950).

Goetzinger, C. P. Word discrimination testing. In J. Katz (Ed.), *Handbook of Clinical Audiology.* Baltimore: Williams & Wilkins (1972).

Harris, J. D.; Haines, H. L.; and Myers, C. K. A new formula for using the audiogram to predict speech hearing loss. *Arch. Otolar., 64,* 447 (1956).

Hughson, W., and Thompson, E. Correlation of hearing acuity for speech with discrete frequency audiograms. *Arch. Otolar., 36,* 526–540 (1942).

Kreul, E. J.; Bell, D. W.; and Nixon, J. C., Factors affecting speech discrimination test difficulty. *J. Speech Hearing Res., 12,* 281–287 (1969).

Palmer, John M., The effect of speaker differences on the intelligibility of phonetically balanced word lists. *J. Speech Hearing Dis., 20,* 192–195 (1955).

Resnick, D. M. Reliability of the twenty-five word phonetically balanced lists. *J. Aud. Res., 2,* 5–12 (1962).

Sieganthaler, B. M., and Strand, R. Audiogram average methods and SRT scores. *J. Acoust. Soc. Am., 36,* 589–593 (1964).

Silverman, S. R., and Hirsh, I. J. Problems related to the use of speech in clinical audiometry. *Ann. Otol. Rhin. Laryng., 64,* 1,234–1,244 (1955).

Thornton, A. R., and Raffin, M. J. M. Speech discrimination scores modeled as a binomial variable. *J. Speech Hearing Res.,* **21,** 507–518 (1978).

Tillman, T. W., and Olsen, W. O. Speech audiometry. In J. Jerger (Ed.), *Modern Developments in Audiology.* New York: Academic Press (1973).

33

Writedown Versus Talkback Scoring and Scoring Bias in Speech Discrimination Testing

DAVID A. NELSON, Ph.D.
Associate Professor, Departments of Otolaryngology and Communication Disorders, University of Minnesota, Minneapolis, Minnesota
JOSEPH B. CHAIKLIN, Ph.D.
Supervisor, Audiology Section, VA Medical Center, New Orleans, Louisiana

Writdown and talkback responses to 500 Hz low-pass filtered CID W-22 words were obtained from eight listeners, and their talkback responses were scored by eight experienced and eight inexperienced examiners. Four of the experienced and four of the inexperienced examiners monitored at 70 dB SPL; four experienced and four inexperienced examiners monitored at 60 dB SPL. Comparison of talkback discrimination scores (DSs) with corresponding writedown DSs revealed: (1) Inexperienced examiners awarded significantly higher mean talkback DSs than the mean writedown DS; i.e., they showed a mean correct bias. (2) Experienced examiners produced talkback DSs that were not significantly different from the mean writedown DS. (3) Decreasing the monitoring level from 70 to 60 dB SPL increased inexperienced examiners' mean correct bias but the experienced examiners' mean talkback DSs did not change significantly with monitoring level. (4) Inexperienced examiners made more scoring errors than experienced examiners at both monitoring levels. (5) Most examiners in both groups made both correct bias and incorrect bias scoring errors to produce a net effect on the talkback DS. (6) Distributions of DS differences show individual differences between talkback and writedown DSs as large as +16 percent and −20 percent and frequent differences of ±6 percent, even when the mean DS difference between scoring methods was negligible.

Lovrinic, Burgi, and Curry's (1968) recent investigation of five speech discrimination tests led them to suggest, ". . . verbal responses should be abandoned in favor of written responses." They found differences between discrimination scores (DSs) obtained clinically with verbal (talkback) scoring procedures and DSs obtained experimentally from the same subjects with written (writedown) scoring procedures. The DS differences were in excess of 10 percent in

"at least three" of the 30 cases examined, and in those three cases talkback response scores were higher than writedown scores. They concluded, ". . . it seems possible that the tester is more inclined to hear a correct than an incorrect response in questionable instances. . . ." We will use the term *correct scoring bias* to describe the inclination to overestimate correct responses and the term *incorrect scoring bias* to describe the tendency to score correct responses incorrectly.

Lovrinic, Burgi, and Curry are not alone in their observation of correct scoring bias. Merrell and

Reprinted by permission of the authors from *J. Speech Hearing Res.*, **13**, 645–654 (1970).

Atkinson (1965) compared DSs obtained with both writedown and talkback scoring procedures. They had a 25-member panel (two audiologists and 23 inexperienced examiners) score the tape-recorded talkback responses of a 64-year-old male patient who had responded to recordings of CID W-22 test words. They found that DSs obtained with a talkback scoring procedure were an average of 8.88 percent higher than DSs obtained with a writedown procedure—a result suggesting a correct scoring bias for their predominantly inexperienced scoring panel. An examination of the Merrell and Atkinson data reveals individual talkback-writedown DS differences as great as 20 percent. Merrell and Atkinson also found fewer scoring errors when their examiners viewed a printed list of the stimulus words during the scoring process.

It is possible that Merrell and Atkinson's 8.88 percent mean DS difference was influenced by the fact that the majority of their examiners were inexperienced with the scoring procedures and stimulus words, in contrast with the usual clinical situation in which examiners are familiar with stimulus and scoring procedures.

In addition, Merrell and Atkinson's results may have been influenced by their examiners' monitoring (scoring) levels. Each of their examiners adjusted the monitoring level to his own "comfort level." The resulting levels were not reported, but if some examiners scored the talkback responses at less than optimum listing levels, they might have been more prone to make listening errors, including both correct and incorrect bias errors.

Finally, an emphasis on talkback-writedown mean DS differences in the studies discussed above, may have obscured the relative effects of correct and incorrect scoring bias on individual DSs. To illustrate, if an examiner exhibits correct bias on four words (+8 percent) and incorrect bias on another four words (−8 percent) in the same list, the net biasing effect on the talkback DS would be zero because the two types of bias cancel each other. Although the resulting talkback DS is numerically equal to the true DS (i.e., the writedown DS), considerable bias operated to produce the paradoxically correct but invalidly derived DS.

In an attempt to answer some of the questions raised by previous research, the study reported here investigated correct and incorrect scoring bias through comparison of talkback and writedown scor-

ing procedures used by experienced and inexperienced examiners who monitored talkback responses at two different intensity levels.

METHOD

General Plan. Both talkback and writedown responses were obtained from eight normal-hearing young adult listeners who responded to low-pass filtered recordings of CID W-22 word lists. The listeners performed the task commonly performed by patients during speech audiometry. Their talkback responses were stored on magnetic tape.

Eight experienced and eight inexperienced examiners individually scored the tape-recorded talkback responses of the listeners. The resulting talkback DSs derived by the examiners were then compared to the writedown DSs of the listeners. Mean differences between talkback and writedown DSs, differences between types of scoring bias, and distributions of talkback-writedown DS differences were analyzed.

Listener's Responses. Tape-recorded dubs of Technisonic Studios disc recordings of CID W-22 lists 1A and 2A (Hirsh et al., 1952) were passed through a 20 dB per octave, 500 Hz, low-pass filter (Peekel, TF823) as they were presented to four male and four female adult (18–26 years) listeners who had normal hearing (15 dB HL or better, ISO 1964) at 500, 1,000, and 2,000 Hz. Stimuli were presented 40 dB above each listener's 1,000 Hz threshold as he sat in a double-wall sound-treated booth (Industrial Acoustics Co., 1202 A). The listeners responded to each of the 50 stimulus words of list 1A or list 2A by writing their responses on a score sheet, and by saying the same word aloud. Four listeners gave the writedown response before the talkback response; two of the four responded to list 1A and two responded to list 2A. The other four listeners gave the talkback response first; two of them responded to list 1A and two to list 2A. The average writedown DS for all the listeners were 49.75 percent (range = 40 percent to 62 percent).

Listeners were asked to clarify spelling errors or illegible writedown responses at the end of each test session. The writedown DS was determined for each listener by comparing writedown responses to a typewritten master list of the W-22 words.

Talkback Response Tapes. The listeners' talkback responses were recorded with an Ampex tape recorder (Model 1460) fed by a condenser microphone (Altec, 150 BR). Each talkback response recorded on the talkback tapes was preceded by an unfiltered recording of the stimulus word to which the listener had responded. Thus, the talkback response tapes later provided a stimulus format similar to the common clinical format in which a clinician (examiner) hears a recorded W-22 stimulus word in his monitor phone and then hears the patient's (listener's) talkback response to the word. The tapes contained a total of 400 stimulus-response pairs—50 pairs from each of the eight listeners.

Average maximum peak levels of the talkback responses were determined with a VU meter (Weston Electric Instrument Corp., N4-862) and a graphic level recorder (Bruel and Kjaer, 2305). The sound pressure level (SPL) of the speech peaks was estimated with a 1,000 Hz pure tone adjusted to zero VU.

Examiner Groups. Sixteen normal-hearing (see above) individuals were selected to serve as examiners to score the talkback response tapes. Eight of the examiners were highly experienced with the test words and with talkback scoring (the Experienced group), and eight were completely inexperienced with the words and talkback scoring (the Inexperienced group). The Experienced group consisted of clinical audiologists who ranged from approximately 24 to 34 years of age and had between one and eight years of full-time clinical experience involving frequent speech discrimination testing. The eight Inexperienced examiners were university students who ranged from approximately 19 to 24 years of age.

Each examiner listened individually to the talkback tapes through a single TDH-39 dynamic earphone in an MX-41/AR cushion with a dummy phone and cushion on the opposite ear as he sat in a control room that had an ambient A-weighted sound level of 40 dB and a C-weighted sound level of 58 dB measured with a sound level meter (Bruel and Kjaer, 2203). During a single session, each examiner listened to and scored four of the eight talkback response lists, received a 15-minute break, and then listened to the other four response lists.

The talkback tapes were presented at 70 dB SPL to four members of the Experienced group and to four members of the Inexperienced group, and at 60 dB SPL to the remaining examiners. Thus, the exam-

iners were divided into four groups, each group containing four examiners: Experienced-70, Experienced-60, Inexperienced-70, and Inexperienced-60.

Standard instructions were read to each examiner instructing him to compare each talkback response to its preceding unfiltered W-22 stimulus word and to make a mark for "incorrect" or "correct" on the score sheet which contained blanks numbered from 1–50; stimulus words were not printed on the score sheet. This listening arrangement is analogous to a clinical test situation in which the clinician uses an earphone to monitor the stimuli as the test progresses, but unlike the clinical situation, there was no opportunity for our examiners to use lipreading cues or to request repetition and clarification of talkback responses that were spoken or heard unclearly.

RESULTS

Mean Talkback-Writedown Differences. Mean talkback DSs and talkback-writedown mean DS differences (talkback minus writedown) for the different examiner groups are shown in Table 33–1. Since each examiner group was treated as a sample from an independent population, a t test for independent means ($df = 24$) was used to assess mean differences.

All talkback-writedown mean DS differences and intercondition differences were small (see Table 33–1), reaching statistical significance ($p = 0.05$) only for the two Inexperienced examiner groups. The 1.62 percent talkback-writedown mean DS difference exhibited by the Inexperienced-70 group increased to 4.25 percent for the Inexperienced-60 group. The 2.63 mean difference between the Inexperienced-60 and Inexperienced-70 groups was also significant ($t = 2.88$). These results indicate that as the monitoring task was made more difficult by decreasing the monitoring level from 70 dB to 60 dB SPL, the talkback-writedown mean DS difference increased, but only for the Inexperienced group.

In addition, Inexperienced examiners awarded a significantly higher mean talkback DS than Experienced examiners at both monitoring levels—2.5 percent higher at 70 dB ($t = 3.42$), and 5.25 percent higher at the 60 dB monitoring level ($t = 5.0$).

Examiner Scoring Bias. As indicated earlier, analysis of mean differences between DSs obtained with talkback and writedown scoring procedures may not tell the whole story. Underlying these differences are

TABLE 33-1. MEAN TALKBACK DISCRIMINATION SCORES (DSs), MEAN DIFFERENCES
BETWEEN TALKBACK AND WRITEDOWN DSs, STANDARD ERRORS (SE) OF THE MEAN
DIFFERENCES AND t RATIOS (df = 24) OBTAINED FROM THE FOUR EXAMINER GROUPS
(N = 4 EXAMINERS PER GROUP).

Examiner Group	Mean Talkback DS (%)	Talkback-Writedown Mean DS Difference (%)†	SE Diff.	t
Inexperienced-70	51.37	1.62	0.49	3.33**
Inexperienced-60	54.00	4.25	0.79	5.52**
Experienced-70	48.88	−0.87	0.54	1.65*
Experienced-60	48.75	−1.00	0.69	1.47*

*$p > 0.05$
**$p < 0.005$
†Mean writedown DS, 49.75 percent; writedown DS ranged from 40 percent to 62 percent.

two types of bias that have an important influence on DSs. The talkback DS reflects the net effect of these two types of bias. For example, consider the correct and incorrect bias of the Inexperienced-60 examiner group as shown in the second row of Table 33-2. Each of the four Inexperienced-60 examiners scored eight 50-item talkback tapes—a total of 400 talkback responses scored by each examiner, or 1,600 talkback responses in all. Of the 1,600 talkback responses, 112 were incorrectly scored as correct against the writedown validity criterion (7 percent correct bias). Similarly 44 of the 1,600 talkback responses were correct with the writedown method but incorrect with the talkback method (2.75 percent incorrect bias). Thus, the Inexperienced-60 group had a total of 156 scoring

bias errors; i.e., they made incorrect decisions on a total of 9.75 percent of the 1,600 talkback responses they monitored. Despite the 9.75 percent total scoring bias, the net mean difference between talkback and writedown DSs was only 4.25 percent, a discrepancy attributable to the cancelling effects of the two types of scoring bias.

An inspection of Table 33-2 shows clearly that both correct and incorrect bias were obtained from Experienced as well as Inexperienced examiners. At each monitoring level, Inexperienced examiners produced more total bias (sum of correct and incorrect bias) than Experienced examiners. Figure 33-1 shows the total bias obtained from each of the examiner groups at each monitoring level.

TABLE 33-2. SUMMARY OF SCORING BIAS OBTAINED FROM THE FOUR EXAMINER GROUPS
(N = 4 EXAMINERS PER GROUP). CORRECT BIAS IS BASED ON THE NUMBER OF RESPONSES
THAT WERE SCORED AS INCORRECT WITH WRITEDOWN SCORING BUT CORRECT WITH
TALKBACK SCORING AND IS STATED AS A PERCENTAGE OF THE TOTAL 1,600 RESPONSES
PER GROUP. INCORRECT BIAS IS BASED ON THE NUMBER OF RESPONSES THAT WERE
SCORED AS CORRECT WITH WRITEDOWN SCORING BUT INCORRECT WITH TALKBACK, AND
IS ALSO STATED AS A PERCENTAGE OF 1,600 RESPONSES PER GROUP. TOTAL BIAS IS THE
SUM OF BOTH CORRECT AND INCORRECT BIAS. NET BIAS IS THE ALGEBRAIC DIFFERENCE
BETWEEN CORRECT AND INCORRECT BIAS.

Examiner Group	Correct Bias	Incorrect Bias	Total Bias	Net Bias
Inexperienced—70 dB	4.25% (68)*	2.63% (42)	6.88% (110)	+1.62% (26)
Inexperienced—60 dB	7.00% (112)	2.75% (44)	9.75% (156)	+4.25% (68)
Experienced—70 dB	1.94% (31)	2.81% (45)	4.75% (76)	−0.87% (−14)
Experienced—60 dB	3.31% (53)	4.31% (69)	7.62% (122)	−1.00% (−16)

*Numbers in parentheses are total errors for each group per 1,600 responses.

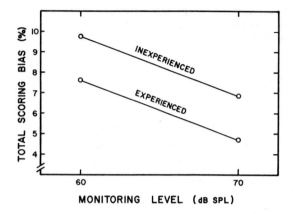

FIGURE 33-1. Total scoring bias (percent of total responses per group) obtained from the Inexperienced and Experienced examiner groups. Total scoring bias is the sum of correct and incorrect scoring bias disregarding the opposite effects the two types of bias have on the talkback discrimination score.

It can be seen in Figure 33-1 that, regardless of monitoring level, Inexperienced examiners made consistently more errors than Experienced examiners in making decisions about the correctness of talkback responses. Figure 33-1 also shows that examiners consistently made more errors at the more difficult 60 dB SPL monitoring level, regardless of their experience.

The effect of the two types of scoring bias on "net scoring bias" is slightly more complicated. It appears from the data in Table 33-2 that two bias patterns underlie the Inexperienced examiners' net bias: (1) Inexperienced examiners made more correct bias errors than incorrect bias errors—more so at 60 dB than at 70 dB SPL; and (2) Inexperienced examiners' incorrect bias remained small and nearly constant with monitoring level. Since their incorrect bias remained nearly constant with monitoring level, and their correct bias increased at the 60 dB monitoring level, there was proportionately greater net correct bias at the 60 dB level.

On the other hand, Experienced examiners produced nearly equal amounts of correct and incorrect bias at both the 60 dB and 70 dB monitoring levels. The effect of decreasing monitoring level from 70 dB to 60 dB was to increase both types of scoring bias almost equally so that the net scoring bias was very small and nearly identical at both monitoring levels. Thus, the net effect of the 3.31 percent correct bias and the 4.31 percent incorrect bias for the Expe-

rienced-60 examiners was only −1.0 percent, and the net effect of the 1.94 percent correct bias and the 2.81 percent incorrect bias for the Experienced-70 group was −0.87 percent.

From the results presented above, one can make inferences only about the types of talkback scoring errors to expect from groups of examiners, rather than from single examiners. In application, one is frequently concerned with a particular examiner and how he scores a particular patient's talkback responses. The following analysis of the distribution of talkback-writedown DS differences obtained by the examiners in this study gives some indication of the discrepancy one might expect between talkback and writedown scoring procedures for a single speech discrimination test.

Distribution of Talkback-Writedown Differences. The frequency histograms in Figure 33-2 summarize the distributions of talkback-writedown DS differences for each examiner group. Recall that each examiner group produced 32 talkback-writedown difference scores, i.e., the four examiners of each group scored one test from each of eight listeners. A positive sign on the abscissa indicates that the talkback DS was higher than the writedown DS and that there was a net correct scoring bias. A negative sign indicates a net incorrect scoring bias. For example, Figure 33-2 shows that the Experienced-70 group yielded 0 percent talkback-writedown difference on only 7 of the 32 tests they scored, and the Inexperienced-70 group yielded 0 percent difference on 5 of the 32 tests they scored.

There is considerable spread in the talkback-writedown DS differences, especially for the examiners who monitored at the most difficult monitoring level. The range of differences was 18 percent for examiners who monitored at 70 dB SPL and 26 percent for examiners who monitored at 60 dB SPL. Interestingly, the ranges were identical for the Inexperienced and Experienced groups. Note that all examiner groups, even the Experienced groups had talkback-writedown differences greater than ±10 percent and that differences of ±6 percent were common even though the mean talkback-writedown difference was relatively small.

The talkback-writedown differences were distributed among all of the examiners in each examiner group, and were not simply the product of only one or two examiners consistently making large scoring bias errors. For example, the thirteen +6 per-

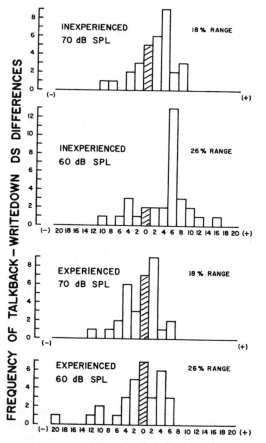

FIGURE 33-2. Distributions of talkback-writedown discrimination-score (DS) differences. A DS difference is the difference between a DS obtained with the talkback scoring procedure and the corresponding DS obtained with the writedown procedure. Each of four examiners in a group scored talkback responses from each of eight listeners to obtain a total of 32 possible DS differences per examiner group. A positive sign on the abscissa indicates that the talkback DS was higher than the writedown DS (the net correct scoring bias); a negative sign on the abscissa indicates net incorrect scoring bias. The range of talkback-writedown differences is shown for each examiner group.

cent-writedown differences produced by the Inexperienced-60 group were distributed among the four examiners as follows: 3, 4, 2, 4; the nine +4 percent talkback-writedown differences produced by the Inexperienced-70 group were distributed: 3, 2, 2, 2.

DISCUSSION

The mean differences between talkback and writedown DSs in this study (−0.87 percent to 4.25 percent) are smaller than the 8.88 percent mean difference reported by Merrell and Atkinson (1965). Our results indicate that differences in monitoring level may account for a portion of the interstudy difference; hence it seems reasonable to conjecture that other sources of increased discrimination-task difficulty, such as a patient's poor articulation, or noise in a talkback monitoring system, might increase the inexperienced examiners' talkback-writedown DS differences in the same direction.

Our results support Merrell and Atkinson's finding that correct bias occurs in speech discrimination testing when a talkback scoring procedure is used. While Merrell and Atkinson reported that their inexperienced examiners did not perform differently from their experienced examiners, we found that correct bias occurred more often and to a greater extent with our inexperienced examiners. However, since experienced examiners usually administer clinical discrimination tests, the preponderance of correct bias shown by our inexperienced examiners probably does not constitute sufficient evidence for complete abandonment of talkback scoring procedures. In addition, we found little *average* difference between talkback and writedown results when our experienced examiners scored talkback responses in relatively ideal acoustic conditions (a monitoring system with a high signal-to-noise ratio, and stimuli at or above 70 dB SPL).

But one should not conclude that a single talkback DS will not be biased when an experienced examiner scores the talkback responses, even under ideal acoustic monitoring conditions. The distributions of talkback-writedown differences shown in Figure 33-2 illustrate the difficulty of generalization to an individual talkback DS. Some DSs were influenced by a preponderance of either correct or incorrect bias, occasionally as great as 16 percent or 20 percent and frequently between 4 percent and 10 percent, even in the Experienced group. In a clinical setting, bias of this magnitude is a serious source of error to add to the inherent unreliability of the test itself.

On the basis of the distributions of talkback-writedown differences discussed here, one may conclude that there is danger of clinically significant scoring bias even with experienced examiners. The range of net scoring bias is large enough to cause serious concern about the clinical use of talkback responses.

An examiner probably can minimize the effects of talkback scoring bias if he requests patients to repeat, spell, or clarify in some other manner, all talkback responses that sound even slightly ambiguous. The poorer a patient's articulation, the more urgent the need for caution with the talkback method. On the other hand, effective use of clarification through repetition presumes an examiner who has a keen respect for test validity, a strong appreciation of the fallibility of his own perceptions, and more than average patience. The need for repetition may be reduced by eliminating examiner distractions, favorable placement of the patient's microphone, adequate monitoring levels, and by watching the patient's face as he responds.

A factor not investigated in this study is the effect of the absolute value of the writedown DS on scoring bias. If an examiner has a tendency to give the patient the benefit of the doubt (correct scoring bias), he has an opportunity to do this only on those talkback responses which are incorrect by the writedown scoring procedure. As the writedown DS increases from 50 percent to 90 percent for a 50-item test, the number of talkback responses on which the examiner has an opportunity to make a correct bias error decreases from 25 to 5. Similarly, the number of talkback responses on which he has an opportunity to make an incorrect bias error increases from 25 to 45. If one assumes that his inherent tendency to make one type of bias error as opposed to another remains constant, i.e., that his criterion for making the correctness decision about the talkback response does not change, then the relative amounts of correct and incorrect bias obtained might change markedly depending upon the absolute value of the writedown DS. The mean writedown DS in this study was 49.75 percent, as close to 50 percent as we could obtain. We suggest that further investigation is needed to determine the constancy of examiner bias for different values of writedown DSs.

With the evidence at hand, the talkback versus writedown scoring controversy is not completely settled. We have shown examiner experience and monitoring level to be critical variables. Merrell and Atkinson have shown that mean scoring bias is influenced by the examiner having the test words in front of him while he scores TB responses. Visual cues (lipreading) may also be valuable in reducing testing bias, particularly when the acoustic monitoring conditions are poor. These variables should be, but sometimes are not, accounted for in a clinical setting.

ACKNOWLEDGMENT

This article is based on a master's project completed by Nelson under the direction of Chaiklin at the University of Minnesota, Department of Speech Science, Speech Pathology and Audiology.

REFERENCES

Hirsh, I. J.; Davis H.; Silverman, S. R.; Reynolds, E. G.; Eldert, E.; and Benson, R. W. Development of materials for speech audiometry. *J. Speech Hearing Dis.*, **17**, 321–337 (1952).

Lovrinic, J. H.; Burgi, E. J.; and Curry, E. T. A comparative evaluation of five speech discrimination measures. *J. Speech Hearing Res.*, **11**, 372–381 (1968).

Merrell, H. B., and Atkinson, C. J. The effect of selected variables upon discrimination scores. *J. Aud. Res.*, **5**, 285–292 (1965).

part IV

MASKING

Masking is generally defined as the temporary elevation of a listener's threshold for one sound or signal by the presence of a second sound (a masker). The need for masking in clinical audiometry is based on two facts: (1) an intense stimulus delivered to an earphone applied to one ear may cross to the opposite ear via bone conduction, via air conduction, or via both routes; and (2) bone-conducted signals tend to stimulate both cochleas simultaneously, frequently at equal or nearly equal intensities. These two circumstances sometimes make it difficult to know which ear is being stimulated. Fortunately, a considerable body of empirical and experimental data defines the bases for determining when signals intended for one ear have reached the opposite ear and for applying masking noises to counteract the unintended stimulation.

Clinical masking is one of the most complex audiometric procedures to understand and execute because it involves so many variables that often operate simultaneously. Masker spectrum, minimum masking levels, interaural attenuation, central masking, and the occlusion effect represent a partial listing of the variables that must be considered. The six articles in this section address most of the important variables that one must understand in order to carry out masking procedures during basic audiologic evaluations. On the other hand, even careful study of the six selections is unlikely to enable a novice to mask confidently. Intensive classroom discussion and one-to-one clinical supervision must supplement the reading, but even then clinical masking will not become automatic. On the contrary, the more one understands the sources of error in clinical masking the less chance there is that it will become perfunctory.

Sanders and Rintelmann's study, retained from the first edition, introduces the basic problem confronted in clinical masking and examines the relative efficiency of three basic maskers—sawtooth noise, white noise, and narrow-band noise. Sawtooth noise was a far more common noise source in 1964 than it is now, but understanding the reason for its inefficiency is still useful for theoretical understanding and because there are many portable audiometers in use that have, as their only masking source, sawtooth noise or a noise with a similar low-frequency spectrum.

Chaiklin's study of interaural attenuation during air-conduction pure-tone audiometry is included again because it provides normative data on interaural attenuation for all the standard octave and interoctave air-conduction frequencies. These data are essential to determine the need for masking in air-conduction audiometry and to estimate maximum permissible masking levels for air- and bone-conduction tests. In this regard, Chaiklin emphasizes the importance of knowing the substantial range of intersubject differences for interaural attenuation and the need to use the low end of this range to gauge when cross-hearing (or overmasking) *may* occur, a principle that recurs in other selections in this part. This article is also of interest because of its treatment of the mechanism of cross-hearing and interaural attenuation, showing that during air-conduction audiometry, stimuli cross to the opposite ear via bone conduction when the stimuli reach critical high intensities. In effect, the earphone becomes simultaneously an air- and bone-conduction transducer, but Chaiklin cautions that data from his study and from other normative studies should be generalized only in relation to comparable measurement variables such as type of earphone and earphone cushion, physical status of the opposite ear, and whether one or both ears are covered by earphones.

The next selection, Coles and Priede's comprehensive treatment of the serious implications of errors in clinical masking, provides additional normative data on interaural attenuation. It discusses the relative merits of different paradigms for clinical masking, with special emphasis on Hood's (1960) shadowing method. Coles and Priede present the essence of clinical masking without the common oversimplifications that can produce grossly inaccurate results.

Studebaker's article on clinical masking of the nontest ear is included again for its orderly delineation of the way in which research data define the mechanisms, interactions, and limitations of specific patient and signal parameters in clinical masking. An important feature of the article is Studebaker's discussion of the relative merits of three threshold-shift masking procedures and his rationale for a method that employs initial masking levels that are higher than the starting levels in Hood's shadowing method. Greater detail concerning Studebaker's method is contained in an earlier publication by Studebaker (1964).

The next selection is Naunton's frequently-cited article concerning one of the most perplexing clinical masking problems: the patient with *apparent* bilateral conductive loss whose unmasked air- and bone-conduction thresholds dictate the need for minimum masking levels intense enough to stimulate both cochleas simultaneously. This creates a ''masking dilemma'' in which the test ear may receive the masker that should be confined to the nontest (masked) ear. Naunton's thought-provoking discussion and empirical data deserve careful study. The reader exposed to the concept of the masking dilemma for the first time should recognize that in some cases the masking dilemma can be resolved. Consequently, an apparent masking dilemma should not lead the clinician to dismiss masking as futile.

The final selection in this part is Studebaker's schematic representation of the variables that influence isolation of the nontest ear during clinical masking. His brief article, although not easy reading, will reward the student or teacher who carefully studies its concise presentation of the variables that influence clinical masking. It is an article that bears rereading and discussion. As Studebaker points out, his article does not present a clinical method for masking but, rather, presents a framework that may be used to contemplate or devise clinical masking methods. The schematic itself should prove to be a valuable teaching and learning tool for unraveling an inherently complex process.

We have not included any articles concerning masking during basic speech audiometry. There have been curiously few articles published specific to masking procedures for threshold and suprathreshold speech audiometry, but a useful general background for understanding this important topic is contained in George Miller's (1947) tutorial article concerning the effects of various maskers on the intelligibility of speech.

Finally, although the emphasis in this part has been masking for basic hearing measurement, the same principles apply to advanced measurement procedures in which signals are delivered monaurally at intensities capable of crossing to the nontest ear.

REFERENCES AND ADDITIONAL READINGS

Bilger, R. C. and Hirsh, I. J. Masking of tones by bands of noise. *J. Acoust. Soc. Amer.,* **28,** 623–630 (1956).

Dirks, D. D. and Malmquist, C. W. Changes in bone-conduction thresholds produced by masking in the nontest ear. *J. Speech Hearing Res.,* **7,** 271–278 (1964).

Hawkins, J. E. and Stevens, S. S. The masking of pure-tones and of speech by white noise. *J. Acoust. Soc. Amer.,* **22,** 6–13 (1950).

Hood, J. D. The principles and practice of bone-conduction audiometry. *Laryngoscope,* **70,** 1211–1228 (1960).

Konig, E. The use of masking noise and its limitation in clinical audiometry. *Acta. Otolaryng. Suppl.,* **180** (1962).

Miller, G. A. The masking of speech. *Psych. Bull.,* **44,** 105–129 (1947).

Sanders, J. W. Masking. In *Handbook of Clinical Audiology,* 2nd ed., ed. J. Katz. Baltimore: Williams and Wilkins (1978).

Studebaker, G. A. Clinical masking of air- and bone-conducted stimuli. *J. Speech Hearing Dis.,* **29,** 23–35 (1964).

Studebaker, G. A. Clinical masking. In *Hearing Assessment,* ed. W. F. Rintelmann. Baltimore: University Park Press (1979).

34

Masking in Audiometry*

JAY W. SANDERS, Ph.D.

Professor of Audiology, Vanderbilt University, and Research Audiologist, Bill Wilkerson Hearing and Speech Center

WILLIAM F. RINTELMANN, Ph.D.

Professor and Chairman of Audiology, Department of Otorhinolaryngology and Human Communication, University of Pennsylvania School of Medicine.

THE PROBLEM

One of the major problems in audiometry is that of determining thresholds in monaural and asymmetrical binaural hearing losses. The clinician confronted with a patient whose two ears differ in acuity may have serious difficulty in obtaining accurate measures of hearing for the poorer ear. Under such circumstances, the clinician may arrive at estimates of hearing for the poorer ear that are better than the actual thresholds in that ear. Such erroneous results may even lead to attempted middle ear surgery on an ear having a profound sensorineural hearing loss.

When the two ears differ sufficiently in acuity, the intensity of the tone presented to the poorer ear may be raised to such a level that it is heard in the better ear, either across the head by air conduction or through the head by bone conduction. A number of investigators (Hood, 1960; Liden, 1954; Liden et al., 1959a; Liden et al., 1959b; Zwislocki, 1953) have shown that pure tones may cross the head by air conduction when the air conduction thresholds differ by 50 to 60 dB. On the other hand, in bone conduction testing the interaural attenuation is essentially zero (Hood, 1960; Liden, 1954; Liden et al., 1959a; Naunton, 1962; Palva, 1954). Indeed, false bone conduction thresholds for the poorer ear may be obtained at approximately the same hearing levels as the bone conduction thresholds in the better ear. Thus it is possible to obtain responses to a bone conduction stimulus at the 0 dB hearing level in a dead ear if the opposite ear has normal sensorineural acuity.

The problem is complicated still further by the fact that false air conduction thresholds at the 50 to 60 dB hearing level can be obtained in the poorer ear even when the better ear exhibits a 50 to 60 dB air conduction loss if bone conduction thresholds in the better ear are at about the 0 dB hearing level. In this instance, the test tone presented to the poorer ear by air conduction at a hearing level of 50 to 60 dB has reached an intensity level sufficient to stimulate the nontest cochlea by bone conduction.

As a result of crossover of the test tone an audiogram may be obtained for the poorer ear showing an air-bone gap with both air and bone thresholds considerably better than actual acuity in that ear.

The answer to the problem, of course, is to eliminate responses from the better ear through the use of masking noise in that ear while attempting to obtain bona fide responses from the poorer ear. The presence of a masking noise in the good ear shifts the threshold in that ear to a higher hearing level, permitting test tones of greater intensities to be presented to the poorer ear without danger of crossover. The degree of threshold shift produced in the good ear varies with the intensity of the masking noise. However, as Carhart (1960) and Naunton (1962) have pointed out, certain cases, notably patients with a conductive impairment in the better ear, pose a

This study was supported by grant NB-01310, grant NB-5329, and grant NB-1048, all from the National Institutes of Health, Public Health Service.

Reprinted by permission of the authors from *Arch. Otolaryngol.*, **80**, 541–556 (1964). Copyright 1964, American Medical Association.

special problem in masking. The effect on the cochlear sensitivity and thus on the bone conduction threshold of a masking noise applied to a conductively deafened ear is reduced by the amount of the air-bone gap present in that ear. A masking noise at a 50 dB effective level for the normal ear[1] when put into an ear with a 40 dB conductive loss will shift the air conduction threshold in that ear to a hearing level of 50 dB but will only shift the bone conduction threshold to a hearing level of 10 dB. Since many commercially available audiometers do not produce much more than 50 dB of effective masking, false threshold measurements for a poorer ear may be obtained in conductive hearing losses even when the maximum amount of masking available is applied to the better ear. Thus it may be seen that the problem of obtaining true threshold responses from a poorer ear might not be overcome in many cases simply by putting a noise into the opposite ear. In order to avoid being misled by false audiometric results, the clinician needs to understand the relative effectiveness and the limitations of the various kinds of masking noise.

PURPOSE

The effectiveness or masking efficiency of a particular noise depends not only upon the intensity but also upon the nature of the noise. For example, previous studies (Egan and Hake, 1950; Wegel and Lane, 1924) have shown that a pure tone can be used to mask other pure tones but that over a range of test frequencies the masking efficiency of a single frequency is low compared to the efficiency of a noise composed of many frequencies. Consequently, the masking noise produced by the commercially available audiometer is usually some form of noise composed of many frequencies.

The two types of masking noise that have been used most commonly in clinical audiometry are saw-tooth noise and white noise. Recently, a third type, narrow band noise, has become available.[2] The purpose of the present study was to compare these three types of masking noise and to determine their relative efficiencies in solving the problem of eliminating false threshold responses. First, the physical characteristics of the noises were compared in order to form

a basis for understanding the masking effectiveness of each noise. Second, a comparison was made of the degree to which each type of noise shifted threshold in a normal ear. Finally, pure tone audiograms were obtained for a number of persons with impaired hearing who presented special problems in masking. In each case four audiograms were obtained, one with no masking and one with each of the three types of masking noise.

THE MASKING NOISES

Saw-Tooth Noise

Saw-tooth noise, one of the two most commonly used for masking in pure tone audiometry, is a noise in which the basic repetition rate (the fundamental frequency) is usually that of the line voltage (60 or 120 cps) and which contains only those frequencies that are multiples of the basic repetition rate. The intensities of these multiple frequencies decrease as their frequencies increase. The acoustic spectrum of the saw-tooth noise used in this study is shown in Figure 34–1. As can be seen in the figure, the fundamental frequency for this particular noise was 78 cps, and the additional frequencies present are multiples of that fundamental (156 cps, 234 cps, etc). The figure also shows that the energy systematically decreases as the frequency increases.

Noises referred to as "complex" or "square wave" noise are similar to saw-tooth noise in that they are composed of a fundamental frequency plus the components that are multiples of the fundamental.

White Noise

White noise, sometimes referred to as thermal noise, and also frequently used as a masking noise in pure tone audiometry, is a noise containing all of the frequencies in the audible spectrum at approximately equal intensities. However, as with any other sound delivered by a transducer, the spectrum is limited at the ear by the frequency response of the earphone. As shown in Figure 34–2, the acoustic spectrum through the TDH-39 earphone is essentially flat out to 6,000 cps but drops rapidly beyond that point.

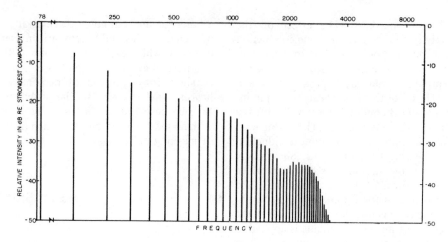

FIGURE 34-1. The acoustic spectrum of a saw-tooth noise through a PDR-8 earphone.

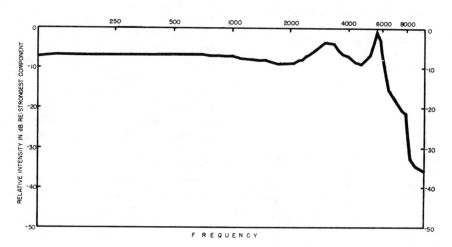

FIGURE 34-2. The acoustic spectrum of a broad band white noise through a TDH-39 earphone.

Narrow Band Noise

Although narrow band noise has only recently become available on American audiometers, a number of investigators (Dirks, 1963; Egan and Hake, 1950; Jerger et al., 1960; Liden et al., 1959b; Studebaker, 1962) have used narrow bands of noise for masking in experimental studies. Actually, the concept of masking with narrow bands of noise was suggested by Fletcher's work in the formulation of the critical band hypothesis (Fletcher, 1940; Fletcher and Munson, 1937). Fletcher pointed out that in masking with thermal noise, the only components of the noise that have any masking effect are those whose frequencies lie within a narrow band around the frequency of the test tone and that, when the tone is just audible against the noise background, the total acoustic power of the components within that narrow band is the same as that of the pure tone. Fletcher defined this restricted range of frequencies as the critical band. The results of further investigations (Bilger and Hirsh, 1956; Egan and Hake, 1950;

Hawkins and Stevens, 1950) have supported the critical band hypothesis.

Narrow band noise is produced by selectively filtering white noise and may be defined as a cluster of frequencies encompassed in a restricted range. The frequency around which the cluster is grouped and the width of the frequency range are matters of choice. A given narrow band of noise may be described in terms of its band width and its rejection rates. The width of the band is defined as the span of frequencies whose energies are no more than 3 dB below that of the peak component, and the rejection rate is defined as the decrease in intensity over a one-octave range on either side of the band.

For maximum masking efficiency, a narrow band must be at least as wide as the critical band defined by Fletcher. As the band width increases beyond the critical width, masking efficiency decreases in that the additional energy present does not contribute to masking. Although the overall level of the noise is raised by the energy present in frequencies beyond the critical band width, the level of masking produced by the noise remains the same. The band widths and rejection rates of the six narrow bands used in this study are shown in Figure 34–3. The band widths, determined at the level 3 dB down from the peak intensity, are all greater than the critical band widths for the different frequencies.

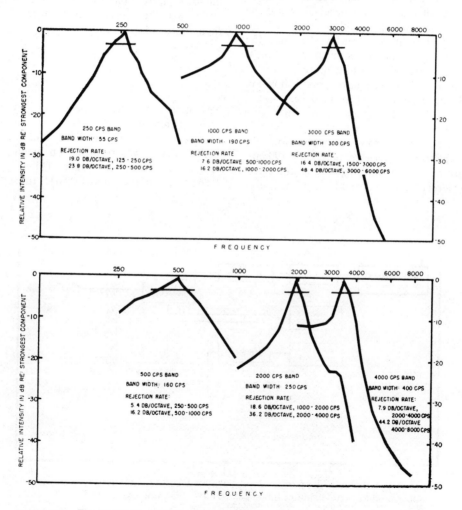

FIGURE 34-3. The acoustic spectra of six narrow bands of noise through a hearing aid type receiver.

Comment

A comparison of the acoustic spectra shown in Figures 34–1 and 34–2 leads to the theoretical expectation that white noise has greater masking efficiency than saw-tooth noise, at least in the highest frequencies. As shown in the figures, most of the energy in the saw-tooth noise is concentrated in the lower portion of the frequency range, whereas white noise has its energy spread uniformly throughout the range from 100 to 6,000 cps. A consideration of Figure 34–3 leads to the further theoretical expectation that, for equal energy delivered to the ear, narrow band noise is more efficient than either of the other two types when the narrow band is matched in frequency to the pure tone it masks. This occurs because the narrow band noise concentrates all of its energy into a limited range of frequencies clustered around the frequency of the pure tone to be masked. To illustrate, suppose we take the white noise shown in Figure 34–2 and the 1,000 cps narrow band shown in Figure 34–3 and produce each at an overall sound pressure level of 80 dB. The energy of the white noise would be distributed over a range of approximately 6,000 cps, whereas the narrow band noise would be the same energy spread over essentially only 190 cps. According to the critical band hypothesis, the effective masking level of a noise depends upon the energy present in a restricted band of frequencies, the critical band, around the test tone, and not upon the total energy of the noise. Since the critical band width is the same for white noise and narrow band noise, the determining factor in masking is the level per cycle, that is, the intensity of each one-cycle band, rather than the overall intensity. Moreover, since the level per cycle is determined by dividing the overall intensity by the width of the noise band, it can be seen that for equal overall intensity a narrow band of noise will have a higher level per cycle than will a broad band of white noise, because the same amount of energy is spread over a much smaller range of frequencies in the narrow band. Thus, for equal overall intensity, narrow band noise with a higher level per cycle might be expected to produce more masking than white noise.

APPARATUS

The apparatus used in the present study is shown schematically in Figure 34–4. The saw-tooth noise from a commercially available audiometer (Maico, model MA-8) was recorded on magnetic tape and fed from a tape reproducer (Magnecorder, type PT63AN, amplifier model PT63J) through the auxil-

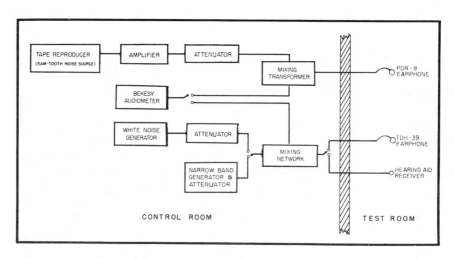

FIGURE 34-4. Schematic diagram of the apparatus used to obtain pure tone thresholds in quiet and in the presence of three different masking noises.

iary circuit of a noise generator (Grason-Stadler, model E-5539A) which served as an amplifier. The noise level was controlled with an attenuator set (Hewlett-Packard, model 350A) with impedance matching networks. A mixing transformer was used to mix the signal from the tape with the test stimulus (pulsed pure tone) from a Békésy audiometer (Grason- Stadler, model E-800). The combined signal was then transduced by a PDR-8 earphone.

The white noise used in the study was produced by a noise generator (Grason-Stadler, model E-5539A) and controlled by an attenuator set (Hewlett-Packard, model 350A) with impedance matching networks. A mixing network was used to combine the white noise with the pulsed stimulus from the Békésy audiometer, and the composite signal was then transduced by a TDH-39 earphone.

A narrow band noise generator (Amplivox prototype, not available commercially) was used to provide the narrow band noise. The noise was combined in the mixing network with the pulsed stimulus from the Békésy audiometer, and the combined signal was then transduced by a hearing aid type receiver fitted with a rubber tipped insert.

Acoustic measurements of the various masking noises and of the audiometer stimuli were made with an artificial ear assembly. The NBS-9A coupler (6 cc) was used with the PDR-8 and TDH-39 earphones, and the NBS-type 2 coupler (2 cc) was used with the insert receiver. Regular calibration checks were made throughout the period of analysis and testing to insure the stability of the equipment.

MASKING AUDIOGRAMS

To determine the relative efficiencies of the three types of noise employed in this study, masking audiograms were obtained at three different intensity levels for each type of noise with ten young, normal hearing subjects. The apparatus shown in Figure 34–4 was used in this portion of the study. For each type of noise, the masking noise and the pulsed pure tone stimuli from a Békésy audiometer were mixed into the same receiver. The subject traced his threshold for fixed frequencies in quiet and at each of three intensity levels for each type of noise. The noise levels used were 50 dB, 70 dB, and 90 dB sound pressure

level. The mean shifts in threshold were expressed as threshold shifts re: the NBS norms.

The results are shown in Figure 34–5. The curves shown in the figure are the hearing levels to which the normal ears studied were shifted by each type of noise at three different intensity levels. For instance, when the overall intensity level for each type of noise was 50 dB sound pressure level, subjects with normal hearing had their thresholds for pure tones shifted by each type of noise to the hearing levels shown in *audiogram I* of Figure 34–5. Of course, a person with impaired hearing would have his air conduction thresholds shifted to the same hearing levels as those shown for the normal ear, providing his air conduction thresholds in quiet were better than the masked thresholds.

Saw-Tooth Noise

As can be seen in Figure 34–5, saw-tooth noise produced a much greater shift in the lower frequencies than in the highs. This is reasonable when one remembers the acoustic spectrum of the saw-tooth noise. As Figure 34–1 shows, most of the energy in the saw-tooth noise was concentrated in the lower frequencies. By 3,000 cps the noise level is 43 dB below that of the peak intensity at the fundamental.

Also shown in Figure 34–5 is the non-linearity of obtained masking with saw-tooth noise. That is, a given increase in the intensity of the masking noise does not produce an equal increase in masking.

Since the frequency of the fundamental in a saw-tooth noise may vary from one noise generator to another, thus varying the spectrum, one might expect two different saw-tooth noises to give somewhat dissimilar masking results. To examine this possibility, the results obtained in the present study were compared with the masked thresholds for saw-tooth noise obtained by Liden (1954) and with those obtained by Palva (1954). The masking obtained with two levels of saw-tooth noise produced by four different audiometers is shown in Table 34–1. The table shows that audiometers A, B, and D produced quite similar results through 1,000 cps, whereas audiometer C produced lesser amounts of masking at these frequencies. For the higher frequencies, audiometer A produced the most masking, audiometers B and D were similar in results, and audiometer C produced the least masking.

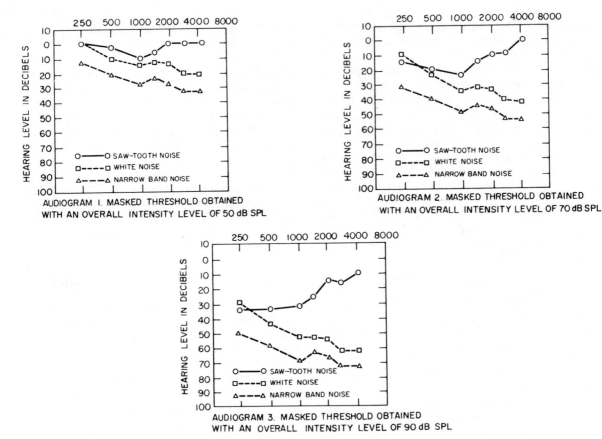

FIGURE 34-5. Masking audiograms obtained with three types of masking noise at three intensity levels.

The variability in the results obtained with four different noise generators suggests that it would be dangerous to generalize regarding masking effectiveness from one saw-tooth noise to another. However, the results of the comparison do indicate that the saw-tooth noise used in the present study (audiometer D) was not too unlike that produced by different audiometers.

White Noise

The masked audiograms obtained with white noise shown in Figure 34–5 demonstrate that white noise tends to be least effective in the lower frequencies. This occurs because the human ear is less acute in the lower frequencies.

A comparison of the masked thresholds for white noise shown in audiograms, 1, 2, and 3 of Figure 34–5 suggests that, unlike saw-tooth noise masking, the masking obtained with white noise is linear. That is, beyond a certain minimum level, each additional decibel of masking noise produces an additional 1 dB shift in threshold. This one-to-one linear relationship between noise intensity and threshold shift is not unexpected. According to Fletcher (1937), when a pure tone is just audible against the noise background, the total acoustic power of the components within the critical band surrounding the tone is the same as that of the pure tone. The effective level of the noise is the total acoustic power within the band minus the pure tone threshold in quiet. Beyond a certain minimum level we would expect to find a one-to-one relation

TABLE 34-1. SAW-TOOTH NOISE MASKING* OBTAINED IN THE PRESENT STUDY
(AUDIOMETER D) COMPARED WITH MASKING REPORTED BY LIDEN (1954) (AUDIOMETER A)
AND PALVA (1954) (AUDIOMETERS B AND C).

	250	500	1,000	2,000	3,000	4,000
Masking noise at 70 dB SPL						
Audiometer A	13.0	17.5	21.8	13.0	16.4	11.7
Audiometer B	11.3	20.0	22.2	6.0	†	5.6
Audiometer C	11.2	12.9	8.9	0.0	†	0.1
Audiometer D	13.7	20.3	23.8	10.1	9.9	0.6
Masking noise at 90 dB SPL						
Audiometer A	24.0	30.0	32.6	25.0	28.9	24.0
Audiometer B	25.8	35.2	33.1	13.3	†	11.4
Audiometer C	24.8	23.6	23.6	9.0	†	0.0
Audiometer D	32.7	33.8	32.8	15.6	17.9	11.6

*Threshold shift in decibels in a normal ear.
†Measurement not made.

between the effective level of the noise and masking, the threshold shift produced by the noise.

Figure 34–6 shows the relation between the masking obtained with ten normal hearing subjects in the present study and the effective levels of the noise used. As can be seen in the figure, the data from the present study are in good agreement with those reported by Hawkins and Stevens (1950) and give further support to the critical band hypothesis.

The relation between masking and effective level is shown in another way in Figure 34–7. In this fugure one set of curves shows the masking actually obtained with normal hearing subjects, at three different noise intensity levels. The second set of curves shows the predicted masking for the same intensity levels determined by computation using the critical band data.[3] The mean differences averaged over all frequencies between obtained and predicted masking are 0.2 dB at the 50 dB level, 0.2 dB at the 70 dB level, and 0.8 dB at the 90 dB level. The close agreement between obtained and predicted masked thresholds indicates that high degree of accuracy with which masking by white noise can be predicted.

Narrow Band Noise

As shown in Figure 34–5, the masked audiograms for narrow bands of noise are similar to those for white noise in two respects. First, the greatest shifts in threshold were obtained at those frequencies where the ear is the most sensitive. Second, narrow band masking shows the same one-to-one linearity between

masking and noise intensity as does white noise masking.

The relation between masking and the effective level of narrow band noise is shown in Figure 34–8 with the data compared to the relation reported by Hawkins and Stevens (1950) for white noise. The results of the present study suggest that the masking-to-effective-level relation is essentially the same for the two types of noise. This finding is in agreement with that reported by Bilger and Hirsh (1956) for the 1,000–1,420 cps noise band.

Since narrow band noise appears to have the same masking-to-effective-level relation as white noise, the critical band data should be just as applicable in the prediction of masked thresholds with narrow band noise. Figure 34–9 compares masked thresholds obtained with normal hearing subjects to the masked thresholds predicted through computation based upon the critical band data. As can be seen in the figure, the thresholds agree closely. The mean differences are 0.3 dB at the 50 dB level, 0.1 dB at the 70 dB level, and 0.1 dB at the 90 dB level. From these results it would appear that the critical band hypothesis is as valid for narrow bands of white noise as it is for a wide spectrum white noise, providing the narrow bands are at least as wide as the critical bands. This finding does not seem unreasonable in light of Fletcher's (1940) concept of equivalance of energy —namely, that when a pure tone is just audible in the presence of noise, the total acoustic power of the components within the critical band surrounding the tone is the same as that of the pure tone. Although the results of the present study are in agreement with

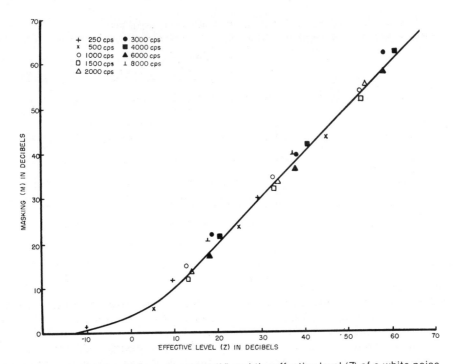

FIGURE 34-6. Relation between masking (M) and the effective level (Z) of a white noise used for masking. M is the change in the threshold of a pure tone in the presence of the noise. Z is the number of decibels that the total energy in a critical band is above the threshold energy for a pure tone whose frequency is at the center of the band. The solid line is the relation reported by Hawkins and Stevens (1950).

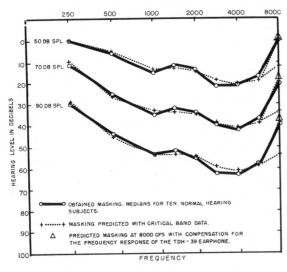

FIGURE 34-7. A comparison of the masking obtained with white noise at three different intensity levels for ten normal hearing subjects and the masking predicted with the critical band data of Fletcher (1940).

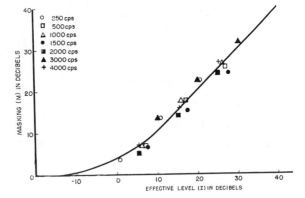

FIGURE 34-8. Relation between masking (M) and the effective level (Z) of six narrow bands of noise used for masking. M is the change in the threshold of a pure tone in the presence of the noise. Z is the number of decibels that the total energy in a critical band is above the threshold energy for a pure tone whose frequency is at the center of the band. The solid line is the masking-to-effective-level for white noise reported by Hawkins and Stevens (1950).

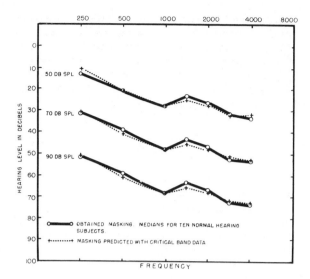

FIGURE 34-9. A comparison of the masking obtained with narrow bands of noise at three different intensity levels for ten normal hearing subjects and the masking predicted with the critical band data of Fletcher (1940).

and the results of the present study suggest that the mean discrepancy averaged over six frequencies is less than 1 dB.

Comment

As shown by the masking audiograms in Figure 34–5, when the noises are equated in terms of overall level, saw-tooth noise is the least efficient of the three types of masking noise, because of its dearth of energy in the higher frequencies; white noise is substantially more efficient than saw-tooth noise in the middle and higher frequencies; and narrow band noise is the most efficient of the three types at all of the frequencies tested.

Table 34–2 shows the advantage of narrow band noise over saw-tooth and white noise at each of the three masking noise levels used at each test frequency. As might be expected, the advantage over saw-tooth noise is greatest in the higher frequencies, whereas the advantage of narrow band noise over white noise is greatest in the lower frequencies. It may be noted in Table 34–2 that at 250 cps the advantage of narrow band noise over white noise seems to increase at higher noise levels. Actually, the difference in advantage at different noise levels is an artifact. Because of the poorer sensitivity of the ear at 250 cps, no threshold shift was produced by white noise at 50 dB sound pressure level. At those noise levels and frequencies where both noises produced threshold shifts, the masking advantage of narrow band over white noise reflects the linearity of the masking produced by each.

A greater advantage of narrow band over white noise in the lower frequencies results from the fact that, although both types of noise have less efficiency in the lows, narrow band noise wastes relatively less

those reported by Bilger and Hirsh, they are at variance with the findings of several other investigators. Egan and Hake (1950), testing at 410 cps, found masking to be 3 dB less than the effective level of a narrow band of noise. Schafer and others (1950), testing at three frequencies, found masking to be 1 to 2 dB less than the effective levels of narrow bands of noise. Palva (1954, 1958), commenting on these findings, repeated Garner's (1952) explanation that when a single band of noise is used, some of the energy "spills over" onto the adjacent frequency areas of the basilar membrane. Actually, discrepancies of 3 dB or less are not of great importance clinically,

TABLE 34–2. THE MASKING ADVANTAGE IN DECIBELS OF NARROW BAND NOISE OVER SAW-TOOTH NOISE AND WHITE NOISE AT THREE MASKING NOISE LEVELS.

	250	500	1,000	1,500	2,000	3,000	4,000
Advantage* of narrow band noise over saw-tooth noise							
At 50 dB SPL of noise	12.7	18.7	18.1	18.4	26.7	32.5	33.8
At 70 dB SPL of noise	18.0	18.7	24.6	28.9	36.6	42.6	53.2
At 90 dB SPL of noise	19.0	25.2	24.1	37.9	51.1	54.6	62.2
Advantage† of narrow band noise over white noise							
At 50 dB SPL of noise	12.7	14.7	13.6	11.9	13.2	11.1	12.5
At 70 dB SPL of noise	20.2	15.7	14.1	11.9	13.2	13.1	12.0
At 90 dB SPL of noise	21.7	15.7	14.6	11.9	11.7	10.1	11.5

*Obtained masking with narrow band noise minus obtained masking with saw-tooth noise.
†Obtained masking with narrow band noise minus obtained masking with white noise.

energy in components outside the critical bands. Although the critical bands at 250 and 500 cps are narrower than those in the middle frequencies, it is more feasible to produce narrow bands in the lows that are only slightly wider than the critical bands. The narrow bands used in the present study are much closer to the critical band widths in the lower frequencies than in the higher.

Previous studies (Feldman, 1961; Hood, 1960; Liden et al., 1959b; Studebaker, 1962) have suggested a greater efficiency for narrow band noise as compared with broad band white noise. The masking audiograms in the present study, shown in Figure 34–5, support this finding and confirm the theoretical expectation stated earlier in this study; namely, that for equal energy delivered to the ear,

narrow band masking is more efficient than sawtooth or white noise. Consequently, the clinician faced with a patient who presents a masking problem should expect to find that narrow band masking is considerably more effective than the other two types in eliminating the danger of obtaining false threshold responses in the poorer ear.

CLINICAL APPLICATION

The final step in the present study, after analysis of the physical characteristics of the three types of noise and measurement of the masking produced by each type in a normal ear, was a return to the original problem of eliminating false threshold responses re-

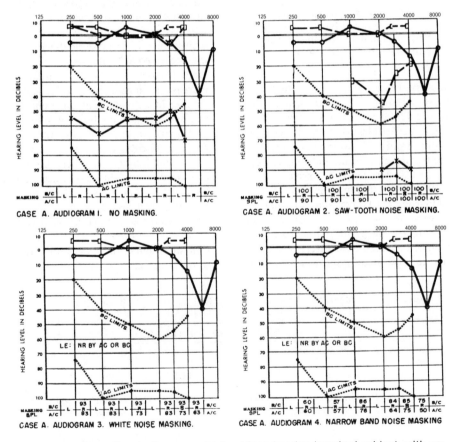

FIGURE 34-10 (case A). Audiograms obtained for a hearing impaired subject, with no masking and with each of three types of masking noise.

sulting from crossover of the test stimulus in hearing-impaired subjects. Three cases were selected to illustrate serious masking problems, and each case was tested with no masking and with each of the three types of masking noise under consideration. Because narrow bands of noise were available only at 250, 500, 1,000, 2,000, 3,000, and 4,000 cps, thresholds for the poorer ear were obtained only at those frequencies. For each case, all audiometric results were obtained during a single testing session. The Hood technique (1960) of masking was employed with each type of noise.

Case A. The patient was a 66-year-old female. This patient had normal hearing in the right ear except for a moderate sensorineural loss in the higher frequencies. She had a complete loss of hearing in the left ear due to surgical intervention for labyrinthine hydrops.

Figure 34–10 shows the results of pure tone audiometry with this patient when no masking was used and when the better ear was masked with each of the three types of noise. *Audiogram 2* shows that saw-tooth noise did not prevent crossover of the test tone in the higher frequencies, even at the maximum masking intensity available, whereas *audiograms 3* and *4* show that responses from the nontest ear were eliminated at all frequencies by both white noise and narrow band noise.

It is worth noting that when the test tone was presented to the left ear (the dead ear) by air conduction with no masking or with saw-tooth noise in the right ear, the patient could not tell in which ear she heard the tone. When the tone was presented to the left ear by bone conduction with no masking or with saw-tooth noise in the right ear, the patient was convinced she heard the tone in the left ear—the dead ear. This confusion is not unusual and illustrates the fact that the clinician must not place too much reliance on a patient's report as to the ear in which the test tone is heard.

Case B. This patient was a 40-year-old female with a diagnosis of bilateral clinical otosclerosis. After middle ear surgery, the patient's left ear developed a complete loss of hearing. Surgery was not performed upon the right ear; thus this ear retained a conductive hearing loss with a sensorineural component in the higher frequencies.

The audiometric results obtained for this case with no masking and with each of the three types of mask-

ing noise are shown in Figure 34–11. *Audiograms 2* and *3* show that in this case neither saw-tooth nor white noise was successful in preventing crossover of the test tone by air conduction and by bone conduction from the poorer ear to the better ear evenw hen the maximum masking intensities available were used. However, as *audiogram 4* shows, masking was successfully accomplished with narrow band noise even with lower intensity levels at all but two frequencies than those used for saw-tooth and white noise.

Case C. This 58-year-old male also had a diagnosis of bilateral clinical otosclerosis. Postsurgical serous labyrinthitis had left this patient with a profound sensorineural hearing loss in the left ear. The unoperated right ear had a conductive loss with a sensorineural component in the higher frequencies.

The audiometric results for this case are shown in Figure 34–12. In this case, too, although white noise again showed a greater efficiency in masking than did saw-tooth noise, neither was successful in eliminating false responses in the poorer ear due to crossover of the test tone to the better ear. However, as in case B, the better ear was successfully masked with narrow band noise. The presence of a response by air conduction at 3,000 cps with a narrow band masking noise of 105 dB sound pressure level in the right ear suggests that this is actually a true left ear response rather than a false response due to crossover of the test tone. With no air-bone gap present in the right ear at that frequency, a narrow band noise of 105 dB sound pressure level would have shifted the right ear threshold to a hearing level of approximately 90 dB, thus effectively ruling out the possibility of a crossover response in the right ear at a hearing level of 95 dB.

Comment

The audiometric results for case A shown above illustrate that when air conduction acuity is good in the better ear, masking sounds are not reduced in their capacity to produce threshold shifts in that ear. Although saw-tooth noise did not prevent false responses in this case, it was possible to achieve full protection with white noise. The results for cases B and C, however, illustrate that, as pointed out by Carhart (1960) and Naunton (1962), a conductive hearing loss in the better ear does increase the diffi-

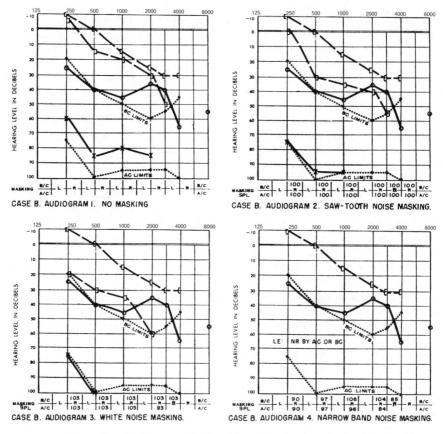

CASE B. AUDIOGRAM I. NO MASKING

CASE B. AUDIOGRAM 2. SAW-TOOTH NOISE MASKING.

CASE B. AUDIOGRAM 3. WHITE NOISE MASKING.

CASE B. AUDIOGRAM 4. NARROW BAND NOISE MASKING.

FIGURE 34-11 (case B).   Audiograms obtained for a hearing impaired subject, with no masking and with each of three types of masking noise.

culty of obtaining true responses from the poorer ear. In these two cases, false responses could be eliminated only with narrow band noise.

A further consideration of the results shown for the three clinical cases might lead to the suggestion that successful masking could have been accomplished with white noise masking in all three cases if higher intensities of white noise had been available. This is possibly true and requires further comment.

One difficulty in the use of white noise at high intensity levels is the problem of patient discomfort. This would not have been a problem in cases B and C above, since the noise level would be substantially reduced by the conductive block, but it is a problem in certain other cases. It is of no use to the clinician to have a high level of white noise available if the pa-

tient will not tolerate it. In this respect, too, narrow band noise has an advantage. Studebaker (1962), using a loudness balancing method with white noise and narrow band noise, has shown that when the two types of noise are equated by subject adjustment to the same loudness, narrow band noise at that level produces considerably more masking than does white noise. This means that for equal masking with the two kinds of noise, narrow band noise subjects the patient to less loudness, thereby reducing patient discomfort and fatigue. An even more important advantage is with the patient who will not tolerate sound at high loudness levels. With these cases it is often possible to mask successfully with narrow band noise when it would not be possible with white noise.

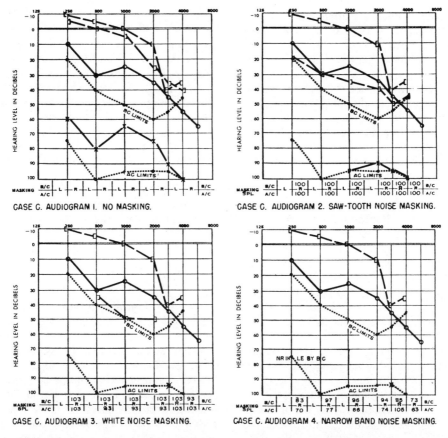

CASE C. AUDIOGRAM I. NO MASKING.

CASE C. AUDIOGRAM 2. SAW-TOOTH NOISE MASKING.

CASE C. AUDIOGRAM 3. WHITE NOISE MASKING.

CASE C. AUDIOGRAM 4. NARROW BAND NOISE MASKING.

FIGURE 34-12 (case C). Audiograms obtained for a hearing impaired subject, with no masking and with each of three types of masking noise.

Also, while it is true that successful masking might have been accomplished with white noise in all three of the clinical cases reported here if higher levels of white noise had been available, it should be remembered that levels beyond approximately 105 dB SPL are often not available on pure tone audiometers; and, regardless of the maximum intensities available, a given level of narrow band noise will produce more masking than the same overall level of white noise.

Although the problem of overmasking did not arise in the present study, it is always a danger when masking noise is used at high intensity. Just as the pure tone test stimulus might cross the head and be heard in the nontest ear, so might the masking noise cross the head and interfere with threshold determination in the test ear. Various studies (Naunton,

1962; Palva, 1958; Palva and Palva, 1962) have shown that white noise transduced through an earphone in a standard cushion crosses over at a level of about 50 dB above threshold in the test ear. The use of narrow band noise does not bring greater interaural attenuation (Naunton, 1962), since the determining factor in overmasking is the level per cycle transmitted across the head, rather than the overall level. However, the danger of overmasking can be decreased by delivering the noise through an insert receiver—a small hearing aid type receiver with a rubber tipped insert that fits into the ear canal. A number of studies (Feldman, 1961; Hood, 1960; Naunton, 1962; Palva, 1958; Palva and Palva, 1962; Studebaker, 1962; Wegel and Lane, 1924) have shown that use of such a receiver can bring about a substantial increase in interaural attenuation. Several investigators (Feldman, 1961; Hood, 1960; Zwislocki, 1953) have reported attenuation of 80 to 90 dB, thereby practically eliminating the problem of overmasking.[4]

One further comment is necessary at this point. The results of this study should not be interpreted as implying that narrow band masking is a panacea that will end all problems in masking. Although false responses were eliminated with narrow band noise in the clinical cases shown, it is certainly possible to obtain false responses due to crossover of the test tone even when using high levels of narrow band noise. To illustrate, suppose we have a patient with a profound sensorineural loss in the left ear and a 50 dB conductive loss in the right ear. At 500 cps, a narrow band noise of 120 dB SPL will shift the air conduction threshold in the right ear to 90 dB hearing level. However, the bone conduction threshold in the right ear would be shifted to a hearing level of only 40 dB because of the 50 dB conductive block in that ear. As a result of crossover of the test tone by bone conduction, it would be possible in this case to obtain false responses from the poorer ear to air conduction presentation at about the 95 dB hearing level and to bone conduction presentation at about the 45 dB hearing level. Thus, although narrow band noise will produce greater masking than either of the other two types, it will not completely eliminate the problem of false responses in all cases, at least with the maximum levels now available. In such cases the clinician's only recourse is to employ the Hood method of masking (1960) to demonstrate that the thresholds obtained are actually false responses.

CONCLUSION

The results obtained in this study[5] indicate that of the three types of noise studied, narrow band noise is the most efficient as a masking noise in pure tone audiometry. The masking audiograms for normal hearing subjects and the clinical results for hearing-impaired subjects show that for equal intensity levels, narrow band noise produces greater threshold shifts than does either of the other two types and thereby affords the clinician greater protection from false responses due to crossover of the test tone. The advantage of narrow band noise over the other two types is great enough to make it distinctly preferable, at least for the special problem cases.

SUMMARY

Three types of masking noise (saw-tooth, broad band white, and narrow band noise) were compared to determine their relative efficiencies as masking noises in pure tone audiometry. The physical characteristics of each type of noise were examined and the noises were used to obtain masking audiograms for ten normal-hearing subjects. Three hearing-impaired subjects, considered critical cases for masking, were tested with each type of noise. The results show that at equal overall intensity levels, white noise has greater masking efficiency than does saw-tooth noise but narrow band noise is considerably more efficient than either of the other two types.

ENDNOTES

1. A masking noise at a 50 dB effective level for the normal ear would shift the pure tone threshold in the normal ear to a hearing level of 50 dB.

2. Actually, narrow band noise is not a third type of noise per se but is rather a restricted frequency band of white noise. Although white noise and narrow band noise are the same except for band width, in the present study the terms "white noise" and "narrow band noise" will be used to differentiate between white noise of unlimited spectrum and white noise in a limited band.

3. The predicted masking at a given noise level is equal to the total energy in the critical band minus the pure tone threshold in quiet.

4. In the present study the narrow band noise was presented through an insert receiver, although danger of overmasking was not a problem. The results obtained with narrow band masking would have been essentially the same if a standard earphone had been used.

5. Dr. George E. Shambaugh, Jr., Dr. Raymond Carhart, Dr. Tom W. Tillman, and Mr. Robert Johnson gave assistance.

REFERENCES

Bilger, R. C., and Hirsh, I. J. Masking of Tones by Bands of Noise, *J. Acoust. Soc. Amer.,* **28:** 623–630, 1956.

Carhart, R. Assessment of Sensorineural Response in Otosclerosis, *Arch. Otolaryng.,* **71:** 141–149, 1960.

Dirks, D. D. Factors Related to Reliability of Bone Conduction, PhD Dissertation, Northwestern University, 1963.

Egan, J. P., and Hake, H. W. On Masking Pattern of Simple Auditory Stimulus, *J. Acoust. Soc. Amer.,* **22:** 622–630, 1950.

Feldman, A. S. Problems in Measurement of Bone Conduction, *J. Speech Hearing Dis.,* **26:** 39–44, 1961.

Fletcher, H. Auditory Patterns, *Rev. Mod. Physics* **12:** 47–65, 1940.

Fletcher, H., and Munson, W. A. Relation Between Loudness and Masking, *J. Acoust. Soc. Amer.,* **9:** 1–10, 1937.

Garner, W. R. Hearing, *Ann. Rev. Psychol.* **3:** 85–104, 1952.

Hawkins, J. E., Jr., and Stevens, S. S. Masking of Pure Tones and of Speech by White Noise, *J. Acoust. Soc. Amer.,* **22:** 6–13, 1950.

Hood, J. D. Principles and Practice of Bone Conduction Audiometry, *Laryngoscope* **70:** 1,211–1,228, 1960.

Jerger, J. F.; Tillman, T.W.; and Peterson, J. L. Masking by Octave Bands of Noise in Normal and Impaired Ears, *J. Acoust. Soc. Amer.,* **32:** 385–390, 1960.

Liden, G. Speech Audiometry, *Acta Otolaryng* (Stockholm), suppl. **114:** 72–76, 1954.

Liden, G. Nilsson, G; and Anderson, H. Masking in Clinical Audiometry, *Acta Otolaryng.* (Stockholm), **50:** 125–136, 1959*a*.

Liden, G.; Nilsson, G.; and Anderson, H. Narrow Band Masking With White Noise, *Acta Otolaryng.* (Stockholm), **50:** 116–124, 1959*b*.

Naunton, R. F. Masking Dilemma in Bilateral Conduction Deafness, *Arch. Otolaryng.,* **72:** 753–757, 1962.

Palva, T. Masking in Audiometry, *Acta Otolaryng.* (Stockholm), suppl. **118:** 156–172, 1954.

Palva, T. Masking in Audiometry: Further Studies, *Acta Otolaryng.* (Stockholm), **49:** 229–239, 1958.

Palva, T., and Palva, A. Masking in Audiometry, *Acta Otolaryng.* (Stockholm), **54:** 521–531, 1962.

Schafer, T. H., et al. Frequency Selectivity of Ear as Determined by Masking Experiments, *J. Acoust. Soc. Amer.,* **22:** 490–496, 1950.

Studebaker, G. A. On Masking in Bone Conduction Testing, *J. Speech Hearing Res.,* **5:** 215–227, 1962.

Wegel, R. L., and Lane, C. E. Auditory Masking of One Pure Tone by Another and Its Probable Relation to Dynamics of Inner Ear, *Physic Rev.,* **23:** 266–285, 1924.

Zwislocki, J. Acoustic Attenuation Between Ears, *J. Acoust. Soc. Amer.,* **25:** 752–759, 1953.

35

Interaural Attenuation and Cross-Hearing in Air-Conduction Audiometry

JOSEPH B. CHAIKLIN, Ph.D.
Supervisor, Audiology Section, Veterans Administration Medical Center, New Orleans

DEFINITION OF TERMS

A frequent problem in air-conduction audiometry is the undesired transfer of intense stimuli from one ear to the other. As the stimuli cross the head they are attenuated (i.e., weakened), hence the term "interaural attenuation" (IA) has been used to refer to reduction of a signal's intensity as it passes between ears by one means or another. For example, a 60 dB (SPL) 1,000 cps tone presented to one ear may be subjected to 55 dB IA before it reaches the other ear as a 5-dB (SPL) signal and will stimulate hearing there only if the cochlea receiving it is sensitive to 5-dB signals. When IA is increased, a stronger signal is required to reach the opposite ear; when IA is decreased, a weaker signal is required.

A term sometimes confused with IA is "interaural threshold difference" (often "interaural difference") which refers to threshold differences between ears at the same frequency. "Cross-hearing," "transcranial hearing" and "shadow hearing" are terms used to describe sensation resulting from stimuli crossing the head during air-conduction audiometry. A shadow curve is an air-conduction threshold curve that results from cross-hearing.

EXPLANATIONS FOR CROSS-HEARING

There has been considerable interest in identifying the route or routes signals follow in cross-hearing. According to Békésy (1948) the bow of the earphone headset does not appear to be a significant route, at least for dynamic earphones in rubber cushions. Békésy concluded that around-the-head (air-conduction) leakage is the primary cross-hearing mechanism in air-conduction audiometry, but most authors appear to favor a through-the-head (bone-conduction) explanation (Feldman, 1963; Fletcher, 1953; Littler, Knight, and Strange, 1952; Sparrevohn, 1946; Studebaker, 1962; Wegel and Lane, 1924; Zwislocki, 1953).

Feldman (1963) found that when unilaterally deaf subjects had both ears covered with TDH-39 phones in MX-41/AR cushions, they evidenced 5- to 15 dB less mean IA at 125, 250 and 500 cps and approximately 1 dB less at 1,000 cps (personal communication) than they did when the better ear was open. If cross-hearing had been by air conduction in this range, signals leaking around the head should have been attenuated further by the phone over the better ear and thus IA should have increased rather than decreased. Feldman attributed this reduction of low-frequency IA to the occlusion effect's apparent enhancement of sensitivity for low-frequency stimuli crossing the head by bone conduction (Goldstein and Hayes, 1965; Naunton, 1957). On the other hand, he found approximately 9 dB increased IA at 4,000 cps (the only other frequency sampled) in the covered state, a finding he attributed to the phone blocking air-conduction leakage around the head.

NORMATIVE DATA

Interaural attenuation norms are important in evaluating the need for masking in air-conduction audiometry, in estimating maximum permissible masking levels for air- and bone-conduction audiometry and in evaluating test validity.

Reprinted by permission of the author from *J. Aud Res.,* **7,** 413–424 (1967).

Previous literature reflects sizeable differences among IA estimates at specific frequencies. For example, Sparrevohn's (1946) report of 57 dB IA at 8,000 cps contrasts sharply with Zwislocki's (1953) mean value of 74 dB reported in his Figure 3–6.

A variety of factors may account for some of the differences referred to above, but earphone and external canal variables are among the most prominent. For example, IA can be increased by using insert phones (Feldman, 1963; Studebaker, 1962) or by deep plugging of the external canal of the nontest ear (Zwislocki, 1953). It can be increased, also, by decreasing the size of the stimulus phone, thus reducing the area of the head stimulated (Feldman, 1963; Studebaker, 1962; Zwislocki, 1953), by increasing the volume of air under the nontest earphone, and, perhaps, by plugging the ear canal of the test ear (Tschiassny, 1952).

Measurement method and subject selection may account for some interstudy differences. For example, Zwislocki (1953) had normal-hearing listeners judge when a strong signal presented to one ear reduced the loudness of a weak signal presented 180° out of phase to the other ear. He found generally higher IA than Miller (1959) and Feldman (1963) found for monaurally deaf patients. Possibly a major source of these normative differences is inherent intersubject variability (Sparrevohn, 1946).

Previous reports on IA have usually been limited to relatively few points in the audiometric range and often have failed to describe measurement procedures adequately. The purposes of the present study were to extend previous data by sampling IA under two conditions at all octave and inter-octave points available on the typical clinical audiometer and to relate the findings to clinical considerations.

METHOD

Subjects

Subjects were three female and two male college students with total unilateral deafness. Their ages ranged from 18 to 23 years, with a mean of 19 years. Four had hearing sensitivity in the better ear within ±5 dB of zero HL (ISO 1964) for most of the audiometric range and one had a 30 to 40 dB loss above 3,000 cps. Mumps in early childhood was the probable etiology for four subjects and etiology was unknown for the other. Otoscopic examination and history for each subject's better ear were negative. Pure-tone Stenger results were negative. Hearing in the poorer ear was ruled out with white noise masking.

General Plan

After conventional pure-tone audiometry, history and otoscopy each subject was scheduled for two additional test sessions (five to ten days apart) consisting of two sets of threshold measurement for each ear at the 11 audiometric frequencies from 125 cps through 8,000 cps. Thresholds were measured with Békésy procedure under two conditions: first, with both ears covered by TDH-39 earphones in MX-41/AR cushions, and second, with both ears covered as in the first condition, but with an individually-made medium-soft plug extending into the bony external meatus of the better ear. The plug produced 40 to 50 dB attenuation for most air-conduction signals delivered to the better ear and also reduced the occlusion effect to negligible values by occupying most of the external canal. Interaural attenuation values with the plug in place may be considered roughly analogous to values obtained with some conductively impaired patients (those without an occlusion effect). Data for the "phones only" condition may be viewed as representative of results obtained with mild sensory-neural impairment or normal hearing.

In each condition (plug vs no plug) the better ear was tested first. The following order was used for each set of threshold measurements for each condition: 125 cps, 250 cps, 500 cps, 750 cps, 1,000 cps, 1,500 cps, 2,000 cps, 3,000, cps, 4,000 cps, 6,000 cps, 8,000 cps, 125 cps, 250 cps, 500 cps and 1,000 cps. Both sessions started with practice tracking, first at 1,000 cps for one minute and then at 500 cps for one minute.

Stimuli were 250-msec tone pulses with 20-msec rise-decay time, separated by 250-msec silent intervals, and delivered for 30 seconds at each frequency at an attenuation rate of 4 dB per second. Threshold was defined as the mean of the pen excursion midpoints.

Apparatus

The system used to measure thresholds consisted of the following components in sequence: Hewlett-Packard 201 CR audio oscillator, Grason-Stadler

829C Electronic Switch, Grason-Stadler E 3262A Recording Attenuator, MacIntosh MC 30 amplifier, Hewlett-Packard 350-B Step Attenuator, Telephonics TDH-39 earphones in MX-41/AR cushions and a Grason-Stadler subject switch with which subjects controlled stimulus intensity. Impedance-matching transformers were used when necessary. Subjects were seated in an Industrial Acoustics Company 1202-A test booth. The experimenter and equipment were located outside the booth. During test conditions the booth had a sound level of 23 dB on the A-Scale and 48 dB on the C-Scale of a Bruel and Kjaer 2203 Sound Level meter. The input to the earphones was monitored with a Ballantine 300B vacuum-tube voltmeter. Earphone output was checked periodically with a Bruel and Kjaer Model 158 audiometer calibration unit with a NBS type 9A coupler.

RESULTS

The data reported below are from the second test session. The first session served to accustom subjects to the experimental task and to reduce practice effects in the second session.

Table 35–1 summarizes mean thresholds (rounded to the nearest 1-dB interval) for each ear with and without the plug in the better ear, differences between means for each condition, and dispersion data. Figure 35–1 shows mean threshold data for each condition plotted in SPL re 0.0002 microbar. Mean IA for each condition can be visualized in Figure 35–1 by noting the differences between plotted points for the better and poorer ears. Similarly, differences between the plugged and phones only conditions can be observed by comparing mean points for the two poorer ear curves. Means above 3,000 cps do not include data from the subject who had elevated thresholds above 3,000 cps. An inspection of Table 35–1 and Figure 35–1 reveals that mean IA varied with frequency and test conditions.

IA With Phones Only

When the ears were covered only with phones mean IA ranged from 38 dB at 125 cps to 70 dB at 4,000 cps; 8 of the 11 means were greater than 58 dB. Table 35–1 shows that differences among subjects were greater above 1,000 cps for this condition, with the largest difference (31 dB) at 1,500 cps. The largest differences were well distributed among subjects.

TABLE 35–1. MEAN THRESHOLDS (RE 0.0002 μBAR) FOR EACH EAR WITH PHONES ONLY AND WITH PHONES PLUS PLUG IN BETTER EAR, AND COMPARISON OF INTERAURAL ATTENUATION (IA) WITH AND WITHOUT PLUG (ALL VALUES ROUNDED TO CLOSEST 1-dB INTERVAL). N = 5 THROUGH 3 KC/S; N = 4 ABOVE 3 KC/S.

	.125	.25	.5	.75	1	1.5	2	3	4	6	8
Phones Only											
Deaf Ear Means	87	77	70	74	66	73	69	75	73	83	76
Better Ear Means	49	26	11	5	5	6	8	7	3	18	19
Phones plus Plug in Better Ear											
Deaf Ear Means	106	95	90	85	71	70	67	73	75	85	75
Better Ear Means	83	66	55	54	52	47	51	52	50	68	65
Attenuation Means and Extremes											
IA, Phones Only	38	51	59	69	61	67	61	68	70	65	57
Most IA	45	58	65	71	66	76	72	72	85	76	69
Least IA	32	44	54	62	57	45	55	56	61	56	51
Change in IA with Plug in											
Better Ear	19	18	20	11	5	−3	−2	−2	2	2	−1
Most IA Change	33	31	36	16	14	−7	−4	−14	14	14	−11
Least IA Change	6	10	11	7	3	2	−1	−1	−1	−1	0
IA with Plug in Better Ear	57	69	79	80	66	64	59	66	73	67	56
Most IA	65	75	93	85	79	77	68	81	81	77	59
Least IA	51	66	65	76	56	38	54	54	60	65	52
Attenuation of Plug	34	40	44	49	47	41	43	45	47	50	46
Most Attenuation	37	48	49	54	51	60	48	53	50	63	57
Least Attenuation	29	33	41	46	40	32	38	34	44	38	37

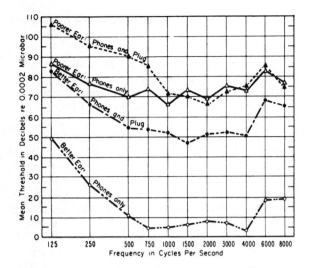

FIGURE 35-1. Mean thresholds in SPL for each ear with phones only and with phones plus plug in better ear. N = 5 through 3,000 cps; N = 4 above 3,000 cps.

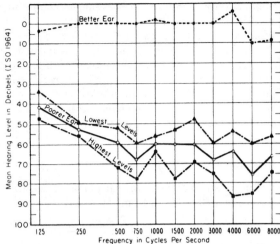

FIGURE 35-2. Mean thresholds for "phones only" condition plotted in hearing level (ISO 1964) and composites of lowest and highest hearing levels at which tones presented to the poorer ear were heard in the better ear. N = 5 through 3,000 cps; N = 4 above 3,000 cps.

IA With Plug in Better Ear

With the solid plug in the better ear and both ears covered with phones, mean IA increased substantially below 1,500 cps; that is, stronger signals had to be applied to the deaf ear to elicit responses in the normal ear. The largest mean increases (18 to 20 dB) were at 125 cps, 250 cps, and 500 cps and were probably related to reduction of the occlusion effect present when the better ear was covered only with a phone (Feldman, 1963).

There was a trend toward decreased IA (hence lower cross-hearing levels) above 1,000 cps in the plugged condition, but the mean decreases were small and there were large differences among subjects and frequencies, thus underscoring the variable effects of plugging the external canal. Zwislocki (1953) also observed instances of slightly decreased IA above 1000 cps when he plugged the bony external auditory meatus. The reason for these changes is not entirely clear but impedance alteration in the external meatus is a possible explanation.

Clinical Cross-Hearing Levels

Figure 35-2 displays mean hearing levels (ISO 1964) for the "phones only" condition to illustrate average audiometric levels at which cross-hearing might occur when a patient's better ear thresholds are very close to Zero hearing level (HL) for most of the audiometric range. The mean HL at which cross-hearing occurred at most frequencies corresponds closely to the interaural differences and IA means. It should be kept in mind, however, that the primary clinical consideration in estimating the likelihood of cross-hearing is the difference between the better ear's best hearing (often bone-conduction thresholds) and the air-conduction level at the poorer ear (Studebaker, 1962). Thus, in a hearing level context, a 250 cps tone presented to a patient's poorer ear at 40 dB (ISO 1964) may appear too weak to cause cross-hearing, but if the patient's better ear threshold is −10 dB the interaural difference is 50 dB, which is within the range of IA values shown in Table 35-1.

Knowledge of the average HLs at which cross-hearing occurs may be less useful clinically than knowledge of the lowest levels at which it occurs. Figure 35-2 contains a composite of the lowest ISO hearing levels at which cross-hearing occurred. Values ranged from 34 dB at 125 cps to 60 dB at 6,000 cps. Figure 35-2 also shows a composite of the highest HLs at which cross-hearing occurred in the "phones only" condition. Values ranged from 47 dB at 125 cps to 85 dB at 4,000 cps. Some of the apparent disparities between the highest and lowest HLs in Figure 35–2 can be understood by comparing the better-and poorer-ear thresholds of individual subjects represented in the composite. This comparison reveals that better-ear thresholds lower than the mean are frequently associated with the lowest poorer-ear levels and *vice versa*.

Attenuation of Plug

The mean attenuation of the ear plugs was 34 dB at 125 cps and 40 to 50 dB from 250 to 8,000 cps. Plug attenuation was fairly homogeneous across subjects with only four deviations from the mean greater than 8 dB. All deviations in excess of 8 dB were at 6,000 and 8,000 cps.

Test-Retest Agreement

All intrasession retests (125 cps to 1,000 cps) for both conditions and both ears were well within ±5 dB of the first measurements. The number of retests that were lower than first tests was nearly equal to the number that were higher. Approximately 20 percent of the retests were identical (i.e., ±.5 dB) to first tests. It should be recalled that all tests and retests were conducted with a single phone or plug placement, hence the data do not reflect variability that might result from placement and replacement.

DISCUSSION

Some clinical texts advise masking when the air-conduction interaural threshold difference at any frequency equals or exceeds a uniform criterion level (Newby, 1964; Saltzman, 1949). To the casual observer, this may suggest that IA is uniform at all frequencies, a notion not supported by the data reported above. Furthermore, when the better ear has a conductive component, interaural comparison of air-conduction thresholds is often not meaningful in evaluating IA. In these instances comparison must involve the bone-conduction thresholds of the better ear. If these limitations are kept in mind, however, a

single estimate of IA might be useful as a rough guide to deciding when masking must be applied in air-conduction audiometry.

Although no single figure will predict IA at all frequencies for all patients, a single figure could define the lower limits of IA for most frequencies and most patients. An inspection of Table 35–1 reveals that in the 250 to 8,000 cps range, the smallest IA values are 44 and 45 dB, although most exceed 50 dB. This suggests that 45 dB may be a reasonable, if somewhat conservative, estimate of the minimum IA that occurs before cross-hearing begins in the 250 to 8,000 cps range. At 125 cps, 35 dB would be a safer estimate. While these estimates are conservative in terms of the present study's results as well as the results of most previous studies, it is highly probable that additional sampling will reveal patients with less IA than the smallest values reported above. On the other hand, data from this study and other studies suggest that IA usually exceeds the limits proposed above. Consequently, some clinicians may prefer a 50-dB estimate for IA in the 250 to 8,000 cps range. A 50-dB estimate would probably result in error only at isolated frequencies and for relatively few patients.

The use of insert receivers to deliver test stimuli and masking signals has been advocated as a method for increasing IA of stimuli, by reducing the area of the head under the masking phone (Feldman, 1963; Hood, 1960; Studebaker, 1962). It is also possible that a deep insert in the nontest ear may increase IA by reducing the occlusion effect in normal ears or ears with sensory-neural loss. Insert receivers introduce a unique set of problems that have probably discouraged their wide-spread use. Wide individual variations in canal size, the need to clean the inserts between tests, frequency response limitations of the insert system, and calibration problems are some of the variables that have retarded general adoption of insert receivers.

There has been a tendency to consider the mechanism of cross-hearing in "either-or" terms—either sound crosses the head by air conduction or it crosses by bone conduction. Clearly, strong air-conduction signals presented to one ear do get to the opposite ear by bone conduction, but they also get there by air conduction. The critical issue, therefore, is the order in which two types of transmission occur. For most of the audiometric range cross-hearing probably proceeds by bone conduction before it occurs by air-conduction, but under special conditions the reverse may be true, at least for a limited portion of the range. Recall, for example, that Feldman (1963) suggested that when the better ear is not covered, cross-hearing occurs at 4,000 cps via air-conduction leakage before it occurs via bone-conduction. In the present study, however, above 750 cps mean cross-hearing values with the plug in the better ear were within a few decibels of values without the plug, which suggests that the same processes were probably operating in each condition. Since cross-hearing in the plugged condition was clearly via bone conduction it follows that the minimum levels for around-the-head transmission probably exceed the IA values reported in the present study.

In a recent personal communication Feldman suggested that his 4,000 cps results were probably attributable to more intense radiation from the earphone case at 4,000 cps than at the other frequencies sampled. Actual measurement of sound radiating from a TDH-39 phone confirms this speculation: There is approximately 20 dB greater radiation at 4,000 cps and closely adjacent frequencies than at other points usually sampled in audiometry. (Mr. Clayton Mullin of Maico Laboratories, Minneapolis, was kind enough to carry out the physical measurements necessary to clarify this issue.) Further confirmation was obtained by testing two unilaterally-deaf subjects as Feldman had done, first with the better ear covered, then open. Results similar to his were obtained at 4,000 cps, but at 1,500 cps, 2,000 cps, 3,000 cps, 6,000 cps and 8,000 cps there was essentially no difference between the covered and uncovered conditions.

Absolute IA values are a product of many measurement variables, hence statements about absolute values must relate to specific measurement conditions and specific diagnostic categories. Minimum specifications should include measurement method, the status of both middle ear mechanisms, the status of both external canals, and the type of earphone and cushion used for each ear.

Similarly, changes in IA are relative to specific reference measurement conditions. For example, the fact that low-frequency IA is greater with an insert phone (or plug) in the nontest (better) ear than it is with a standard phone is attributable to the difference in measurement conditions: Low-frequency

bone-conduction thresholds tend to be raised by the insert's reduction of the occlusion effect, therefore calculation of IA must relate to the better ear's elevated bone-conduction thresholds. Although hearing level at the poorer ear may appear to increase with the insert, absolute IA may not increase at all when the better ear's bone-conduction status is used to compute IA.

Future study of IA should be directed to expanding data on intersubject variability, particularly to discovering and investigating additional variables that may account for some of this variability. There may be merit, also, in studying the variability of IA in repeated test sessions to determine whether differences between subjects for various measurement conditions are stable differences or merely reflect random intersession variation.

SUMMARY

Interaural attenuation (IA) was investigated in 5 subjects with total monaural deafness. Air-conduction Békésy audiometry was performed at each ear at 11 audiometric frequencies under two conditions—first, with both ears covered by TDH-39 phones in MX-41/AR cushions, and second, with both ears covered as in the first condition but with a deep plug in the meatus of the better ear. Mean IA in the first condition ranged from 38 dB at 125 cps to 70 dB at 4,000 cps; at frequencies below 1,500 cps IA means in the plugged condition were 5–19 dB higher than means without the plug. The increased IA in the lower frequencies probably was a function of the plugs' reduction of the occlusion effect. It was recommended that 45 dB be used as a conservative clinical estimate of minimum IA in the 250–8,000 cps range, and that 35 dB be used as an estimate at 125 cps.[1] Discussion emphasized variables that affect IA and the importance of specifying measurement conditions and methods.

ACKNOWLEDGMENT

This research was supported by a grant-in-aid from the Graduate School of the University of Minnesota.

ENDNOTE

1. Considering the many variables that affect interaural attenuation, it probably would have been more appropriate for me to have recommended an AC-BC interaural difference of 40 dB as the criterion for potential cross-hearing effects from 250 Hz through 8,000 Hz. This conservative recommendation is consistent with most other authors' advice, including those whose work is included in this section. Nonetheless, cross-hearing occurs very seldom with interaural differences smaller than 45 dB, as evidenced by research data published during the last thirty years. Similarly, a 30-dB AC-BC interaural difference criterion at 125 Hz would probably be more appropriate than the 35 dB criterion recommended in the article (Note that one of my subjects experienced cross-hearing with a 32 dB interaural difference at 125 Hz.) In any case, masking with the revised criteria should embrace almost all of the isolated cases in which cross-hearing occurs with small interaural difference (April 1981).

REFERENCES

Békésy, G. V. Vibration of the head in a sound field and its role in hearing by bone conduction. *J. Acoust. Soc. Amer.,* 1948, **20,** 749–760.

Feldman, A. S. Maximum air-conduction hearing loss. *J. Speech Hearing Res.,* 1963, **6,** 157–163.

Fletcher, H. *Speech and Hearing in Communication.* Princeton: D. Van Nostrand, 1953, 157–159.

Goldstein, D. P. and Hayes, C. S. The occlusion effect in bone conduction hearing. *J. Speech Hearing Res.,* 1965, **8,** 137–148.

Hood, J. D. The principles and practice of bone conduction audiometry: A review of the present position. *Laryngoscope,* 1960, **70,** 1211–1228.

Littler, T. S.; Knight, J. J.; and Strange, P. H. Hearing by bone conduction and the use of bone-conduction hearing aids. *Proc. Royl. Soc. Med.,* 1952, **45,** 783–790.

Miller, M. H. Transmission loss across the skull in a patient with known total monaural deafness. *Laryngoscope,* 1959, **69,** 100–102.

Naunton, R. F. Clinical bone-conduction audiometry. *Arch. Otolaryngol.,* 1957, **66,** 281–298.

Newby, H. A. *Audiology.* New York: Appleton-Century Crofts, 1964, pp. 98–99.

Saltzman, M. *Clinical Audiology.* New York: Grune & Stratton, 1949, p. 155.

Sparrevohn, U. R. Some audiometric investigations of monaurally deaf persons. *Acta Otolaryngol.,* 1946, **34,** 1–10.

Studebaker, G. On masking in bone-conduction testing. *J. Speech Hearing Res.,* 1962, **5,** 215–227.

Tschiassny, K. The mechanism of shadow hearing. *Arch. Otolaryngol.,* 1952, **55,** 22–30.

Wegel, R. L. and Lane, C. E. The auditory masking of one pure tone by another and its probable relation to the dynamics of the inner ear. *Phys. Rev.,* 1924, **23,** 266–285.

Zwislocki, J. Acoustic attenuation between the ears. *J. Acoust. Soc. Amer.,* 1953, **25,** 752–759.

36

On the Misdiagnoses Resulting from Incorrect Use of Masking

R. R. A. COLES, M.D.
Professor and Consultant in Audiological Medicine, University of Southampton, Southampton, England

VILIJA M. PRIEDE, Ph.D.
Audiologist in Charge of Wessex Regional Audiology Centre, University of Southampton, Southampton, England

Over the past three years, the authors' clinical research material has been comprised of patients referred by otologists from the Wessex Region, Armed Services, and further afield for comprehensive audiological and/or vestibular investigation, with the object of determining the site of the lesion in the ear or its central connections. The special tests applied fall into two general groups according to whether the hearing loss is conductive or perceptive (sensorineural), and in order to know which tests to apply the type of hearing loss has to be known. Further, for correct interpretation of the results of the special diagnostic tests performed, it is essential to know not only the full extent of the air- and bone-conduction loss at one or two frequencies but also the degree to which such factors as cross masking may have limited the scope or reliability of the basic audiometric and masking procedures employed.

In fact, about 15 percent of the cases referred have come with major errors in their basic audiograms and it would appear that we are not alone in such experience either in this country (Hood, personal communication, 1968) or abroad (Feldman, 1961; Studebaker, 1967). All too frequently the errors lead to patients being mismanaged either by hearing aids which would be useless in a completely deaf ear or by wasteful, disappointing and possibly even harmful surgery. This paper is intended therefore to draw attention to defects in audiometric techniques that cause such errors and what is needed to prevent them.

Reprinted from *J. Laryngol. and Otol.*, **84**, 41–63 (1970) by courtesy of the authors and the editor of the *Journal of Laryngology and Otology*.

Although the audiometric misdiagnoses encountered have all been due to inadequacy or lack of masking, the original audiometric results conflicted in many cases with the general clinical picture and the results of the otologist's tuning fork tests. From the latter observation a moral might be drawn that it is better to rely on clinical acumen and tuning fork tests than on audiometry, if the necessary masking techniques are not fully understood and correctly applied. To accept this moral alone, however, is to ignore the advantages given by audiometry in scientific measurement of hearing loss and by the more recent audiological techniques for differential diagnosis of the site of hearing loss. It would seem, therefore, that more systematic attention to basic audiological techniques is necessary if the full benefits from even conventional air and bone-conduction are to be obtained, and that a general review of the problems and techniques involved would be a timely and worthwhile contribution.

I. AUDIOMETRIC MISDIAGNOSES AND THEIR CAUSES

The misdiagnoses encountered have in general been due either to failure to detect a very severe hearing loss or to exhibition of a false air/bone gap.

A. Underestimated Severity of Air-Conduction Hearing Loss

(i) Non-use of Masking. In some instances misdiagnosis arose from a failure to recognize the necessity for masking. In turn, this may have resulted

from the frequently occurring misconception that masking of an air-conduction (a/c) threshold is only needed where the difference in thresholds between the ears is 50–60 dB. Even Littler et al. (1952) have advised masking where the differences are '40 dB or more,' but later (1968) Littler modified his rule by adding the words 'if there is the likelihood of conductive deafness on one side . . . masking is necessary even if the two air conduction audiograms are closer together.' For instance, by the 50 dB criterion, masking would be needed only for the right ear of Case B of the two cases illustrated* in Figure 36–1.

The possible need for masking in order to test the right ear of Case A can best be understood by considering, as an example, only one of the possible diagnoses. Take the case of a 30 dB conductive loss in the left ear and a total deafness (e.g., congenital or traumatic) in the right ear. Without masking, the test tones of 60 dB hearing level directed into the non-hearing right ear would just be detected by the unimpaired left cochlea and an apparent threshold in the right ear of about 60 dB would result. This would happen because the sounds derived from the earphone would set the whole bony structure of the skull

into vibration, the average earphone-to-bone transmission loss being about 60 dB (see Table 36–1). Thus, resulting from unmasked a/c audiometry, the right ear of Case A would be misdiagnosed as having only 60 dB of hearing loss and under certain circumstances (not helped by the difficulty of masking out a false negative Rinne test where there is conductive loss in the ear to be masked) might then be selected for a stapedectomy or correction of an ossicular discontinuity, which would of course result in no improvement in hearing.

Whether or not masking of an a/c threshold is needed depends on the possibility of it being a shadow of the *bone conduction* (b/c) threshold of the *opposite* ear, i.e., in cross-hearing the sound reaches the non-test ear by air-to-bone conduction and not, as is sometimes thought, by pericranial air conduction. In effect, this leads to the following rules:

1. When the difference at any frequency between the left and right ears is 40 dB or more (see Case B), masking must be used.
2. When the difference between the ears is less than 40 dB but the a/c threshold of the worse ear is 40 dB or more (see Case A), masking may be needed. In this situation, an unmasked unoccluded b/c test should be performed; then, if the gap between the worse a/c threshold and the unmasked b/c threshold is 40 dB or more, masking must be used. Only if this gap is less than 40 dB can masking of the a/c measurements be omitted with safety.

---

*For sake of clarity, all audiograms and masking functions illustrated in this paper have been modified to remove confusing deviations from straight-line configurations. Apart from the actual shapes of audiogram and variations due to minor inaccuracies in their measurement, further irregularities can occur in bone-conduction audiograms due to such factors as the Carhart notch and occlusion effects caused by the insert telephones or earphones used for masking.

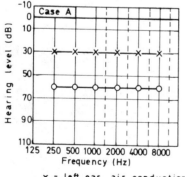

x = left ear, air conduction

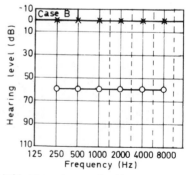

o = right ear, air conduction

FIGURE 36-1. For which ears is masking needed? Common misconception: masking needed for the test of the right ear of Case B but not for Case A, because the difference between left and right ears of Case A is only 30 dB. Fact: masking may be needed for test of right ear of Case A also (i.e., if the bone conduction threshold of the left ear was between 0 and 20 dB).

TABLE 36-1. DATA ON INTERAURAL TRANSMISSION LOSS FOR TONES DELIVERED BY AIR CONDUCTION IN CASES OF UNILATERAL DEAFNESS.

	125 Hz	250 Hz	500 Hz	1,000 Hz	2,000 Hz	4,000 Hz	8,000 Hz	250–4,000 Hz average
					Transmission loss (dB)			
Mean								
Present authors								
(*N* = 20)	—	61	63	63	63	68	(60)*	63
Gyllencreutz and Lidén (1967)								
(*N* = 50)	—	54	60	62	64	70	—	62
Littler et al. (1952)								
(*N* = 4)	46	48	55	48	65	58	55	53
Range								
Present authors	—	50–80	45–80	40–85	45–75	50–85	(60)*	
Littler et al.	45–50	45–55	45–60	30–60	50–80	40–90	35–70	

*Data from one patient only.

Note: The present authors' data and those of Gyllencreutz and Lidén were obtained with an audiometer using receivers mounted in MX = 41/AR cushions, as in the case with most audiometers used in this country. The generally lower figures obtained in the four cases illustrated by Littler et al. (1952) may have been due to their use of an audiometer whose receivers were mounted in ADC cushions which were made (Knight, 1968; personal communication) of a harder material and possibly covered a greater area of the ear. Similar considerations are probably relevant to the data of Fletcher (1953) who went on to point out that the value of 50 dB is dependent upon the type of telephone receivers used.

In order to provide up-to-date information on levels of cross-hearing, the authors have presented in Table 36-1 data from a series of twenty persons with severe unilateral deafness. Whereas the average interaural transmission loss for sound delivered by an earphone is about 60 dB, it is the 40 dB minima which should be considered when assessing the possibility of cross-hearing in any one patient at any one frequency. Thus 40 dB was taken as the critical figure for the rules on need for masking, as set out above.

Returning to Case A, if the unmasked b/c thresholds were between 0 and 20 dB, then the 60 dB a/c thresholds of the right ear could be a shadow of the left cochlea. On the other hand if the unmasked b/c thresholds had been 30 dB, then the unmasked 60 dB a/c thresholds must have been the true hearing level of that ear.

It may be argued that tuning fork and other clinical tests would indicate the general nature of the hearing loss and whether masking of the audiogram was needed. Whilst not decrying the immense value of such tests when very carefully performed, it has been pointed out by Hinchcliffe and Littler (1961) that little quantitative information is obtained and that the Weber test has a test-retest coefficient of only 0.75, and by Groen (1962) that the Weber test should not be used at frequencies above 1,000 Hz.

Patients' responses to fork tests in general are likely to be considerably less reliable than with the 'heard' or 'not heard' tasks of audiometry, and the

authors have noted that even the basic concept of lateralization seems to be meaningless in the majority of patients with severe unilateral perceptive deafness of long standing. Every effort should therefore be made to ensure that the diagnostic evidence provided by the pure-tone audiogram is complete in itself; the latter must include masking as and when indicated by audiometric considerations.

(ii) Insufficient Masking. On other occasions, misdiagnosis arose from use of insufficient levels of masking. One probable reason for this was too faithful reliance on the nominal 'level of masking' provided by many of the older audiometers. Whilst the level of masking dial may be quite accurate in one part of the frequency range, the level may be wholly inaccurate at other test frequencies. For instance, in one popular clinical audiometer employing narrowband noise for masking, the 30 dB masking level was found to be quite accurate at 2,000 Hz and above but at 250 Hz the same nominal level of noise was not even audible. Thus with this audiometer, if a single level of masking was used (a most unsatisfactory but, regrettably, widely used masking technique), then a 30 dB level of masking might be considered adequate to mask all frequencies of an ear with normal hearing, e.g. of Case B. In fact though, there would have been no masking effect at all at 250 Hz and considerably less than the nominal 30 dB effect at 500 and 1,000 Hz.

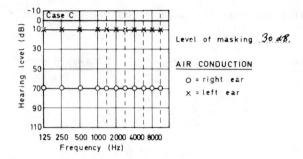

FIGURE 36-2. Case C, as referred for speech audiometry prior to fitting of hearing aid.

When white noise, modified mains hum, or saw-tooth noise is used for masking, even a check on its audibility is no safeguard as to its effectiveness. This is demonstrated by Figure 36-2 of the paper by Denes and Naunton (1952) in which no masking effect on tones of 250 Hz was produced until the white noise masker reached a level of 30 dB above its threshold (i.e. sensation level of the masker was 30 dB).

Another cause of insufficient masking is that one dial setting of masking level is used for all frequencies regardless of differences in hearing level between one frequency and the next in the ear to be masked. This error is probably related to a long outdated feature on the audiogram forms used in many E.N.T. departments. The feature criticized is the notation:

'Level of Masking . . . '

'Setting of Masking Control . . . '

This implies that one setting is satisfactory for all frequencies, which clearly it can only be in the rare instances when the audiogram of the ear to be masked corresponds in shape to the relative effectiveness of the masking noise at each test frequency. The only way to use the notation 'Level of Masking . . . '

is to adjust the level in relation to the threshold of the ear to be masked at each frequency and to record the level of masking as so many decibels sensation level (e.g. '30 dB S.L.'). The adjustment should, of course, include any corrections necessary for variations from frequency to frequency in the threshold levels of the masking noise previously measured in persons with normal ears. An example of how to do this is shown in Table 36-2, but the reader is referred to the Appendix A for a more detailed account of the methods by which the effectiveness of an audiometer's masking noises may be checked.

Whilst the calibration of masking noises as delivered by audiometer earphones has improved in recent years and may often be found to be correct for all frequencies, the advantages of insert-type telephones in reducing the problems of cross-masking have resulted in their wide-spread use for delivering the masking noise. Unfortunately, due largely to variations in their placement in individual ear canals, the actual sound field introduced into the patient's ear from an insert telephone cannot be relied upon and the audiometrician must resort to measuring the threshold of the masking noises for each and every insertion of the telephone.

(iii) Failure to Use More than One Level of Masking. The notations referred to above contribute to misdiagnosis not only because one level of masking noise is seldom the correct one for all test frequencies but also because of its general implication that for any given test frequency one level of masking is sufficient.

This is not to say that use of only one level is always wrong or that there is an error in the measurement when so plotted on the audiogram, e.g., that a hearing level of x dB was measured when a masking control setting of y dB was used. A serious error may

TABLE 36-2. EXAMPLE OF A TABLE FOR ACHIEVING STATED SENSATION LEVELS OF MASKING NOISE.

Sensation level of masking noise desired	Set the masking dial to the hearing level of the ear to be masked, plus the amounts below				
	250 Hz	500 Hz	1,000 Hz	2,000 Hz	4,000 Hz
0 dB*	35	20	10	0	0
30 dB	65	50	40	30	30
60 dB	95	80	70	60	60
90 dB	—	—	100	90	90

*Note: Calibration errors in the nominal levels of the masking noise (as measured by differences in threshold for the pure tones and the masking noises) are indicated by the 0 dB S.L. figures.

creep in, however, if the plotted hearing level of *x* dB is later read off the audiogram as the true threshold of that ear; it is liable to be read off in this way because, after all, the audiogram is intended to be a representation of the auditory thresholds. In fact, it is quite likely that if the full range of masking levels had been used the tone threshold might have been found to be considerably in excess of *x* dB. Examples of diagnostic mistakes of this kind are illustrated by Case C below.

Case C was referred for speech audiometry in relation to possible hearing-aid usage. In accordance with our usual practice, the audiogram was repeated with detailed attention being given to the masking of just a few selected test frequencies. Masking charts of the kind illustrated in Figure 36-3 were used and the masking procedure employed followed the shadowing principle first described by Hood (1957).

The masking function shown was for a/c tests of the right ear at 2,000 Hz. The unmasked tonal threshold of 55 dB was recorded outside the chart above the arrow indicating 'NIL' masking. Next, the hearing threshold (M) for the masking noise in the left ear (that to be masked) was established[1]; this was at the 0 dB reading of the masking dial, indicated as the 'nominal masking level.'

Masking of the non-test ear followed, first at a nominal masking level of M + 10 dB (i.e., at a masking noise sensation level of 10 dB) and subsequently at M + 30 dB, M + 50 dB and M + 70 dB. These resulted in thresholds of 60, 80, 100 and over 110 dB respectively, which were recorded on the masking chart.

It can be seen from Figure 36-3, that the hearing levels recorded in the right (test) ear rose steadily on a one-for-one basis with every increase of masking level in the left (non-test) ear, and that when sufficient masking was used not even the maximum 110 dB output of the audiometer could be heard. In fact, the threshold of 70 dB recorded in the original audiogram (see Figure 36-2) with 30 dB nominal level of masking from their audiometer was in fair agreement with our own results at a 30 dB masking dial setting; but the recording of 70 dB on the original audiogram was misleading, implying as it did that this was the tone threshold. If 10 dB higher or lower levels of masking had been used, the apparent thresholds would likewise have been 10 dB higher or lower. Thus, in this type of case, if a single level of masking is used the threshold recorded is purely a function of the level of masking applied to the non-test ear and entirely fails to measure the true threshold.

One other frequency, 500 Hz, was tested in the same way and the same fully masked hearing level of over 110 dB was recorded. The audiogram of C, as remeasured, is shown in Figure 36-4.

Clearly there was no useful hearing in the speech range, which obviated the requirement for speech audiometry, nor would the patient have benefited from a hearing aid.

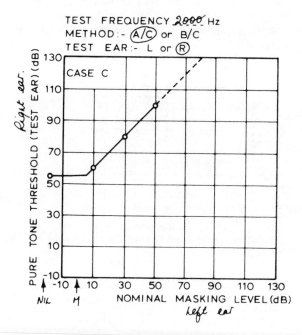

FIGURE 36-3.   A masking function in Case C.

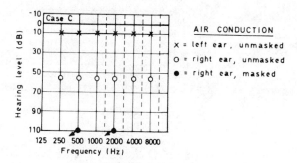

FIGURE 36-4.   Case C, as re-recorded after use of full range of masking.

Incorrect Measurement of Air/Bone Gap

Case D illustrates misdiagnosis of a persistent air/bone gap following a left stapedectomy, for which a revision operation was offered. The audiogram, at referral for absolute impedance measurements prior to operation with the object of finding out what had gone wrong with the original operation, is shown in Figure 36-5. In obtaining the air-conduction thresholds of the left ear the right ear had not been masked, the omission presumably being due to the left-to-right a/c difference being less than 50 dB. The b/c thresholds of around 20 dB that were recorded on the original audiogram had resulted from a single (50 dB) level of masking of the non-test ear.

For the sake of illustration concerning the true air/bone gap, one of the b/c masking functions performed by the authors is shown in Figure 36-6. The same masking procedure, as described in connection with Figure 36-3 with a/c tests, was employed for the b/c tests.

Again, the apparent thresholds recorded depended entirely on the degree to which the non-test ear was masked. In the original tests the 50 dB nominal level of masking from their audiometer resulted in an apparent b/c threshold of 20 dB and an apparent air/bone gap of 40 dB but, from study of the full masking function shown in Figure 36-6, it can now be seen that if 30 or 70 dB nominal levels of masking had been used (in the original tests) the apparent b/c thresholds recorded would merely have been 20 dB

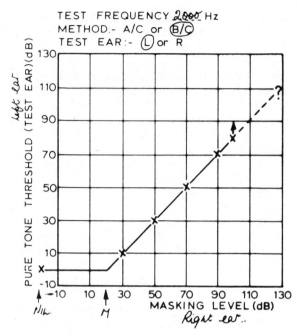

FIGURE 36-6. A bone conduction masking function in Case D.

lower or higher and apparent air/bone gaps of 60 or 20 dB respectively would have resulted. Again, the cause of misdiagnosis was the use of a single level of masking.

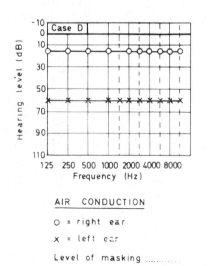

AIR   CONDUCTION

o = right ear

x = left ear

Level of masking ....

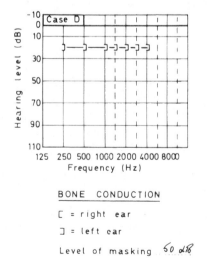

BONE   CONDUCTION

[= right ear

] = left ear

Level of masking   60 dB

FIGURE 36-5. Case D, as referred for impedance measurements prior to revision of stapedectomy.

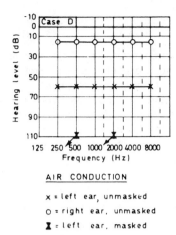

AIR CONDUCTION

x = left ear, unmasked
o = right ear, unmasked
𝕀 = left ear, masked

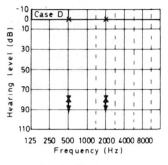

BONE CONDUCTION

Same symbols as for air conduction
but recorded in red (and, in our
practice, with separate audiograms
for left (a/c and b/c) and for
right (a/c and b/c))

FIGURE 36-7. Case D, as re-recorded after use of full range of masking.

The true hearing state of this patient could have been measured by full-range masking tests at just one or two selected frequencies. Indeed, as will be seen from our final audiogram Figure 36-7, if the need for masking of the a/c tests had been recognized, properly masked a/c tests alone would have given the information essential to the surgeon, i.e., that there was a profound loss of hearing in the left ear. It is noteworthy also that the inadequate masking of the b/c tests yielded an apparent 'mixed deafness' spread over all the frequencies so tested; in fact, a fixed level of masking technique will inevitably lead to a high proportion of cases of wholly perceptive deafness being misdiagnosed as 'mixed deafness.'

II. DEFINITION OF WHEN MASKING IS NEEDED

A. Masking in Conventional Air-Conduction Tests

Rules for deciding when masking is needed for these tests have already been described in Section I.A.(i).

B. Masking in Bone-Conduction Tests

Although the interaural transmission loss by b/c may amount to 5-15 dB (Gyllencreutz and Lidén, 1967; Studebaker, 1967), the only safe rule for clinical practice is to regard it as zero. Masking should therefore be used for b/c tests of the ear with the worse hearing by a/c at all the frequencies where an appar-

ent gap of 10 dB or more is found between its a/c threshold and the previously obtained unmasked b/c threshold (which should have been measured without occlusion of either ear, e.g., by an earphone or insert telephone). If this masking results in a shift of threshold of 10 dB or more, then the unmasked b/c threshold at that frequency can be attributed to the better hearing ear: if such a shift does not occur, then it would be advisable to conduct further b/c tests whilst masking the worse-hearing ear.

In agreement with the above rule, it can be seen that there is one important type of case where no masking of b/c tests is required. This is where there is a more or less symmetrical a/c loss in the two ears and the unmasked b/c threshold pattern is essentially similar.

Finally it should be noted that adaptation of the Weber test, for the purpose of deciding whether masking is needed and which ear to mask, is too unreliable a method and should not be used.

C. Masking in Other Forms of Air-Conduction Tests

The rules for masking of conventional audiometric a/c tests apply equally to most of the special topo-diagnostic tests, notably Békésy audiometry, tone decay tests, and speech audiometry. Loudness balance and acoustic reflex threshold (Metz) tests are not masked, although account must be taken of the true (masked) thresholds in assessing the degree of recruitment present. The S.I.S.I. test must also be masked whenever there is a possibility that the test tones reaching the non-test cochlea may be 25 dB or more above the latter's threshold.

The techniques of masking in these procedures is beyond the scope of this paper. Suffice to say that they require an even higher degree of understanding and experience than with masking in conventional audiometric tests.

III. INSTRUMENTATION REQUIREMENTS FOR MASKING

A. Types of Masking Noise

(i) In Pure-Tone Tests. The advantages of narrow-band noise as a masker of tonal signals are sufficiently great for the use of wide-band noise, modified mains hum or saw-tooth noise to be regarded as obsolete. Restricted-band noises are provided in some audiometers and are better than wide-band noise though not having the full advantages of narrow-band noises.

The advantages themselves are twofold. Firstly, for a given amount of effective masking a considerably lower intensity of narrow-band noise is needed than would be the case with a wide-band noise; that is, the 'masking efficiency' (Denes and Naunton, 1952) of narrow-band noise is greater. The lesser loudness of the noise results in less general disturbance of the listener and less central masking, when the ability of the brain to detect weak signals coming from one ear is reduced by the presence of stronger signals coming from the other ear: also, due to intolerance of intense sounds the dynamic range of effective masking is wider in the case of the less loud narrow-band noises. Secondly, a single wide-band masking noise of a given level is apt to produce major differences in amount of effective masking at different test frequencies, whilst the minimum effective level (E.L.) of a range of narrow-band noises can more readily be adjusted to correspond to the calibration at each and every test frequency of the tones they are designed to mask.

(ii) In Speech Tests. As the frequency spectrum of speech covers a large proportion of the audio range, a wide-band noise is needed to mask it. Any audiometer used for both pure-tone and speech tests should, therefore, have a facility for selection of either narrow-band or wide-band noise for masking.

B. Maximum Intensity of Masking Noise

To obtain maximum diagnostic information from masking procedures, a considerably greater intensity range of masking noises is needed than is available with many audiometers. Both tones and masking noises can be delivered by air conduction up to hearing levels of 110 dB, or even 120 dB, in the middle frequencies and such intensities are useful.

C. Means of Delivery of Masking Noise

(i) By an Insert Telephone. Use of an insert as a means of delivery of a sound to the ear results in a considerable increase in the interaural transmission losses shown in Table 36–1. Therefore, if an insert is used for delivering the test tone the need for masking is often obviated, whilst if it is used for delivering the masking noise, as first recommended by Littler et al. (1952), the level at which cross-masking occurs is increased by about 15 dB according to the data published by Gyllencreutz and Lidén in 1967. The latter can be an enormous advantage in those difficult masking problems where there is an extensive bilateral a/c hearing loss and an air/bone gap in one or both ears.

The difficulties with insert telephones lie in (1) their acoustic calibration; (2) differences in shape of frequency response of audiometer earphones and insert telephones such that they are not readily interchangeable; and (3) the wide test/retest variations in sound pressure level developed in the ear that result from minor variations in placement of the insert in the ear and in the shape and size of different people's ear canals. For use in masking, however, both disadvantages are overcome if the masking dial readings are regarded as purely nominal and a masking procedure such as that described in connection with Figure 36–3 is adopted. (Note, however, that if an insert telephone is buttoned on to a headset with an earphone cushion as provided with some audiometers or if an earphone is placed over the insert telephone then the result will be a return to the cross-masking levels appropriate to earphones.)

(ii) By an Earphone. The advantages here are of simplicity of equipment, relatively easy calibration, fair test/retest repeatability and consequently greater speed. A further advantage has recently been described by Littler (1968) whereby the greater cross-

masking effects of earphone masking can sometimes be utilized to diagnostic advantage: an example of this is illustrated in Figure 36–8 and is described in more detail later.

(iii) By Either Earphone or Insert Telephone. Ideally an audiometer should provide both means of delivering masking noise for either a/c or b/c tests; the choice at the time of test depending on the requirements of each particular audiometric problem.

(iv) By the Bone-Conduction Vibrator. This is used in the Rainville (1955) and S.A.L. or sensorineural acuity level (Jerger and Tillman, 1960) tests. As these are not regularly used in this country and have particular problems which render them of doubtful advantage over conventional masking techniques with narrow-band noise and insert telephones, they will not be discussed here.

IV. PROCEDURES USED FOR MASKING

To emphasize the importance of having a proper masking procedure, fully understood and carefully carried out, one cannot do better than to quote Studebaker (1967) in his criticism of audiological practice in America. He said that 'many audiologists know far less about masking procedures than about any other commonly used clinical technique. Clinical masking procedures often consist of unsystematic guesswork for which there is little or no defence.'

Distinctly the most reliable technique has already been mentioned here in description of Figures 36–3 and 36–6. This is usually known as the shadowing technique and was first reported from this country by Hood (1957). We have found it helpful to chart the complete masking function by measuring the tonal threshold of each of a series of masking levels: apart from being useful in judging the true thresholds of hearing in difficult or uncertain cases, it has great advantages for all concerned in learning to understand the effects of masking and also for the otologist in charge by rendering him less vulnerable to mistakes of procedure or interpretation by the technician. More commonly though, the full procedure is simplified in order to conserve time, and the methodology for this will be outlined.

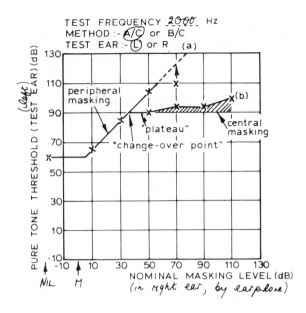

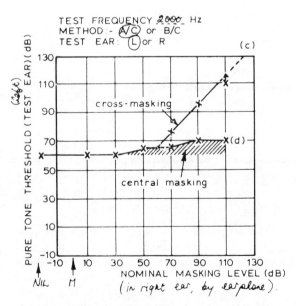

FIGURE 36–8. Four common configurations of masking function. (Illustrated by a case of unilateral hearing loss measured without masking at 60 dB hearing level.) Conclusions: (a) over 110 dB deafness with perceptive element of 50 dB or more; (b) 95 dB deafness with perceptive element of 30 dB or more; (c) 60 dB deafness with little or no perceptive element; (d) 60 dB deafness with perceptive element of about 50 dB or more.

A single level of masking is far more frequently applied in this country. This has advantages in speed and apparent simplicity, but as already indicated by the misdiagnoses described earlier, it is subject to much greater possibility of error due to the risk of either under- or over-masking. An added difficulty with the method in practice though is that neither audiology technician nor otologist gain from it a sufficient familiarity with the wide variety of masking functions occurring in clinical practice to enable them to recognize the frequent and serious limitations of the method. With such understanding of its limitations and with care, it can, however, be used in a number of cases and this section will therefore include a discussion of this method also.

It is important not to overstress the time taken in applying the shadowing technique as compared to a single level of masking. All too frequently the latter is used over an unnecessarily wide range of frequencies with results of very uncertain meaning, whereas the time used would have been better spent in using a full range of masking levels for just one or two test frequencies. As illustrated in Case D, Figure 36–7, masking at only one or two frequencies is all that was needed for diagnosis, which is the principal object of audiometry, and even if this means performing audiometry on a slightly smaller proportion of patients it is much more worthwhile to arrive at the right diagnosis in selected patients rather than perform tests in a greater number of patients over a greater frequency range but with doubtful reliability. If at a later date a more comprehensive audiogram is required prior to some surgical procedure then this could usually be arranged by appointment at some more convenient and less rushed time.

A. The Correct Method: Shadowing

The basic procedure has already been outlined in its application to cases (C and D) of complete hearing loss in one ear. The linear patterns of masking shown in Figures 36–3 and 36–6 resulted, but many other patterns can arise and the principles of their interpretation need further description. To do this, let us consider the possible outcome of masking in a case initially found to have 60 dB of unilateral a/c hearing loss.

Four common configurations of masking function are shown in Figure 36–8. Configuration (a) has already been illustrated in Figures 36–3 and 36–6; in this case the true hearing loss of the left ear was in ex-

cess of the maximum 110 dB output of the audiometer. Note that there is a 1 dB shift in threshold with every 1 dB increase in masking which is the one-for-one pattern typical of peripheral masking, i.e., the masking noise mixes with the tonal signal in the peripheral sense organ.

The opposite extreme is shown in configuration (d); apart from some central masking, characterized by a much less than one-for-one slope, the masking function is essentially flat: this shows that the apparent 60 dB threshold in the left ear was in fact the true one.

In configuration (b), the threshold rose with a one-for-one slope until the tonal level in the left ear reached 90 dB; the plateau of tonal thresholds at the 90 dB level indicated the true threshold of that ear. Thereafter, with further increases in masking noise delivered to the right ear there was no further increase in threshold, apart from some small central masking effects.

The third configuration shown, (c), shows cross-masking which, like peripheral masking, also has a one-for-one slope. In fact it is due to peripheral masking as, in this case, the masking is affecting the left ear as well as the right, i.e. the masking noise has been transmitted across the head from the masking earphone on the right ear to the cochlea of the left ear. When this happens at a level of masking that corresponds roughly to the level at which cross-hearing is to be expected (see Table 36–1), then this means that the masking noise is being heard by the cochlea of the test ear at levels corresponding to normal threshold, i.e., in the case shown by configuration (c) the left ear has 60 dB a/c loss and 0 dB b/c loss. Thus, as mentioned earlier here and as described by Littler in 1968, the cross-masking effect in a/c tests can in fact yield information on the b/c threshold also.

Likewise, the lack of cross-masking in configuration (d) up to levels of 110 dB infers that the masking noise of 110 dB less the expected interaural transmission loss (60 dB), i.e., reaching the left ear at 50 dB level, has not in fact been heard and the hearing loss in this ear is largely if not wholly perceptive in type. Conclusions on type of deafness can also be drawn from configurations (a) and (b). In these cases, the peripheral masking would not have originated at such low levels of masking if any part of the 60 dB tones delivered had been heard by the left cochlea; as, in configuration (a), they were not heard even at 110 dB there must have been about 50 dB (i.e., 110 dB less 60 dB interaural transmission loss) or more of perceptive element in the hearing loss.

Once experience with the shadowing method has been obtained, the detailed technique can often be speeded up by not charting the masking function or measuring the tonal threshold with each increment of masking. With the tone at its apparent threshold level, the masking level is set to a S.L. of 10 dB when the tone is usually effectively masked; alternate increments, commonly of 10 dB, of tone and noise are then applied and the successive reappearances and disappearances of the tones are noted if and when the plateau is reached, and a further 20 dB of noise fails to mask the tone by more than 5 dB or so, the level of the plateau indicates the true threshold. If the initial 10 dB S.L. of masking fails to cause masking (as it may do—see Table 36A-1), a further 20 dB of noise should also be applied before any definite conclusions are drawn regarding the true threshold.

B. An Unreliable Method: Single Level of Masking[2]

One only needs to look at the possible configurations shown in Figure 36-8 and to consider the various ramifications possible with other degrees of hearing loss in one or both ears to realize the gross inadequacy and uncertainty that is inherent in use of only one level of masking in a large proportion of cases. It is also apparent that even in the most simple types of case, e.g. those of configurations (c) and (d) where a single 40 dB level of masking would show the true a/c threshold to be 60 dB, diagnostic information obtained from presence or absence of cross-masking is lost if the full range of masking levels is not employed.

Apart from this loss of information and uncertainty of interpretation of results, there is the most difficult question of what level of masking to use at each frequency. Any ruling that can be really reliable must of necessity be so complicated that it fails to provide a practicable answer to this question. The difficulty lies in choosing a level that does not result in either under-masking (i.e., below the 'change-over point') or over-masking (i.e., including elements of central masking or cross-masking). For instance, 40 dB of masking in cases with configurations (a) and (b) would result in apparent hearing levels of 95 or 90 dB; this would correspond to the true threshold only in the second case. Likewise, 90 dB of masking with configurations (b) and (c) would both yield apparent

hearing levels of 95 dB; in Case (B) this would be fairly correct, but in Case C a patient with an actual 60 dB of purely conductive deafness would be misdiagnosed as having 95 dB hearing loss which would include a sizeable element of cochlear loss also (because the average air-to-bone conduction transmission loss averaged across frequencies is about 50–70 dB see Table 36-1, it is unusual to measure with conventional earphones on air/bone gap greater than about 70 dB, Feldman, 1963).

With these limitations in mind, the best ruling that can be offered for use of a single level of masking is to try the effect of masking levels of 10–40 dB E.L. (effective level) or 20–40 dB S.L. (sensation level) for the masking noise, i.e., at M + 20 dB to M + 40 dB. Even then there are a number of provisos:

1. It can only be applied safely at this level if the a/c hearing in the ear being masked is within normal limits, otherwise there is the risk of cross-masking;
2. The calibration of the masking source must have been checked with sufficient accuracy to ensure that the E.L. of the noise is correct, or the threshold (M) of the narrow-band masking noises has to be measured at each frequency (as it has to be anyway, whenever insert telephones are used for delivering the masking noises) in order to set the dials to the desired S.L.;
3. Further levels of masking are used if there is more than 10 dB of shift in threshold induced by the masking, i.e., if configurations (a) or (b) are becoming apparent. The masking procedure can only be regarded as sufficient if no shift in threshold results from delivery of masking noise of a quite certain degree of effectiveness.

It is evident that this technique is liable to so many complications and uncertainties, that it is really easier to proceed with the shadowing technique in the first place and to regard use of a single level of masking as obsolescent.

C. An Acceptable Compromise: Synchronous Masking

Various other forms and procedures for masking have been described from time to time, but in the authors' opinion there is only one that is reasonably satisfactory and does not introduce further problems of its own; it is 'synchronous masking,' a method first described in the English language by König in

1962. This is in fact a still more time-saving simplification of the shadowing technique. It involves adjusting the masking level dial synchronously with the hearing level dial, either by an automatic locking as in some of the more elaborate audiometers or by manual adjustment as can be done with any audiometer.

The hearing level control is set to the unmasked threshold of the test ear and the masking level control is set to a level corresponding to the threshold of the non-test ear and sufficiently far above it to be certain that it would be effectively masked; the latter step involves accurate prior calibration of the effectiveness of the masking noises at each frequency and application of a +10 dB allowance in order to be certain, or setting a level at least 20 dB above the threshold of the masking noise (see Table 36A–1). If the tone is not then heard it is turned up in 5 or 10 dB steps with synchronous 5 or 10 dB rises in masking level until the level is found at which the tone may become audible in spite of the masking. This tonal level corresponds to the plateau in the masking function and thereby identifies the true threshold.

Whilst this method is a compromise between speed and accuracy, it should not be adopted for routine usage until the audiometrician is thoroughly familiar with the usage and interpretation of the shadowing technique. In the most difficult cases it would still be wise to determine and plot the detailed masking function over a full range of masking levels.

V. USEFUL SYMBOLS AND NOTATIONS

Various organizations have from time to time published recommendations with intent to achieve some general standardization in the detail of forms used for recording audiogram. On the other hand, it is left to each otologist to make the final decision on the forms to be used in his own department.

Ideally, an audiogram should show only the true thresholds of hearing. But in fact these can often be obtained only after a most careful and exhaustive series of masking tests for which, in a busy clinic, there is not always time or sufficient expertise. It is essential therefore to indicate on the form precise details of the masking used and to which of the recorded thresholds these details apply.

To this end, it is most worthwhile to record on the audiogram both the thresholds measured initially without masking and those measured later with masking. The shifts in threshold between the two then enable a more reliable assessment to be made as to whether the thresholds recorded are the true ones or whether they may still be simply a function of the amount of masking used. As this takes up rather too much space on an audiogram if it shows left and right ears together, in our own practice we plot left and right ears on separate audiograms and have adopted ideas on symbols given us by Dr. A. Boothroyd (recently of Department of Audiology and Education of the Deaf, University of Manchester):

X = left ear, unmasked
O = right ear, unmasked
B = binaural (used for unmasked b/c tests and
    in some forms of speech audiometry)
𝐗 = left ear, masked
● = right ear, masked

A different colour code for the a/c and b/c thresholds is also used. The advantages of this in ease of reading are obvious and easily outweigh the one disadvantage, that is when carbon copies are required: the carbon is then used for a/c tests (recorded in black or blue) only and it is not a great labour to mark in the relatively few b/c thresholds on the copies at a later date.

It is most important of course to use either the shadowing technique, or a masking noise calibrated and stated precisely in terms of sensation level or effective level. The notations 'Level of masking . . .' or 'Setting of masking control . . .' would then be completed by addition of such words as 'shadowing,' 'x dB S.L.,' or 'y dB E.L.' If more than one level is used, or different levels used for a/c and b/c tests these will have to be indicated also by lettering on the audiogram in the former case or by colour coding in the latter case.

Only by care in use of masking and in recording of the results obtained can audiometry become systematic and thus yield results that are both reliable and capable of proper interpretation.

SUMMARY

Errors in basic air and bone conduction due to nonuse or incorrect use of masking still arise all too frequently. Examples are given of the sort of misdiagnoses that occur.

The most common cause of such diagnostic errors is due to the prevalent practice of using just one level of masking, a malpractice encouraged by the notation 'Level of masking . . .' or 'Setting of masking control . . . ,' which appears on many audiogram forms. Not only should the level be adjusted from frequency to frequency to allow for variations in the hearing level of the non-test ear and also in the calibration of the masking noise, but often more than one level of masking is needed at individual frequencies if the true thresholds are to be determined and indicated on the audiogram.

A plea is made for restriction of the number of frequencies to be tested with masking: one or two frequencies properly masked and the results carefully interpreted yield more accurate information than a range of frequencies masked at one level only.

Details of when masking is needed, means of delivering masking, type of masking noise, procedures for masking, useful symbols and an appendix on checking the calibration of the masking noise provided by an audiometer are all intended to make the paper one of constructive criticism.

ENDNOTES

1. Although the nominal level at which effective masking should start could have been calculated from a masking calibration table, in practice it seems worthwhile to spend a few seconds in checking the actual level of M for each frequency to be masked, and indicating this on the masking chart. Further, as already indicated and to be discussed in more detail later, measurement of M is essential when an insert telephone is used for delivering the masking noise.

2. This method does not of course mean the use of one level of masking for all frequencies, but rather a series of separate settings of the masking dial, the settings being determined by the threshold of the ear to be masked and the calibration of the masking noise at each frequency.

REFERENCES

Denes, P., and Naunton, R. F. (1952) *Proceedings of the Royal Society of Medicine,* **45**, 790.

Elliott, E. (1958) *Nature (London),* **181**, 1076.

Feldman, A. S. (1961) *Journal of Speech and Hearing Disorders,* **26**, 39.

Feldman, A. S. (1963) *Journal of Speech and Hearing Research,* **6**, 157.

Fletcher, H. (1953) *Speech and Hearing in Communication,* Princeton: D. Van Nostrand, Chapter 10.

Groen, J. J. (1962) *The value of the Weber test. Proceedings of Henry Ford Hospital International Symposium on 'Otosclerosis.'* Published by Little, Brown & Co. Inc.

Gyllencreutz, T., and Lidén, G. (1967) *Acta oto-laryngologica (Stockholm),* Supplement **224**, 229.

Hawkins, J. E., and Stevens, S. S. (1950) *Journal of the Acoustical Society of America,* **22**, 6.

Hinchcliffe, R., and Littler, T. S. (1961) *Journal of Laryngology and Otology,* **75**, 201.

Hood, J. D. (1957) *Proceedings of the Royal Society of Medicine,* **50**, 689.

Hood, J. D. (1960) *Laryngoscope (St. Louis),* **70**, 1211.

Jerger, J., and Tillman, T. W. (1960) *Archives of Otolaryngology,* **71**, 948.

König, E. (1962) *Acta oto-laryngologica (Stockholm),* Supplement **180**, 1.

Littler, T. S. (1968) *Sound,* **2**, 11.

Littler, T. S.; Knight, J. J.; and Strange, P. H. (1952) *Proceedings of the Royal Society of Medicine,* **45**, 783.

Rainville, M. J. (1955) *'Nouvelle methode d'assourdissement pour le releve des courbes de conduction osseuse.' Journal français d'oto-rhino-laryngologie et chirurgie maxillo-faciale,* **4**, 851.

Studebaker, G. A. (1964) *Journal of Speech and Hearing Disorders,* **29**, 23.

Studebaker, G. A. (1967) *Journal of Speech and Hearing Disorders,* **32**, 360.

APPENDIX A: SUBJECTIVE METHODS FOR CHECKING SENSATION LEVEL OR EFFECTIVENESS OF AN AUDIOMETER'S MASKING NOISES

There is a simple means of checking that the narrow-band masking noises provided by most modern audiometers have a degree of effectiveness similar to their nominal level (i.e., as indicated by the masking level dial). This is to measure in a small group of persons with flat audiograms their earphone thresholds for pure tones and for the corresponding narrow-band noises. In theory, a narrow-band noise that is just audible will be sufficient to mask out a pure-tone that is otherwise just audible; thus the accuracy of the masking level dial can then be judged in terms of sensation level of masking noise at each test frequency by the size of any differences between averaged tonal and masking-noise thresholds. From this, a calibration table (such as in Table 36–2) can be constructed and the dial setting for any required *sensation level* of masking can easily be calculated.

From data collected by the authors with a good quality commercial audiometer, it was found, however, that the sensation level of a masking noise may not in practice be an entirely reliable indication of masking effectiveness. In twenty cases of severe unilateral deafness, it was possible to study the relationship between thresholds for the masking noises and their actual masking efficiency by plotting masking functions of the sort illustrated in Figures 36–3 and 36–7(a). The results given in Table 36A–1 show that for the noises to have their expected masking effect they had to be 0–20 dB more intense than would be indicated by the sensation level method described above.

The average discrepancies between the thresholds of audibility and of effectiveness of the masking noises apparent in Table 36A–1 might be regarded as being particular to the audiometer employed. It is relevant, therefore, to mention four possible causes for discrepancies of the sort found. First, the band width of the narrow-band noises provided by an audiometer may be considerably greater than the critical band width, especially if they are of 'restricted band' (e.g., 1 or 2 octaves wide); second, the noise bands may not be centred very precisely on the frequencies of the corresponding pure-tones (though this was not true of the audiometer used in obtaining the data of Table 36A–1); third, the shape of the narrow-band of noise may not be as flat as it should be; fourth, the threshold of hearing varies by 6–12 dB with about 60 Hz differences in frequency (Elliott, 1958) and a band of noise is, therefore, more likely than any one tone within the band to coincide with peaks of auditory sensitivity, with the result that the masking effect of the noise may be somewhat less

TABLE 36A–1. RELATIONSHIP BETWEEN THRESHOLD OF NARROW-BAND MASKING NOISE AND EFFECTIVE MASKING LEVEL IN 20 CASES OF UNILATERAL DEAFNESS.

Level of masker at which effective one-for-one* masking began	Number of masking functions demonstrating the relationships Frequency (Hz)					
	250	500	1,000	2,000	4,000	Total
M − 5 dB	0	0	0	0	0	0
M	0	3	4	9	4	20
M + 5 dB	2	3	8	5	0	18
M + 10 dB	1	2	6	4	3	16
M + 15 dB	2	5	0	1	1	9
M + 20 dB	4	2	1	1	0	8
M + 25 dB	0	0	0	0	0	0
Total	9	15	19	20	8	71
Median	M + 14	10	6	5	6	M + 6·7

M = Auditory threshold of the masking noise in the non-test ear; both masking noise and test tones delivered by earphones.

*Often there was an initial rise of threshold by one or two 5 dB attenuator steps before the main linear masking effect commenced. In these cases, the one-for-one peripheral masking function was extrapolated back to the original unmasked threshold level in order to find the minimum effective level of the masking noise. Similar curvilinear origin to masking functions were shown by Hawkins and Stevens in 1950 and by Studebaker in 1967, and the latter stressed the importance of allowing for this in order to avoid overestimation of the masking efficiency of a noise.

than its sensation level. Whatever may be the true cause or causes of the ineffectiveness of the first 0–20 dB sensation level of masking, the fact remains that in some audiometers available commercially such discrepancies occur and users of audiometers should be aware of this possibility.

The scatter about the average also deserves comment: it is attributed to the inherent ±5 dB unreliability of threshold audiometry, which applies to both tonal and masking-noise thresholds, and to the approximations to threshold inherent in the use of 5 dB attenuator steps.

A more elaborate but more accurate procedure for subjective checking on the calibration of masking noises has been described by Studebaker (1964). To carry out this, minor instrumental modifications may be needed but the method has the advantage of providing a direct measure of the actual masking effectiveness of the masking noises as delivered by the audiometer, rather than relying on a slightly uncertain (see Table 36A–1) relation between masking-noise thresholds and masking effectiveness. In the case of masking noises other than narrow-band ones either the Studebaker type of calibration technique or masking tests in cases of unilateral deafness must be used for making subjective checks on the actual effectiveness of masking noise delivered by an audiometer. The calibration of masking noise is then in terms of *effective level*.

37

Clinical Masking of the Non-Test Ear

GERALD A. STUDEBAKER, Ph.D.
*Professor of Speech and Hearing Science,
Memphis State University*

The application of a masking noise to the nontest ear is a daily clinical activity. Yet many audiologists know far less about masking procedures than about any other commonly used clinical technique. Clinical masking procedures often consist of unsystematic guesswork for which there is little or no logical defense.

Current texts (Davis and Silverman, 1961; Glorig, 1965; Jerger, 1963; Newby, 1964; O'Neill and Oyer, 1966; Sataloff, 1966) used in beginning and intermediate audiology classes imply by omission that little, or nothing, appears in the journals on the subject of clinical masking. The procedures given in these texts are often presented without reference and, in some instances, the procedures contradict available evidence. The bibliography at the end of this discussion is presented, in part, to illustrate that there is a substantial body of literature on, or closely related to, clinical masking. A review of these references reveals that there are, indeed, some areas of disagreement. However, on many important procedural aspects there is substantial consensus among those who have studied masking methods most thoroughly.

DEFINITIONS

Masking is best defined operationally as an elevation in the threshold of one signal produced by the introduction of a second signal. The first signal is called the maskee or the test signal and the second signal is called the masker. The level to which the threshold of test signal is shifted by the masker is the effective level of the masker. Effective level can be expressed in sound pressure level, hearing level, or any other level depending upon the reference above which the level of the test signal is expressed. The effective level

of a masker at a given intensity level varies across different test signals. That is, a given noise intensity elevates the thresholds of various test signals to different intensity levels.

An efficient masker is one which produces a high effective level at a given intensity level. A given masker may be a more efficient masker of some test signals than others.

Minimum masking equals masker intensity minus effective level (effective level equals the level of a just masked test signal). When the masker is expressed in effective level, minimum masking equals 0 dB. Alternatively, minimum masking may be defined as the masking level which is just sufficient to mask the test signal in the ear to which the masker is presented.

Maximum masking is the masker level at the masked ear which is just insufficient to mask the test signal in the test ear. It is also equal to minimum masking plus interaural attenuation plus the test signal level at test ear cochlea.

Interaural attenuation is the reduction in the physical intensity of an acoustic signal in passing from a transducer on one side of the head to the opposite cochlea.

THE MASKING NOISE

It is generally agreed (Denes and Naunton, 1952; Hood, 1960; Liden, Nilsson, and Anderson, 1959a; Sanders and Rintelmann, 1964; Studebaker, 1962, 1964; Zwislocki, 1951) that narrow-band noises which center at the test signal frequency are the most efficient maskers of pure tones; that is, they produce a given effective level with the least intensity and, therefore, the least loudness. The use of narrow-band noises offers the further convenience that each band can be calibrated in effective level independently. Thus, the numerical masking dial reading equals the test signal intensity that will be just masked at all test tone frequencies.

Reprinted by permission of the author from *J. Speech Hearing Dis.*, **32**, 360–371 (1967).

Palva (1954, 1958) and Palva and Palva (1962) opposed the trend toward the use of narrow-band noises. However, his principal objection is that the gain in efficiency over broad-band noise is not sufficient to justify the additional cost and complexity of narrow-band noise generators. But, narrow-band noise generators have become relatively inexpensive and, in fact, simplify the clinical procedure by permitting the calibration of the noise in effective level for each test tone frequency.

Before clinical masking can begin, it is necessary to determine the minimum masking level for each masker and test signal combination used in the evaluation of patients. A satisfactory procedure is the following one. Introduce the masker and the test signal into the same ear by a single earphone. Each signal must be independently controlled by its own attenuator. With most two-channel clinical audiometers, this is accomplished with ease. The simple combining network shown in Figure 37–1 can be used with portable audiometers or independent noise sources. This network reduces the output of the earphone by 8 or 9 dB. The reduction is equal for all frequencies and for both masker and test signal. The minimum masking levels obtained, therefore, are unaffected by the network.

The next step is to obtain the threshold of each test signal in the presence of various levels of the appropriate masker in the same ear. Six to 10 subjects with normal hearing or with known sensorineural hearing loss may be used. Minimum masking for a particular test signal and masker combination is equal to the difference between noise level and test signal threshold in the presence of that noise, averaged across subjects and noise levels.

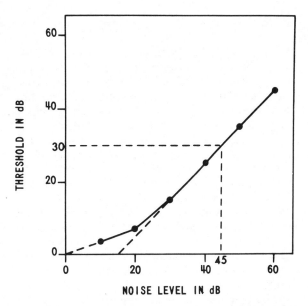

FIGURE 37-2. The relationship between masker level and test signal threshold when the test signal frequency is within the noise band. Minimum masking equals 15 dB in this example.

Figure 37–2 illustrates the relationship between masker level and test signal threshold when the test signal frequency is within the noise frequency band. This condition is highly desirable because a one to one relationship between noise level and test signal threshold is observed with this relationship. As Figure 37–2 shows, low levels of masker produce some threshold elevation. As the noise level is increased, the rate of threshold elevation increases until a given increment in noise level produces an equal increment in threshold. The difference between the two signals (minimum masking) then remains constant for all higher noise levels within the expected variability of all threshold measurements. In determining minimum masking levels, it is necessary to exclude the curvilinear portion of the curve from the calculation. Inclusion of these results produces an overestimation of masking efficiency.

Calibration of the noise source is essential when a broad-band noise is used. However, narrow-band noise generators calibrated in effective level should be similarly checked for accuracy since the clinician must assume the responsibility for the calibration of the equipment he uses.

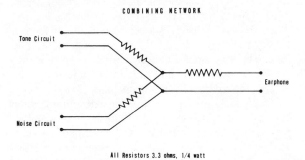

COMBINING NETWORK

Tone Circuit

Earphone

Noise Circuit

All Resistors 3.3 ohms, 1/4 watt

FIGURE 37-1. A combining network for the purpose of directing test signal and masker to the same earphone. A loss of 8 or 9 dB can be expected with this network.

WHEN TO MASK?

Virtually all audiology texts (Glorig, 1965, p. 117; Jerger, 1963, p. 251; Newby, 1964, p. 76; O'Neill and Oyer, 1966, p. 64; Sataloff, 1966, p. 305) which discuss clinical procedures state or imply that during air-conduction testing masking should be applied to the opposite ear whenever the difference between ears exceeds a specified number of decibels, usually 40 or 50 dB. Hood (1960) also makes this statement. However, available research (König, 1962a, 1962b, and Littler, Knight, and Strange, 1952; Luscher and König, 1955; Naunton, 1960; Palva, 1954, 1958; 1962, 1964; Zwislocki, 1951, 1953) indicates that this rule is inadequate and can result in significant error.

It is impractical to discuss here whether air conduction or bone conduction is the pathway of least attenuation of an earphone-presented signal to the opposite cochlea of a normal listener (Zwislocki, 1953). However, when the opposite ear exhibits a conductive loss, there is little question that bone conduction is the pathway of least attenuation, because the conductive loss raises the attenuation in the air-conduction pathway around the head and into the opposite ear by the amount of the air-bone gap (Naunton, 1960; Studebaker, 1962, 1964). In clinical practice, the clinician must assume that an earphone-presented signal reaches the opposite cochlea by passing through the bones of the head. The air-conduction threshold of the opposite ear, therefore, is irrelevant to the determination of when to mask.

Either one of two rules may be applied in air-conduction testing. Palva (1954, 1958) and Palva and Palva (1962) proposed masking the opposite ear whenever the air-conduction presentation level exceeds the smallest expected interaural attenuation value (usually 40 dB). The application of this rule results in unnecessary masking at times but never results in failure to mask when required. A second acceptable rule (Studebaker, 1964) is to mask the opposite ear whenever the air-conduction presentation level at the test ear exceeds the bone-conduction threshold of the opposite ear by more than the smallest expected interaural attenuation value (usually 40 dB). Application of the first rule results in some unnecessary masking. The second occasionally requires a return to air-conduction testing after the completion of bone-conduction testing. However, use of either rule enables the clinician to avoid the errors which must result from the use of a simple comparison of air-conduction to air-conduction.

Both preceeding rules specify test-signal presentation level and not the apparent threshold of the tested ear. In threshold finding procedures, these two values will not differ greatly. However, in suprathreshold presentations it is apparent that the presentation level is the significant variable. For example, in speech discrimination testing, masking should be used whenever the *presentation level* is more than 40 dB above the bone-conduction threshold of the opposite ear (40 dB is used because average interaural attenuation for speech is about 50 dB). When speech is presented to the poorer ear at 40-dB SL, contralateral masking is almost always indicated. This is particularly true when the discrimination score of the test ear is below that of the opposite (better) ear. Speech arriving at the opposite ear (at presentation level minus interaural attenuation) may be more intelligible than the speech arriving at the tested ear; or, the speech signal at the better ear may contribute enough to improve the apparent test ear discrimination score, even though the sensation level at the opposite ear is considerably less than that at the test ear.

Masking should be applied to the opposite ear during SISI testing on the poorer ear whenever the signal arrives at the nontest ear at a level of 25- to 30-dB HL or above; that is, a presentation at the test ear of about 70-dB HL or more. In tone-decay and Bekesy testing, the opposite ear should be masked when the presentation level is more than 40 dB above the opposite ear bone conduction threshold or, if following Palva's rule, whenever the presentation level is above 40-dB HL.

During bone-conduction testing, most investigators (Hood, 1960; König, 1962b; Liden, Nilsson, and Anderson, 1959b; Luscher, and König, 1955; Naunton, 1957; Palva, 1958; Sataloff, 1966; Studebaker, 1962, 1964; Zwislocki, 1951) agree that the decision when to mask must not depend upon the difference between the bone-conduction thresholds of the two ears. The very small interaural attenuation of vibrator-presented signals makes it impossible to use an interear comparison for this purpose.

One widely used procedure for determining when to mask and which ear to mask during bone-conduction tests is based on the Weber test (Liden, Nilsson, and Anderson, 1959b; Markle, Fowler, and Molonquet, 1952; Naunton, 1960). If the patient lateralizes the Weber test tone to one ear, the masking noise is applied to that ear. If the tone is reported to be in the center of the head, masking is not used. Clinical experience and research evidence (Fournier, 1954; König, 1962b) indicate that lateralization results can be misleading. Even the advocates of this procedure suggest that lateralization should be disregarded if the results appear improbable (Liden, Nilsson, and Anderson, 1959b; Naunton, 1957).

Another commonly applied rule states: "Always mask when testing by bone conduction." While this rule obviously never results in a failure to mask when needed, it does result in considerable wasted effort since it is unnecessary to mask the opposite ear when the unmasked bone-conduction threshold of the tested ear is already as poor as the air-conduction threshold of the same ear. Therefore, a more efficient rule is to apply masking to the opposite ear during bone-conduction tests whenever an air-bone gap is observed.

Placement of the vibrator at the forehead does not change this procedure. The clinician simply assumes that the unmasked threshold obtained from the forehead represents the unmasked bone-conduction threshold of each ear.

HOW MUCH MASKING?

Clinical masking is basically an effort to avoid the presentation of too much or too little noise. Avoidance of improper masking intensities requires consideration of a number of factors, including the test signal level, effective level, interaural attenuation, occlusion effect, and the air-bone gap of each ear. Few clinicians find it feasible to manipulate this number of variables in day-to-day clinical practice. Therefore, various writers have presented procedures designed to simplify the clinician's task. Unfortunately, the simplest procedures provide the greatest opportunity for error. For example, the use of a single masking noise intensity level (Harbert and Sataloff, 1955; Hawkins and Stevens, 1950; Hood, 1960) must result in over- and under-masking in many cases. The masking effectiveness of a given level of saw-tooth or white noises varies as a function of test-signal frequency by 30 dB or more (Sanders and Rintelmann, 1964). This factor, plus the influence of the hearing loss in each ear, requires frequent adjustments of masker intensity. The procedure is improved substantially if the proposed single level is a single effective level rather than a single intensity level. However, even under this condition adjustments must be made when the presentation level

exceeds 40-dB HL by bone conduction and about 80-dB HL by air conduction.

Another widely used procedure (Liden, Nilsson, and Anderson, 1959b; Markle, Fowler, and Molonguet, 1952; Naunton, 1957) is based upon lateralization of the test tone. As mentioned earlier, the noise is applied to the ear to which the tone is lateralized in the Weber test. The masker level is increased until the patient reports that the test signal has shifted from the masked ear to the tested ear. While this procedure appears adequate in most cases, it does depend upon the judgment of the patient. Even those who have used this method, express an unwillingness to rely upon it exclusively in all instances (Liden, Nilsson, and Anderson, 1959b; Naunton, 1957).

Threshold shift is the basis for a number of solutions to the clinical masking level problem. Three of the methods based on this phenomenon are presented in the next section. Figure 37–3 illustrates threshold shift in a hypothetical patient. In the figure the course of the apparent bone-conduction threshold of one ear is plotted as a function of noise level in the opposite ear. It is assumed, in this example, that the actual bone-conduction threshold of the test ear is above the bone-conduction threshold of the ear to be masked, that interaural attenuation is 0 dB, and that the masked ear is normal. Without masking in the opposite ear, threshold is obtained at 0-dB HL. Threshold improvement is noted due to the occlusion effect when an earphone is placed on the ear to be masked. Low noise effective levels increase the apparent threshold, because threshold in this instance is determined by the masked ear. As the noise level is increased further, the threshold of the masked ear is elevated above that of the test ear. Threshold is then determined by the test ear. Since the noise is not yet strong enough to mask the test ear, further noise increases produce little threshold increase, forming a plateau in the masking curve (a slight increase is seen due to central masking). When the noise level is increased further, the noise crosses the head with sufficient intensity to elevate the threshold of the tested ear, again increasing the observed threshold. This procedure was labeled a "control test" by Zwislocki (1951). Hood (1960) labeled the shifting threshold "shadowing," and the point of change to the plateau as the "change-over" point.

A number of factors influence minimum and maximum masking levels. The first factor is the presentation level of the test signal. The second is the interaural attenuation of the test signal for each

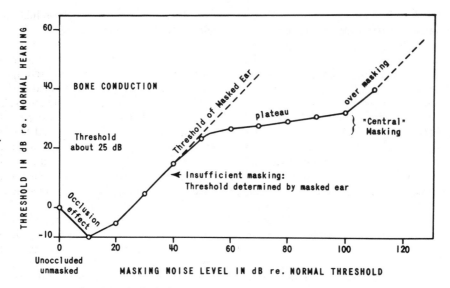

FIGURE 37-3. An example depicting the course of the apparent bone-conduction threshold as a function of noise level. Assumed are normal hearing for the masked ear and about a 30 dB actual bone-conduction threshold for the test ear.

mode of presentation. The third is the noise level required to mask the test signal. The fourth is the occlusion effect. The fifth are the air-bone gaps exhibited by each ear.

The test signal presentation level is simply the audiometer dial setting. Interaural attenuation for earphone-presented stimuli ranges from about 45 dB at low frequencies to about 65 dB at the highest frequencies. Interaural attenuation for vibrator-presented stimuli ranges from about 0 dB to 250 Hz to about 15 dB at 4,000 Hz (with forehead placement interaural attenuation is, in effect, 0 dB at all frequencies). The third factor, effective level, was discussed earlier.

Considering only these factors for a moment, it is apparent that the least masking one can use is an effective level equal to the presentation level minus interaural attenuation (of the test signal to the masked cochlea). The greatest permissible level is an effective level equal to the presentation level plus the interaural attenuation (of the masking noise to the test ear). The occlusion effect and air-bone gap complicate this picture.

The influence of the occlusion effect is illustrated in Figure 37-4. The occlusion effect, produced by placing an earphone over the ear to be masked,

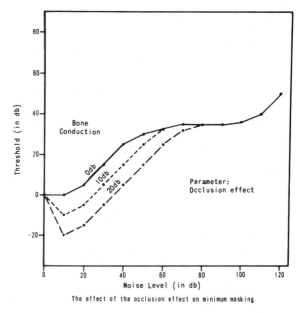

The effect of the occlusion effect on minimum masking

FIGURE 37-4. The relationship between masker level and apparent bone-conduction threshold for occlusion effects of three magnitudes on the masked ear. Assumed are normal hearing for the masked ear and about a 35 dB actual bone-conduction threshold for the test ear.

increases the intensity of the test signal at that ear (it does not modify cochlear sensitivity). Therefore, the minimum-masking intensity is increased by the amount of this factor. An air-bone gap in the masked ear also increases the minimum required level. The conductive loss decreases the intensity of the noise reaching the cochlea to be masked, but does not decrease the test-signal level arriving from the test ear side.

Both occlusion effect and masked ear air-bone gap increase the minimum required level but do not affect the maximum permissible level. Thus, each decreases the size of the plateau. However, the two factors are mutually exclusive and do not summate as illustrated in Figure 37–5. It is apparent that a large masked ear air-bone gap reduces the plateau to the vanishing point under some circumstances (i.e., during bone-conduction testing and also during air-conduction testing if the test ear also exhibits an air-bone gap).

An air-bone gap on the tested ear affects the maximum permissible masking when the test signals are presented by earphone. With no air-bone gap in the test ear, maximum masking during air-conduction tests equals the test-signal level, plus the interaural attenuation of the masking noise. That is, the noise can be presented safely at effective levels up to 40 dB above the test signal level. A conductive loss in the test ear reduces the test signal level but not the noise level at the test cochlea. Therefore, the maximum permissible level is decreased by the amount of the air-bone gap. In the case of an air-bone gap of about 45 to 50 dB or more, the maximum permissible level for air-conduction tests is equal to the maximum level for bone-conduction tests. It is for these reasons that the "masking dilemma" described by Naunton (1960) occurs with bilateral conductive losses and why it applies equally to both air- and bone-conduction tests.

A further consideration in the development of a clinical procedure is intersubject variability. It is not satisfactory to use the measures of central tendency for interaural attenuation, effective level, or occlusion effect values. The value used for interaural attenuation should be the smallest value expected across subjects. The effective-level value should be as low as expected across subjects when low effective levels are used. Occlusion effect, on the other hand, should always be assumed to be as high as expected with any subject. Only by considering the appro-

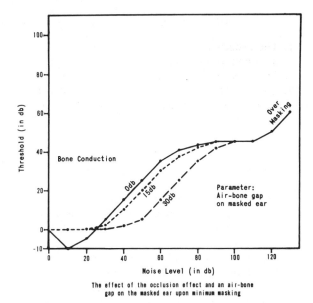

The effect of the occlusion effect and an air-bone gap on the masked ear upon minimum masking

FIGURE 37-5. The relationship between masker level and apparent bone-conduction threshold with air-bone gaps of three magnitudes on the masked ear. Assumed are normal bone-conduction thresholds for the masked ear and about a 45 dB actual bone-conduction threshold for the test ear.

priate extreme of each distribution, is the clinician reasonably assured that he is not over or under masking.

THRESHOLD SHIFT PROCEDURES

A usable clinical procedure must be devised either to avoid or compensate for each of the factors discussed above. Each of the following three masking methods do this or can be so adapted by slight modification.

A procedure based solely on the threshold shift observation was first presented by Hood in 1957. His procedure is as follows: First, find the unmasked threshold. Second, apply a masking noise to the non-test ear at an effective level of 10-dB SL. If no threshold shift is observed, threshold is the value obtained without contralateral masking. If the apparent threshold increases, then raise the noise in 10-dB steps, finding threshold at each step until further increases result in no further threshold shifts. The threshold of the tested ear is the value which does not increase with noise level.

This procedure has the following advantages:

1. The procedure involved is simple and requires a minimum of calculation.
2. The noise levels used are not loud.
3. Masking of air-conduction tests can be carried out without a knowledge of the bone-conduction thresholds.

Disadvantages:

1. The procedure, as originally presented, does not compensate for the occlusion effect. (The occlusion effect should be added to the first noise level used. The value used must be at least as large as the largest occlusion effect expected across individuals and not an average value.)
2. Intersubject variability of effective level and of the occlusion effect may, in individual cases, be sufficient to produce undermasking at the low effective levels used. Therefore, masking should be at least applied at two levels to insure that the 10-dB SL effective level is not insufficient.
3. If more than the lowest levels are used, there is danger of overmasking in the presence of an air-bone gap in the masked ear. While other procedures have the same limitation, this method does not give the clinician the information necessary to recognize the danger of overmasking.

A second procedure is one reported by Luscher and König in 1955 based on earlier work by Zwislocki (1951). This method was published by König in English (1962b). With this method, an audiometer is used which automatically presents to the nontest ear a narrow-band noise which centers on the test tone. The noise level is coupled to the test-signal attenuator so that the noise level at the opposite ear is always just above the test-signal level, minus interaural attenuation, plus occlusion effect. A secondary attenuator is used to increase the noise level above this value in order to compensate for an air-bone gap in the masked ear. In practice, the masking is presented at a just-sufficient level automatically, except for the addition of the masked ear air-bone gap by the examiner. The masked ear conductive component is estimated when testing the first ear by bone-conduction by noting the difference between the apparent bone-conduction threshold of the tested ear obtained with the first contralateral masking level and the air-conduction threshold of the masked ear. It is recommended by Luscher and König (1955) that an additional 5 to 15 dB be added to compensate for individual variability and that, if there is any doubt, threshold shift procedures should be carried out using 5-dB noise level steps.

Advantages:

1. The procedure is largely automatic and simple to use in practice.
2. The occlusion effect and air-bone gap are considered.
3. The noise levels used are not loud.

Disadvantages:

1. The use of low effective levels requires additional noise-level increases of 5 to 15 dB, nullifying some of the advantage of the automatic procedure.
2. Special equipment is required.

A method published by the present writer in 1964 based on Zwislocki's and Luscher and König's work is as follows. First, the unmasked threshold is obtained. Second, a noise is presented at an effective level of 40 dB above the bone-conduction threshold of the tested ear. Third, the noise is increased by an amount equal to any observed threshold shift. If a sizable air-bone gap is observed in the masked ear, a threshold shift procedure is used with the calculated noise level as the starting point. Threshold is the presentation level which does not shift upon masker application or masker-level increase.

Advantages:

1. The 40-dB effective level produces relatively large threshold shifts avoiding the sometimes equivocable outcomes associated with low effective-level presentations.
2. The occlusion effect and smaller masked ear air-bone gaps need not be considered.
3. The noise level is always at a level equal to the interaural attenuation, minus 40 dB, below the smallest average maximum-masking level.
4. The procedure can be used with automatic equipment of the type used by Luscher and König (1955).

Disadvantages:

1. The basis for the procedure is more difficult to understand.
2. The noise levels used are relatively loud.
3. It is necessary to have bone-conduction results before precise masking levels for air-conduction tests can be determined.

SUMMARY

In contrast to the impression gained from audiologic texts, a considerable body of literature exists on the subject of clinical masking. Most writers now agree that narrow-band noise is the most satisfactory for masking pure-tone test signals. However broad-band noises are still required for the masking of speech signals.

Masking should be applied to the nontest ear when testing by air-conduction whenever the test-signal presentation level exceeds the bone-conduction threshold of the nontest ear by 40 dB or more. When testing by bone-conduction, masking should be applied to the nontest ear whenever an apparent air-bone gap is observed in the tested ear.

Various methods have been proposed to determine the proper masking intensity. Of these, those based on the threshold shift phenomenon seem most satisfactory. Three methods based on this phenomenon are presented including the major advantages and disadvantages of each. The Luscher and Konig procedure requires equipment not generally found in this country. The Hood method is the simplest of the two remaining procedures. This method has disadvantages associated with the use of low effective levels (as does the Luscher and Konig procedure). The present writer has presented a method which uses higher effective levels in order to solve these problems. This procedure can be used equally well with both air- and bone-conducted stimuli and with suprathreshold, as well as threshold, test-signal presentations.

BIBLIOGRAPHY

Burgemeestre, A. J. Auditory masking in continuous audiometry. *Acta Otolaryng.*, **43**, 506 (1953).

Békésy, G. A new audiometer. *Acta Otolaryng.*, **35**, 411 (1947).

Davis, H., and Silverman, S. R. *Hearing and Deafness.* New York: Holt, Rinehart and Winston (1961).

Dean, C. E. Audition by bone conduction. *J. Acoust. Soc. Amer.*, **2**, 281 (1930).

DeBoer, E. Clinical masking. *Pract. ORL.*, **24**, 351 (1962). (dsh #72, Jan. 1963).

Denes, P., and Naunton, R. F. Masking in pure tone audiometry. *Proc. Roy. Soc. Med.*, **45**, 790 (1952).

Dirks, D. Bone conduction measurements. *Arch. Otolaryng.*, **79**, 594 (1964).

Dirks, D., and Malmquist, C. Changes in bone-conduction thresholds produced by masking in the non-test ear. *J. Speech Hearing Res.*, **7**, 271 (1964).

Dirks, D. D., and Malmquist, C. Shifts in air-conduction thresholds produced by pulsed and continuous contralateral masking. *J. Acoust. Soc. Amer.*, **37**, 631 (1965).

Dirks, D. D., and Norris, J. N. Shifts in auditory thresholds produced by ipsilateral and contralateral maskers at low intensity levels. *J. Acoust. Soc. Amer.*, **40**, 12 (1966).

Elpern, B., and Naunton, R. F. The stability of the occlusion effect. *Arch. Otolaryng.*, **77**, 376 (1963).

Feldman, H. Masking the test-tone by the test-tone. *Inter. Aud.*, **1**, 240 (1962). (dsh, #1031, July 64).

Fletcher, H. Auditory patterns. *Rev. Modern Physics*, **12**, 47 (1940).

Fournier, J. E. The "false-bing" phenomenon. Some remarks on the theory of bone conduction. *Laryngoscope*, **64**, 29 (1954).

Glorig, A. *Audiometry: Principle and Practice.* Baltimore: The Williams & Wilkins Co. (1965).

Goetzinger, C. P.; Proud, G. O.; and Embry, J. E. Masking and bone conduction. *Acta Otolaryng.*, **54**, 287 (1962).

Harbert, F. Masking levels for clinical use. *Arch. Otolaryng.*, **66**, 214 (1957).

Harbert, F. The clinical masking level. *Ann. Oto. Rhino. Laryng.*, **67**, 332 (1958).

Harbert, F., and Sataloff, J. A. Clinical applications of recruitment and masking. *Laryngoscope,* **65**, 113 (1955).

Hardy, W. G. Masking in testing for otosclerosis. In H. F. Schuknecht (Ed.), *Otosclerosis.* Boston: Little, Brown, 199 (1962).

Hart, C., and Naunton, R. F. Frontal bone conduction tests in clinical audiometry. *Laryngoscope,* **71**, 24 (1961).

Hawkins, J. E., and Stevens, S. S. The masking of pure tones and of speech by white noise. *J. Acoust. Soc. Amer.*, **22**, 6 (1950).

Hood, J. D. The principles and practice of bone conduction audiometry. A review of the present position. *Proc. Roy. Soc. Med.*, **50**, 689 (1957), and *Laryngoscope*, **70**, 1211 (1960).

Huizing, E. H. Bone conduction. The influence of the middle ear. *Acta Otolaryng. Supp.*, **155** (1960).

Jerger, J. *Modern Developments in Audiology.* New York: Academic Press (1963).

Jerger, J.; Tillman, T. W.; and Peterson, J. L. Masking by octave bands of noise in normal and impaired ears. *J. Acoust. Soc. Amer.*, **32**, 385 (1960).

Jerger, J., and Wertz, M. The indiscriminate use of masking in bone-conduction audiometry. *Arch. Otolaryng.*, **70**, 419 (1959).

König, E. On the use of hearing-aid type earphones in clinical audiometry. *Acta Otolaryng.,* **55,** 331 (1962*b*).

König, E. The use of masking noise and its limitation in clinical audiometry. *Acta Otolaryng. Supp.,* **180,** 1 (1962*b*).

Liden, G.; Nilsson, G.; and Anderson, H. Narrow band masking with white noise. *Acta Otolaryng.,* **50,** 116 (1959*a*).

Liden, G.; Nilsson, G.; and Anderson, H. Masking in clinical audiometry. *Acta Otolaryng.,* **50,** 125 (1959*b*).

Littler, T. S.; Knight, J. J.; and Strange, P. H. Hearing by bone conduction and the use of bone conduction hearing aids. *Proc. Roy. Soc. Med.,* **45,** 783 (1952).

Luscher, E., and König, E. Die Vertaubung des Gegenhores bei audiometrischen Bestimmerng der Knochenlertung. *Arch. Ohr.-Nas. u. Kehlk.-Heilk,* **168,** 68 (1955).

Markle, D. M.; Fowler, E. P., Jr.; and Molonquet, H. The audiometric Weber test as a means of determining the need for and the type of masking. *Ann. Oto. Rhino. Laryng.,* **61,** 888 (1952).

Martin, F. N.; Bailey, H. A. T., Jr.; and Pappas, J. J. The effect of central masking on threshold for speech. *J. Aud. Res.,* **5,** 293 (1965).

Menzel, O. J. Masking noise in audiometers. *EENT Monthly,* **43,** 93 (1964).

Miller, M. H. Clinical application of paired masking enclosures in pure tone air and bone conduction testing. *Arch. Otolaryng.,* **69,** 315 (1959).

Miller, M. H. Transmission loss across the skull in a patient with a known total monaural deafness. *Laryngoscope,* **69,** 100 (1959).

Naunton, R. F. Clinical bone conduction audiometry. The use of frontally applied bone-conduction receiver and the importance of the occlusion effect in clinical bone-conduction audiometry. *Arch. Otolaryng.,* **66,** 281 (1957).

Naunton, R. F. A masking dilemma in bilateral conduction deafness. *Arch. Otolaryng.,* **72,** 753 (1960).

Newby, H. A. *Audiology.* New York: Appleton-Century-Crofts (1964).

O'Neill, J. J., and Oyer, H. J. *Applied Audiometry.* New York: Dodd, Mead & Company (1966).

Palva, T. Masking in audiometry. With special reference to the non-thermal type of noise. *Acta Otolaryng. Supp.,* **118,** 156 (1954).

Palva, T. Masking in audiometry, Further studies. *Acta Otolaryng.,* **49,** 229 (1958).

Palva, T., and Palva, A. Masking in audiometry. III. Reflections on the present position. *Acta Otolaryng.,* **54,** 521 (1962).

Saltzmann, M., and Ersner, M. S. Masking and shadow hearing in bone conduction. *Arch. Otolaryng.,* **51,** 809 (1950).

Sanders, J. W., and Rintelmann, W. F. Masking in audiometry. *Arch. Otolaryng.,* **80,** 541 (1964).

Sataloff, J. *Hearing Loss.* Philadelphia: J.B. Lippincott Co. (1966).

Shuel, J. Masking in pure tone audiometry. Its use and its limitations. *J. Laryng.,* **72,** 959 (1958).

Studebaker, G. A. On masking in bone-conduction testing. *J. Speech Hearing Res.,* **5,** 215 (1962).

Studebaker, G. A. Clinical masking of air- and bone-conducted stimuli. *J. Speech Hearing Dis.,* **29,** 23 (1964).

Veniar, F. A. Individual masking levels in pure tone audiometry. *Arch. Otolaryng.,* **82,** 518 (1965).

Watson, N., and Gales, R. Bone conduction threshold measurements: Effects of occlusion, enclosures, and masking. *J. Acoust. Soc. Amer.,* **14,** 207 (1943).

Welsh, L. W., and Welsh, J. J. Clinical problems in masking. *Arch. Otolaryng.,* **73,** 342 (1961).

Zwislocki, J. Acoustic attenuation between the ears. *J. Acoust. Soc. Amer.,* **25,** 752 (1953).

Zwislocki, J. Eine verbesserte Vertaubungsmethode fur die Audiometrie. *Acta Otolaryng.,* **39,** 338 (1951). *Trans. Beltone Inst. Hear. Res.,* No. 19, April 1966.

38

A Masking Dilemma in Bilateral Conduction Deafness

RALPH F. NAUNTON, M.D.

Professor of Surgery, and Head, Section of Otolaryngology, University of Chicago

There are theoretical grounds for believing that, in testing the hearing of some subjects with bilateral conduction deafness, it is impossible adequately to mask the hearing of the opposite ear without at the same time masking the hearing of the test ear.

Discussion of this problem will be facilitated by a preliminary definition of a number of familiar audiological terms.

DEFINITIONS

Test Ear

The ear whose performance is under investigation in a monaural hearing test.

Opposite Ear

The ear whose performance is *not* under investigation in a monaural hearing test.

Auditory Stimulus

Any sound, simple or complex, fed to a listener's ear during a hearing test.

Test Stimulus

The auditory stimulus to whose presence or arrival a listener's response is being examined during a hearing test.

Reprinted by permission of the author from *Arch. Otolayngol.*, **72**, 753–757 (1960). Copyright 1960, American Medical Association.

Overheard Stimulus

Any auditory stimulus fed into one ear will also stimulate the other ear; the stimulus may, for the sake of clarity of definition, be said to travel from the transducer (headphone, loudspeaker, bone-conduction receiver, etc.) into one ear then "across the head" to the other ear. The stimulus "crossing" the head and arriving at the other ear may still be of sufficient magnitude to evoke a sensation of hearing at that ear; the stimulus is then said to be overheard. It has been shown that when air-conduction receivers are in use, the overheard stimulus "crosses" largely by bone conduction (Zwislocki, 1953).

Mask Ear

Under some circumstances in monaural hearing tests the opposite ear must be actively prevented from hearing a test stimulus "crossing the head" from the test ear; this end must be achieved in such a way that the performance of the test ear remains unaffected. Taking an analogy from the telephone company, detection of the overheard test stimulus is prevented by creating a "busy line" state—the opposite or overhearing ear being kept busy listening to another auditory stimulus. The hearing of the opposite ear for the test stimulus "crossing" the head is said to be masked, and that ear is thereafter described as the *mask ear*.

Masking Stimulus

The auditory stimulus referred to above that keeps the mask ear in a busy line state. The masking stimulus will usually be an electronically generated noise whose audible character will be clearly different from that of the test stimulus (tone or speech). The masking stimulus operates by raising the threshold of the mask ear for the test stimulus, the magnitude of the masking stimulus required to insure a "busy line" effect being dependent upon the magnitude of the overheard test stimulus. In subsequent discussion it will be assumed that, for any given test stimulus, "X" dB of masking stimulus will raise the threshold of the mask ear by "X" dB (i.e., "X" dB of masking stimulus will be assumed to have a *masking effect* of "X" dB).[1]

Interaural Attenuation

In "crossing" from one ear to the other an auditory stimulus will usually be reduced in intensity (or attenuated) en route. This intensity reduction (in decibels) is described as the "interaural attenuation"; its magnitude will depend upon the frequency of the stimulus and the type of transducer (headphone, loudspeaker, bone-conduction receiver, etc.) delivering the stimulus to the head. The test stimulus and the masking stimulus are both auditory stimuli and both will "cross the head," being attenuated by the amount of the interaural attenuation en route. Masking will be required when a test stimulus is overheard; but the masking stimulus will "cross the head" and, if it is overheard by the test ear to a sufficient extent, will mask the test ear and distort the hearing test results.

INDICATIONS FOR MASKING

The situations in air conduction tests where masking is required are often described by quoting the simplest type of masking problem, the case with a large (40 to 50 dB or more) disparity between the air conduction losses in a listener's two ears. This description, correct as far as it goes, is based upon the general recognition that when using standard headphones the interaural attenuation is approximately 50 dB. There are other cases where masking is desirable but where there may, for example, be as little as zero difference between the two ears.

Application of available information to two theoretical situations will clarify the "indications for masking" and illustrate a theoretical dilemma.

The rule, quoted above, indicates that, in this theoretical case, the right ear must be masked when the air-conduction thresholds of the left ear are determined because there is a disparity between the air-conduction thresholds of the two ears of more than 40 or 50 dB. It is, however, more practical to arrive at the same conclusion by what may appear to be an unnecessarily laborious process of deduction. Thus the sound entering the left ear or test ear when its threshold is reached is 55 dB; this sound will "cross the head," losing 50 dB en route, and will be heard by the right or opposite ear at a level of 5 dB (It is assumed that the interaural attenuation is 50 dB and that the bone-conduction hearing of the right ear is normal.) Masking is therefore necessary to exclude the right ear from the test.

The maximum amount of masking that can be delivered to the right or mask ear without raising the threshold of the test ear can similarly be deduced. Any masking stimulus entering the mask ear will "cross the head," losing 50 dB en route, since the interaural attenuation is 50 dB; but, if the test ear is to remain unaffected by it, the masking stimulus must be at 0 dB (re normal threshold) when it reaches the test ear; if it arrives at 0 dB, having lost 50 dB en route, it must have started at 50 dB. The maximum permissible intensity of the masking stimulus entering the right or mask ear must therefore be 50 dB above normal threshold.

The masking effect of this 50 dB masking stimulus will be 50 dB because the air conduction threshold of the mask ear is normal (*see* section above, "Definitions": Masking Stimulus).

Three conclusions have thus been reached concerning the theoretical case, Type I:

1. The right ear must be masked when the air conduction threshold of the left ear is determined.
2. No more than a 50 dB masking stimulus may be used for this purpose.
3. The masking effect of the 50 dB masking stimulus will be 50 dB.

The steps described leading to the three conclusions above appear to be laborious, but the process is often a very necessary one, both in carrying out hearing tests and in interpreting their results; with very little practice these steps become far easier to apply than to describe.

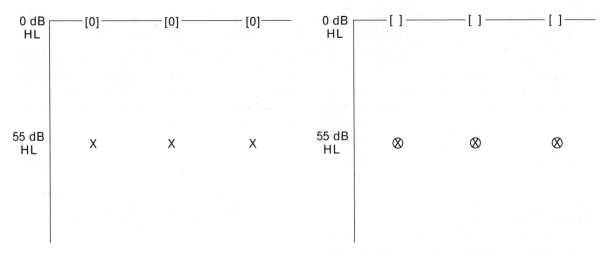

FIGURE 38-1. Stylized pure-tone audiogram of theoretical case Type 1: unilateral conduction deafness.

FIGURE 38-2. Stylized pure-tone audiogram of theoretical case Type 2: bilateral conduction deafness.

A second type of theoretical situation may be examined in the same way.

The 55 dB test stimulus entering the left ear or test ear at its threshold will "cross the head" and stimulate the opposite ear at a level of 5 dB (i.e., 55 − 50 dB). The bone-conduction threshold of the opposite ear is assumed to be normal; therefore the test stimulus will be overheard by the opposite ear at a level of 5 dB. Masking is therefore necessary, when testing the left ear, to exclude the right ear from the test.

Any masking stimulus entering the right or mask ear (regardless of the state of air-conduction or bone-conduction hearing in the mask ear) will "cross the head" losing 50 dB en route; but, if the test ear is to remain unaffected by it, the masking stimulus must be at zero dB (re normal threshold) when it reaches the test ear. If it arrives at 0 dB (re normal threshold) when it reaches the test ear, having lost 50 dB en route, it must have started at 50 dB. The maximum permissible intensity of the masking stimulus entering the mask ear must therefore be 50 dB above normal threshold.

The masking effect of this 50 dB maximum masking stimulus will, however, be zero because the air-conduction threshold loss of the mask ear is 55 dB; thus the masking stimulus will not be heard by or elevate the threshold of the mask ear.

Three conclusions have been reached concerning the theoretical case, Type 2:

1. The right ear must be masked when the threshold of the left ear is determined.
2. No more than a 50 dB masking stimulus may be used for this purpose.
3. The masking effect of the 50 dB masking stimulus will be zero.

Theoretical case Type 2 thus serves to illustrate a theoretical dilemma where masking is necessary but impossible to achieve without at the same time affecting the test ear.

It will be recognized that the general type of audiogram illustrated in theoretical case Type 2 is commonly found in otosclerosis and other types of bilateral middle ear deafness and that the dilemma, if in fact it does occur, will be found in clinical cases of this type. The existence of the dilemma will be proven if, in a clinical case, a masking stimulus fed to one ear masks both ears simultaneously and to equal extents.

EXPERIMENTAL INVESTIGATION

The intensity of a broad-spectrum white noise masking stimulus required to mask a 500 cps tone, 10 dB above the listener's threshold of hearing for that tone, was determined for a group of 20 adults suffering from bilateral otosclerosis. The air-conduction losses of the patients tested in this series ranged between 25 and 65 dB at 500 cps.

Matched PDR 10 receivers covered with small rubber cushions were used for all tests. Complete unmasked air- and bone-conduction threshold audiograms were first made; then measurements of the threshold of hearing for a 500 cps pulsed tone, in the presence of noise, were made under each of two conditions. Each listener's two ears will be identified as Ear 1 and Ear 2 for purposes of description.

Condition A (Figure 38–3): Pure tone and white noise mixed and fed to Ear 1. Experimental measurement: Intensity of white noise required to mask a 500-cps tone 10 dB above the threshold of Ear 1. Condition B (Figure 38–4): White noise delivered to Ear 1; pure tone delivered to Ear 2. Experimental measurement: Intensity of white noise required to mask a 500-cps tone 10 dB above the threshold of Ear 2.

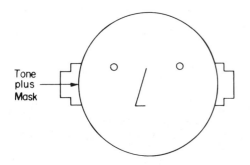

FIGURE 38-3. Test condition A.

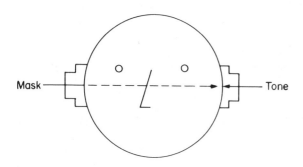

FIGURE 38-4. Test condition B.

It can be stated, on the basis of the preceding discussion, that the audiometric dilemma illustrated theoretically practically if, in the experimental investigation outlined, examples occur where little or no difference can be found between the intensities of the direct (Condition A, Figure 38–3) and overheard (Condition B, Figure 38–4) masking stimuli required to mask the 10 dB 500 cps tones.

RESULTS

The differences observed in the 20 experimental subjects between the intensities of the direct and the overheard masking stimuli required to mask the 10 dB test stimuli at the two ears were as follows:

24.6 dB	17.4 dB	8.4 dB	3.8 dB
23.4	16.9	8.3	3.1
20.1	15.0	8.1	2.6
19.3	14.8	7.8	−3.7
17.5	13.6	4.8	−12.4

Positive values indicate that the ear receiving the masking stimulus directly, mixed with the tone, required less noise to mask the 10 dB tone than the opposite ear required when receiving the masking stimulus by conduction "across the head"; negative values indicate the reverse, that the masking stimulus fed directly to one ear was masking the opposite ear by cross conduction more effectively.

COMMENT

The investigation described has served to indicate that an audiometric dilemma, predicted on a theoretical basis, does in fact occur in clinical cases of otosclerosis. There clearly are cases within the group studied conforming with the theoretical case Type 2 in which a masking stimulus fed to one ear masks the opposite ear to an almost equal extent. There were two cases where a masking stimulus fed to one ear produced a greater masking effect on the opposite ear than on the ear receiving the mask directly.

The figures listed can, without introducing any serious error, be assumed to represent the differences between the *masking effects* produced at a listener's two ears by a masking stimulus fed to one ear. Clearly, if this assumption is made, the experimental results indicate that it would be impossible in practice to carry out a monaural hearing test on approximately half of the subjects examined because any stimulus used to produce a useful degree of masking in the mask ear will also mask the test ear. The magnitude of this problem will be increased as above-threshold and bone-conduction tests are attempted because the overheard test stimuli will be greater and will require more intense masking stimuli to prevent their being heard by the untested ear.

The limiting factor in the theoretical and practical problems discussed is the interaural attenuation, whose value is determined by the nature of the headphones or other devices used to deliver auditory stimuli to the listeners' ears during audiometric testing. Zwislocki (1953) has examined this aspect of the problem in detail and indicated that the acoustical isolation between a listener's ears (interaural attenuation) depends upon the area of contact between the listener's head and the headphone or other device delivering the auditory stimuli; when this area of contact is large (e.g., in orthodox headphones) the interaural attenuation is poor; when the area is small (e.g., when sound-conducting tubes are inserted into the external meatuses) the interaural attenuation will be considerably increased. The dilemma whose occurrence has been demonstrated will be overcome to a considerable degree if masking stimuli are delivered to the mask ear by means of a sound-conducting tube held in the external meatus rather than by an orthodox headphone, because the resulting increase in interaural attenuation will reduce the risk of cross conduction of the masking stimulus. An additional advantage will accrue if air-conduction test stimuli are delivered by a similar system in that there will be fewer occasions when masking is required.

It should be reemphasized that the interaural attenuation, although frequency dependent, is not otherwise related to the type of auditory stimulus "crossing the head." For this reason the interaural attenuation is unaffected by the use of narrow-band masking stimuli in place of broad band white noise; there are advantages in the use of narrow-band noises (Denes and Naunton, 1952), but increased interaural attenuation is not one of them.

It should also be noted that, in examining the need for the use of masking in a clinical hearing test, the determining factor is the difference between the air-conduction threshold of the tested ear and the bone-conduction threshold of the opposite or untested ear.

SUMMARY

There are theoretical grounds for believing that in some subjects with bilateral middle ear deafness it is impossible adequately to mask the hearing of the untested ear without at the same time masking the hearing of the tested ear. Measurements of the masking effect of white noise made on a series of 20 listeners with bilateral otosclerosis have indicated that the problem is encountered in practice and is therefore more than a theoretical concept without foundation in fact.

ENDNOTE

1. It should be noted that this relation between the intensity of the masking stimulus and its masking effect, while being near true for narrow band noises (Denes and Naunton, 1952), does not hold for the commonly used broad-spectrum white noise.

REFERENCES

Zwislocki, J.: Acoustic Attenuation Between the Ears, *J. Acoust. Soc. America* **25**:752–759, 1953.

Denes, P., and Naunton, R. F.: Masking in Pure Tone Audiometry, *Proc. Roy. Soc. Med.* **45**:790–794, 1952.

39

A Schematic Representation of the Nontest Ear Masking Problem

GERALD A. STUDEBAKER, Ph.D.
Professor of Speech and Hearing Science,
Memphis State University

Figure 39–1 depicts a simplified schematic representation of the major factors which affect the nontest ear masking problem. It is intended that this figure will be of some assistance to those who find visual representations more readily understood and remembered than formulas, graphs or printed or verbal statements. The figure does not represent a method or procedure for contralateral ear masking. Instead it reveals those factors which must be considered in developing or evaluating such a procedure. It obviously cannot be used as a part of a clinical routine. Rather, it is hoped that those who teach audiological methodology will find the diagram useful as a basis for concretizing for their students those factors which influence the transcranial conduction of acoustic energy. The diagram may also prove useful to those who might wish to develop an electronic "artificial masking head" which could be used to provide practice for students; and finally, it also may prove useful to those attempting the development of computer programs for routine audiometric testing. Any elaboration needed for this latter application can be easily appended to the basic schematic.

The lines in the figure represent acoustical pathways. The resistance symbols represent the acoustic attenuation in these pathways. The representation is "simplified" in that the actual acoustic attenuation in the various pathways is not entirely frequency independent as implied by the resistance symbols. However, the addition of other symbols to improve the accuracy of the representation does not appear justified in view of the very considerable increase in pictorial complication which results.

The various resistance symbols are labeled **A** through **F**. These represent the following attenuation sources:

A represents the attenuation of sound which occurs as it passes through the air from one side of the head to the other. It does not include the attenuation produced as a sound leaks out from under an earphone cushion or emanates from the back of the earphone. It is a headshadow effect. It increases gradually but continuously as frequency is increased.

B_1 and B_2 together represent the attenuation between the two sides of the head for bone-conducted (bc) sound energy. The attenuation value is very small but somewhat larger in the high frequencies. The attenuation is arbitrarily split into two parts so that the forehead bc vibrator (**VF**) placement can be placed symmetrically between the two cochleas.

C represents the difference between forehead and mastoid bc thresholds. It is a moderately frequency-dependent factor, being somewhat larger at the lower frequencies.

D_1 and D_2 represent the attenuation of a sound which occurs at the air-tissue interface. It is the pathway through which air-borne sound energy is transmitted to the skull bone. This attenuation is relatively large and probably accounts for the major portion of the interaural attenuation associated with signals presented by earphone.

E_1 and E_2 represent the acoustic attenuation produced by conductive hearing losses. (Actually represented is the excess attenuation in a diseased middle ear over and above any losses associated with sound conduction in the normal

This article has been expanded slightly from the original and is reprinted by permission of the author from *J. and Res.*, **11**, 345–350 (1971).

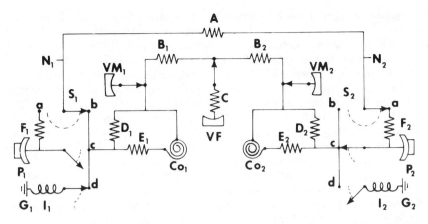

FIGURE 39-1. A simplified schematic representation of those factors which affect the nontest ear masking problem.

middle ear). A conductive loss can be large or small, of course, and may be somewhat frequency dependent, usually greater at the lower frequencies.

F_1 and F_2 represent the acoustic attenuation produced by earphones and cushions in place over the ear. Like the other attenuations depicted, these attenuations function in both directions. That is, sound is attenuated whether passing out from under (or through) the cushion or passing in from the outside through or under the cushion and earphone into the ear canal.

The remaining symbols in alphabetical order are as follows:

Co_1 and Co_2 are the two cochleas.

G_1 and G_2 are grounds; that is, ambient atmospheric pressure.

I_1 and I_2 are inertances which provide a low-pass filter pathway to ground when the earphone is *not* on the ear.

N_1 and N_2 are ambient noise sources which may arrive from any side.

S_1 and S_2 are switches. Each has poles a, b, c and d. These will be explained in succeeding paragraphs.

P_1 and P_2 are earphones.

VF is a bc vibrator placed at the forehead.

VM_1 and VM_2 are bc vibrators placed on the respective mastoid processes.

A factor requiring further explanation than given above is the function of the switches S_1 and S_2. These switches are used to depict the situations when the earphone is off the ear (shown in S_1) and on the ear (shown in S_2). Each switch has three poles to represent the three major things that occur when an earphone is placed over the external ear. These are (1) the earphone-produced signal is presented to the ear canal (S_{2c} is closed), (2) the earphone cushion attenuation (F_2 in this case) is inserted between the ambient noise (N_1 and N_2) and the ear canal (S_{2b} is opened and S_{2a} is closed, and (3) the occlusion effect is produced (S_{2b} is disconnected).

The occlusion effect in the diagram is represented as follows: The situation without earphone occlusion is shown on the #1 (Left) side of the figure. Here a connection is shown at S_{1d} (ear canal open) which provides a pathway to ground through the low-pass filter I_1. Low frequency acoustic energy in the #1 ear canal can "escape" to the ambient atmosphere through this pathway. When this pathway to ground is interrupted, as when an earphone covers the ear as shown at S_{2d}, there is an increase in the low frequency energy level in the ear canal. Hence, the thresholds for low frequency bc sound appear to improve with occlusion of the ear canal. It must be noted here that the occlusion effect is considerably more complicated than this depiction would imply. It is intended here only that the major effect (i.e., the low frequency intensity increase) should be illustrated simply. The figure should not be taken to represent a theoretical statement concerning the mechanism which produces the occlusion effect.

This completes the identification, and basic explanation, of the elements shown in Figure 39–1. Two potentially important acoustic pathways which are now shown are the acoustic radiations from the backs of the earphones and the cases of the bc vibrators into the air. Radiation from the outer case of an earphone is probably an insignificant factor except possibly when the opposite ear is uncovered. However, even in this instance the presence of this pathway in no way changes the basic arrangement shown in Figure 39–1, because it simply represents a pathway parallel to attenuation factor F (attenuation of earphone). Radiation from the back of a bc vibrator is normally only a problem at 4 Kc/s and is strong enough to have an effect only on the uncovered tested ear during bc testing. This is particularly true with the bc vibrator placed at the mastoid position.

Virtually all acoustical factors influencing nontest ear masking problems can be considered using the diagram. As an example, consider the question often posed as to whether acoustic energy from an earphone on one ear gets to the opposite ear by air conduction (ac) or by bc. Consideration of the figure should reveal that this is not exactly the correct question. The fact is that acoustic energy crosses to the opposite cochlea via both pathways simultaneously. The more nearly correct question is "Which pathway provides the least attenuation of the acoustic signal under any given set of circumstances?" The diagram shows two parallel pathways (there may be others) for sound energy to arrive at one cochlea (Co_1) from the earphone (P_2) at the opposite ear (Ear #2). Tracing from P_2, the ac pathway is $F_2 + A$, i.e., the sum of the attenuation produced by the earphone and cushion (F_2) and the attenuation produced by the headshadow (A). If the earphone (P_1) is on Ear #1, then add the attenuation (F_1) of that earphone and cushion. If there is a conductive loss in Ear #1, add the value of the loss (E_1) to the total. The bc pathway passes from P_2 through D_2 (the acoustical losses at the air-tissue interface when sound passes from the air under the earphone cushion into the bone of the skull) and then through B_2 and B_1 (the interaural attenuation for bc signals) and into the opposite cochlea (Co_1). A certain amount of energy may arrive in the conductive mechanism (ear canal and middle ear system) through D_1. If Ear #1 is not occluded, some low frequency energy will be lost into the atmosphere (G). If the ear is occluded this energy will be retained to influence Ear #1.

Keeping the components of these two parallel pathways in mind, consider the influence of the addition of an earphone over Ear #1. Obviously this move should increase the attenuation in the air pathway by the amount of F_1 while decreasing the attenuation in the bc pathway in the low frequencies by the amount of the occlusion effect. Other factors such as a conductive loss in Ear #1 serve to reduce the influence of the occlusion effect, but nevertheless it should be apparent from the diagram that covering the opposite ear should produce opposite effects on the attenuation in the two parallel pathways. It should also be evident that a conductive loss on the opposite ear (Ear #1 in this case) elevates the attenuation in the ac pathway by the amount of the conductive loss, but should have relatively little effect on the attenuation in the bc pathway except, perhaps, as influenced by the occlusion effect produced.

Figure 39–1 may also be used to consider how the various depicted elements affect the required masking noise intensity level. Before proceeding with examples, however, four points require brief exposition: (1) It is the signal-to-noise (S/N) ratio at each of the two cochleas that is the variable of fundamental significance. Assume that the noise level is expressed in effective level. The goal in the nontest ear masking problem then is to maintain a positive S/N ratio in the tested ear while producing a negative S/N ratio in the masked ear. (Accepting the assumption in the first sentence of this paragraph means, by definition, that the signal becomes just audible at an S/N ratio of 0 dB provided that the signal level is above the absolute threshold of the listener.)

(2) It is the S/N ratio in the cochlea and not the S/N ratio in the ear canal or on the audiometer dials that matters. Whether a test signal is masked is determined by the S/N ratio in the cochlea, nowhere else.

(3) The individual's hearing threshold level, as such, is not the variable of significance in the masking problem; rather, it is the presentation level of the test signal that is the relevant variable. Of course, most often the presentation level is close to threshold, but often it is much higher in level. Contralateral masking of suprathreshold tests poses absolutely no additional conceptual difficulties when the student

has been taught from the outset that it is presentation level and not threshold *per se* that is the variable of relevance. it should be obvious that a masking value calculated to be just adequate on the basis on the of the intensity at threshold cannot be adequate for test signals presented 5, 20 or 40 dB above threshold.

(4) For nontest ear masking purposes there are two kinds of hearing losses, sensorineural and conductive, which differ very significantly in their effect on the required masking noise levels. A sensorineural loss has only an indirect influence on the required masking level; i.e., the magnitude of the sensorineural hearing loss influences the presentation level. The presentation level, in turn, dictates the masking levels required. The sensorineural loss in no way affects the intensity level in the cochlea except in this indirect way. A conductive loss on the other hand physically reduces the acoustical energy delivered to the ipsilateral cochlea. With sensorineural losses the energy level in the cochlea is equal to the presentation level (except for the "normal" energy losses in the normal conductive system). In case of conductive losses the energy level in the cochlea is equal to the presentation level minus the attenuation produced by the conductive loss. It is this factor that is responsible for the very difficult masking problem inherent in audiometric evaluations of persons with conductive hearing losses.

Numerical problems can be worked particularly well using Figure 39–1. Fixed values may be assigned to those factors not under the control of the clinician, such as attenuations **A**, **B** and **C** (also, the influence of different values for these attenuations may be evaluated.) Problems then can be constructed by assigning various numerical values to the conductive losses and occlusion effects in each ear. Certain factors may have differing values depending upon the equipment used. For example, D_1 and/or D_2 can be increased by using insert earphones, and F_1 and F_2 as well as the size of the occlusion effect can be affected by the quality of the seal provided by the earphone cushion. With particular equipment and at particular frequencies, however, these factors can be considered as fixed at some specified value. The purpose of a numerical problem solution is to check on a student's comprehension of the concepts involved in solving the problem. These calculations cannot form a clinical method, at least not one for human use. However, if the influence of the various factors are

better understood by the clinician, then the consequences of various simplifying assumptions and the limitations and dangers associated with the various methods that have been proposed will be better understood. Also, note that while such a formula or circuit-based approach may be too complicated for direct clinical application by human clinicians, this aspect does not preclude its use in computer-directed testing procedures.

A calculation example follows: Assume that at a particular frequency, **A** (headshadow effect) = 50 dB; B_1 and B_2 (bc interaural attenuation effects) = 2 dB each; **C** (forehead vs. mastoid bc threshold effects) is unrelated to the problem; D_1 and D_2 (attenuation at the air-tissue interface which together with B_1 and B_2 create the total interaural attenuation for signals presented by earphones) = 50 dB each; E_1 (conductive loss at Ear #1) = 25 dB; E_2 (conductive loss at Ear #2) = 10 dB; F_1 and F_2 (acoustic attenuation produced by earphones and cushions) = 15 dB each; and OE_1 and OE_2 (occlusion effects at each ear) = 0 dB and 8 dB respectively. (We will assume that the occlusion effects differ in the two ears and are small because of the conductive hearing losses.) Question: What are the minimum and maximum masking effective levels relative to the test signal presentation level when the test signal is presented to Ear #1 by ac? (Because effective level is called for, expressed relative to the presentation level of the test signal, neither the presentation level nor the nature of the test signal need be specified.) Solution: The least noise required is an effective level in the masked cochlea equal to the test signal presentation level (**PL**) minus the interaural attenuation (**IA**) for the earphone-presented test signal being used. That is, in this case, minimum effective level = $PL - (D_1 + B_1 + B_2) + E_2$. The maximum masking level = $PL + (D_2 + B_1 + B_2) - E_1$. (The items in parentheses together represent the interaural attenuation.) Substituting the numerical values given above into the formula results in minimum effective level = $PL(50 + 2 + 2) + 10 = PL - 44$. Maximum effective level = $PL + (50 + 2 + 2) - 25 = PL + 29$ dB. Note that the expected plateau size is Max. $-$ Min. or $+29 - (-44) = 73$ dB. One can show that for earphone-presented test signals the plateau size, in the absence of conductive losses, is equal to 2 **IA**. But the size of the plateau is reduced by the conductive components in each ear. The maximum effective level = **PL** plus the **IA** minus the air-bone gap on the test ear. The minimum effective level = **PL** minus **IA** plus the air-bone gap on the masked ear. Hence the plateau width equals 2 **IA** minus (E_1 + E_2) or, in this case, its width equals 108 − (25 + 10) = 73 dB.

Similar procedures can be followed for stimuli presented by bc vibration where the principal differences from the above formulations are that (1) the conductive loss on the test ear has no influence on the problem and (2) the occlusion effect must be considered. (The fact that the **IA** for the test signal is very small is not a special consideration but only calls for a different numerical value.)

Taking the same hearing loss given above, the minimum effective level = **PL** − (B_1 + B_2) + E_2 + **OE**$_2$ or **PL** − (4) + 10 + 8 = **PL** + 14. The 10 dB is added to overcome the small conductive loss and the 8 dB is added to overcome the increased test signal input to the masked cochlea (#2) produced by occluding ear #2 with the masking earphone. The maximum effective level = **PL** + (D_2 + B_2 + B_1) or **PL** + (50 + 2 + 2) = **PL** + 54 dB. The plateau size in this case equals 40 dB (Max. − Min.). This can be calculated in another way by adding the IA for bc stimuli (4) to the **IA** for ac stimuli (54) and subtracting from that the conductive loss and the occlusion effect on Ear #2, 58 − 18 = 40.

The way in which these various factors affect Rainville-type bc procedures can also be dealt with using Figure 39-1. A noise input at **VF** passes through attenuation **C** and then B_1 and B_2 to arrive at the two cochleas at equal intensity. The tones are delivered via earphones through E_1 and E_2. Recalling that it is the physical S/N ratios at the cochleas that matters in a masking problem it should be apparent that conductive losses will reduce the intensity of the test tones while sensorineural losses will not (i.e., if there is a 50-dB output from P_2 with a 50-dB sensorineural loss, then the physical intensity of the test signal in Cochlea #2 is analogous to 50 dB. If, on the other hand, there is a 50-dB conductive loss at E_2, then the physical intensity of the test signal in Cochlea #2 is analogous to 0 dB.) A noise from **VF** presented at a 50-dB **EL** would just mask the tone 50 percent of the time in the one case but in the other the tone could not be heard. In order to be made just audible, the test tone in the latter case must be raised to 100 dB which will deliver a 50 dB signal to the test cochlea.

The above few paragraphs represent only a very few of the many problems that can be dealt with using Figure 39–1. Should more be desired, the reader may contact the author who will supply problems and solutions for both traditional bc and Rainville (SAL) procedures upon request.

part V

IMPEDANCE AUDIOMETRY

The first edition of this book, submitted for publication in 1969, did not include any articles on impedance audiometry. Commercial instrumentation for impedance measurements was being produced, but it was not generally available in clinics and, at that time, few people considered that this form of evaluation eventually might prove valuable in screening programs as well as in diagnostic audiology. Today, impedance audiometry is considered almost as important as pure-tone and speech audiometry; often it is included as part of the standard audiometry battery, and it sometimes provides important diagnostic information when behavioral measurements are impossible to obtain.

The first article in this part, by Jerger, presents an excellent introduction to the use of impedance audiometry. He demonstrates its value in the diagnosis of a variety of auditory problems, conductive as well as sensorineural, and emphasizes the need for interpretation of the overall pattern of the impedance test battery since the results of individual tests may be ambiguous. In the next article, Feldman describes the use of otoadmittance audiometry (the reciprocal form of expressing impedance measurements) to indicate its diagnostic capability, particularly in conductive disorders. Students should find the two tables in Feldman's article to be particularly helpful in the interpretation of tympanograms.

Commercial instrumentation for measuring acoustic impedance typically includes a low-frequency probe tone such as 220 Hz, but some units also make available a higher-frequency probe signal (often 660 Hz) which Liden et al. (1970) first associated with W-shaped tympanometric configurations in patients with healed perforations of the tympanic membrane. The third reading, also by

Feldman, further investigates the effects of healed perforations on tympanograms obtained with high- and low-frequency probe tones, particularly with respect to static compliance. Feldman reports that for both probe tones, the presence of a healed perforation tended to alter static compliance. He concludes that static impedance measurements are of little value in ears with healed perforations when the purpose of the test battery is to seek evidence of middle ear abnormalities. An additional finding reported by Feldman was that the W-shaped pattern occurred in many ears with healed perforations, particularly with the 660-Hz probe tone.

A major cause of otitis media in children is Eustachian tube dysfunction. Harford's article illustrates this point and stresses the usefulness of impedance audiometry in assessing Eustachian tube efficiency. He emphasizes the value of impedance measurements for identifying preclinical pathology of the middle ear and for monitoring the effects of medical treatment.

To what extent does impedance audiometry indicate effusion in the middle ear? We have selected from the literature on this topic a reading by Orchik, Morff, and Dunn. They performed impedance audiometry on patients shortly before the patients were to undergo myringotomies for suspected otitis media. Tympanograms and acoustic reflex measurements, when considered together, provided a better predictor of effusion than either test by itself. The authors also present data indicating expected false-positive and false-negative rates for each test and for the battery, and they discuss the implications of the study for hearing screening programs.

Niemeyer and Sesterhenn (1974) made a major contribution to clinical audiology when they suggested that acoustic reflex thresholds might be used to estimate hearing thresholds. Jerger, Burney, Mauldin, and Crump (1974) further elaborated on this technique. Theoretically, individuals with normal hearing should have lower acoustic reflex thresholds for complex signals, such as white noise, than for pure tones. A sensorineural hearing loss might be indicated when no difference is found between reflex thresholds for these signals. Particularly in children, disparities between expected relationships can be employed to determine the possibility of sensorineural hearing impairment. The paper by Margolis and Fox is included here since it evaluates the relative efficiency of three methods for using reflex thresholds to estimate sensorineural loss. The authors were especially concerned with the false-positive rate associated with each method. They suggest a modified method that seemed to be effective in identifying losses greater than 32 dB (re ANSI, 1969) while simultaneously minimizing false-positive classifications.

Impedance audiometry is most often used to assess middle ear function, to determine the possibility of hearing impairment in children and, on occasion, to identify nonorganic hearing loss. The last article in this section, by Olsen, Noffsinger, and Kurdziel, discusses a further use of acoustic reflex measurements in the differential diagnosis of sensorineural hearing loss. Their study showed that patients with eighth nerve lesions are most likely to have no acoustic reflex, but if a reflex is observed, it often decays long before the eliciting stimulus is terminated.

The selections we have included provide a basic introduction to impedance audiometry. More extensive treatments of this subject may be found in such texts as Jerger and Northern (1980), Feldman and Wilber (1976), and Harford, Bess, Bluestone, and Klein (1978).

REFERENCES AND ADDITIONAL READINGS

Feldman, A. S. and Wilbur, L. A. *Acoustic Impedance and Admittance.* Baltimore: Williams and Wilkins Inc. (1976).

Harford, E. R.; Bess, F. H.; Bluestone, C. D.; and Klein, J. O. *Impedance Screening for Middle Ear Disease in Childhood.* New York: Grune and Stratton (1978).

Jerger, J.; Burney, P.; Mauldin, L.; and Crump, B. Predicting hearing loss from the acoustic reflex. *J. Speech Hearing Dis.,* **39,** 11–22 (1974).

Jerger, J. F. and Northern, J. S. *Clinical Impedance Audiometry,* 2nd ed. Acton, Mass.: American Electromedics Association (1980).

Lidén, G.; Peterson, J; and Bjorkman, G. Tympanometry. *Arch. Otolaryng.,* **92,** 248–257 (1970).

Niemeyer, W. and Sesterhenn, G. Calculating the hearing threshold from the stapedius reflex threshold for different sound stimuli. *Audiology,* **13,** 421–427 (1974).

40

Clinical Experience with Impedance Audiometry

JAMES F. JERGER, Ph.D.
Professor of Audiology, Baylor College of Medicine

Impedance audiometry was performed as part of the routine clinical examination in a consecutive series of more than 400 patients with various types and degrees of hearing impairment. An electroacoustic bridge (Madsen, ZO 70) was used to carry out the measurement of tympanometry, acoustic impedance, and threshold for the acoustic reflex. Results indicate that, while individual components of the total impedance battery lack diagnostic precision, the overall pattern of results yielded by the complete battery can be of great diagnostic value, especially in the evaluation of young children.

The development of impedance audiometry during the past decade has added new scope and dimension to clinical audiology. Based on the pioneering efforts of Metz (1946), subsequent workers have refined instrumentation, technique, and interpretation to produce an invaluable tool for differential diagnosis.

The development of contemporary instrumentation for impedance audiometry has, in the main, followed two essentially parallel paths. In the United States, Zwislocki (1961) and his colleagues (Feldman, 1963, 1964, 1967; Zwislocki and Feldman, 1969) developed an electromechanical bridge. In Europe, Thomsen, Terkildsen, Møller, and others (Thomsen, 1955; Terkildsen, 1957; Terkildsen and Nielsen, 1960; Møller, 1960), pioneered the application of the electroacoustic approach, culminating in the present commercially available electroacoustic bridge.

The present paper reports our clinical experience with the latter instrument based on its routine administration to well over 400 successive patients over a one-year period. Our aim was to assess the efficacy of the electroacoustic approach as a routine clinical procedure and to evaluate its diagnostic value in a typical audiologic case load.

Reprinted by permission of the author from *Arch. Otolaryng.*, **92**, 311–324 (1970). Copyright 1970, American Medical Association.

In general we found that the testing procedure was easily mastered, even by audiologically unsophisticated personnel, that valid and meaningful results could be obtained for almost every patient, and that, with certain reservations, the data of impedance audiometry constitute extremely valuable diagnostic information.

Subsequent sections present statistical information when patients are grouped according to age and type of hearing loss, and individual case reports illustrating the diagnostic value of impedance audiometry.

METHOD

Apparatus

Impedance audiometry was carried out by means of an electroacoustic impedance bridge (Madsen, type ZO-70) and an associated pure-tone audiometer (Beltone, type 10D). Figure 40–1 shows a schematic diagram of the principal components of the impedance bridge.

A probe tip containing three tubes is sealed in the external meatus, forming a closed cavity bounded by the inner surface of the probe tip, the walls of the external meatus, and the tympanic membrane. One tube is used to deliver, into this closed cavity, a probe

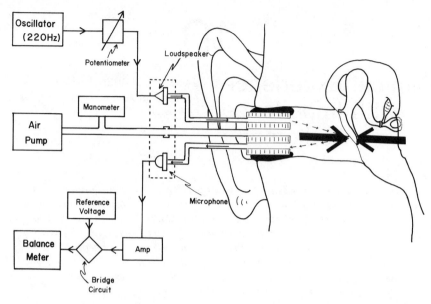

FIGURE 40–1. Schematic diagram of principal components of the electroacoustic impedance bridge.

tone generated by a 220-hertz oscillator driving a miniature receiver. The second tube is connected to a miniature probe microphone which monitors the sound pressure level of the 220-Hz probe tone in the closed cavity and delivers the transduced voltage through an amplifier to a bridge circuit and balance meter. The balance meter is nulled by an SPL of exactly 95 dB in the closed cavity. A potentiometer on the output of the 220-Hz oscillator permits variation of the SPL over a range corresponding to a compliance variation (equivalent volume) of 0.2 to 5.0 cc. The third tube is connected to an airpump which permits variation in air pressure in the closed cavity over a range of ±400 mm (water). Air pressure is read on an electromanometer.

The receiver and probe microphone are contained in a small housing mounted at the end of a conventional headband. They are connected to the probe tip by small rubber hoses. A third rubber hose delivers air to the probe tip. At the opposite end of the headband a conventional earphone is mounted. When connected to a suitable sound source it delivers signals to the ear opposite the one in which the probe tip is sealed, in order to measure threshold for the acoustic reflex. In our project the sound source was a standard clinical audiometer (Beltone, type 10D) feeding an earphone (Telephonic TDH-39) mounted in a cushion (MX 41/AR). When the headband is positioned on the patient's head, the earphone cushion covers one ear and the probe tip, attached to the housing on the headband by the three rubber hoses, may be conveniently sealed in the external meatus of the opposite ear.

With this instrumentation the three basic components of impedance audiometry—tympanometry, acoustic impedance, and acoustic reflex threshold—may be carried out.

Tympanometry

Tympanometry describes how eardrum compliance changes as air pressure is varied in the external canal. The basic datum is the pressure-compliance function, a graph relating compliance change to pressure variation. The shapes of pressure-compliance functions fall into three basic types—A, B, and C. The three types are illustrated, in idealized form, in Figure 40–2.

The type A function is characterized by a relatively sharp maximum at or near 0 mm. Type A func-

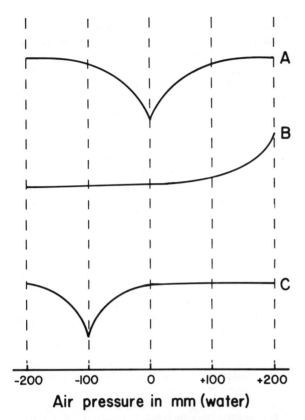

FIGURE 40-2. The three types of tympanometry curves (pressure-compliance functions): Type A curves are found in normal and otosclerotic ears; type B curves are found in serous and adhesive otitis; type C curves are due to negative pressure in the middle ear.

tions are found in normal and otosclerotic ears. The type B function shows little or no maximum. Compliance remains essentially unchanged over a large range of pressure variation. Type B functions are found in ears with serous or adhesive otitis media.

In the type C function the maximum is shifted to the left of zero by negative pressure in the middle ear. Slight negative pressure is quite common in many otherwise normal ears, but when the maximum equals or exceeds approximately 100 mm (water) significant negative pressure in the middle ear may be presumed.

Lidén (1969a, 1969b) describes a fourth type of function characterized by a double maximum at or near 0 mm. Such functions are found, according to Lidén (1969b), in cases with discontinuity of the ossicular chain. In our experience with the bridge we have never encountered this function. All of our cases of ossicular chain discontinuity show relatively deep type A functions, indicating considerable compliance change, but we have not observed the double maximum described by Lidén. This discrepancy is undoubtedly due to the difference in probe frequency used in tympanometry. Lidén has used a probe frequency of 800 Hz, whereas the bridge we employ uses a probe frequency of 220 Hz. Indeed, in recent still unpublished work by Lidén, Peterson, and Björkman (made available to us by Dr. John Peterson, Louisiana State University School of Medicine) the authors demonstrate, in a case of hypermobile tympanic membrane that whereas a probe frequency of 800 Hz shows a clearly defined Lidén function, the double maximum is greatly attenuated by changing the probe frequency to 625 Hz and entirely abolished by shifting to 220 Hz. It is not surprising, therefore, that one does not observe Lidén's function with the bridge we use. Instead, cases of ossicular discontinuity typically show exceedingly deep type A functions.

In the unit we employ acoustic impedance is derived from two input potentiometer settings, Z_1 and Z_2 (expressed in equivalent air volume or acoustic ohms). Z_1 is obtained by introducing a positive air pressure of 200 mm and adjusting the probe tone oscillator potentiometer until the balance meter is nulled. Z_2 is obtained by setting the air pressure to the value which yields maximum compliance and rebalancing the meter.

Impedance, in acoustic ohms, is given by the relation:

$$Z = \frac{Z_1 Z_2}{Z_1 - Z_2}.$$

Acoustic Reflex Threshold

In the measurement of the acoustic reflex threshold the electroacoustic bridge is used only to show relative changes in impedance. The balance meter is first nulled to zero. Then an acoustic signal is introduced to the opposite ear. If the signal is sufficient to elicit the bilateral acoustic reflex, the resulting contraction of the stapedius muscle in the ear containing the probe tip will increase the impedance at the eardrum, resulting in an upward deflection of the balance meter. In order to determine the reflex threshold the tester varies the signal level until he has identified the lowest level capable of eliciting an observable deflection of the balance meter.

Procedure

The bridge we employ was used to carry out impedance audiometry as a routine procedure on virtually every patient tested by the Audiology Service of the Methodist Hospital during 1969. Of the more than 400 patients on whom the procedure was attempted, successful results were obtained in approximately 96 percent of the cases. The primary reason for failure was inability to achieve a lasting airtight seal of the probe tip in the external canal. This problem could undoubtedly have been overcome, in this small number of cases, by special measures, such as inflatable cuffs, custom molding, or extraordinary sealing procedures, but our purpose was to evaluate the efficacy of the test as a routine clinical procedure. From this standpoint it is noteworthy that in the overwhelming majority of patients (96 percent) an airtight seal was achieved without particular difficulty.

The second most common reason for failure arose from very young children who could not maintain the requisite degree of immobility for a period sufficient to obtain complete data (usually five to ten minutes). Some of these children were retested under sedation (chloral hydrate), usually with successful results.

In order to carry out impedance audiometry, the patient was seated in a comfortable chair and the headband was carefully positioned so that the test earphone covered one ear. The probe tip was then sealed into the external canal of the opposite ear by means of an ear tip. During the first six months of the project we used the hard rubber ear tips supplied with the instrument. More recently, however, we have abandoned the hard rubber tip in favor of a tip made from a silicone material. We have found that the latter greatly facilitates the establishment of an adequate seal.

After the adequacy of the seal had been verified by the introduction of positive air pressure in the external canal, the tester proceeded to plot the pressure-compliance function (tympanometry). Compliance, in arbitrary units, was plotted as a function of varying air pressure. The latter was varied in steps of

10 to 20 mm (water) until the shape of the pressure-compliance function, and the position of its maximum, had been defined.

The second step in the examination was the measurement of acoustic impedance. Compliance values, in acoustic ohms, necessary to balance the null meter, first with air pressure at +200 mm (Z_1), then with air pressure at the maximum value of the pressure-compliance function (Z_2), were determined.

The final step in the examination was the measurement of the acoustic reflex. With the balance meter set to maximum sensitivity and nulled to zero, pure tones were introduced to the opposite ear by means of the audiometer. The intensity of the pure tone was varied until the tester had identified the lowest hearing level (HL) at which a deflection of the balance meter, synchronous with the onset and offset of the tone (making suitable allowance for the latency of the reflex response), could be observed. This level was recorded as the acoustic reflex threshold HL. In this fashion reflex thresholds were measured for signals of 500, 1,000, 2,000 and 4,000 Hz.

It should be noted that the acoustic reflex phase of the total procedure tests the ear opposite to the ear in which tympanometry and impedance measures have been carried out. For tympanometry and impedance the left ear is tested by inserting the probe tip in the left ear. For reflex thresholds, however, the left ear is tested by introducing sound to the left ear while the probe tip is inserted in the right ear.

As a result of this reversal there is some confusion in the literature over the appropriate symbol to indicate that sound is presented to one ear and the reflex is detected in the contralateral ear. Some investigators (Jepsen, 1963) feel that they are testing the right ear when the bridge is connected to the right ear and sound is introduced to the left ear. Others (Anderson et al., 1969) feel that they are testing the right ear when sound is introduced to the right ear and the bridge is connected to the left ear.

The present paper conforms to the latter convention. The symbol "O" indicates the lowest hearing level at which sound presented to the right ear elicited an acoustic reflex as detected by the bridge in the left ear. The symbol "X" indicates the lowest hearing level at which sound presented to the left ear elicited an acoustic reflex as detected by the bridge in the right ear.

When testing had been completed on the first ear, headband, earphone, and probe tip were reversed, and the entire procedure was repeated on the opposite ear. Typically the entire procedure on both ears required five to ten minutes of testing time. Longer testing time was occasionally required when an adequate seal could not be readily obtained on one or both ears.

Subjects

The total group of patients tested constituted a relatively representative sampling of a typical hospital audiologic case load. Patients ranged in age from 10 months to 81 years, and included virtually every type and degree of loss. Approximately 32 percent of the total sample showed a purely sensorineural audiometric configuration. Conductive and mixed patterns accounted for 28 percent and 22 percent respectively. The remaining 18 percent showed normal sensitivity.

RESULTS

Results are presented in two sections. The first section summarizes statistical data on the distribution of the various measures of impedance audiometry. The second section presents a series of case reports illustrating the diagnostic value of impedance audiometry.

Distributions

In order to analyze distributions as functions of age and type of loss, a subsample was formed from the total sample according to the following criteria: (1) age greater than 2 years; (2) audiometric pattern consistent with normal hearing, pure conductive loss (excluding ossicular discontinuity), or pure sensorineural loss; and (3) no history of middle ear surgery.

Patients with either suspected or confirmed retrocochlear disorder and patients with either suspected or confirmed functional hearing problems were excluded from the analysis. These criteria yielded usable data for 554 ears of 316 patients. Table 40–1 summarizes the breakdown of these subjects and ears by age and type of loss.

Tympanometry. Figure 40–3 shows the percent of ears in each age and type-of-loss category yielding either type A, B, or C pressure-compliance functions.

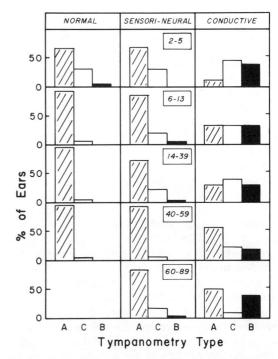

FIGURE 40-3. Distributions of types of tympanometry curves are functions of age and type of audiometric configuration.

TABLE 40-1. NO. OF SUBJECTS AND EARS BY AGE AND TYPE CATEGORIES.

| Age (yr) | Type Category | | | | | |
| | Normal | | Sensorineural | | Conductive | |
	Subjects	Ears	Subjects	Ears	Subjects	Ears
2–5	19	35	22	41	15	27
6–13	25	49	25	44	19	33
14–39	19	38	25	47	30	43
40–59	10	20	22	41	30	47
60–89	—	—	35	61	20	28
Total	73	142	129	234	114	178

Roughly, the distributions in Figure 40-3 are according to expectation. In ears with either normal or sensorineural audiometric patterns, the type A curve predominates. In ears with conductive audiometric findings, however, types B and C curves predominate. It is instructive, however, to study the distributions in the age category of 2 to 5 years. Here we observe that, in both the normal and sensorineural groups, there appears to be a higher incidence of types B and C patterns than would be predicted from the distributions for older children and adults. This is especially true of the children from 2 to 5 years with normal audiograms. The appearance of some B and a fair number of C curves in this group suggests the presence of undetected middle ear problems in children without obvious audiometric evidence of a conductive component.

In the sensorineural group, like the normal group, the type A function predominates, but the type C curve occurs in an alarming 31 percent of ears in the 2 to 5 age group. This percentage gradually declines with increasing age.

In the conductive group it is interesting to observe a gradual increase in the percentage of ears showing type A functions as age increases. This change perhaps reflects the differing distributions of middle ear pathological abnormality characterizing the various age groups. In very young children one might anticipate that otitis media and faulty eustachian tube function would account for the majority of middle ear problems, thus accounting for the predominance of types B and C. In adults, however, one would anticipate a relatively lower incidence of such problems but a relatively higher incidence of stapes fixation due to otosclerosis. Hence, the increase in the type A curve and the decrease in the B and C curves is not unexpected.

Impedance. Figure 40-4 shows the distribution of acoustic impedance values for the various groups. The solid horizontal bar in each vertical box is the median value. The box itself encompasses the semi-interquartile range or middle 50 percent of the impedance distribution.

No data are shown for normal groups in the age categories of 40 to 59 and 60 to 79 years, since we have not tested numbers of patients with truly normal sensitivity in these age categories sufficient to ensure stable medians and semi-interquartile ranges.

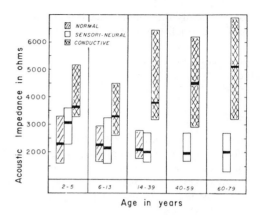

FIGURE 40-4. Distributions (median and semi-interquartile ranges) of acoustic impedance as functions of age and type of audiometric configuration.

The primary message of Figure 40-4 is a point made by previous investigators (Terkildsen and Nielsen, 1960; Bicknell and Morgan, 1968) namely that there is considerable overlap between the impedance distributions of normal and disordered middle ears. As a very rough rule of thumb, one might say that the highest 20 percent of normals overlap the lowest 20 percent of conductives. This overlap limits the diagnostic value of the impedance score when viewed in isolation. As we shall attempt to show in subsequent sections, however, the impedance may have substantial diagnostic value when considered within the framework of complete impedance audiometry.

It is also interesting to note in Figure 40-4 that in the 2 to 5 age group both the normal and sensorineural distributions are displaced upward relative to the adult distributions. The shift is especially obvious in the sensorineural group. These shifts are consistent with the high incidence of types B and C tympanometry functions noted earlier, and furnish added evidence of middle ear problems in these very young children (Brooks, 1969).

Using the distributions of the normal and sensorineural ears in the 14 to 39 age group as a standard we can form the rough rule of thumb that most normal middle ears will yield impedance scores in the range from 1,000–3,000 ohms, but that occasionally scores as low as 800 or as high as 4,200 ohms can be expected.

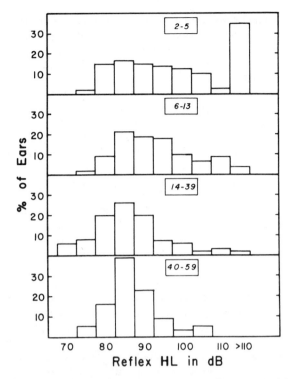

FIGURE 40-5. Distributions of acoustic reflex threshold hearing levels as function of age in subjects with normal hearing.

Acoustic Reflex. Figure 40–5 shows the distribution of the hearing level necessary to elicit the acoustic reflex. The analysis is limited to ears with normal audiometric configurations. Data for all four frequencies—500, 1,000, 2,000, and 4,000 Hz—have been pooled, since preliminary analysis failed to suggest a significant frequency effect.

Three significant factors emerge from Figure 40–5. First, the modal reflex HL is 85 dB in all age groups. Second, the distribution is about 40 dB wide. Third, there is a fairly high incidence of ears in which the reflex could not be elicited (>110 dB) in the 2 to 5 age group. This is consistent with the previous findings of Robertson et al. (1968). The distributions exhibit two relatively systematic trends with age. First, there is a tendency toward narrowing and sharpening of the distribution as age increases. Second, there is a decreasing incidence of ears that fail to show a reflex response. These trends could be inter-

preted to support a hypothesis of maturation of the reflex arc, up to perhaps early adulthood. On the other hand, one cannot exclude the possibility that the high incidence of no-response in the 2 to 5 age group merely reflects the middle ear problems suggested by the B and C tympanometry types and shifted impedance distributions noted earlier.

Although the acoustic reflex to pure tones occurs at a sensation level of approximately 85 dB in the average normal ear, the reflex SL is reduced by the presence of loudness recruitment (Jepsen, 1963; Metz, 1952; Ewertsen et al., 1958; Klockhoff, 1961; Lamb et al., 1968). This occurs because the reflex is apparently mediated by the loudness of the sound signal. In the normal ear this loudness level is reached for pure tones at sensation levels of 70 to 100 dB (Jepsen, 1963). In the ear with loudness recruitment, however, the loudness level required to elicit the reflex will be reached at a much lower level above the impaired threshold.

Figure 40–6 shows how the reflex SL declines as a function of increasing hearing loss in patients with loudness recruitment. The data are taken from the test results of sensorineural patients in the age range from 14 to 59 years.

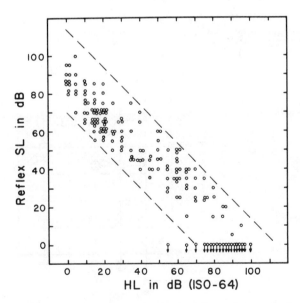

FIGURE 40-6. Relation between reflex SL and degree of hearing loss in patients with sensorineural (presumably cochlear) loss.

Figure 40–6 shows that, as sensorineural hearing loss increases, the reflex SL decreases in regular, one-to-one fashion. The relationship is linear and of unit slope. Note, also, that for any particular level of hearing loss, the range of variability among patients is about 40 dB, a range comparable to the distribution of reflex levels in normal ears.

Analysis of the trend in Figure 40–6 suggests two conclusions. First, when the reflex SL is less than 60 dB, the presence of loudness recruitment may be reasonably inferred. Second, most sensorineural losses with recruitment should yield reflex responses until the hearing level exceeds about 80 dB. This means that, when a reflex is observed at a particular frequency, the hearing level at that frequency must lie somewhere between 0 and 80 dB. Eighty decibels is, to be sure, a fairly substantial range, and well illustrates the principle that the reflex threshold level cannot be used to predict the absolute threshold level with any degree of precision. Nevertheless, the rule that reflex response means a hearing level of 80 dB or better can be extremely useful in the evaluation of very young children.

Illustrative Case Reports

Figure 40–7 shows conventional and impedance audiometry in a 7-year-old boy with serous otitis media. Results are consistent with mass lesions in the middle ears. Tympanometry curves are type B, impedance values are well above the normal range of 1,000 to 3,000 ohms, and acoustic reflexes cannot be elicited.

Figure 40–8 shows results in a 54-year-old man with bilateral otosclerosis. Tympanometry curves are type A, impedance scores are above the normal range, and acoustic reflexes are absent.

Figure 40–9 shows results in a 59-year-old woman with a unilateral loss due to endolymphatic hydrops. Tympanometry curves are type A, and impedance values are within normal limits on both ears. In this case acoustic reflexes occur at the expected normal hearing levels on both ears. The reduced sensation levels at which the reflex occurs on the right ear at 500 and 1,000 Hz are due to the loudness recruitment phenomenon.

Figure 40–10 summarizes results in a 60-year-old man with a right acoustic neurinoma. As expected, tympanometry curves are type A in both ears, and impedance values are within the normal range. The value of 4,125 ohms on the right ear is high, but, as noted earlier, a very small number of normal ears may show impedances as high as 4,200 ohms. On the left ear, reflexes are observed at the expected sensation levels of 85 to 90 dB, except at 4,000 Hz where loudness recruitment due to the high-frequency coch-

SEROUS OTITIS MEDIA

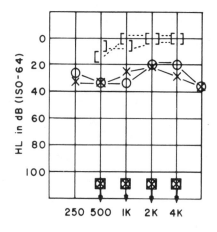

EAR	TYMP. TYPE	IMPEDANCE
R	B	7500 Ω
L	B	11667 Ω

	R	L
AC	○	×
BC	[	]
SAL	⊱	⊰
AR	▣	⊠

FIGURE 40-7. Impedance audiometry in a 7-year-old boy with serous otitis media. Note type B tympanometry curves, very high acoustic impedance scores, and bilateral absence of acoustic reflex.

OTOSCLEROSIS

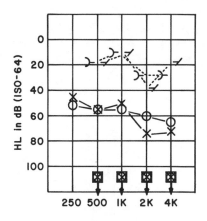

EAR	TYMP. TYPE	IMPEDANCE
R	A	4680 Ω
L	A	5525 Ω

	R	L
AC	O	X
BC	[	]
SAL	>-	-<
AR	▢	⊠

FIGURE 40-8. Impedance audiometry in a 54-year-old man with otosclerosis. Note type A curves, relatively high impedance scores, and bilateral absence of acoustic reflex.

LABYRINTHINE HYDROPS

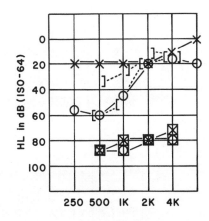

EAR	TYMP. TYPE	IMPEDANCE
R	A	844 Ω
L	A	1784 Ω

	R	L
AC	O	X
BC	[	]
SAL	>-	-<
AR	▢	⊠

FIGURE 40-9. Impedance audiometry in a 59-year-old woman with labyrinthine hydrops. Note type A curves, normal impedances, and reduced reflex SL at 500 and 1,000 Hz on right ear (due to loudness recruitment).

lear loss causes the reflex to appear at a sensation level of only 50 dB. On the right ear reflexes are absent at all frequencies. Since eighth nerve disorders, such as acoustic neurinoma, are not accompanied by loudness recruitment, sounds presented to this patient's right ear never attain sufficient loudness to elicit the reflex.

Figure 40-11 shows how facial nerve lesions central to the branch supplying the stapedius muscle abolish the acoustic reflex (Ewertsen et al., 1958). The patient had a left facial nerve paralysis due to Bell's palsy. When sound was presented to the left ear, and the probe tip was sealed in the uninvolved right ear, reflexes appeared at normal levels. How-

RIGHT ACOUSTIC NEURINOMA

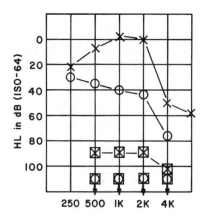

EAR	TYMP. TYPE	IMPEDANCE
R	A	4125 Ω
L	A	2250 Ω

	R	L
AC	O	X
BC	[	]
SAL	>—	—⊣
AR	◻	⊠

FIGURE 40-10. Impedance audiometry in a 60-year-old man with a right acoustic neurinoma. Note type A curves. Impedance is high (4,125 ohms) on the right ear but is still within the normal range. Absence of reflexes on the right ear indicates that recruitment is not present.

TOTAL LEFT FACIAL PARALYSIS — BELL'S PALSY

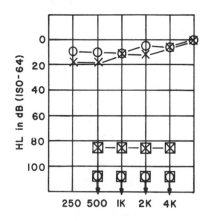

EAR	TYMP. TYPE	IMPEDANCE
R	A	2338 Ω
L	A	2057 Ω

	R	L
AC	O	X
BC	[	]
SAL	>—	—⊣
AR	◻	⊠

FIGURE 40-11. Impedance audiometry in a 22-year-old woman with left-sided facial paralysis. Absence of reflexes on right ear is due to loss of innervation to left stapedius muscle.

ever, when sounds were presented to the right ear, and the probe tip was sealed in the left ear, reflexes were not observed becaue the left stapedius muscle could not contract.

Figure 40-12 illustrates the value of impedance audiometry in very young children. The audiogram of this 3-year-old child suggested a mild unilateral loss. Properly masked bone conduction thresholds were difficult to obtain because of the child's age. Impedance audiometry clearly demonstrated, however, the conductive basis for the reduced sensitivity on the left ear. The left tympanometry curve was type B and the impedance on the left side was more than double the impedance on the right. This finding illus-

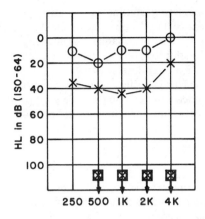

EAR	TYMP. TYPE	IMPEDANCE
R	C	1737 Ω
L	B	3619 Ω

	R	L
AC	O	X
BC	[	]
SAL	>-	-<
AR	⃞	⊠

FIGURE 40-12. Impedance audiometry in a child of 37 months. Type B curve, higher impedance on left than on right ear, and bilateral absence of acoustic reflex indicate conductive loss on left ear.

trates the diagnostic value of the absolute impedance score in spite of the overlap problem described earlier. Here the value of 3,619 ohms is within the normal range, but the fact that it is so much larger than the right ear value of 1,737 ohms adds support to the overall picture of left middle ear involvement suggested by the type B tympanometry function. Finally, the fact that acoustic reflexes are absent in both ears yields still more support for a left middle ear disorder. Failure to elicit reflexes when sound is introduced to the left ear results from the fact that

the conductive loss attenuates the loudness of the input signal to such an extent that, even at the maximum output of the audiometer, 110 dB HL, the loudness is not sufficient to trigger the reflex. Failure to elicit reflexes when sound is presented to the normal right ear results from the fact that, even though the loudness in the right ear is sufficient to elicit a reflex, the probe tip in the left ear will fail to detect the contraction because of the middle ear disorder.

This particular configuration of results has con-

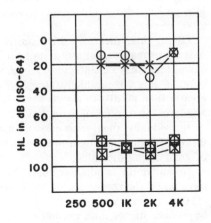

EAR	TYMP. TYPE	IMPEDANCE
R	A	1710 Ω
L	A	1636 Ω

	R	L
AC	O	X
BC	[	]
SAL	>-	-<
AR	⃞	⊠

FIGURE 40-13. Impedance audiometry in a child of 27 months. Type A curves, normal impedances, and normal acoustic reflexes confirm behavioral impression of normal hearing.

siderable diagnostic value. It means, in effect, that the combination of unilateral loss and bilateral absence of the acoustic reflex can only mean unilateral middle ear disorder. In unilateral cochlear disorder one would always see the reflex on the good ear and, if the loss did not exceed 80 dB, on the bad ear as well. In unilateral eighth nerve disorder one would at least see the reflex on the good ear. Only unilateral middle ear problems abolish the reflex bilaterally.

In the case of this 3-year-old boy the results of impedance audiometry pointed unequivocally to a unilateral conductive problem. Subsequent medical examination and treatment confirmed the accuracy of this conclusion.

The value of impedance audiometry in this patient lay in the fact that it led to an unequivocal diagnosis of conductive impairment without the need for bone conduction audiometry. The clinician who has attempted to measure bone conduction thresholds on children in this age range, while simultaneously masking the ear not being tested, will, perhaps, appreciate the value of such diagnostic support.

Figure 40-13 shows the result of impedance audiometry in a child of 27 months. The audiogram suggested reasonably normal sensitivity in both ears, but, again, one does not always feel comfortable about the validity of threshold estimates in children so young. In this case impedance audiometry served to confirm the impression of normal hearing. The fact that all results were normal gave, at least to us, valuable confirmation of our impression that the child suffered no significant ear pathological abnormality.

Figure 40-14, *top* and *bottom,* illustrates how impedance audiometry can be carried out under sedation in the very young child. Figure 40-14, *left,* shows the result of our first examination of a child of 10 months. Orienting responses to familiar speech sounds in a sound field (SFSP) suggested a threshold sensitivity level of about 30 dB. Impedance audiometry, carried out under chloral hydrate sedation, showed type C tympanometry functions in both ears. On the left ear impedance was well within the normal range (2,150 ohms), but on the right ear a value of 6,000 ohms, well above the normal range, was noted. In addition, there was no reflex bilaterally. We interpreted these findings to indicate a right middle ear disorder. After two months of medical treatment the child was retested (Figure 40-14, *right*). The speech awareness level had improved only slightly, to 15 dB, but changes in impedance audiometry were dramatic. Although the tympanometry curve was still type C,

indicating continuing negative pressure, the impedance had dropped from 6,000 to 2,000 ohms on the right ear. Impedance was unchanged on the left ear. In addition, reflexes could be elicited from both ears at expected levels.

This case illustrates the value of impedance audiometry in detecting middle ear problems in the child too young for conventional play audiometry.

COMMENT

In our experience, impedance audiometry represents an invaluable diagnostic tool in clinical audiology. It has become, in our clinic, a routine part of the audiologic assessment of every patient. We frankly wonder how we ever got along without it.

Equally clear, however, is the fact that the technique is useful only as a complete battery and that diagnostic judgments must be based on the overall configuration of tympanometry, acoustic impedance, and the acoustic reflex.

Tympanometry alone is useful only to a limited degree. Types B and C curves strongly suggest middle ear disorder but, as illustrated in Figure 40-3, type A curves also occur in a large percentage of conductive losses, especially in older adults.

The acoustic impedance score, per se, is simply too variable for accurate diagnosis. As shown in Figure 40-4, there is an overlap of about 20 percent between normals and conductives. An impedance in the vicinity of 4,000 ohms is quite ambiguous. It may be normal or it may indicate a considerable increase in a patient whose impedance is normally less than 2,000 ohms.

Of the three measures the acoustic reflex thresholds are probably most useful individually. But here, again, there may be ambiguity. Absence of the reflex may be due to conductive loss, to cochlear loss greater than 80 dB, to eighth nerve loss at virtually any level, or to a facial nerve lesion.

Individually, then, each measure has serious limitations. In combination, however, they yield patterns of great diagnostic value.

In unilateral conductive loss, for example, we have noted the recurrence of the following pattern: (1) tympanometry of types B or C on the bad ear; (2) impedance higher than normal on the bad ear; and (3) acoustic reflex absent in both ears.

This pattern points, unequivocally, to the presence of middle ear disorder on the bad ear. There are

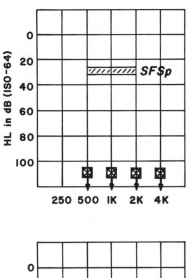

EAR	TYMP. TYPE	IMPEDANCE
R	C	6000 Ω
L	C	2150 Ω

	R	L
AC	O	X
BC	[	]
SAL	>—	—<
AR	▢	⊠

EAR	TYMP. TYPE	IMPEDANCE
R	C	2000 Ω
L	C	2111 Ω

	R	L
AC	O	X
BC	[	]
SAL	>—	—<
AR	▢	⊠

FIGURE 40-14. Top: Impedance audiometry carried out under sedation in a child of 10 months. Behavioral observation suggests relatively normal sensitivity, but high impedance (6,000 ohms) and bilateral absence of acoustic reflex suggest conductive loss on right ear. Bottom: Same child two months later after medical treatment for otitis media. Decrease of impedance from 6,000 to 2,000 ohms and appearance of acoustic reflex bilaterally indicate that middle ear problem has been resolved.

only two common exceptions to this pattern. Otosclerotics will usually give a type A function rather than a B or C. Cases of ossicular discontinuity may give unusually deep type A functions and lower than normal impedance. Also, in the latter group, there may be an observable acoustic reflex at high levels when sound is introduced to the good ear.

In unilateral cochlear loss with loudness recruitment the following pattern recurs: (1) tympanometry of type A on both ears; (2) impedance normal on both ears; and (3) acoustic reflex elicited at normal HL in both ears (i.e., at reduced SL in the bad ear).

The only common exception to this pattern occurs when the loss on the bad ear exceeds about 80 dB. Then the reflex is absent on the bad ear, but still present on the good ear.

In unilateral eighth nerve loss the following pattern recurs: (1) tympanometry of type A on both ears; (2) impedance normal on both ears; and (3) acoustic reflex elicited at normal HL on the good ear, but absent on the bad ear.

The only exception to this pattern occurs when the loss on the bad ear is very mild. Under this circumstance the sound may reach a loudness sufficient to elicit a reflex at a normal or greater than normal SL on the bad ear. Under this circumstance the reflex amplitude decay test of Anderson et al. (1969) may be applied for further confirmation of the retrocochlear site.

Using these recurring patterns as a frame of reference, we have employed the results of impedance audiometry to great advantage diagnostically. It must be reemphasized, however, that there will always be exceptions to the expected outcomes of individual components of the impedance battery. As illustrated in Figure 40–3, some normals and many sensorineurals will give type C tympanometry functions. And, as we have emphasized earlier, acoustic impedance values may be difficult to interpret unless they easily exceed the normal range. Finally, there is a very small percentage of otherwise normal individuals who simply do not show the acoustic reflex at any level (Robertson, 1968).

Nevertheless, the expected patterns recur with sufficient regularity so that we find them distinctly advantageous in clinical work. They are especially useful in the evaluation of very young children. Here we find that impedance audiometry is valuable in either confirming or denying the diagnostic impressions gained from observation and behavioral audiometry.

Table 40–2 shows how the overall pattern of impedance data can be helpful in confirming the tester's clinical impression based on behavioral observation. Table 40–2 is also useful in denying the likelihood that one's clinical impression is correct. If, for example, one cannot observe response to sound at any level, yet acoustic reflexes occur at normal levels bi-laterally, it is unlikely that the behavioral impression of total deafness is correct. One must then seek other reasons for the child's failure to respond behaviorally. Similarly, if the child seems to be responding behaviorally at moderate sound levels, yet the reflex is bilaterally absent in spite of normal impedance and type A tympanometry, then the validity of the behavioral responses is rendered suspect. Finally, the results of impedance audiometry can be extremely valuable in identifying middle ear disorders in children whose bone conduction levels cannot be validly measured either because of age and cooperation factors or because the sensorineural loss is too severe (Farrant and Skurr, 1966; Brooks, 1968; Djupesland, 1969). In our clinical experience the combination of play or conditional orienting reflex (COR) audiometry and impedance audiometry yields a reasonably accurate estimate of both degree and type of loss in all but a small percentage of the children referred to our service.

Many studies published in the American literature (Feldman, 1963, 1964; Zwislocki and Feldman, 1969) have dwelt on the value of impedance audiometry in distinguishing between stapes fixation and ossicular discontinuity. As a result, there is a feeling in many quarters that this is the principle application of impedance audiometry. Otologic surgeons have, therefore, questioned whether the results of impedance audiometry are of more than academic interest since surgical intervention is indicated in either event.

Our own experience certainly concurs with the results of previous investigators in demonstrating that the distinction between fixation and discontinuity is dramatically revealed in both the pressure-com-

TABLE 40–2. SHOWING HOW RESULTS OF IMPEDANCE AUDIOMETRY HELP TO CONFIRM AUDIOMETRIC IMPRESSION IN THE EVALUATION OF YOUNG CHILDREN.

Tympanometry	Impedance	Acoustic Reflex	Confirm Behavioral Audiometric Impression of
A in both ears	Normal in both ears	Normal bilaterally	Bilateral normal hearing or bilateral mild-moderate sensorineural loss or unilateral mild-moderate sensorineural loss
A in both ears	Normal in both ears	Absent bilaterally	Severe bilateral sensorineural loss
A in one ear; B or C in other ear	Normal in A ear; high in B or C ear	Absent bilaterally	Unilateral conductive loss
B or C in both ears	High in both ears	Absent bilaterally	Bilateral conductive loss

pliance function and the acoustic impedance. We have, however, purposely avoided extensive discussion of this issue in the present paper in order to emphasize, to the clinician, that impedance audiometry has far broader implications for the diagnostic evaluation of hearing disorder.

ACKNOWLEDGMENT

This study was supported by grant FR-05425 from the Public Health Service.

Mrs. Phyllis Segal, supervising audiologist, the Methodist Hospital, Houston, assisted in the collection of data.

REFERENCES

Anderson, H.; Barr, B.; and Wedenberg, E. Intra-aural reflexes in retrocochlear lesions, in Hamberger, C., and Wersall, J. (eds): *Disorders of the Skull Base Region.* Stockholm, Almqvist & Wiksell, 1969.

Bicknell, M. and Morgan, N. A clinical evaluation of the Zwislocki acoustic bridge. *J Laryng* **82:** 673–691, 1968.

Brooks, D. An objective method of detecting fluid in the middle ear. *Int Aud* **7:** 280, 1968.

Brooks, D. The use of the electro-acoustic impedance bridge in the assessment of middle ear function *Int Aud* **8:**563–569, 1969.

Djupesland, G. Use of impedance indicator in diagnosis of middle ear pathology. *Int Aud* **8:**570–578, 1969.

Ewertsen, H.; Filling, S.; Terkildsen, K. et al. Comparative recruitment testing. *Acta Otolaryng* **140**(suppl):116–122, 1958.

Farrant, R. and Skurr, B. Measuring the acoustic impedance of severely deaf ears to test for conductive component. *J Otolaryng Soc Aust* **2:**49–53, 1966.

Feldman, A. Impedance measurements at the eardrum as an aid to diagnosis. *J Speech Hearing Res* **6:**315–327, 1963.

Feldman, A. Acoustic impedance measurements as a clinical procedure. *Int Aud* **3:**1–11, 1964.

Feldman, A. Acoustic impedance studies of the normal ear. *J Speech Hearing Res* **10:**165–176, 1967.

Jepsen, O. Middle-ear muscle reflexes in man, in Jerger, J. (ed): *Modern Developments in Audiology.* New York, Academic Press Inc., 1963, pp. 193–239.

Klockhoff, I. Middle ear muscle reflexes in man: A clinical and experimental study with special reference to diagnostic problems in hearing impairment. *Acta Otolaryng.* suppl 164, 1961.

Lamb, L.; Peterson, J.; and Hansen, S. Application of stapedius muscle reflex measures to diagnosis of auditory problems. *Int Aud* **7:**188–199, 1968.

Lidén, G. The scope and application of current audiometric tests. *J Laryng* **83:**507–520, 1969a.

Lidén, G. Tests for stapes fixation. *Arch Otolaryng* **89:** 215–219, 1969b.

Metz, O. The acoustic impedance measured on normal and pathological ears. *Acta Otolaryng,* suppl **63,** 1946.

Metz, O. Threshold of reflex contractions of muscles of middle ear and recruitment of loudness. *Arch Otolaryng* **55:**536–543, 1952.

Møller, A. Improved technique for detailed measurements of the middle ear impedance. *J Acoust Soc Amer* **32:**250–257, 1960.

Robertson, E.; Peterson, J.; and Lamb, L. Relative impedance measurements in young children. *Arch Otolaryng* **88:**70–76, 1968.

Terkildsen, K. Movements of the eardrum following intraaural muscles reflexes. *Arch Otolaryng* **66:**484–488, 1957.

Terkildsen, K. and Nielsen, S.S. An electroacoustic impedance measuring bridge for clinical use. *Arch Otolaryng* **72:**339–346, 1960.

Thomsen, K. Employment of impedance measurement in otologic and oto-neurologic diagnostics. *Acta Otolaryng* **45:**159–167, 1955.

Zwislocki, J. Acoustic measurement of the middle ear function. *Ann Otol* **70:**1–8, 1961.

Zwislocki, J. and Feldman, A. *Acoustic Impedance of Pathological Ears,* technical report LSC-S-5 of the Laboratory of Sensory Communication. Syracuse, N.Y., Syracuse University, 1969.

41

Diagnostic Application and Interpretation of Tympanometry and the Acoustic Reflex

ALAN S. FELDMAN, Ph.D.

Director, Communication Disorders Unit, State University of New York, Upstate Medical Center, Syracuse, N.Y.

Abstract. Tympanometry and the acoustic reflex constitute a powerful middle ear measurement battery. Together, these measurements provide us with direct objective information about the integrity and mobility of the middle ear system and the status of the sensorineural auditory function. A descriptive analysis of tympanograms involves a consideration of the amplitude and shape of the tympanogram as well as the location of the peak along the air pressure axis. The differential effect of pathology on tympanogram pressure peak location, amplitude and shape as well as on the acoustic reflex provides the capability for the application of this battery in the differential diagnosis of auditory disorders.

Acoustic impedance measurements in the clinical evaluation of auditory problems have now been applied, in one or another form, for three decades. Over this period, we have seen dramatic changes in instrumentation and measurement approaches. Some of these changes are the direct result of the accumulation of data from basic and applied research, while others grew out of clinical experience (Metz, 1946; Terkildsen and Scott Nielsen, 1960; Zwislocki, 1963; Feldman, 1964). All of these have led to the development of what may be referred to as an acoustic impedance battery. This battery utilizes the direct objective measurement of various aspects of middle ear function. It provides us with information about the ability of the middle ear to behave as an efficient impedance-matching transformer and reveals abnormalities contributing to its malfunction. It also serves as an inferential basis for the evaluation of sensorineural function.

While there can be no question that we have yet to reach the ultimate level of sophistication with this form of measurement of the auditory system, its present stage of development is such that it can provide a major contribution to the differential diagnosis of auditory problems. The acoustic impedance battery can provide us with a variety of both direct and indirect objective measures of function of the various components of the auditory system and, further, can help localize where in the system abnormality can exist. This localization can extend from the ear canal, itself, to the central auditory network. At the same time, it is worth noting that this battery, as is true for most other tests, is not infallible, and one must not be tempted to view the results in isolation.

The intent of this paper is to provide some examples of how the acoustic impedance battery may be applied and the results interpreted in the evaluation and identification of some of the clinical abnormalities that may exist at the eardrum, in the middle ear space and its various structures, and in the sensorineural system.

Paper presented at the Round Table Conference on Advances in Acoustic Impedance Measurements at the 13th International Congress of Audiology in Florence, Italy, on October 19, 1976.

Reprinted by permission of the author from *Audiology,* **16,** 294–306 (1977).

THE ACOUSTIC IMPEDANCE BATTERY

The outline and application of the acoustic impedance battery consists of tympanometry, intra-aural reflex testing and Eustachian tube testing.

Tympanometry. This measurement offers information about (1) the air pressure status of the middle ear; (2) the static acoustic impedance and admittance (the source establishing parameters of stiffness or flaccidity at the eardrum); (3) the integrity and mobility of the eardrum; (4) the integrity and mobility of the ossicular chain, and (5) the resonant point of the middle ear system.

Intra-Aural Reflex Testing. (1) Acoustic reflex measurements are a source of information about the mobility and integrity of the ossicular chain and the sensorineural system and (2) the non-acoustic reflex test results are a source of information about the mobility and integrity of the ossicular chain and the Vth and VIIth cranial nerves.

Eustachian Tube Testing. This is a means of evaluating: (1) the patency of the tube and (2) the function of the tube.

In some individual evaluations some components of the battery may not be necessary. The basic tympanogram and acoustic reflex would constitute the components of the basic battery. For the purposes of this presentation, direct consideration of Eustachian tube patency and function will not be considered.

TYMPANOMETRY

The measurement of the changing flow of energy into or through the middle ear as air pressure is modified across the plane of the tympanic membrane may be displayed as a tympanogram. Tympanometry is effective in identifying and differentiating various abnormalities of the middle ear system. It has not yet been proven to be of clinical significance in individual sensorineural problems, although some studies have suggested there are group differences that can be demonstrated (Rezen and Lloyd, 1975; Wilber et al., 1976). All tympanograms, regardless of instrumentation, possess certain basic features that may be analyzed to permit interpretation.

INTERPRETATION OF TYMPANOGRAMS

The identifiable features of tympanograms are demonstrated in Figure 41-1. They are: a definable air pressure peak, a definable amplitude and a definable shape. The location of the pressure peak addresses the question of middle ear ventilation; the amplitude addresses the question of the static impedance of the ear. The shape of the tympanogram may be viewed as a revelation of altered resonance or internal noise in the middle ear system. Pathology and other abnormalities of the middle ear system variably influence these features of the tympanogram as outlined in Table 41-1.

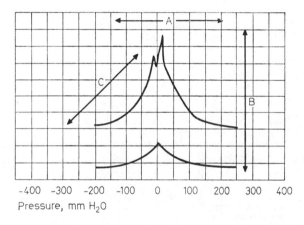

-400 -300 -200 -100 0 100 200 300 400
Pressure, mm H$_2$O

FIGURE 41-1. Parameters of a tympanogram. A = Pressure peak; B = amplitude; C = shape.

TABLE 41-1.

Pressure peak effects of middle ear abnormalities
  Negative
  Normal
  Positive
  Absent
Amplitude effects of middle ear abnormalities
  Increased
  Decreased
  Normal
Shape effects of middle ear abnormalities
  Slope
    Increased
    Decreased
  Smoothness

TABLE 41–2.

Pressure peak (pressure-related pathologies)
  Pathologies with negative pressure peak
    Blocked Eustachian tube
    Serous otitis media
  Pathologies with normal pressure peak
    Ossicular bony fixation
    Adhesive fixation
    Ossicular discontinuity
    Middle ear tumor
    Eardrum abnormality
  Pathologies with positive pressure peak
    Early acute otitis media
  Absence of pressure peak
    Middle ear effusion
    Open tympanic membrane
    Cholesteatoma
    Artifact
Amplitude (pathologies influencing amplitude)
  Pathologies with increased tympanogram amplitude
    Eardrum abnormality
    Ossicular discontinuity
  Pathologies with decreased tympanogram amplitude
    Ossicular fixation bony or adhesive
    Serous otitis media
    Cholesteatoma, polyps, granuloma
    Glomus tumors
  Pathologies not influencing tympanogram amplitude
    Blocked Eustachian tube
    Early acute otitis media
Shape (pathologies altering tympanogram shape)
  Slope
    Pathologies which flatten or decrease slope
      Serous otitis
      Ossicular fixation
      Tumors of middle ear
    Pathologies which increase slope
      Eardrum abnormality
      Ossicular discontinuity
  Smoothness
    Eardrum abnormality
    Ossicular discontinuity
    Vascular tumors
    Patulous Eustachian tube

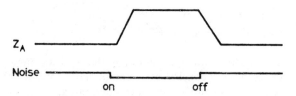

FIGURE 41–2. Y-T recording of impedance (Z_A) change coinciding with introduction (on) and removal (off) of a noise stimulus.

THE INTRA-AURAL REFLEX

A change in the flow of energy (admittance or impedance) at the eardrum of the normal ear occurs as a consequence of contraction of one or the other of the middle ear muscles and the consequent stiffening of the middle ear system. This can be revealed in a number of ways, most commonly as a meter deflection or in a Y-T recording, as shown in Figure 41–2. The presence of the reflex is generally interpreted as indicating mobility of the ossicular chain. Most middle ear pathologies will obliterate the ability to monitor a reflex. Notable exceptions would be Eustachian tube obstruction without effusion and interruption of the ossicular chain with ossicular or fibrous continuity maintained through the insertion of the stapedial tendon. The normal sensation level of the acoustic reflex (70–95 dB) may be altered in sensorial or neural pathologies. Anticipated results of the acoustic reflex with various pathologies are illustrated in Figure 41–3.

CLINICAL EXAMPLES

The following examples are illustrations of the applications of acoustic impedance measurements using a descriptive analysis of the results in the evaluation of the middle ear system.

Findings Related to the Eardrum

Pressure Peak. The only factor at the eardrum influencing the location of the air pressure point of peak flow is whether or not the drum is intact. The

The interpretation of tympanograms using a descriptive analysis of pressure, amplitude and shape would consider the differential effects of pathology listed in Table 41–2.

It is important to keep in mind that any of the pathologies may exist in conjunction with another. Otosclerotics, for example, could have a blocked Eustachian tube and exhibit negative pressure as well as decreased amplitude.

Possible Pathologies	Results of Monitored Acoustic Reflex: Contralateral Stimulation	Results of Monitored Acoustic Reflex: Ipsilateral Stimulation
Unilateral Conductive (C) 	● Absent both ears	● Absent in ear with conductive loss Present in normal ear
Bilateral Conductive (C) 	● Absent both ears	● Absent both ears
Unilateral Cochlear (SN) 	● Present in impaired ear May be present in normal ear if sufficient residual hearing in impaired ear	● Present in normal ear May be present in impaired ear if sufficient residual hearing in that ear
Unilateral Neural (NR) 	● Present in impaired ear ● Normal ear reflex may be 1. Absent 2. Present in response to elevated RSL 3. Present but with decay	● Present in normal ear ● Abnormal ear reflex may be 1. Absent 2. Present but with elevated RSL 3. Present but with decay
Unilateral Central (CNT) 	● Absent in ear contra-lateral to lesion Present in ear ipsilateral to lesion	● Present in both ears

FIGURE 41-3. Anticipated results of contralateral and ipsilateral acoustic reflex measurements with various pathologies.

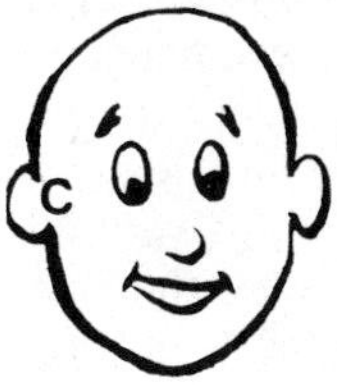

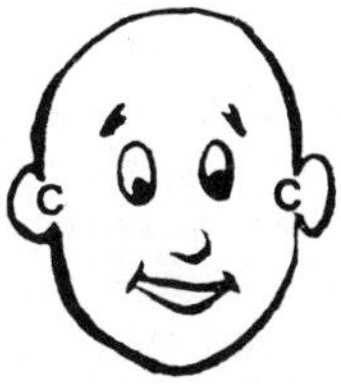

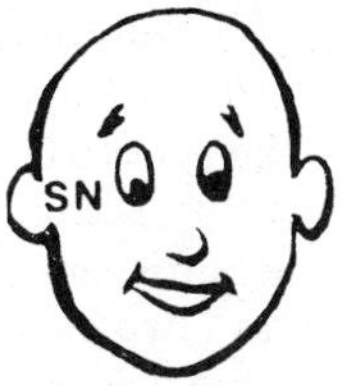

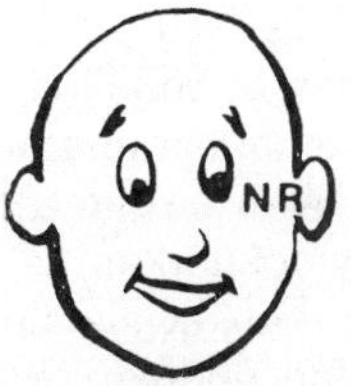

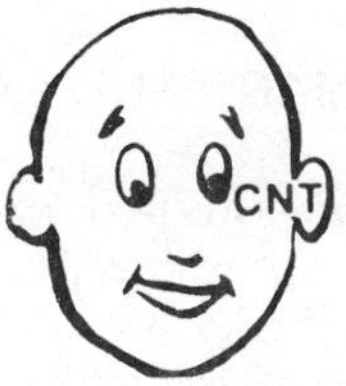

energy flow across the membrane will only change with ear canal air pressure modification when that air pressure is different on the two surfaces of the eardrum. Thus, a perforation will be revealed by a flat tympanogram without a pressure peak.

Amplitude. It has been shown that for any type of electro-acoustic measuring system the presence of eardrum abnormality results in tympanograms of excessive amplitude which misrepresents the true static impedance of the middle ear (Feldman, 1974).

Shape. In addition to exaggerating amplitude, when the impedance of the eardrum is low enough, it will also result in shape alteration. Figure 41-4 illustrates the increasing slope and notching commonly observed as a direct consequence of eardrum abnormality (Williams et al., 1975).

Findings Related to the Middle Ear

Pressure. Perhaps the most commonly observed tympanometric deviation is the presence of a tympanogram peak at a negative ear canal pressure. The extreme of the condition would be a flat tympanogram which could suggest a negligible air space in the middle ear.

Amplitude. Reduction in amplitude implies increased stiffness and may be consistent with a reduced middle ear air space (effusion) or a fixed ossicular chain. The differentiating feature would be the location of the tympanogram peak on the pressure axis. Figure 41-5 compares tympanograms of otosclerotic and middle ear effusion ears. Increases in amplitude would be attributable to either eardrum abnormality or ossicular discontinuity.

Shape. Increased amplitude implies lower impedance and lower resonance of the system. Consequently, notching aberrations of shape which occur when stiffness influence is minimal or absent will be a common observation with probe tones of 500 Hz and above. There are those who feel that the presence of this notching confuses the interpretation of tympanograms. In actuality, it often helps to clarify the picture. Not only does it provide information which can validate or invalidate estimates of static impedance obtained with low frequencies, the notching also reveals much about the middle ear ossicular integrity. Most eardrum notching is very different in appearance from that observed with ossicular discontinuity. As was noted in Figure 41-4, the former is usually quite spiking, whereas the latter, as demonstrated in Figure 41-6, is typically multiple, broad and undulating. This is not to deny that a major problem in tympanometry is the flaccid tympanic membrane. When the impedance of the eardrum is lower than the impedance of the middle ear, accurate assessment of static impedance is impossible (Møller, 1965). This is true for all probe tone frequencies.

Because amplitude and shape aberrations occur with both eardrum and ossicular discontinuities it may sometimes be important to establish the basis for these aberrations. Møller (1965) and then Lidén et al. (1974) first suggested a means of minimizing the undesirable eardrum effect. We have studied this further and validated the effectiveness of increasing eardrum impedance with colloidin to eliminate its interference with the measurement of the middle ear system. Figure 41-7 shows two ears before and after colloidin application. One has a flaccid tympanic membrane with a normal middle ear resulting in increased amplitude and notching of the usual smooth bell-shaped tympanogram. The other ear has an ossicular discontinuity as well as some eardrum abnormality. Application of colloidin in the former instance results in a tympanogram that is normal in all respects. In the ear with an interruption, however, the post-colloidin tympanogram is only slightly reduced in amplitude with negligible shape changes. The typical broad and undulating multiple notches characteristic of interruption remain.

SUMMARY AND CONCLUSIONS

Two features of the acoustic impedance battery, tympanometry and the acoustic reflex, have been reviewed with case examples provided demonstrating the application of this battery in the differential diagnosis of auditory disorders. The emphasis has been primarily focused on middle ear disorders and the

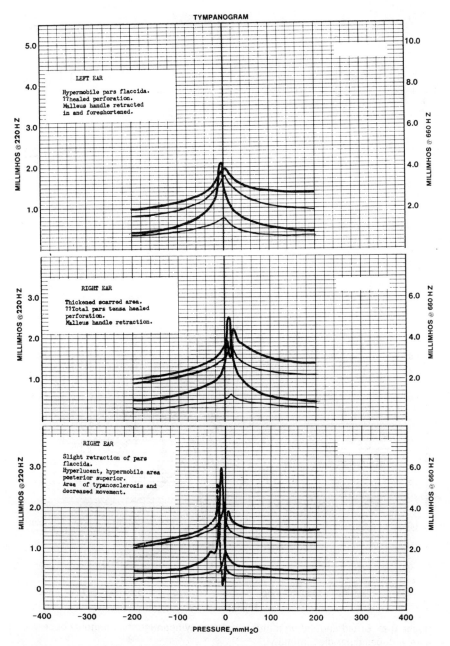

FIGURE 41-4. Increasing amplitude and shape changes in tympanograms of ears with tympanic membrane abnormality.

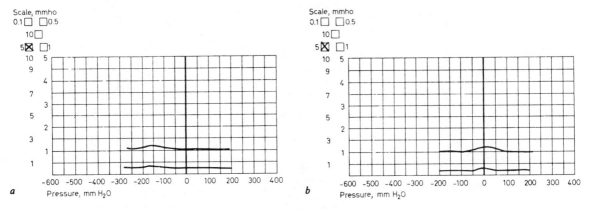

FIGURE 41-5. Tympanograms of ears with middle ear effusion (a) showing reduced amplitude and negative pressure and otosclerosis (b) showing reduced amplitude and normal pressure.

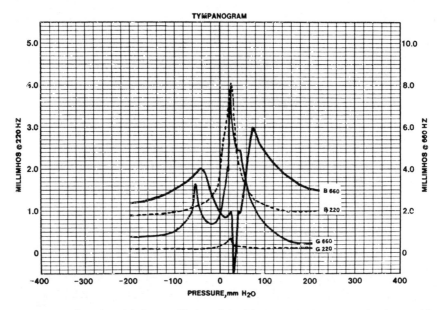

FIGURE 41-6. Broad undulating multiple notched tympanogram commonly observed in ears with ossicular discontinuity.

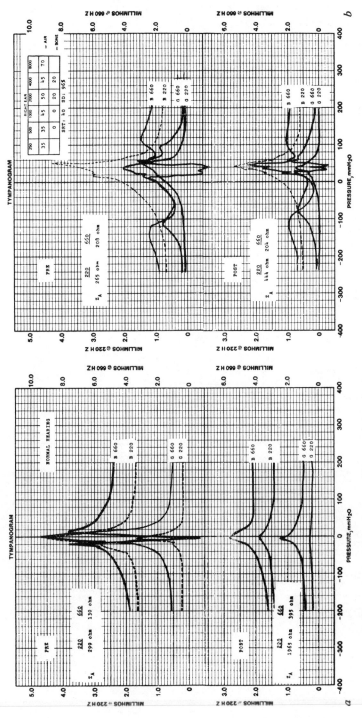

FIGURE 41-7. Changes in tympanogram features and acoustic impedance (Z_A) when a flaccid tympanic membrane is stiffened with colloidin. a = 'Pre' and 'post' are in an otherwise normal ear. b = 'Pre' and 'post' are in an ear with ossicular discontinuity in addition to a healed perforation.

examples given are by no means all inclusive. They were chosen to demonstrate the value of a descriptive analysis in the interpretation of tympanograms which

when used in conjunction with the results of tests of the intra-aural muscle reflex, provide a powerful clinical diagnostic tool.

REFERENCES

Feldman, A. S. Acoustic impedance measurements as a clinical procedure. *Int. Audiol.,* **3:** 156 (1964).

Feldman, A. S. Eardrum abnormality and the measurement of middle ear function. *Arch. Otolaryng.,* **99:** 211 (1974).

Lidén, G.; Harford, E.; and Hallen, O. Tympanometry for the diagnosis of ossicular disruption. *Arch. Otolaryng.,* **99:** 23 (1974).

Metz, O. The acoustic impedance measured on normal and pathological ears. *Acta Otolaryng.,* suppl., **63** (1946).

Møller, A. R. An experimental study of the acoustic impedance of the middle ear and its transmission properties. *Acta Otolaryng.,* **60:** 129 (1965).

Rezen, S. V. and Lloyd, L. An investigation into the use of impedance measurements in the diagnosis of Menière's disease. Impedance Newsletters American Electromedics Corp. *Dobbs Ferry,* **4:** 3 (1975).

Terkildsen, K. and Scott Nielsen, S. An electroacoustic impedance measuring bridge for clinical use. *Arch. Otolaryng.,* **72:** 339 (1960).

Wilber, L. A.; Goodhill, V.; and Bettsworth, A. H. In Feldman and Wilber, Acoustic impedance and admittance: The measurement of middle ear function. Baltimore: Williams & Wilkins, 1976.

Williams, P. G.; Hunt, W.; and Rodriguez, D. Eardrum variables influencing tympanometry. *ASHA,* **17:** 609 (1975).

Zwislocki, J. An acoustic method for clinical examination of the ear. *J. Speech Hearing Res.,* **6:** 303 (1963).

42

Eardrum Abnormality and the Measurement of Middle Ear Function

ALAN S. FELDMAN, Ph.D.

Director, Communication Disorders Unit, State University of New York, Upstate Medical Center, Syracuse, New York

Ranges of static impedance in two "normal" middle ear populations are compared. One population (100 ears) showed no audiometric evidence of middle ear abnormality, and tests showed normal function. History and otologic findings also showed a normal middle ear system. The second group (29 ears) also had no audiometric evidence of conductive abnormality, but did have healed perforations of the tympanic membranes.

Ranges for resistive and reactive measurements with a 220-Hz and 660-Hz probe-tone were computed. Healed perforations markedly lowered measured acoustic impedance and strongly suggested that both low and high frequency tympanograms are contaminated by eardrum abnormality. These results account for previously observed but unexplained overlap between some presumably stiff pathological eardrums and normals and restrict use of static acoustic impedance in differential diagnosis of middle ear abnormality to ears with normal tympanic membranes.

The evaluation of middle ear function by the measurement of static acoustic impedance involves a measurement of parameters of a probe signal reflected off the intact tympanic membrane. The flow of acoustic energy introduced into the ear canal by an impedance measuring instrument is affected by mechanical factors encountered at the eardrum. The eardrum characteristics are generally presumed to be related primarily to its attachments. The mobility of the ossicles and the size and state of the air in the middle ear and mastoid space as well as the resistance of the cochlear fluid are presumed to be the primary factors that affect the impedance of the middle ear system (Moller, 1961, 1963, 1965; Onchi, 1949, 1961; Zwislocki, 1957a, 1957b, 1962). The presence of fluid, space-occupying tumors, adhesive or ossicular fixation, as well as interruption of the ossicular chain result in changes of the mechanical transmission system and are revealed by changes in static acoustic impedance that can be measured at the plane of the tympanic membrane (Feldman, 1963, 1964; Nilges et al., 1969; Zwislocki and Feldman, 1970). However, overlap, particularly of ears with an abnormality that should induce stiffness in the middle ear system, has been felt by some to impose serious limitation on the diagnostic application of static acoustic impedance in individual cases (Bicknell and Morgan, 1968; Jerger, 1970).

The effect of abnormality of the eardrum itself has been reported, but not accurately measured. Terkildsen and Thomsen (1959) demonstrated the effect of eardrum abnormality in the very earliest stages of tympanometry by pointing out the change in shape it causes in the tympanogram with a low frequency (220 Hz) probe-tone. Wilber et al. (1970) sug-

From the Department of Otorhinolaryngology, Communication Disorders Unit, State University of New York, Upstate Medical Center, Syracuse, N.Y.

Reprinted by permission of the author from *Arch. Otolaryng.*, **99**, 211–217 (1974). Copyright, 1974, American Medical Association.

gested that eardrum abnormality affects the static acoustic impedance, but offered no definitive documentation of that observation. Lidén et al. (1970) demonstrated the bizarre effect of healed perforations on tympanograms obtained using high frequency (625 Hz and 800 Hz) probe-tones, but because they were concerned with tympanogram shape rather than amplitude and its related static acoustic impedance values, inferred no effect for a 200-Hz probe-tone. They noted a W notching of the 625-Hz and 800-Hz tympanograms in patients with healed perforations. A similar notching was observed in flaccid but unperforated drums with an 800-Hz probe-tone, but only minimally in the 625-Hz tympanogram. This would be a predictable observation because, as a probe-tone frequency approaches the normal resonance point of the ear, mass/stiffness interactions begin to shift and can be expected to be revealed by tympanograms with W patterns even in normal ears. This differential probe-tone frequency effect was noted by Alberti and Jerger (1974), who also related eardrum disease to W patterns when using an 800-Hz probe-tone. They observed that the W pattern diminished as probe-tone frequency was reduced. Again, their major concern was with pattern effects, not actual static acoustic impedance values.

Purpose of This Investigation

Through the use of calibrated tympanometry, this investigation explores the effect on static acoustic impedance of healed perforations of the tympanic membrane. Although tympanograms may be interpreted according to their configuration, this was not the primary focus of this study. Instead, the tympanometry was used to provide the computational basis for the determination of the actual acoustic impedance as measured with both low (220 Hz) and high (660 Hz) probe-tone frequencies.

METHODS

Using an otoadmittance meter (Grason Stadler Model 1720), tympanograms were obtained on a series of subjects with either normal hearing (no less at 250 to 4,000 Hz greater than 10 dB) or sensorineural

hearing loss. In the latter category, no air-bone gap was evident. Subjects were either children or adults who were seen in conjunction with an evaluation of their hearing or were specifically recruited for this investigation. One hundred ears constituted the normal sample.

In addition, a second sample of 29 ears was compared with the normal group. This second sample also displayed no evidence of conductive abnormality by pure-tone audiometry, but notching W patterns with high-frequency tympanometry (660 Hz) did disclose a pattern consistent with a healed perforation of the tympanic membrane, and either otologic examination or history, or both, supported the presence of a healed perforation.

Measurement with the otoadmittance meter provided four tympanograms (Figure 42–1). For each ear tested, a tympanogram was derived for acoustic susceptance (B_A) and acoustic conductance (G_A) at both 220 Hz and 660 Hz. Static values for B_A and G_A were then converted to both the complex acoustic admittance (Y_A) and its reciprocal acoustic impedance (Z_A) using appropriate conversion tables (Burke, 1972; Newman and Fanger, 1973).

RESULTS

Population with Normal Tympanic Membranes

The ranges for B_A and G_A in the normal population are displayed in template form in Figure 42–2. The upper and lower boundaries of each template represent 10th and 90th percentile points at ambient atmospheric pressure. No attempt is made in this representation to adhere to the actual shape of the tympanogram with the eardrum under various states of stress induced by changing air pressure in the ear canal. These same data plus the ranges and medians for the computed Y_A and Z_A are tabulated in Table 42–1. There has been no previous report of similar measurements with the otoadmittance meter, to our knowledge. However, the Z_A data are compared in Table 42–2 to previously reported values on normal subjects when measured with the Zwislocki mechanical acoustic bridge (Lilly, 1972) and an electroacoustic bridge (Madsen ZO 70) (Jerger, 1970; Wilbur et al., 1969). Also included here is the phase angle for

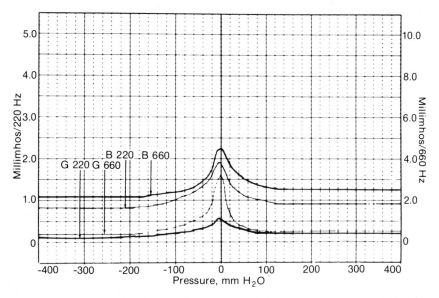

FIGURE 42-1. Normal tympanogram recording with otoadmittance meter showing four measures, conductance (G) and susceptance (B), at 220 Hz and 660 Hz.

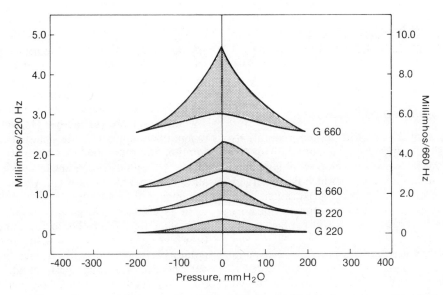

FIGURE 42-2. Ranges of 100 normal ears for conductance (G) and susceptance (B) at 220 Hz and 660 Hz. Values for 220-Hz range refer to left vertical scale and for 660 Hz to right. Difference between upper and lower boundary at 0 mm H_2O pressure and 200 mm H_2O pressure are 90th and 10th percentiles, respectively.

TABLE 42-1. B_A, G_A, Y_A, AND Z_A FOR 100 NORMAL EARS.

Measurement	B_A 220	B_A 660	G_A 220	G_A 660	Y_A 220	Y_A 660	Z_A 220	Z_A 660
80% Range, mmho	.3–.75	.9–2.45	.05–.35	1.0–4.2	.33–.85	1.38–4.5	1.124–3.048	220–715
Medians, mmho	.5	1.3	.15	1.95	.52	2.43	1856	409

TABLE 42-2. NORMAL RANGES FOR ACOUSTIC IMPEDENCE (Z_A).

Probe Frequency	Range Source, Percentile	Madsen ZO 70* (Jerger, 1970) Z_A in Acoustic Ohms	Phase Angle	Madsen ZO 70* (Wilber et al., 1969) Z_A in Acoustic Ohms	Phase Angle	Grason Stadler 1720 (This Article) Z_A in Acoustic Ohms	Phase Angle	Zwislocki (Lilly, 1972) Z_A in Acoustic Ohms	Phase Angle
220/250 Hz	90th	2,750	...	1,890	...	3,048	−70°	2,060	−72.2°
	50th	2,050	...	1,395	...	1,856	−69.5°	1,530	74.1°
	10th	1,750	...	880	...	1,124	−75°	1,075	−74.8°
660/750 Hz	90th	...	...	...	...	715	−44°	798	−37.9°
	50th	...	...	...	...	409	−31°	521	−41.6°
	10th	...	...	...	...	220	−39°	329	−45.6°

*Data approximated from figures in original references. Second frequency and phase angle cannot be measured with Madsen ZO 70.

Z_A. Apart from a greater overall range at 220 Hz in the direction of higher impedance, which is reflected in the data for the otoadmittance meter, the ranges all relate fairly well.

Population with Healed Perforations

The population of 29 ears with healed perforations displayed markedly different values, not only for 660 Hz but for 200 Hz as well. A typical set of tympano-grams is shown in Figure 42–3, which demonstrates two patterns observed with healed perforations. The B 660 tympanogram demonstrates the W notching described first by Lidén et al. (1970) for higher frequency probe-tones, and the very sharp peaking and somewhat exaggerated amplitudes are also evident in the B 220, G 220, and G 660 curves. This latter deviation in shape was first described by Terkildsen and Thomsen (1959), but although it is present in this patient, it is not always observed with a 220-Hz probe-tone. Figure 42–4 compares B_A tympanogram ranges for a 220-Hz probe-tone for the normal population with the 29 ears with healed perforations. It is clearly apparent that the effect of the healed perforation is of major importance for even a 220-Hz probe-tone. The complete picture is shown in Table 42–3 and Figure 42–5, which present tabulation and bar graphs of the 80 percent distribution and medians for B_A, G_A, Y_A, and Z_A at 220 Hz and 660 Hz. When compared to a normal population, the values of the healed perforation group are modified by better than a factor of 1 to 3 for almost all parameters. The greatest overall effect appears to be for G_A, which is the resistive component of acoustic impedance.

In an effort to add greater control to the study, the values for 17 subjects in the sample with confirmed healed perforations were treated as a separate group. Their opposite tympanic membrane was without evidence of a healed perforation. All other factors being equal, the acoustic impedance of the two ears of the same subject are highly correlated (Feldman, 1967; Fausti et al., 1973). As seen in Figure 42–6 and Table 42–4, the results with this control group were similar to those observed above. The me-

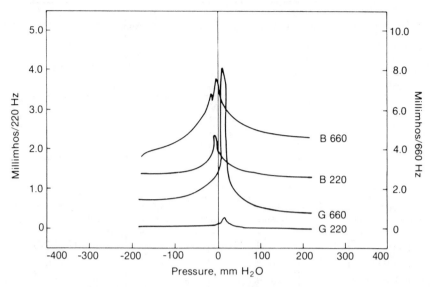

FIGURE 42-3. Tympanogram of one ear with healed perforation showing a W pattern at B 660 and sharp peaking and exaggerated amplitude at B 220, G 220, and G 660.

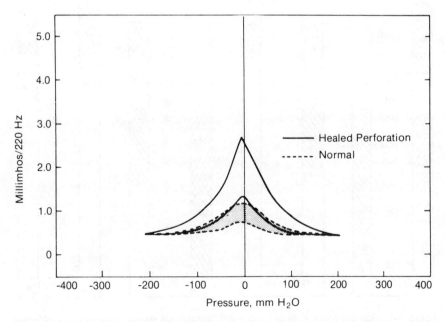

FIGURE 42-4. Comparison of susceptance ranges for 29 ears with and 100 ears without healed perforations for B 220 measurements.

Tympanogram	80% Range, mmho		Medians, mmho	
	TM Abnormality	Normal	TM Abnormality	Normal
B_A 220	1.0–2.5	.3–.75	1.50	.5
G_A 220	.2–.85	.05–.35	.5	.15
B_A 660	.60–4.55	.9–2.45	2.70	1.3
G_A 660	4.25–10.1	1.0–4.2	6.80	1.95
Y_A 220	.95–2.6	.33–.85	1.6	.52
Y_A 660	4.55–11.1	1.38–4.5	7.9	2.43
Z_A 220	380–1,054	1,124–3,048	625	1,856
Z_A 660	90–220	220–715	135	409

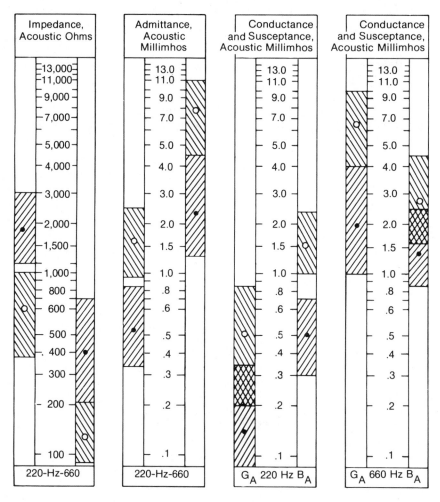

FIGURE 42-5. Ranges and medians of acoustic conductance (G_A), acoustic susceptance (B_A), acoustic admittance (Y_A), and acoustic impedance (Z_A) for normal population (right diagonal) and 29 ears with healed perforations (left diagonal). Cross-notched area is overlap. Filled circles show median normal values, and open circles median for 29 ears with healed perforations.

TABLE 42–4. B_A, G_A, Y_A, AND Z_A FOR 17 PATIENTS.*

Tympanogram	80% Range, mmho		Medians, mmho	
	TM Abnormality	Normal	TM Abnormality	Normal
B_A 220	.75–2.25	.45–1.25	1.40	.7
G_A 220	.1–.9	.05–.40	.45	.15
B_A 660	2.3–4.55	.8–3.65	2.70	1.65
G_A 660	4.25–10.75	1.45–5.3	6.80	2.50
Y_A 220	.8–2.4	.45–1.25	1.5	.75
Y_A 660	4.55–11.6	1.65–6.45	7.4	3.4
Z_A 220	412–1,235	798–2,223	656	1,333
Z_A 660	86–220	155–602	135	295

*Patients with one normal eardrum and one eardrum with evidence of healed perforation.

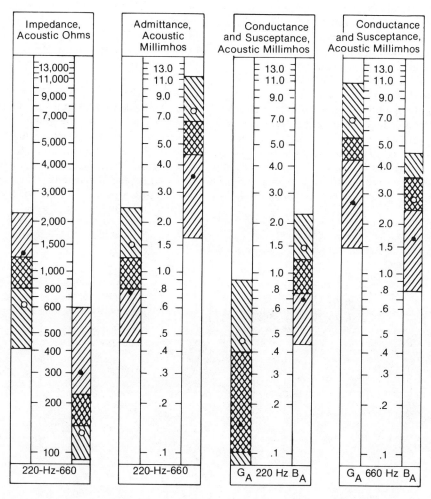

FIGURE 42-6. Ranges and medians of acoustic conductance (G_A), acoustic susceptance (B_A), acoustic admittance (Y_A), and acoustic impedance (Z_A) for 17 normal ears (right diagonal) and 17 ears with healed perforations (left diagonal). Cross-notched area is overlap. Filled circles show median normal values, and open circles median for 17 ears with healed perforations.

dian values for the ears with healed perforations differ from the normal tympanic membranes by a factor approaching or exceeding 2 for all parameters. The results for the two ears of these subjects do not correlate, and the difference must be attributed to the presence of a healed perforation on one tympanic membrane.

COMMENT

The results of this investigation strongly suggest that the status of the tympanic membrane is an important factor that affects the measurement of static acoustic impedance. Not only does a healed perforation contribute to major modifications of the shape of the tympanogram with higher frequency probe-tones, and on occasion a peaking of lower frequency tympanograms, but there is also a gross effect on the amplitude of the tympanogram and, consequently, the static acoustic impedance measurement at even the lowest used probe-tone frequencies. As a consequence, *the presence of a healed perforation would invalidate the use of static acoustic impedance as one of the tests in the impedance battery as it is used in the differential diagnosis of middle ear abnormalities.*

It is generally acknowledged that otosclerosis is a stiffening abnormality that will be revealed by an increase in acoustic impedance (Feldman, 1963; Zwislocki and Feldman, 1970). However, some overlap between otosclerotic and normal populations has been a factor that could not always be easily explained. Figure 42–7 displays both the otoadmittance tympanogram and measurements with a Zwislocki acoustic bridge of the left ear of a patient with confirmed otosclerosis. Both 660-Hz curves show the notching W pattern, and the 220-Hz curves present a sharply peaked, large amplitude tympanogram. The static acoustic impedance values are suggestive of a loose, rather than stiff, middle ear system. This is further corroborated by the mechanical acoustic bridge values, which are well within normal limits, despite the fact that it is an unoperated otosclerotic ear. The reason is revealed by the shape of the tympanogram, which discloses the effect of the large, multiple, healed perforations of the tympanic membrane. Consequently, the static values derived by either tympanometry or with a mechanical acoustic bridge yield misleading information about the middle ear. The healed perforation actually obscures the stiff middle ear system and a measurement results that is more a measure of the eardrum abnormality than anything else.

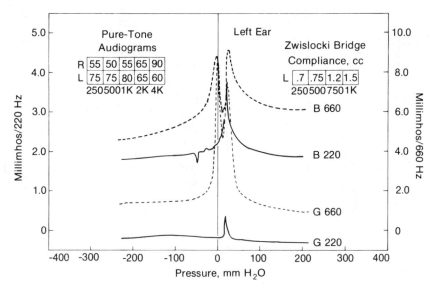

FIGURE 42-7. Tympanogram of patient with otosclerosis and healed perforation of tympanic membrane. Also shown are compliance measures obtained with Zwislocki mechanical acoustic bridge and bilateral air-conduction threshold tests.

One of the real problems this poses to the clinician is that eardrum abnormality is often ignored or invisible in routine otoscopic examinations. It does not generally affect the overall mobility of the system to gross pneumatic massage and is of minimal consequence in its effect on hearing. As a result, it is often undetected or undisclosed in referral reports. Furthermore, a large number of patients are themselves totally unaware of the existence of healed perforations that may have occurred and been undetected in early infancy. Often the first disclosure of the existence of the healed perforations is with automatic tympanometry that results in alteration of the shape of the tympanogram. Most commonly this is observed by the W pattern with the higher frequency probe-tone, but may sometimes also be revealed by a sharp peaking of an otherwise smooth tympanogram. This latter observation occurs more commonly with the higher frequency probe-tone, but is sometimes observed for lower frequency probe-tones.

When one limits the impedance evaluation to discrete measuring points with a low frequency probe-tone, the presence of the healed perforation and its consequent effect will be overlooked. The use of automatic tympanometry coupled with the use of a probe-tone that approaches, but is below the normal resonance of the ear, provides a most effective means of identifying the presence of a healed perforation and, consequently, validating or invalidating the measurement of the static acoustic impedance. Recognition of this complicating factor on the measurement of static acoustic impedance will reduce the overlap between normal and stiffening pathological conditions. When a healed perforation effect is noted the clinician cannot relate obtained values of static acoustic impedance (or compliance) to any normal population.

CONCLUSIONS

The use of automatic tympanometry employing high-frequency as well as low-frequency probe-tones provides a means of identifying ears with healed perforations of the tympanic membrane. The healed perforation has a dual effect on tympanometry. One is the alteration of the shape of the tympanogram whereby the normal shape is modified either by a W patterning for a high-frequency probe-tone or by an accentuation of the peak of the tympanogram. This latter effect on shape is more commonly observed with a higher frequency probe-tone, but may also be observed in many instances with the traditional 220-Hz probe-tone. The other related effect of the healed perforation is an exaggeration of the amplitude of the tympanogram. It results in a lower impedance for all probe-tone frequencies.

On the basis of these findings the following conclusions may be drawn: (1) Tympanometry is a highly sensitive measurement that discloses minor modifications of function of the tympanic membrane as a consequence of a healed perforation of that structure. (2) It is clearly evident that healed perforations affect measurements at all presently used probe-tone frequencies by resulting in lower static acoustic impedance values than do intact normal eardrums. This may, in large part, account for overlap of diseased ears into normal ranges of static acoustic impedance. (3) Without evidence gathered from higher frequency tympanogram configuration (W patterns or a sharper peak), which is less commonly observed with a lower frequency probe-tone, the interpretation of static acoustic impedance values at 220 Hz is highly tenuous. (4) The use of static acoustic impedance in the differential diagnosis of middle ear abnormality is only appropriate in the presence of a normal tympanic membrane.

REFERENCES

Alberti, P. W, Jerger, J. F. Probe-tone frequency and diagnostic value of tympanometry. *Arch. Otolaryngol.,* **99:** 206–210, 1974.

Bicknell, M. R., Morgan, H. V. A clinical evaluation of the Zwislocki acoustic bridge. *J. Laryngol. Otol.,* **82:** 673–692, 1968.

Burke, K. S. An impedance conversion table (G and B to Z). *ASHA,* **14:** 655–656, 1972.

Fausti, S. A.; Kimmel, B. L.; Jacobson, J. T. An investigation of between-ear tympanometry measures in normal hearing young adults, abstracted. *ASHA,* **15:** 453, 1973.

Feldman, A. S. Impedance measurements at the eardrum as an aid to diagnosis. *J. Speech Hear. Res.,* **6:** 315–327, 1963.

Feldman, A. S. Acoustic impedance measurements as a clinical procedure. *Int. Audiol.,* **3:** 156–166, 1964.

Feldman, A. S. Acoustic impedance studies of the normal ear. *J. Speech Hear. Res.,* **10:** 165–176, 1967.

Jerger, J. F. Clinical experience with impedance audiometry. *Arch. Otolaryngol.,* **92:** 311–324, 1970.

Lidén, G.; Peterson, J. L.; Bjorkman, G. Tympanometry. *Arch. Otolaryngol.,* **92:** 248–257, 1970.

Lilly, D. J. Acoustic impedance at the tympanic membrane, in Katz, J. (ed). *Handbook of Clinical Audiology.* Baltimore, Williams & Wilkins Co., 1972, pp. 434–469.

Møller, A. R. Network of the middle ear. *J. Acoust. Soc. Am.,* **33:** 168–176, 1961.

Møller, A. R. Transfer function of the middle ear. *J. Acoust. Soc. Am.,* **35:** 1,526–1,534, 1963.

Møller, A. R. An experimental study of the acoustic impedance of the middle ear and its transmission properties. *Acta Otolaryngol.,* **60:** 120–149, 1965.

Newman, B. T., Fanger, D. M. *Otoadmittance Handbook #2.* Concord, Mass, Grason Stadler Co, 1973.

Nilges, T. C.; Northern, J. L.; Burke K. S. Zwislocki acoustic bridge: Clinical correlations. *Arch. Otolaryngol.,* **89:** 727–744, 1969.

Onchi, Y. A study of the mechanism of the middle ear. *J. Acoust. Soc. Am.,* **25:** 404–410, 1949.

Onchi, Y. Mechanism of the middle ear. *J. Acoust. Soc. Am.,* **33:** 794–805, 1961.

Terkildsen, K., Thomsen, K. A. The influence of pressure variations on the impedance of the human eardrum: A method for objective determination of the middle ear pressure. *J. Laryngol. Otol.,* **73:** 409–418, 1959.

Wilber, L. A.; Goodhill, V. G.; Hague, A. C. Diagnostic implications of the acoustic impedance measurements, abstracted. *ASHA,* **11:** 417, 1969.

Wilber, L. A.; Goodhill, V. G.; Hague, A. C. Comparative acoustic impedance measurements, abstracted. *ASHA,* **12:** 435, 1970.

Zwislocki, J. Some measurements of impedance at the eardrum. *J. Acoust. Soc. Am.,* **29:** 349–356, 1957*a.*

Zwislocki, J. Some impedance measurements on normal and pathological ears. *J. Acoust. Soc. Am.,* **29:** 1,312–1,317, 1957*b.*

Zwislocki, J. Analysis of middle ear function: I. Input impedance. *J. Acoust. Soc. Am.,* **34:** 1,514–1,523, 1962.

Zwislocki, J., Feldman, A. S. Acoustic impedance of pathological ears. *ASHA Monogr.,* **15:** 1–42, 1970.

43

Tympanometry for Eustachian Tube Evaluation

EARL R. HARFORD, Ph.D.

Professor and Director of Audiology, Department of Otolaryngology, University of Minnesota Medical School, Minneapolis, Minnesota.

Since Metz first suggested in 1946 that impedance measures may detect the status of the eustachian tube as a middle ear ventilator, only a few reports have appeared in the literature on this subject until just recently. This, in spite of the fact that the principle of tympanometry has been gaining a significant role in the differential diagnosis of middle ear pathology in the Scandinavian countries for the past dozen years. The availability of a commercial electro-acoustic impedance bridge was the impetus for a recent surge of interest in the concept of impedance audiometry in the United States. Tympanometry is the segment of impedance audiometry that consists of a graphic measurement of the ear drum's compliance during changes in static pressure in the external ear canal. It is a simple, quick procedure administered by nonmedical personnel on patients of all ages. It has the potential to serve as an adjunct to the diagnosis of eustachian tube insufficiency, to monitor treatment restoring adequate function, and, possibly, as a screening device to detect preclinical pathological conditions of the middle ear.

Dysfunction of the eustachian tube is an important factor in the development of different kinds of middle ear diseases and is a common cause for failure in attempts to correct conductive involvements. An early symptom of an insufficient eustachian tube is the presence of negative pressure in the middle ear. Upon correction of a malfunctioning tube, air pressure in the middle ear should return to atmospheric level. Unquestionably, a simple quantitative technique for the measurement of air pressure in the middle ear should play a worthwhile role in the diagnosis of eustachian tube insufficiency, prognosis for treatment, and evaluation of the effectiveness of treatment of many conductive auditory problems.

Numerous techniques and clinical procedures have been advanced for assessing the adequacy of the eustachian tube. Some require a tympanic membrane perforation, some do not; some are direct measures and others are indirect; but basically all techniques fall into one of the following five categories: (1) transmission of sound through the eustachian tube (Perlman, 1953), (2) fluoroscopy or clearance tests (Compere, 1958), (3) radiographic examination (Parisier and Mansko, 1970), (4) equilibration of negative or positive air pressure introduced to the middle ear (Zöllner, 1942), and (5) impedance measurements (Metz, 1946). We certainly would be remiss not to credit the pioneering efforts of Toynbee, Valsalva, Politzer, Zöllner, Perlman, Fowler, and van Dishoeck. More recent work employing these principles and techniques has been reported by numerous authors. It is not my intent to present an exhaustive historical review of this subject; however, the interested reader may wish to consult Ingelstedt et al. (1963). In spite of the advances already made, there appears to remain the need for a quick, simple,

Read before the Fourth Workshop on Microsurgery of the Temporal Bone, Northwestern University, Thorne Hall, March 25, 1971.

Reprinted by permission of the author from *Arch. Otolaryng.,* **97,** 17–20 (1973). Copyright, 1973, American Medical Association.

and practical method for assessing the sufficiency of the eustachian tube as a middle ear ventilating mechanism—especially in the presence of an intact ear drum. Thus, the objective of this paper is to present the background and current status of a technique based on an impedance measurement which offers a quick, quantitative assessment of air pressure in the middle ear.

Metz (1946) was the first person to advance the hypothesis that changes in acoustic impedance can be used to measure the level of air pressure in the middle ear. A decade later, Thomsen (1955) in Copenhagen, Anderson et al. (1956) in Stockholm, and Terkildsen and Thomsen (1959) published articles on the use of impedance measures as an objective method of testing middle ear function. In the years following these early reports, a technique emerged in the Scandinavian countries which represents a combination and modification of the efforts of Terkildsen and Thomsen and Anderson and his associates. This technique is now referred to as tympanometry and applies an objective measurement to the basic principle of van Dishoeck's subjective pneumophone test; recall that van Dishoeck's technique is based on the principle that a tone fed into the ear canal will be heard most distinctly when the air pressure on both surfaces of

the ear drum is equal. Tympanometry, as it has developed over the past decade, uses an electro-acoustic impedance bridge to indicate changes in the compliance of the ear drum while simultaneously varying the air pressure in a hermetically sealed ear canal of the same ear. This technique permits simultaneous assessment of (1) the mobility of the tympanic membrane, (2) the status of the ossicular chain, including its supporting mechanism, and (3) the air cushion of the middle ear.

For unknown reasons, no systematic research was reported on tympanometry until just recently when Lidén et al. (1970) and Peterson and Lidén (1970) published two excellent articles on this subject. Tympanometry is one segment of impedance audiometry that is rapidly gaining in popularity as a clinical, differential diagnostic tool. Jerger (1970) recently reported the results of impedance audiometry, including tympanometry, on 400 patients with various types and degrees of hearing impairment. He used an electro-acoustic impedance meter (Madsen, model ZO 70) which is the most popular instrument for this clinical measurement. Jerger's description of the Madsen instrument will allow us to understand the principle of this clinical tool; it can be followed in Figure 43–1.

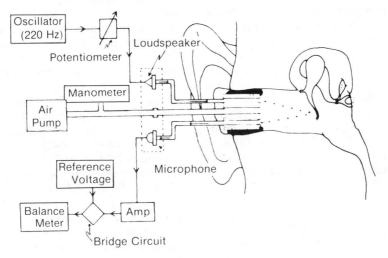

FIGURE 43-1. Functional components of the Madsen electro-acoustic bridge (model ZO 70).

A probe tip containing three tubes is sealed in the external meatus, forming a closed cavity bounded by the inner surface of the probe tip, the walls of the external meatus, and the tympanic membrane. One tube is used to deliver, into this closed cavity, a probe tone generated by a 220 Hz oscillator driving a miniature receiver. The second tube is connected to a miniature probe microphone which monitors the sound pressure level of the 220 Hz probe tone in the closed cavity and delivers the transduced voltage through an amplifier to a bridge circuit and balance meter. The balance meter is nulled by an SPL of exactly 95 dB in the closed cavity. A potentiometer on the output of the 220 Hz oscillator permits variation of the SPL over a range corresponding to a compliance variation (equivalent volume) of 0.2 to 5.0 cc. The third tube is connected to an airpump which permits variation in air pressure in the closed cavity over a range of ± 400 mm H_2O. Air pressure is read on an electromanometer. The receiver and microphone are contained in a small housing mounted at the end of a conventional headband. They are connected to the probe tip by small rubber hoses. A third hose delivers air to the probe tip.

This approach is not to be confused with the electromechanical bridge such as that designed by Zwislocki (1961). It is almost essential to include a strip recorder or x-y plotter for a graphic record of the pressure/compliance function. An automatically controlled airpump is also necessary if one intends to develop a quantitative analysis for the pressure/compliance function, called a tympanogram.

A tympanogram is obtained by varying the air pressure in the sealed ear canal from -200 to $+200$ mm H_2O while simultaneously tracking the level of the probe tone. Figure 43-2 illustrates a typical normal tympanogram obtained with the instrument described above. The abscissa represents time in seconds; a measurement can be obtained in less than one minute. The lower ordinate scale shows the air pressure ranging from -200 mm to $+200$ mm H_2O. The upper, curved line represents the sound-pressure level of the probe tone that indicates how ear drum compliance changes as the air pressure is varied in the external canal. The higher the line, the less compliant the ear drum, and the more intense the tone. A normal tympanogram shows a smooth notch with the deepest point at 0 mm H_2O or where the air pressure on both sides of the tympanic membrane is equal, thus permitting the greatest compliance. As might be expected, it is not uncommon to measure a slight negative pressure in persons with no middle ear or

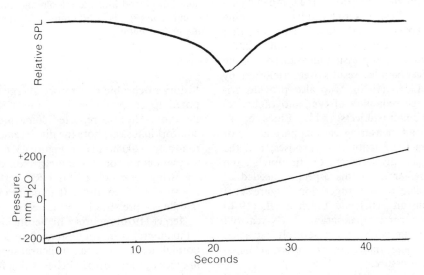

FIGURE 43-2. Type A, normal, tympanogram showing the pressure/compliance function of a normal ear drum and middle ear structure.

eustachian tube problems. It is at this point that the patient reports the tone sounds loudest, as in the pneumophone test. As the ear drum is forced inward by an increase of pressure in the canal, or bulges outward in response to a decrease of pressure, it becomes less compliant or absorbent and the sound level of the probe tone fed to the balance portion of the impedance unit is increased. We expect to see a Type A, or normal, tympanogram in patients with sensorineural damage and stapedial otosclerosis —provided there is no tubal inefficiency. A relatively flat, somewhat depressed Type B curve is obtained on cases with middle ear fluid or massive ossicular fixation. Ossicular discontinuity results in a Type D configuration showing rather large undulations, indicating a highly compliant ear drum. Finally, and most pertinent to the subject of this paper, patients with negative middle ear pressure present a Type C tympanogram with the deepest portion of the notch located in the negative pressure range. Incidentally, a patulous tube will cause fluctuation in the pressure/compliance curve corresponding to respiration and will make it difficult to establish a point of greatest compliance.

The three tympanograms illustrated in Figure 43–3 were obtained from a fresh human temporal bone. The tympanogram labelled A was obtained under normal conditions, type B resulted from introducing +100 mm H_2O pressure to the tympanic cavity, and type C illustrates the results of trapping −100 mm H_2O pressure in the middle ear. Note that the point of greatest compliance corresponds almost exactly to the amount of pressure introduced into the middle ear. Very similar results were reported by Peterson and Lidén (1970), who also provide evidence of the high reliability of tympanographic recordings on human subjects. Also, Lidén et al. (1970) recommend measuring various parameters of a tympanogram for quantitative purposes; eg., the depth, width, and displacement of the notch from 0 mm; more research on this aspect is needed to examine the value of this suggestion. Figure 43–4 was taken from an article by Lidén et al. (1970) illustrating a left ear tympanogram of a 9-year-old boy with recurrent colds and a severely retracted tympanic membrane, indicative of abnormal, negative middle ear pressure.

Figure 43–5 shows a right tympanogram obtained in our Hearing Clinic on a 50-year-old man with a

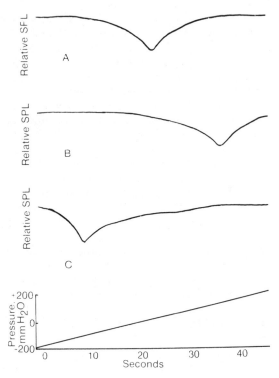

FIGURE 43-3. Three tympanograms obtained from a fresh human temporal bone; pressure/compliance function under normal conditions (A), with +100 mm H_2O pressure introduced into the middle ear through the eustachian tube (B), and −100 mm H_2O pressure trapped in the middle ear (C).

history of chronic respiratory allergy and a superimposed upper respiratory infection (URI) of one-week duration. He also reported some pressure and discomfort in his ear; note the displacement of the notch to nearly −200 mm H_2O. Figure 43–6 shows the right tympanogram for this same person one week later, following remission of his URI, with no feeling of pressure or discomfort. It appears evident that the middle ear pressure has returned to normal.

Jerger (1970) reports a higher incidence of Type C tympanograms in youngsters, 2 to 5 years old with normal hearing and sensorineural hearing loss, than in older age groups. He believes this finding suggests the presence of undetected middle ear problems in children without obvious audiometric evidence of a

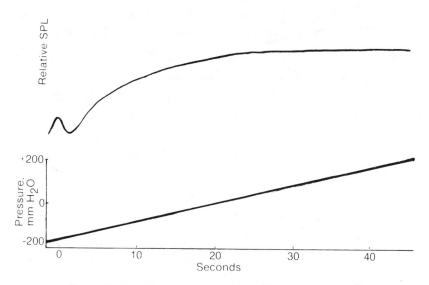

FIGURE 43-4. Tympanogram of a 9-year-old boy indicating reduced middle ear pressure.

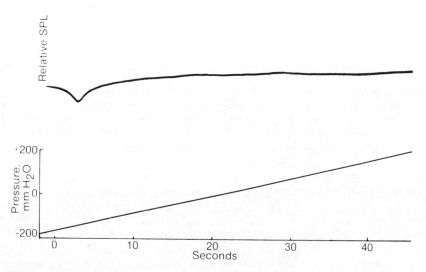

FIGURE 43-5. Type C right tympanogram of a 50-year-old man with chronic respiratory allergy and a superimposed URI.

Britain. His objective was to learn if screening tympanometry could detect the presence of secretory otitis media. One criterion was a displacement of the greatest compliance to negative air pressure in the sealed ear canal. He reported that 20 percent of the conductive component. In fact, the Type C curve occurred in 31 percent of the ears in the younger age group reported in his study.

Brooks (1969) reported the use of tympanometry as a screening technique for school children in Great

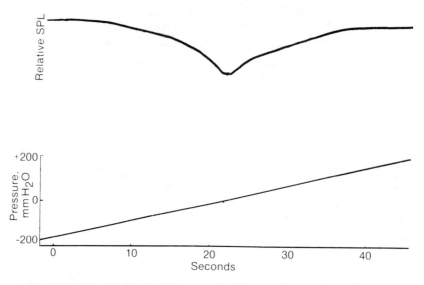

FIGURE 43-6. Type A right ear tympanogram of the same 50-year-old-man taken one week after the first tympanogram (Figure 43-5).

children in the 5-year-old group had clear signs of secretory otitis media based on this criterion. As might be expected, Brooks reports a steady decrease with age in the rate of occurrence of secretory otitis media. In contrast, we find that about 5 percent of the young, school-age children fail pure-tone audiometric screening. Thus, it appears tympanometry has potential as a screening device for early secretory otitis media.

COMMENT

With the availability of a commercial electro-acoustic bridge, impedance audiometry is becoming a popular clinical tool. Concurrently, we can expect more clinical research on this principle in the near future. Because of its simplicity and swift registration of information, the otologist should find the method as easy as routine, pure-tone audiometry. In fact, a complete impedance study can be done by nonmedical personnel faster and with less chance of error than air and bone audiometry on many patients with conductive involvement. Tympanometry has the potential for detecting eustachian tube insufficiency where even microscopic observation of the tympanic membrane may fail to reveal an abnormal conductive system. Clearly, tympanometry is far less complicated than some direct and indirect techniques currently used to evaluate the function or sufficiency of the tube. It can be used on preschool children almost as easily as on adults; this, in my opinion, is one of its most salient features—because of the difficulty of performing other clinical techniques on young children, and the high incidence of tubal insufficiency in these youngsters. It has real potential as a method of monitoring treatment for restoring good tubal function in the pathological conditions of the middle ear and as a prerequisite for tympanoplasty. By using just the air-pump and electromanometer, one can use the deflation and aspiration method of Ingelstedt et al. (1963) in evaluating tubal sufficiency as a prelude to myringoplasty. Finally, it is quite possible that tympanometry may ultimately find its place along with pure-tone audiometry as a more effective identifier of middle ear abnormalities in school screening programs than just pure-tone audiometry alone.

REFERENCES

Anderson, H.; Holmgren, L.; Holst, H. E. Experiments with an objective method of testing the middle ear function. *Acta Otolaryngol.,* **46:** 381–383, 1956.

Brooks, D. N. The use of the electro-acoustic impedance bridge in the assessment of middle ear function. *Int. Audiol.,* **8:** 563–569, 1969.

Compere, W. E. Tympanic cavity clearance study. *Trans. Am. Acad. Ophthalmol. Otolaryngol.,* **62:** 444–454, 1958.

Ingelstedt, S., et al. On the function of middle ear and eustachian tube. *Acta Otolaryngol.* (Suppl.), **182:** 1963.

Jerger, J. Clinical experience with impedance audiometry. *Arch. Otolaryngol.,* **92:** 311–324, 1970.

Lidén, G.; Peterson, J.; Björkman, G. Tympanometry. *Arch. Otolaryngol.,* **92:** 248–257, 1970.

Metz, O. The acoustic impedance measured on normal and pathological ears. *Acta Otolaryngol.* (Suppl.), **63:** 1946.

Parisier, S. C., Mansko, T. K. The roentgenographic evaluation of eustachian tubal function. *Laryngoscope,* **80:** 1210–1211, 1970.

Perlman, H. B. Observation on the eustachian tube. *Arch. Otolaryngol.,* **53:** 370–385, 1953.

Peterson, J. L., Lidén, G. Tympanometry in human temporal bones. *Arch. Otolaryngol.,* **92:** 258–266, 1970.

Terkildsen, K., Thomsen, K. A. The influence of pressure variations on the impedance of the human eardrum. *J. Laryngol. Otol.,* **73:** 409–418, 1959.

Thomsen, K. A. Eustachian tube function tested by employment of impedance measuring. *Acta Otolaryngol.,* **45:** 252–267, 1955.

Zöllner, F. *Anatomie, Physiologie, Pathologie und Klinik der Ohrtrompete.* Berlin, Springer Verlag, 1942.

Zwislocki, J. Acoustic measurement of middle ear function. *Ann. Otol. Rhinol. Laryngol.,* **70:** 1–8, 1961.

44

Impedance Audiometry in Serous Otitis Media

DANIEL J. ORCHIK, Ph.D.
Associate Professor of Speech and Hearing Science, Memphis State University
ROSEMARY MORFF, M.S.
Audiologist at the East Texas Rehabilitation Center, Kilgore, Texas, when this article was prepared
JAMES W. DUNN, M.D.
In private practice in Denton, Texas

The relationship between the results of impedance audiometry and middle ear effusion in serous otitis media was examined in 76 ears immediately prior to myringotomy. Tympanometry and acoustic reflex threshold showed the highest correlation with the operative findings relative to middle ear effusion. The combination of tympanometry and acoustic reflex threshold was superior to the use of either component alone. Results are discussed in terms of clinical implications with specific consideration of hearing screening programs.

The most common cause of hearing loss in children of preschool- and elementary school-age levels is serous otitis media (Goin, 1975). In recent years, impedance audiometry has been advocated as a more efficient means of screening for serous otitis media in children when compared with conventional pure-tone methods (Bluestone et al., 1973; McCandless and Thomas, 1974; Orchik and Herdman, 1974; Cooper et al., 1975). In most applications of impedance audiometry to screening, tympanometry has been the major component of the hearing conservation program designed to detect serous otitis media (McCandless and Thomas, 1974; Cooper et al., 1975).

Assessing the validity of impedance screening has traditionally followed one of two approaches. Either the findings of impedance audiometry are compared with otoscopic findings (McCandless and Thomas, 1974), or the impedance results are compared with postoperative findings at myringotomy (Bluestone et al., 1973). Recent evidence suggests that agreement between tympanometry and otoscopy is not as strong as once thought (Roeser et al., 1977).

When postoperative data have been employed, the results of tympanometry are usually evaluated on the basis of the ability to predict the presence or absence of effusion in the middle ear (Bluestone et al., 1973; Beery et al., 1975; Paradise et al., 1976; Orchik et al., 1978). Although the presence or absence of effusion is not the only clinically significant finding from the viewpoint of the otolaryngologist, it is a relatively objective finding when compared with routine otoscopic examination.

The relationship between the results of tympanometry and the presence of middle ear effusion has been examined by a number of researchers (Bluestone et al., 1973; Paradise et al., 1976; Orchik et al., 1978; Jerger, 1974). Although certain tympanometric types, i.e., type B as described by Jerger et al. (1974) have been shown to indicate a high probability of middle ear effusion, sufficient variability exists to suggest that single tympanometric screening may not be the most efficient means of predicting middle ear effusion common to serous otitis media (Jerger et al., 1974; Lewis et al., 1975).

Our investigation was designed to assess whether any combination of components in the impedance audiometry test battery (tympanometry, static compliance, acoustic reflex testing) might prove to be a better indicator of significant middle ear effusion. If the sensitivity could be so enhanced, the efficiency of impedance screening might be likewise improved.

METHOD

Subjects

The sample for this investigation included 76 ears of patients who underwent myringotomy for suspected serous otitis media. Subjects ranged in age from 6 months to 14 years, with a mean of 4½ years.

Experimental Procedure

Each subject was brought to the operating room area approximately 30 minutes prior to surgery. The patient's transport bed was placed in a position adjacent to a cart that contained an electroacoustic impedance bridge (Madsen 70–72), which was used to gather the impedance data. The following information was obtained for each ear:

1. A tympanogram was plotted from +200 to −400 mm/H_2O in 100 mm/H_2O steps, including the point of maximum compliance. In addition, the points at ±50 mm/H_2O, in reference to the point of maximum compliance, were plotted.
2. The measurement of static compliance was obtained for the middle ear.
3. The acoustic reflex threshold was examined at 500 through 4,000 Hz.

Tympanograms were classified as either type A, B, or C since the use of these symbols was thought to represent an easily recognized classification system (Jerger, 1970). In addition, type C tympanograms were further subdivided into three categories on the basis of the magnitude of negative pressure. A C_1 classification was applied to those curves whose point of maximum compliance fell within the negative pressure range of −100 to −150 mm/H_2O. The point of maximum compliance for a C_2 tympanogram fell between −151 and −200 mm/H_2O. Those tympanograms with a point of maximum compliance greater than −200 mm/H_2O were classified as C_3 curves. In

this manner, tympanograms could be rated on a five-point scale from normal through increasing abnormality. The type A indicated normal function while a type B represented the opposite extreme. Types C_1, C_2, and C_3 described the intermediate points on the scale.

Static compliance was recorded in cubic centimeters by subtracting the volume measure that was obtained with a positive pressure of 200 mm/H_2O from the volume measure that was obtained at the point of maximum compliance (Northern and Downs, 1974). The acoustic reflex threshold was taken at the lowest level in decibels of the hearing threshold level (HTL) (ANSI-1969), where a consistent deflection of the balance meter could be observed. For the purpose of this analysis, acoustic reflex thresholds were recorded for the probe ear so that they could be analyzed with the tympanometric and static compliance data for the same ear.

The patient was then taken to the operating room where the myringotomy was performed. The surgeon (J.W.D.) had no prior knowledge of the impedance data. During the surgery, data relative to the status of effusion in the middle ear were recorded by a second observer, as noted by the operating physician.

The presence or absence of effusion was rated by the operating physician on a four-point scale as none, minimal, moderate, or impaction. A rating of no effusion indicated that the middle ear was dry on examination after myringotomy, whereas a rating of impaction indicated that the middle ear space was completely filled with effusion. The ratings of minimal and moderate were somewhat more subjective but were used to establish a boundary for significant effusion. A rating of minimal was employed to indicate an ear where a very slight amount of fluid was found, while a rating of moderate was used to indicate an ear with a significant amount of effusion but some remaining air space in the middle ear. The operating physician was satisfied with this four-point-rating scale since it provided a means of differentiating to a somewhat greater degree the status of effusion in the middle ear. The same rating scale had been used in a previous investigation (Orchik et al., 1978).

The data were then subjected to a computer analysis that yielded Pearson's r's and multiple correlations (R's) between components of the impedance battery and the status of middle ear effusion at myringotomy.

RESULTS

Tympanometry and Middle Ear Effusion

Of the 76 ears that were examined, 55 were found to have fluid present in the middle ear at myringotomy. Of these, 32 ears were impacted, and seven ears were judged to have moderate amounts of fluid in the middle ear. The remaining 16 ears displayed minimal amounts of middle ear effusion. As shown in Table 44–1, a significant correlation ($r = .66$, $P < .01$) was found between the tympanogram type and the amount of effusion in the middle ear. Table 44–2 displays the ears according to tympanogram type and the amount of fluid present in the middle ear.

With the use of the designations of "moderate" and "impacted" as indicative of significantly abnormal findings at myringotomy (Orchik et al., 1978), 39 ears displayed significant amounts of middle ear effusion. Twenty-one (54 percent) of those with significant fluid exhibited type B tympanograms. Of those remaining, 15 ears (38 percent) were type C tympanograms, and three ears (8 percent) were type A tympanograms.

No effusion or an insignificant amount was found in 37 ears. Twenty-four of those ears (65 percent) showed type A tympanograms, 11 ears (30 percent) showed type C curves, and two ears (5 percent) showed type B tympanograms.

As noted earlier, the 26 type C tympanograms were further differentiated into three categories according to the amount of negative middle ear air pressure. Table 44–3 presents a breakdown of the type C tympanograms as a function of the amount of effusion present in the middle ear at myringotomy.

Fifteen type C tympanograms displayed significant amounts of effusion. Of these, one ear (6 percent) was a C_1 curve, ten ears (67 percent) were C_2 curves, and four ears (27 percent) were C_3 curves.

Static Compliance and Middle Ear Effusion

A small yet significant negative correlation was shown to exist between the static compliance measurement and the amount of middle ear effusion, i.e., as the amount of effusion increased, static com-

TABLE 44-1. CORRELATION COEFFICIENTS FOR TYMPANOMETRY, STATIC COMPLIANCE, ACOUSTIC REFLEX THRESHOLD, AND STATUS OF EFFUSION IN MIDDLE EAR AT MYRINGOTOMY.

Variable	Static Compliance	Reflex Threshold, Hz				Middle Ear Effusion
		500	1,000	2,000	4,000	
Tympanogram	−.44*	.39*	.42*	.45*	.38*	.66*
Static compliance	...	−.11	−.12	.13	−.10	−.37*
Reflex threshold, 500 Hz	...	...	.91*	.91*	.48*	.61*
Reflex threshold, 1,000 Hz	...	...	...	.95*	.51*	.62*
Reflex threshold, 2,000 Hz	...	...	...	...	.54*	.62*
Reflex threshold, 4,000 Hz	...	...	...	...	...	.52*
Middle ear effusion	...	...	...	...	...	...

*Significant at the .01 level.

TABLE 44-2. STATUS OF EFFUSION IN MIDDLE EAR AS FUNCTION OF TYMPANOGRAM TYPE.

Tympanogram Type	No. (%) of Ears				
	Insignificant Effusion		Significant Effusion		
	None	Minimal	Moderate	Impacted	Total
A	14 (52)	10 (37)	...	3 (11)	27
C	5 (19)	6 (23)	4 (15)	11 (42)	26
B	2 (9)	...	3 (13)	18 (78)	23

TABLE 44-3. STATUS OF EFFUSION AS FUNCTION OF MAGNITUDE OF NEGATIVE PRESSURE IN MIDDLE EAR.

Tympanogram Type*	No. (%) of Ears			
	Insignificant Effusion		Significant Effusion	
	None	Minimal	Moderate	Impacted
C_1	5 (56)	3 (33)	...	1 (11)
C_2	...	3 (23)	2 (15)	8 (62)
C_3	...	...	2 (50)	2 (50)

*C_1 = negative pressure of 100 to 150 mm H_2O; C_2 = negative pressure of 151 to 200 mm H_2O; C_3 = negative pressure of 200 mm H_2O.

TABLE 44-4. STATUS OF MIDDLE EAR EFFUSION AS FUNCTION OF MEASURED STATIC COMPLIANCE.

Static Compliance	No. of Ears			
	Insignificant Effusion		Significant Effusion	
	None	Minimal	Moderate	Impacted
Normal (≥ 0.28 cc)	9	6	1	3
Reduced (< 0.28 cc)	12	10	6	29

pliance decreased ($r = -.37$, $P < .01$). Table 44-4 presents the relationship between the static compliance value and the amount of effusion present in the middle ear. It is apparent that the relationship is not as strong as that found between the results of tympanometry and the amount of middle ear effusion.

As shown in Table 44-4, of the 76 ears that were examined, 19 had static compliance values within the normal range (0.28 to 1.72 cc), as specified by Brooks (1971). Of these, 15 (78 percent) exhibited insignificant effusion at myringotomy. However, significant effusion was discovered in four (21 percent) of the ears with normal static compliance.

Reduced static compliance values (< 0.28 cc) were evident in 57 ears. Of these, 22 (39 percent) were judged to have insignificant amounts of effusion present at myringotomy. Significant effusion was present in 35 ears (61 percent) with reduced static compliance.

Acoustic Reflex Threshold and Middle Ear Effusion

Acoustic reflex thresholds were examined at the octave frequencies from 500 through 4,000 hz. The correlation coefficients (r's) for reflex threshold and amount of effusion are displayed as follows:

Reflex Threshold, Hz	r
500	.61
1,000	.62
2,000	.62
4,000	.52

Each coefficient was significant at the .01 level of confidence.

The relationship between the acoustic reflex threshold and the amount of effusion at each test frequency yielded similar findings. First, in impacted middle ears, the probability of the reflex being absent (> 110 dB HL) is very high, ranging from 94 percent at 500, 2,000, and 4,000 Hz to 97 percent at 1,000 Hz.

If one considers all the ears that showed moderate effusion, as well as the impacted ears, the probability of an absent reflex is lessened, but remains high. The percentage of absent reflexes in the significant effusion categories range from 87 percent at 500, 2,000, and 4,000 Hz to 90 percent at 1,000 Hz. In contrast, the percentage of absent reflexes in ears with less than significant effusion is quite low, ranging from 23 percent to 30 percent, depending on the test frequency employed.

COMMENT

Tympanometry and Middle Ear Effusion

Correlational analysis supports previously suggested relationships between tympanogram type and the presence or absence of significant effusion (Bluestone et al., 1973; Orchik et al., 1978). Of the type A tympanograms, 89 percent had insignificant effusion while of the ears that demonstrated type B tympanograms, 90 percent had significant effusion. The ears that yielded type C tympanograms were evenly distributed, with 52 percent showing significant effusion and 48 percent showing insignificant effusion.

However, when type C tympanograms were further analyzed as to the magnitude of negative pressure, the relationship was somewhat clarified. Although the subsamples were small, the data suggested that as negative pressure increased, the probability of significant effusion also increased with 82 percent of the ears with negative pressure in excess of 150 mm H_2O exhibiting significant effusion.

Static Compliance and Middle Ear Effusion

The lesser correlation between static compliance and middle ear effusion supports the generally held contention that when used alone, static compliance is the least useful diagnostic tool of the entire impedance battery (Jerger, 1970). In the present sample, almost 40 percent of the ears with reduced static compliance failed to demonstrate significant middle ear effusion while more than 20 percent of the ears with significant effusion demonstrated normal static compliance.

Acoustic Reflex and Middle Ear Effusion

The significant correlations support the use of acoustic reflex measurement in the identification of serous otitis media, as suggested by Brooks (1976). Although similar at all test frequencies, 4,000 Hz demonstrated the smallest correlation. This is in agreement with the suggestion that the acoustic reflex at 4,000 Hz may be absent even though no objective evidence of abnormality can be shown (Jerger et al., 1972). Even though correlations for acoustic reflex measurement and middle ear effusion were significant, approximately 20 percent failed to demonstrate an acoustic reflex in the absence of significant effusion.

Impedance Battery and Middle Ear Effusion

From the preceding discussion, it appears that tympanometry and acoustic reflex measurement show the strongest correlation with the presence or absence of significant middle ear effusion. Furthermore, tympanometry and acoustic reflex measurement appear to be of equivalent power in predicting the presence or absence of significant effusion in serous otitis media. The possibility of improving diagnostic efficiency by combining these two components of the impedance battery was investigated. Multiple correlations were obtained for various combinations of tympanometry and acoustic reflex measurement and are reported in Table 44-5.

As shown in Table 44-5, the combined use of tympanometry and acoustic reflex measurement markedly improves the correlation between the impedance battery and the presence of middle ear effusion. Moreover, it appears that the addition of a single reflex measurement at 500, 1,000 or 2,000 Hz provides as accurate a predictor of middle ear effusion as measurement of reflexes at all test frequencies.

Past research with the use of tympanometry alone has suggested use of type A and C_1 tympanograms, as defined in this study, as normal findings (Brooks, 1971). Use of this criterion in the current population would have resulted in a 10 percent false-negative rate (four ears). However, results of further examination of these four ears showed that all had absent reflexes at all test frequencies.

Use of the acoustic reflex alone to establish normal middle ear function, as recommended by Brooks (1976), would result in false-negative findings in 12 percent (five ears) of this population. Additional analysis of these five ears reveals that all displayed type C tympanograms with negative pressure greater than −150 mm H_2O.

TABLE 44–5. MULTIPLE CORRELATIONS FOR VARIOUS COMBINATIONS OF TYMPANOMETRY AND ACOUSTIC REFLEX THRESHOLDS WITH STATUS OF MIDDLE EAR EFFUSION.

Predictors*	R*	Regression Equation†
Tympanogram; ART, 500 Hz	.76	$-5.9 + 0.50_T + 0.41_{R500}$
Tympanogram; ART, 1,000 Hz	.76	$-4.7 + 0.48_T + 0.42_{R1k}$
Tympanogram; ART, 2,000 Hz	.75	$-4.0 + 0.48_T + 0.40_{R2k}$
Tympanogram; ART, 500 and 1,000 Hz	.76	$-5.7 + 0.48_T + 0.22_{R500} + 0.21_{R1k}$
Tympanogram; ART, 500 and 2,000 Hz	.76	$-5.7 + 0.49_T + 0.31_{R500} + 0.11_{R2k}$
Tympanogram; ART, 1,000 and 2,000 Hz	.75	$-4.7 + 0.48_T + 0.36_{R1k} + 0.06_{R2k}$
Tympanogram; ART, 500, 1,000, and 2,000 Hz	.76	$-5.8 + 0.49_T + 0.24_{R500} + 0.26_{R1k} -0.06_{R2k}$
ART, 500, 1,000, and 2,000 Hz	.62	$-7.4 + 0.18_{R500} + 0.24_{R1k} + 0.22_{R2k}$

*Art indicates acoustic reflex threshold; R, multiple correlations.

†Status of effusion = regression equation. T indicates tympanogram; R500, acoustic reflex at 500 Hz; R1k, acoustic reflex at 1,000 Hz; R2k, acoustic reflex at 2,000 Hz.

TABLE 44–6. COMPARISON OF FALSE-POSITIVE AND FALSE-NEGATIVE RATES WITH USE OF TYMPANOMETRY AND ACOUSTIC REFLEX MEASUREMENT ALONE OR IN COMBINATION.

Rate	Tympanometry Alone	Acoustic Reflex Alone	Combined
False-positive, %	18	22	10
False-negative, %	10	10	0

Further, if failure criterion were defined to include type B tympanograms, type C_2 or C_3 tympanograms, or absent reflexes in this population, all the children with significant middle ear effusion would have been identified. In addition, the 10 percent false-positive rate would represent a significant reduction from previous studies (Roberts, 1976). The data with regard to false-positive and false-negative rates with the use of tympanometry or acoustic reflex measurement alone and in combination are displayed in Table 44–6.

CLINICAL IMPLICATIONS

The results of the present investigations suggest that tympanometry and acoustic reflex measurement are of equal predictive value in the identification of significant middle ear effusion. Further, the combined use of these two impedance test components would significantly enhance the diagnostic efficiency of impedance audiometry in identifying serous otitis media.

The implication has special significance for the application of impedance audiometry to hearing screening programs. While the superiority of impedance audiometry to traditional pure-tone screening programs is generally recognized, a variety of impedance protocols have been suggested (Orchik and Herdman, 1974; Cooper et al., 1975; Brooks, 1976; Roberts, 1976). The results of this investigation suggest the combined use of tympanometry and acoustic reflex measurement is preferable to the use of either component alone. Finally, it should be noted that such a protocol would not rule out the possibility of a sensorineural hearing loss, and thus, the impedance battery must be combined with a single high-frequency pure-tone screening (Cooper et al., 1975) in any hearing conservation program.

It would appear that the combination of negative middle ear pressure in excess of -150 mm H_2O with no discernable acoustic reflex at 110 dB HTL should be highly suspect for significant middle ear effusion. Such a pass-fail criterion should allow for maximal identification of serous otitis media with a minimal false-positive rate.

REFERENCES

Beery, Q. C.; Bluestone, C. D.; Andrus, W. S., et al. Tympanometric pattern classifications in relation to middle ear effusions. *Ann. Otol. Rhinol. Laryngol.,* **84:** 56–64, 1975.

Bluestone, C. D.; Beery, Q. C.; Paradise, J. L. Audiometry and tympanometry in relation to middle ear effusions in children. *Larynoscope,* **83:** 594–604, 1973.

Brooks, D. N. Electroacoustic impedance bridge studies on normal ears of children. *J. Speech Hear. Res.,* **14:** 247–253, 1971.

Brooks, D. M. School screening for middle ear effusions. *Ann. Otol. Rhinol. Laryngol.,* **85** (suppl. 25): 223–228, 1976.

Cooper, J. C.; Gates, G. A.; Owen, J. H., et al. An abbreviated impedance bridge technique for school screening. *J. Speech Hear. Disord.,* **40:** 260–269, 1975.

Goin, D. W. Acute inflammatory diseases of the middle ear and mastoid, in English, G. M. (ed.), *Otolaryngology.* New York, Harper & Row Publishers Inc., 1975.

Jerger, J. Clinical experience with impedance audiometry. *Arch. Otolaryngol.,* **92:** 311–324, 1970.

Jerger, J.; Anthony, L.; Jerger, S., et al. Studies in impedance audiometry: III. Middle ear disorders. *Arch. Otolaryngol.,* **99:** 165–171, 1974.

Jerger, J.; Jerger S.; Mauldin, L. Studies in impedance audiometry: I. Normal and sensorineural ears. *Arch. Otolaryngol.,* **96:** 513–523, 1972.

Lewis, N.; Dugdale, A.; Canty A., et al. Open-ended tympanometric screening: A new concept. *Arch. Otolaryngol.,* **101:** 722–725, 1975.

McCandless, G. A., Thomas, G. K. Impedance audiometry as a screening procedure for middle ear disease. *Trans. Am. Acad. Ophthalmol. Otolaryngol.,* **78:** 98–102, 1974.

Northern, J. L, Downs, P. *Hearing in Children.* Baltimore, Williams & Wilkins Co., 1974.

Orchik, D.; Dunn, J.; McNutt, L. Tympanometry as a predictor of middle ear effusion. *Arch. Otolaryngol.,* **104:** 4–6, 1978.

Orchik, D., Herdman, S. Impedance audiometry as a screening device with school age children. *Audiol. Res.,* **14:** 283–286, 1974.

Paradise, J. L.; Smith, C. G.; Bluestone, C. D. Tympanometric detection of middle ear effusion in infants and young children. *Pediatrics,* **58:** 198–210, 1976.

Roberts, M. E. Comparative study of pure-tone, impedance and otoscopic hearing screening methods: A survey of native Indian children in British Columbia. *Arch. Otolaryngol.,* **102:** 690–694, 1976.

Roeser, R.; Soh, J.; Dunckel, D., et al. Comparison of tympanometry and otoscopy in establishing pass/fail referral criteria. *J. Am. Audiol. Soc.,* **3:** 20–26, 1977.

45

A Comparison of Three Methods for Predicting Hearing Loss from Acoustic Reflex Thresholds

ROBERT H. MARGOLIS, PH.D.
Associate Professor and Director, Hearing Clinic, Division of Special Education and Rehabilitation, Syracuse University, Syracuse, New York

CYDNEY M. FOX, M.A.
Audiologist, UCLA School of Medicine

Previously reported acoustic reflex threshold data from normal and hearing-impaired subjects indicate that the effect of stimulus bandwidth on reflex thresholds is altered by sensorineural hearing loss. It is this change in the "bandwidth effect" that forms the basis for predicting hearing loss from reflex threshold data. Three predictive procedures were compared for 17 normal and 60 hearing-impaired ears.

All methods correctly identified most hearing losses but none of the methods accurately estimated magnitude of hearing loss. Two methods were characterized by a high rate of false positives. The third was tailored to minimize false positives (6 percent) and maintain a high rate (93 percent) of predicting hearing losses greater than 32 dB while making no attempt to make finer discriminations. This more conservative approach minimizes serious predictive errors while identifying a high proportion of clinically significant hearing losses.

The acoustic reflex has recently emerged as a potential method for the objective determination of hearing loss. This reflex is usually measured as a change in the acoustic input impedance to the middle ear concomitant with the presentation of an acoustic stimulus to the opposite ear. In normal ears the threshold of the reflex, the lowest stimulus SPL resulting in a stimulus-locked change in acoustic impedance, is lower for wide-band stimuli than for tonal stimuli (Fisch and von Schulthess, 1963; Dallos, 1964; Franzen, 1970; Peterson and Liden, 1972; Margolis and Popelka, 1975a, b). A number of investigations have demonstrated a "critical bandwidth" effect in reflex-threshold data. That is, reflex thresholds remain relatively constant as stimulus bandwidth increases up to the critical bandwidth. Further increases in bandwidth result in decreasing reflex thresholds (Flottorp, Djupesland, and Win-

ther, 1971; Djupesland and Zwislocki, 1973; Popelka, Karlovich, and Wiley, 1974; Popelka, Margolis, and Wiley, 1976). The difference in reflex sensitivity for narrow-band and wide-band stimuli is reduced in cases of sensorineural hearing loss (Niemeyer and Sesterhenn, 1974; Jerger et al., 1974; Djupesland, Sundby, and Hogstad, 1975; Popelka et al., 1976). It is this reduction in the difference in reflex thresholds for wide-band and narrow-band stimuli that forms the basis for predicting hearing loss from reflex threshold data.

Three procedures for predicting hearing loss from reflex threshold data have been proposed. Niemeyer and Sesterhenn (1974) proposed a method of calculating average hearing thresholds (0.5–4.0 kHz) from measurements of reflex thresholds for tones and wide-band noise. Jerger et al. (1974) estimated the degree of hearing impairment (normal, mild-moderate, severe, or profound) from reflex thresholds. Popelka et al. (1976) presented a method of plotting reflex threshold data that appeared to differentiate

Reprinted by permission of the authors from *J. Speech Hearing Res.*, **20**, 241–253 (1977).

effectively between normal-hearing subjects and subjects with noise-induced sensorineural hearing loss. In the Popelka et al. plotting procedure, the reflex threshold for a tonal stimulus is plotted on the ordinate. The abscissa represents the ratio of the reflex threshold for a wide-band stimulus to the reflex threshold for the tonal stimulus. This plotting procedure takes advantage of two primary differences between reflex-threshold data obtained from normal and pathological ears (Popelka et al., 1976, Figure 3). First, at center frequencies remote from the hearing loss region, pathological subjects fail to demonstrate a "bandwidth effect." That is, reflex thresholds are relatively constant for all bandwidths. Second, at center frequencies near the hearing loss region, in addition to the absent bandwidth effect, reflex thresholds for narrow band stimuli are elevated. The two dimensions of the bivariate plot estimate these two effects. The ratio of two reflex thresholds, one for a narrow-band and one for a wide-band stimulus, is a measure of the bandwidth effect while the reflex threshold for the tonal stimulus estimates the overall position of the function relating reflex thresholds to stimulus bandwidth.

To determine the relative effectiveness of these methods, it is necessary to compare predictions made by the three procedures for the same group of subjects. The sample should include both normal and hearing-impaired subjects and exclude patients with possible middle ear and central nervous system pathologies that may alter acoustic-reflex thresholds without causing hearing loss. This investigation was undertaken to compare these procedures on normal-hearing subjects and subjects with sensorineural hearing loss of varying degree and etiology.

METHOD

Apparatus

Acoustic reflex thresholds were measured by monitoring changes in the acoustic impedance of the middle ear with an acoustic admittance meter (Grason-Stadler 1720B). The probe frequency was 660 Hz. The two outputs of the acoustic admittance meter (with the reflex amplifier switch up) were low pass filtered at 17 Hz, amplified, and displayed on two channels of a polygraph (Beckman Type RB)

with a sensitivity of 0.05 mmhos/mm. A third channel was used as an event marker and recorded each reflex-activating stimulus presentation. Reflex-activating stimuli were generated by an audio-frequency oscillator (Hewlett Packard 200 AB) or noise generator (Grason-Stadler 1285). To produce filtered noise bands, the output of the noise generator was passed through either the high-pass or low-pass section of an active filter (Krohn-hite 315 AR) set to result in identical cutoff frequencies of 2,600 Hz and a rejection rate of 24 dB/octave. Timing, attenuation, and impedance matching were accomplished with modular equipment (Grason-Stadler 1200 series).

Subjects

Normal-hearing subjects were paid volunteers recruited from the UCLA student population or were employees of the Division of Head and Neck Surgery, UCLA School of Medicine. Seventeen subjects ranging in age from 12 to 29 years (mean = 21.6 years) served as the normal sample. Criteria for normal-hearing subjects were: hearing threshold levels not exceeding 15-dB HTL (ANSI-1969) at any audiometric frequency; air-bone gap not exceeding 10 dB at any frequency; normal otoscopic examination; negative otologic history; and normal tympanometry. Subjects with sensorineural hearing loss were recruited from the Audiology Clinic, UCLA School of Medicine. Subjects were eliminated from the study if (1) the difference between air-conduction and bone-conduction thresholds exceeded 10 dB at any frequency; (2) the tympanogram reflected high acoustic impedance at 220 Hz (> 3,000 acoustic ohms); (3) the history and otologic examination suggested the possibility of central nervous system impairment; or (4) the acoustic reflex could not be elicited by wide-band noise stimulation. Only one ear from normal-hearing subjects was tested. Both ears of hearing-loss subjects were tested when time permitted and when both ears met the requirements listed above. This resulted in a total of 60 hearing-impaired ears from 36 subjects. To evaluate predictive procedures on subjects with various magnitudes and configurations of hearing loss, the classification shown in Table 45–1 was developed. Although substantial variations can occur within these groups, this classification allows for examining the effects of

TABLE 45-1. SUBJECT CLASSIFICATION.

Group	Description	Thresholds (dB HTL) for 250–4,000 Hz
1	Normal	< 20 dB HTL
2	Flat except drop at 4,000 Hz	≤ 30 dB HTL (250–2,000 Hz) difference between 2,000 and 4,000 Hz ≥ 25 dB
3	Flat (± 15 dB), slight	Average HTL 15–30 dB (500, 1,000, and 2,000 Hz)
4	Flat (± 15 dB), mild	Average HTL 31–45 dB (500, 1,000, and 2,000 Hz)
5	Flat (± 15 dB), moderate	Average HTL 46–70 dB (500, 1,000, and 2,000 Hz)
6	Sloping, mild	Average HTL 0–32 dB (500, 1,000, and 2,000 Hz)
7	Sloping, moderate	Average HTL 32–58 dB (500, 1,000, and 2,000 Hz)
8	Irregular	"humped" or "trough-shaped" audiograms Average HTL 15–50 dB (500, 1,000, and 2,000 Hz)

various aspects of audiometric configuration like sloping loss, flat loss, and high-frequency loss. Four subjects who could not be categorized with any of these patterns were placed in the "irregular" category. Means and ranges of hearing threshold levels at audiometric frequencies are given in Table 45–2 for each subject group.

Stimuli

Reflex-activating stimuli included four tones (500, 1,000, 2,000, and 4,000 Hz) and three noise bands (high-pass, low-pass, and wide band). All stimuli had two-second durations and 25-msec rise-fall times. The interstimulus interval was three seconds.

TABLE 45-2. MEANS AND RANGES OF HEARING THRESHOLD LEVELS AND ACOUSTIC REFLEX THRESHOLDS FOR EACH SUBJECT GROUP.

Group	N		Hearing Threshold Levels (ANSI-1969)					Acoustic Reflex Thresholds (dB SPL)						
			250	500	1,000	2,000	4,000	500	1,000	2,000	4,000	WBN	LPN	HPN
1	17	Mean	6	4	2	3	4	94	90	92	96	75	79	82
		Range	−5–15	−5–15	0–5	0–10	0–15	78–103	79–99	82–98	84–115	61–89	64–91	68–92
2	12	Mean	11	10	11	18	58	91	89	96	113	87	83	95
		Range	0–25	0–20	0–25	5–30	45–75	83–106	78–100	86–115	93–125	77–96	71–97	88–108
3	8	Mean	15	16	18	24	34	95	93	94	106	83	84	93
		Range	0–30	10–25	5–30	0–40	25–50	82–102	80–106	81–113	86–125	76–97	73–95	81–103
4	2	Mean	30	30	30	40	35	113	107	125	117	103	105	123
		Range	25–35	30–30	30–30	40–40	35–35	108–118	104–109	125–125	113–122	92–114	93–117	121–125
5	12	Mean	49	52	56	53	59	97	96	103	112	95	93	103
		Range	35–65	40–65	50–70	40–75	35–75	85–107	87–103	89–115	87–125	85–102	82–101	85–118
6	13	Mean	16	14	16	43	68	93	92	105	114	91	85	103
		Range	5–25	5–25	0–40	25–75	45–85	76–116	74–107	85–125	95–125	80–107	74–103	85–125
7	9	Mean	28	28	41	62	71	96	94	105	112	93	91	104
		Range	10–55	15–55	10–90	45–100	50–95	83–116	81–114	83–125	94–125	82–125	77–125	89–125
8	4	Mean	45	40	24	29	50	101	91	97	110	93	89	98
		Range	30–60	20–60	5–55	5–40	25–70	98–103	84–96	84–116	93–125	85–102	82–94	86–118

Stimuli were presented to the ear contralateral to the probe by a supraaural earphone (TDH-39 with MX 41/AR cushion). Due to the resonance effects of the earphone and ear canal, the power spectra of the noise bands were not flat. The earphone used in this experiment is characterized by a 12-dB resonance peak at 3,700 Hz as measured in a 6-cc coupler (Zwislocki, 1970). Differences in earphone response may result in different reflex thresholds for wideband activating stimuli.

Procedure

After routine audiometric testing, the acoustic admittance probe was sealed into one ear and the earphone was placed on the contralateral ear. Tympanograms were recorded with a 220-Hz probe for both components of acoustic admittance (susceptance and conductance). Activating stimuli were initially presented at sound pressures sufficient to result in large responses and then reduced in 1-dB steps until no response was observed. Reflex threshold was defined as the lowest SPL in a descending series of trials resulting in a stimulus-locked change in acoustic susceptance or acoustic conductance, or both. Reflex thresholds for normal-hearing subjects were independently determined from the recorder tracings by three judges. The resulting interjudge reliability coefficients computed separately for the seven activating stimuli always exceeded 0.98. Reflex thresholds for hearing-impaired subjects were determined by only one of the three judges.

RESULTS AND DISCUSSION

Table 45-1 presents a description of the subject groups used in this experiment. Means and ranges for hearing threshold levels and acoustic-reflex thresholds are presented in Table 45-2 for all groups. In general, large differences occurred between reflex thresholds for tonal and noise stimuli for normal subjects and this difference was diminished even for subjects with very mild hearing losses.

The results of the Niemeyer and Sesterhenn and the Jerger et al. procedures for 17 normal subjects are summarized in Table 45-3. The mean hearing level computed by the Niemeyer and Sesterhenn method was 7.6 dB with a standard deviation of 19.4 dB. Actual hearing levels (three-frequency pure-tone average) had a mean of 3.0 dB with a standard deviation of 2.7. The variability around the estimated hearing level suggests that many subjects were incorrectly diagnosed as having rather sizeable hearing losses. Five normal subjects had hearing level estimates in excess of 25 dB. The mean difference between hearing level estimates and pure-tone averages was 4.5 dB with a standard deviation of 18.8 reflecting discrepancies between predicted and actual hearing levels as large as 35 dB.

The D statistic used by Jerger et al. to predict hearing loss was computed for the normals in this study and the results are summarized in Table 45-3. By the criteria described in Table 1 of the Jerger et al. (1974) paper, seven of the 17 normal subjects would be included in the mild-moderate hearing loss group. This high rate of false positives is in agreement with the results summarized in Figure 2 of the Jerger et al. paper.

The results of these two procedures for the hearing-impaired subjects are summarized in Table 45-4. In general, hearing levels estimated by the Niemeyer and Sesterhenn procedure increase with hearing loss. The variance associated with the differences between actual and computed hearing levels reflects occasional large errors in prediction. The D statistic computed by the Jerger et al. procedure is smaller, as expected, for the hearing-impaired groups than for the normal-hearing subjects. The D value was used to categorize subjects into normal, mild-moderate, and

TABLE 45-3. MEANS AND STANDARD DEVIATIONS OF PREDICTED HEARING LEVEL (HL) DIFFERENCE (d) BETWEEN HL AND THREE-FREQUENCY PURE-TONE AVERAGE (PTA) (NIEMEYER AND SESTERHENN, 1974) AND D STATISTIC (JERGER ET AL., 1974) FOR 17 NORMAL SUBJECTS.

| Parameter | PTA | Niemeyer and Sesterhenn | | Jerger et al. |
		HL	d	D
Mean	3.0	7.6	4.5	16.0
SD	2.7	19.4	18.8	8.6

TABLE 45–4. MEAN PREDICTED HEARING LEVELS (HL), DIFFERENCE (d) BETWEEN HEARING LEVEL AND THREE-FREQUENCY PURE-TONE AVERAGE (NIEMEYER AND SESTERHENN, 1974), AND D STATISTIC (JERGER ET AL., 1974) FOR THE HEARING-IMPAIRED SUBJECT GROUPS.

Group	N		Niemeyer and Sesterhenn HL	d	Jerger et al. D
2	12	Mean	35.6	22.5	3.1
		SD	13.7	14.2	5.4
3	8	Mean	25.7	6.7	10.3
		SD	11.4	13.6	5.1
4	2	Mean	48.3	15.0	8.4
5	12	Mean	49.2	−4.6	0.8
		SD	10.6	9.7	5.5
6	13	Mean	38.9	15.0	2.7
		SD	14.9	18.0	6.2
7	9	Mean	44.7	1.1	1.9
		SD	22.1	25.1	5.7
8	4	Mean	46.1	15.3	3.0
		SD	5.4	19.3	3.1

TABLE 45–5. NUMBER OF SUBJECTS CLASSIFIED BY THE JERGER ET AL. (1974) PROCEDURE AS NORMAL, MILD-MODERATE, OR SEVERE FOR EACH SUBJECT GROUP.

Group	N	Normal N	%	Mild-Moderate N	%	Severe N	%
1	17	10	59	7	41	0	0
2	12	0	0	9	75	3	25
3	8	0	0	1	13	11	87
4	2	0	0	1	50	1	50
5	12	0	0	3	25	9	75
6	13	0	0	7	54	6	46
7	9	0	0	5	56	4	44
8	4	0	0	1	25	3	75

severe hearing-loss groups (see Jerger et al., 1974, Table 1) and the results are summarized in Table 45–4. The predictions for the normal-hearing group reflect the high rate (41 percent) of false positives referred to earlier. Some subjects with mild hearing losses (Groups 2 and 3) were predicted to have "severe" losses. About 50 percent of the subjects with moderate to severe losses (Groups 4–8) were classified as mild-moderate; the remaining 50 percent were classified as severe.

From the foregoing analysis of the Niemeyer and Sesterhenn and Jerger et al. procedures, we concluded the following. First, both procedures result in a high rate of false positives. Second, although the Niemeyer and Sesterhenn procedure predicts mean hearing level with reasonable precision for some patients, occasional large errors in prediction make this a very dangerous procedure for clinical use. Third, both procedures correctly identify moderate to severe hearing losses with high accuracy. However, neither procedure distinguishes between mild-to-moderate and severe hearing losses with adequate precision.

The data suggest that the relationship between hearing loss and acoustic reflex thresholds is not systematic enough to estimate magnitude of hearing loss with the precision attempted by the Niemeyer and Sesterhenn and Jerger et al. procedures. Accordingly, a more conservative approach, one that identifies both normal hearing and clinically significant hearing loss with few errors, may be more appropriate for clinical use. An attempt to develop such a procedure is described below.

Reflex threshold data for Groups, 1, 4, 5, and 7 are plotted in Figures 45-1 to 45-3 with the bivariate plotting procedure described by Popelka et al. (1976). Acoustic reflex threshold (in dB SPL) for a tonal stimulus is plotted on the ordinate. The

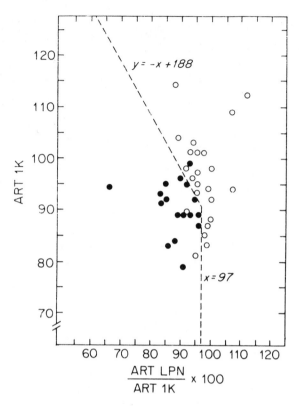

FIGURE 45-2. Bivariate plot of acoustic reflex thresholds for a 1000-Hz tone and low-pass noise. See Figure 45-1 legend.

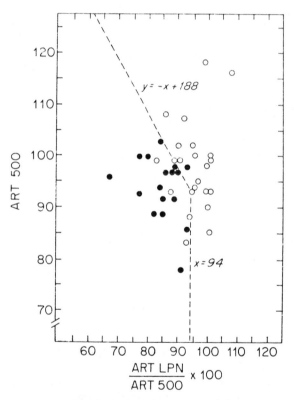

FIGURE 45-1. Bivariate plot of acoustic reflex threshold data. The ordinate shows acoustic reflex threshold for a 500-Hz tone (dB SPL). The abscissa presents 100 times the ratio of the reflex threshold for a low-pass noise to the reflex threshold for the 500-Hz tone (both expressed in dB SPL). The dashed lines define the normal region. Filled circles represent data for normal subjects; open circles, for hearing-impaired subjects (Groups 4, 5, and 7).

abscissa represents a ratio of two reflex thresholds (both in dB SPL), one for a noise band and the other for a tonal stimulus. Note that the low-pass noise threshold was used for the 500- and 1,000-Hz data (Figures 45-1 and 45-2) and the high-pass noise threshold for the 2,000-Hz data (Figure 45-3). This procedure resulted in more distinct separation of normal from pathological subjects than using wideband noise thresholds in all bivariate plots. Initially the high-pass noise threshold was used in a similar bivariate plot using the 4,000-Hz activating stimulus. Due to the greater variability in reflex thresholds for the 4,000-Hz stimulus (see Table 45-2), these data did not contribute to the predictive power of the method. Consequently, the procedure is based on reflex thresholds for three tonal stimuli (500, 1,000, and 2,000 Hz) and two noise stimuli (low-pass and high-pass, filtered at 2,600 Hz).

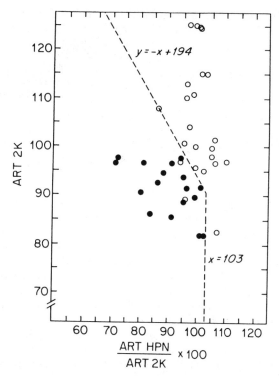

FIGURE 45-3. Bivariate plot of acoustic reflex thresholds for a 2000-Hz tone and a high-pass noise. See Figure 45-1 legend.

The data points for normal-hearing subjects tend to cluster toward the lower left corner of the graph. Data points for hearing-impaired subjects tend to be displaced toward the upper right. The region occupied by the normal subjects is described in each group by the intersection of two line segments (dashed lines). The line segments are of the following forms:

$$x = k_1$$
$$y = -x + k_2$$

The values of k_1 and k_2 for activating signal frequencies of 500, 1,000, and 2,000 Hz are given in Table 45-6 along with the proportion of normal-hearing subjects included within the region described by the two line segments. The k values were selected empirically to include as many normal subjects as possible while excluding as many pathological subjects as possible. The values given in Table 45-6

TABLE 45-6. VALUES OF THE CONSTANTS USED TO DESCRIBE NORMAL REGIONS IN THE BIVARIATE PLOTS. P REFERS TO PERCENTAGE OF NORMAL SUBJECTS CORRECTLY PREDICTED BY THE NORMAL REGION DEFINED BY k_1 AND k_2.

Frequency (Hz)	k_1	k_2	P
500	94	188	94
1000	97	188	94
2000	103	194	100

correctly identified 94 percent of the normals at 500 and 1,000 Hz and 100 percent of the normals at 2,000 Hz.

The proportion of subjects in each group who fall within the normal range is given in Table 45-7. About 50 percent of the subjects with mild hearing losses (Groups 2 and 3) fall within the normal range. Subjects with more severe hearing losses fall outside the normal range with increasing probability. It is interesting to note that a substantial number of the subjects in Groups 2, 3, and 6 had normal hearing at 500 Hz but fell outside the normal range at that frequency. It was suspected that these subjects may have had more high-frequency hearing loss than those who fell within the normal range. However, subjects with normal hearing at 500 Hz who fell within the normal region at that frequency did not, as a group, differ in extent or configuration of hearing loss from those who fell outside the normal region. Consequently no attempt has been made to estimate hearing impairment by frequency region. Instead a two out of three criterion was used to separate subjects into two groups—normal and impaired. Table 45-8 presents the proportion of subjects in each group who fell within the normal region at 0, 1, 2, or 3 of the signal

TABLE 45-7. PERCENTAGE OF SUBJECTS WITHIN THE NORMAL REGION ON THE BIVARIATE PLOTS AT THREE SIGNAL FREQUENCIES.

Group	N	Frequency (Hz) 500	1,000	2,000
1	17	94	94	100
2	12	42	58	50
3	8	50	63	38
4	2	0	0	0
5	12	8	8	17
6	13	8	62	15
7	9	22	11	0
8	4	25	0	25

TABLE 45-8. PERCENTAGE OF SUBJECTS WITHIN THE NORMAL REGION ON THE BIVARIATE PLOTS AT 0, 1, 2, OR 3 OF THE THREE SIGNAL FREQUENCIES ANALYZED (500, 1,000, AND 2,000 Hz).

Group	N	Number of Normal Frequencies			
		0	1	2	3
1	17	0	6	0	94
2	12	33	9	33	25
3	8	38	13	12	37
4	2	100	0	0	0
5	12	83	8	0	9
6	13	39	31	15	15
7	9	78	11	11	0
8	4	50	50	0	0

frequencies—500, 1,000, and 2,000 Hz. Table 45–9 presents the proportion of subjects in each group judged normal by the two out of three criterion. With this procedure the rate of false positives is very low (6 percent). Subjects with mild hearing loss (Groups 2, 3, and 6) are categorized as normal about 50 percent of the time. Subjects with average pure-tone losses greater than 32 dB are correctly identified as impaired with high accuracy (93 percent).

Although the Niemeyer and Sesterhenn and Jerger et al. procedures correctly identify hearing losses for most patients, they are characterized by high rates of false positives reducing the clinical utility of the procedures. The rationale of the procedure described in this paper is as follows. The dependence of reflex thresholds on stimulus bandwidth changes in two ways as a result of hearing loss (Popelka et al., 1976). There is (1) less "bandwidth effect" and (2) the overall position of the function shifts upward reflecting elevated reflex thresholds for narrow-band stimuli. The bivariate plotting procedure takes advantage of these two features of pathological acoustic reflex threshold data. By defining the range occupied by normal-hearing subjects and using a criterion for normality at two out of three frequencies, a low

false-positive rate was achieved. This resulted in correct identification of hearing losses in excess of 32 dB at a rate of 93 percent. Subjects with mild hearing losses or normal hearing through 2,000 Hz with high-frequency hearing losses are categorized as impaired at a rate of approximately 50 percent.

It should be noted that predictive procedures based upon reflex threshold data are based on the assumption that abnormal reflex thresholds are due to peripheral hearing loss. There are, however, other factors, such as brain stem and facial nerve pathologies, that may influence reflex thresholds without altering the pure-tone audiogram. Brain stem lesions, for example, may result in absent contralateral acoustic reflexes (Greisen and Rasmussen, 1970) with no hearing loss. In a sense, these subjects represent a type of false positive for predictive procedures based on the acoustic reflex since absent reflexes would have to place the subject in the hearing-impaired category. The elimination of these subjects from the present study may have reduced the probability of this type of false positive. However, subjects with absent reflexes are probably more commonly due to peripheral hearing losses and thus the exclusion of these subjects would reduce the "hit rate" as well as false alarms.

No attempt was made to study the relative effectiveness of predictive procedures for specific etiologies of sensorineural hearing loss. Future research would be appropriately directed toward determining differential effects of various etiologies and on determining the effectiveness of these procedures on hearing-impaired infants and children. Although normal infants have reflex thresholds that are similar to normal adults (Margolis and Popelka, 1975b), additional research is necessary to determine the predictive ability of these procedures for infants with hearing loss. If the bivariate plotting procedure can be shown to be effective for younger subject groups, this procedure could be valuable for early detection of clinically significant hearing losses while mini-

TABLE 45-9. PERCENTAGE OF SUBJECTS JUDGED NORMAL BY THE TWO OUT OF THREE CRITERION.

Group	1	2	3	4	5	6	7	8
N	17	12	8	2	12	13	9	4
Judged normal (%)	94	58	38	0	9	30	11	0

mizing the rate of false positives. A low false-positive rate not only reduces the risk of undue alarm resulting from the misdiagnosis, but also lends credibility to the correct predictions.

(The predictive procedure originally described in this article was later simplified so that a prediction is made from one bivariate plot instead of three. The ordinate represents the average reflex threshold (in dB SPL) for these tonal stimuli (500, 1,000, and 2,000 Hz). The abscissa represents the ratio of the reflex threshold for wide band noise (in dB SPL) to the average reflex threshold for the tonal stimuli. R. H. M., C. M. F.)

ACKNOWLEDGMENT

This research was supported by USPHS Grants NS 09713 and NS 09823 and by a grant from the Deafness Research Foundation. Computing assistance was obtained from the Health Sciences Computing Facility, UCLA, supported by NIH Special Research Resources Grant RR-3.

REFERENCES

American National Standards Institute. *Specification for Audiometers.* ANSI S3.6–1969. New York: American National Standards Institute (1969).

Dallos, P. Dynamics of the acoustic reflex: Phenomenological aspects. *J. Acoust. Soc. Am.,* **36,** 2,175–2,183 (1964).

Djupesland, G.; Sundby, A.; and Hogstad, K. A study of critical bandwidth in Meniere's syndrome using the acoustic stapedius reflex. *Scand. Audiol.,* **4,** 127–130 (1975).

Djupesland, G., and Zwislocki, J. On the critical band in the acoustic stapedius reflex. *J. Acoust. Soc. Am.,* **54,** 1,157–1,159 (1973).

Fisch, U., and von Schulthess, G. Electromyographic studies of the human stapedial muscle. *Acta Otolaryng.,* **56,** 287–297 (1963).

Flottorp, G.; Djupesland, G.; and Winther, F. The acoustic stapedius reflex in relation to critical bandwidth. *J. Acoust. Soc. Am.,* **49,** 457–461 (1971).

Franzen, R. Threshold of the acoustic reflex for pure tones. Doctoral dissertation, Univ. of Iowa (1970).

Greisen, O., and Rasmussen, P. Stapedius muscle reflexes and otoneurological examinations in brain-stem tumors. *Acta Otolaryng.,* **70,** 366–370 (1970).

Jerger, J.; Burney, P.; Mauldin, L.; and Crump, B. Predicting hearing loss from the acoustic reflex. *J. Speech Hearing Dis.,* **39,** 11–22 (1974).

Margolis, R. H., and Popelka, G. R. Loudness and the acoustic reflex. *J. Acoust. Soc. Am.,* **58,** 1,330–1,332 (1975a).

Margolis, R. H., and Popelka, G. R. Static and dynamic acoustic impedance measurements in infant ears. *J. Speech Hearing Res.,* **18,** 435–443 (1975b).

Niemeyer, W., and Sesterhenn, G. Calculating the hearing threshold from the stapedius reflex threshold for different sound stimuli. *Audiology,* **13,** 421–427 (1974).

Peterson, J., and Liden, G. Some static characteristics of the stapedial muscle reflex. *Audiology,* **11,** 97–114 (1972).

Popelka, G. R.; Karlovich, R.; and Wiley, T. Acoustic reflex and critical bandwidth. *J. Acoust. Soc. Am.,* **55,** 883–885 (1974).

Popelka, G. R.; Margolis, R. H.; and Wiley, T. L. Effect of activating signal bandwidth on acoustic reflex thresholds. *J. Acoust. Soc. Am.,* **59,** 153–159 (1976).

Zwislocki, J. An acoustic coupler for earphone calibration. Syracuse University Laboratory for Sensory Communication, Special Rept., LSC-S-7 (1970).

46

Acoustic Reflex and Reflex Decay
Occurrence in Patients With Cochlear and Eighth Nerve Lesions

WAYNE O. OLSEN, Ph.D.
Consultant in Audiology, Division of Audiology, Department of Otorhinolaryngology, Mayo Clinic, Rochester, Minnesota
DOUGLAS NOFFSINGER, Ph.D.
Associate Professor of Audiology, Northwestern University, Auditory Research Laboratory, Evanston, Illinois
SABINA A. KURDZIEL, M.A.
Audiologist, Audiology Division, Department of Otorhinolaryngology, Mayo Clinic, Rochester, Minnesota

Acoustic reflex and reflex decay tests were administered to 50 normal ears, 50 ears with hearing loss due to noise trauma, 50 ears that had Ménière disease, and 28 ears that had involvement of the eighth nerve. In one normal ear, ten noise trauma ears, 11 Ménière disease ears, and 24 eighth nerve lesion ears no reflexes or reflex decay that were suggestive of retrocochlear lesions were observed. Acoustic reflex and reflex decay results are also compared to tone decay results for these patients.

The Metz test for loudness recruitment that utilizes measurements of the acoustic reflex in response to intense sound stimulation is well known (Metz, 1952; Lidén, 1970; Jerger et al., 1972). In 1969, Anderson et al. (1969) added another clinical dimension to the Metz test by measuring decay of the acoustic reflex amplitude when the sound stimulation was sustained for some time.

Anderson et al. reported that decay of the acoustic reflex was not observed for normal ears in response to 500 and 1,000 Hz stimulation, but was observed for 2,000 and 4,000 Hz stimuli. In addition, they reported that of 17 cases that had confirmed intracranial tumors that affected the eighth nerve, acoustic reflexes could not be elicited from seven of them by intense stimulation of the impaired ear; acoustic reflexes were elicited from the other ten subjects, but when the 500- or 1,000-Hz stimulus was raised 10 dB above the acoustic reflex threshold and sustained for

some time, the magnitude of the observed reflex response diminished to less than half of its original amplitude in less than ten seconds. They further noted that of more than 600 additional patients tested, reflex decay at 500 Hz, 1,000 Hz, or both, was observed in only six patients for whom further medical examination proved negative for eighth nerve involvement.

Support for the observations of Anderson et al. was provided recently by Jerger et al. (1974) who found absence of acoustic reflexes or reflex decay, or both, in 26 of 30 patients who had retrocochlear lesions. However, only four patients in the sample of Jerger et al. revealed reflex decay. The absence of acoustic reflexes was the more common abnormality for their patients. Similarly, Sanders et al. (1974) recently reported that of ten patients with eighth nerve tumors for whom acoustic reflex results could be interpreted as indicative of either the presence or absence of recruitment, four did not yield reflexes; three others showed reflex decay. Sanders et al. also found that of 71 patients with cochlear lesions for whom acoustic reflex results were interpretable in terms of presence or absence of recruitment, four (5.6 percent) had "no recruitment." Reflex decay results were not reported for their patients with cochlear lesions.

While acknowledging the high success ratio of acoustic reflex and reflex decay testing in identifying eighth nerve lesions, Jerger and Jerger (1974) recently cautioned that the reflex decay phenomenon, like its "first cousin," the threshold tone decay test, must be watched for ". . . . a high false-positive rate (i.e., reflex decay in a significant proportion of patients without eighth nerve disorders)." We present data that relate to this concern.

METHOD

Acoustic reflex and reflex decay measurements were completed for 50 normal ears (25 dB hearing level [HL] or better; ANSI, 1969, 250 to 8,000 Hz; mean age, 39.9 years; age range, 16 to 60 years) and for 128 ears that had sensorineural hearing losses. Of the 128 ears with sensorineural hearing loss, 50 had high frequency losses due to noise trauma (mean age, 47.5 years; age range, 16 to 62), 50 had medically diagnosed Ménière disease (mean age, 47.9 years; age range, 28 to 61), and 28 had retrocochlear involvement (mean age, 45.4 years; age range, 17 to 64). For the latter 28 patients, neurilemomas arising from the eighth nerve, or cerebellopontine angle tumors compressing the eighth nerve, were found during subsequent surgery.

Routine pure-tone audiometry and tympanometry were completed for all subjects. Interweaving air and bone curves and normal tympanometric findings bilaterally were required for all subjects participating in this study.

Acoustic reflex thresholds and reflex decay were determined with the aid of either an electro-acoustic impedance bridge or an oto-admittance meter. Conventional audiometers provided the 500 to 4,000 Hz pure-tone stimuli that were used to elicit the reflexes. The changes in acoustic impedance that reflected stapedius muscle contraction were recorded by strip chart devices, coupled to the impedance bridge or oto-admittance units. Reflex decay was measured over a ten-second period, during which the eliciting pure-tone stimulus was presented at 10 dB above the acoustic reflex threshold for the test frequency. When the oto-admittance unit was employed for the

assessment of reflex decay, a custom-built direct current amplifier was inserted between it and the strip chart recorder in order to observe reflex behavior without the decay artifact inherent in that unit.

RESULTS

Acoustic reflexes were obtained for all 50 normal ears at 500, 1,000, and 2,000 Hz, and for all but three of them at 4,000 Hz. Reflex decay to one half or less than one half of the original reflex amplitude in ten seconds for a tone 10 dB above acoustic reflex threshold was not observed for 500 Hz, but was found for one ear at 1,000 Hz, five ears at 2,000 Hz, and for six ears at 4,000 Hz.

The findings of no reflex response to intense 4,000 Hz stimuli, or reflex but with reflex decay at 4,000 and 2,000 Hz, in spite of normal hearing sensitivity, are in agreement with previous reports and support the contention that measurement of acoustic reflex thresholds at 4,000 Hz and reflex decay at 2,000 and 4,000 Hz does not yield clinically differential information (Jerger et al., 1972; Chiveralls and Fitz-Simons, 1973; Habener and Snyder, 1974; Alberti and Kristensen, 1972). Therefore, in the following tabulations of acoustic reflex data for the groups with auditory pathologic findings, all data for 4,000 Hz and reflex decay results for 2,000 Hz have been omitted.

The incidence of the presence and absence of acoustic reflexes and reflex decay is given in Table 46–1. Of the 50 ears that had hearing losses attributed to noise trauma, acoustic reflexes were elicited from all but two of them at 500 and 1,000 Hz, and from all but six ears at 2,000 Hz. The absence of reflexes at all three test frequencies was observed for only one ear; hearing sensitivity was relatively good for this particular ear (15 to 20 dB HL at 500 and 1,000 Hz, and 35 dB HL at 2,000 Hz). The other ear that yielded no acoustic reflexes for intense 500 and 1,000 Hz stimuli did demonstrate acoustic reflex response to a 2,000 Hz tone presented at 100 dB HL. Thus, only one of these ears revealed no acoustic reflexes at any test frequency, and five additional ears failed to show stapedius muscle contraction in response to 2,000 Hz stimuli. The 2,000 Hz threshold sensitivity was not poorer than 50 dB HL for any of these ears. Reflex decay was observed at both 500

TABLE 46-1. ACOUSTIC REFLEX AND REFLEX DECAY IN PATIENTS WITH SENSORINEURAL HEARING LOSS.

Group	Reflex at 500 Hz			Reflex at 1,000 Hz			Reflex at 2,000 Hz	
	Present	Absent	Decay	Present	Absent	Decay	Present	Absent
Noise trauma	48	2	1	48	2	4	44	6
Ménière disease	49	1	0	49	1	7	45	5
Eighth nerve lesion	18	10	3	13	15	4	7	21

and 1,000 Hz for one of the subjects in this group. Reflex decay at only 1,000 Hz was observed for three ears. The reflex decay obtained at 1,000 Hz for one ear in the noise trauma group was observed shortly after the onset of a high frequency hearing loss due to a nearby explosion. Six months later, no reflex decay was observed even though there had been no appreciable improvement in the hearing sensitivity or acoustic reflex thresholds for this patient.

Regarding the 50 ears in this study that had medically diagnosed Ménière disease, acoustic reflexes were obtained for all but one of these ears at 500 and 1,000 Hz, and for all but five of them at 2,000 Hz (Table 46-1). One of these yielded no reflexes at any frequency. One of the five ears that failed to yield a reflex response at 2,000 Hz had a severe hearing loss (75 dB HL at 2,000 Hz). Jerger et al. (1974) suggested that the inference of retrocochlear involvement on the basis of a lack of acoustic reflex response should be made only when the sensorineural hearing loss at the test frequency is less than 70 dB HL. For the other three ears in this group that failed to yield acoustic reflexes in response to 2,000 Hz stimuli, routine pure-tone audiometry revealed 2,000 Hz-thresholds at 10 dB HL, 45 dB HL, and 60 dB HL.

Reflex decay was not observed at 500 Hz for any of the 50 ears with Ménière disease that were tested, but reflex decay to one half or less than one half amplitude in ten seconds was observed at 1,000 Hz in seven of these ears. Review of the pure-tone threshold and acoustic reflex threshold data for these seven ears failed to reveal any pattern of findings that might help explain the 14 percent incidence of reflex decay for this group. Threshold sensitivity at 1,000 Hz was no poorer than 65 dB HL for any of these ears, and acoustic reflex thresholds were elicited at 80 to 90 dB HL. In other words, the levels at which acoustic reflexes were obtained for these ears were neither unusually low nor elevated.

Acoustic reflex and reflex decay results for the eighth nerve lesion group (28 ears) are also reported in Table 46-1. The decreasing incidence of elicitable acoustic reflexes as a function of higher stimulus frequencies is obvious. Whereas acoustic reflexes were absent for ten ears in response to intense 500 Hz stimuli, no reflexes were obtained from 15 of them in response to 1,000 Hz tones, or from 21 of them for 2,000 Hz tones presented at 110 dB HL. However, two ears revealed threshold sensitivity poorer than 65 dB at 1,000 Hz, and seven had thresholds that were greater than 65 dB at 2,000 Hz. Hence, there were ten instances in which the absence of acoustic reflex response at 500 Hz could be interpreted to be suggestive of retrocochlear involvement, 13 such instances at 1,000 Hz, and 14 at 2,000 Hz. In total, 19 of these ears yielded no acoustic reflex at one or more of the three test frequencies when threshold sensitivity was no poorer than 65 dB HL at these frequencies.

Reflex decay was observed at 500 Hz for three of the 18 ears that yielded acoustic reflexes at that frequency, and for four ears at 1,000 Hz when an acoustic reflex could be elicited (13 ears). Reflex decay at both 500 and 1,000 Hz was observed for one of these ears.

Overall, there were 21 ears in the eighth nerve lesion sample that demonstrated either an absence of acoustic reflex or reflex decay, or both, at 500 or 1,000 Hz, when threshold sensitivity was better than 70 dB HL. For three ears, acoustic reflexes and a lack of reflex decay were observed in response to 500 and 1,000 Hz stimuli, but no reflex could be elicited at 2,000 Hz even though threshold sensitivity was decreased to no more than 50 dB HL.

Therefore, by imposing a set of criteria including (1) the absence of acoustic reflexes at 500, 1,000, or 2,000 Hz in spite of pure-tone thresholds no greater than 65 dB at these frequencies, or (2) reflex decay to one half or less than one half amplitude for a 500 or

1,000 Hz tone sustained for ten seconds at 10 dB above acoustic reflex threshold reflex, reflex decay testing suggested retrocochlear involvement for 24 of the 28 ears in this sample that were subsequently found to have intracranial tumors affecting the eighth nerve.

However, as mentioned previously, some of the subjects with either normal ears or ears with cochlear lesions also failed to yield acoustic reflexes, or revealed reflex decay that was suggestive of retrocochlear involvement. Table 46-2 illustrates the incidence of acoustic reflex test results that were suggestive of retrocochlear involvement in all four groups.

As mentioned previously, an absence of acoustic reflexes was more common than an absence of reflex decay for the ears with eighth nerve lesions (68 percent vs. 18 percent). The occurrence of reflex decay and the absence of reflexes was essentially reversed for the two groups with cochlear lesions. There was a 14 percent incidence of reflex decay and an 8 percent incidence of an absence of reflex response in the Ménière disease group, and an 8 percent incidence of of reflex decay and a 12 percent incidence of absence of acoustic reflexes for the noise trauma group.

TABLE 46-2. INCIDENCE OF ACOUSTIC REFLEX TEST RESULTS THAT WERE SUGGESTIVE OF RETROCOCHLEAR INVOLVEMENT.

Group	Reflex		
	Absent (%)	Decay (%)	Total (%)
Normal	0 (0)	1 (2)	1 (2)
Noise trauma	6 (12)	4 (8)	10 (20)
Ménière disease	4 (8)	7 (14)	11 (22)
Eighth nerve	19* (68)	6* (21)	24 (86)

*One patient in common showed no reflex at 2,000 Hz and had reflex decay at 1,000 Hz.

Table 46-3 gives a breakdown (by frequency) of acoustic reflex test results that suggested retrocochlear lesions in the ears that had pure-tone thresholds of 65 dB HL or better in each group. Whereas 3 percent of the ears with cochlear lesions failed to yield acoustic reflexes at 500 and 1,000 Hz, the incidence of an absence of reflex response was 12 times greater at 500 Hz, and 16 times greater at 1,000 Hz for the ears with eighth nerve lesions. At 2,000 Hz, an acoustic reflex could not be elicited from 10 percent of the ears with either noise trauma or Ménière disease, but the incidence in ears with eighth nerve lesions was seven times greater (71 percent).

It is also apparent that reflex decay at 500 Hz was uncommon for all groups (Table 46-3). In those ears that had subsequently confirmed eighth nerve involvement, only three (17 percent) of those for whom acoustic reflexes were elicited at 500 Hz showed reflex decay. Reflex decay at 1,000 Hz was more frequent for all groups; when acoustic reflexes were elicited, reflex decay was about four times more frequent for the eighth nerve lesion group (31 percent) than for the noise trauma group (8 percent). However, 14 percent of the reflex decay tests given to the Ménière disease group at 1,000 Hz also showed reflex decay.

On this basis, one might be tempted to forego reflex decay testing. However, if reflex decay tests had been ignored, five individuals with threshold sensitivity of 65 dB HL or better at 500 and 1,000 Hz would not have been identified has eighth nerve lesion suspects from acoustic reflex threshold testing. Reflex decay at 1,000 Hz also provided confirmatory evidence in one subject who failed to yield reflex response to a 2,000 Hz tone even though threshold sensitivity was not severely impaired at that frequency (50 dB HL).

TABLE 46-3. EARS THAT SHOWED ABSENCE OF ACOUSTIC REFLEXES* OR REFLEX DECAY.†

Group	Absence of Reflex			Reflex Decay	
	500 Hz	1,000 Hz	2,000 Hz	500 Hz	1,000 Hz
Normal	0	0	0	0	2.0
Noise trauma	4	4	12	2.1	8.3
Ménière disease	2	2	8	0	14.2
Eighth nerve	36	48	71	16.7	30.8

*Percentage given only for ears with pure-tone thresholds of less than 70 dB HL.
†Percentage of these patients for whom acoustic reflexes were elicited. See Table 46-1 for number of patients.

COMMENT

The results obtained for the normal ears that were tested in this investigation are in agreement with other reports in the literature of the incidence of acoustic reflexes and reflex decay for normal ears (Jerger et al., 1972; Chiveralls and FitzSimons, 1973; Habener and Snyder, 1974; Alberti and Kristensen, 1972). The absence of reflex response at any frequency for one ear in the noise trauma group and for one ear in the Ménière disease group was somewhat surprising. However, Jerger et al. (1972) reported an absence of reflex response for both ears of one of their normal subjects. Also, in their histologic studies, Hoshino and Paparella (1971) observed ectopic or absent stapedius muscles with no other apparent congenital abnormalities in six of 195 middle ears that were studied.

The absence of reflexes at 2,000 Hz, suggestive of no recruitment at that frequency, for nine other ears with cochlear lesions in this sample agrees reasonably well with the data of Sanders et al. (1974). Four (5.6 percent) of the 71 cochlear lesion ears in the sample for which they could interpret acoustic reflex results as indicating "the presence or absence" of recruitment were judged to show "no recruitment."

Since only one of the normal ears tested in this study had reflex decay, the observation of reflex decay for 11 of the ears with cochlear lesions was somewhat surprising. Colletti (1974) observed reflex decay for one of 24 ears with Ménière disease. Reflex decay results for cochlear lesion patients were not reported by Sanders et al. (1974).

The findings for the group with eighth nerve lesions are in agreement with the data of Jerger et al. (1974). Acoustic reflex and reflex decay testing indicated retrocochlear involvement in 26 of 30 eighth nerve lesion patients in their study, and in 24 of 28 patients in our study. The absence of acoustic reflex response was more common than reflex decay, as was also found in the study by Jerger et al.

In view of the comparison of reflex decay and threshold tone decay as "first cousins," (Jerger and Jerger, 1974) it is of interest to note the tone decay results obtained for the ears with sensorineural hearing loss that were tested in our investigation. Tone decay tests administered in the manner described by Carhart (1957) or by Olsen and Noffsinger (1974) were completed for all but one of the ears with sensorineural hearing loss. In both test methods, tone decay exceeding 30 dB is regarded as a signal of a possible retrocochlear lesion.

None of the ears in the noise trauma sample that showed reflex decay demonstrated tone decay in excess of 30 dB at any frequency tested, including 4,000 Hz. Excess tone decay was noted only at 3,000 Hz for both ears of one patient in this group; absences of acoustic reflexes bilaterally were also observed for this patient at 2,000 Hz, even though threshold sensitivity at 2,000 Hz was not less than 50 dB HL for either ear.

With regard to the Ménière disease group, excess tone decay was observed for three ears, all at only 4,000 Hz. One of these ears revealed reflex decay at 1,000 Hz, one yielded no reflex at 2,000 Hz in spite of good hearing sensitivity at that frequency, and the other one demonstrated reflex response at all frequencies and no reflex decay.

Three of the six ears in the eighth nerve lesion group that exhibited reflex decay also showed excess tone decay. Of the 19 ears in this group that did not yield acoustic reflexes at one or more frequencies, excess tone decay was found at one or more frequencies for 13 of them. Both absence of reflexes at 2,000 Hz and reflex decay at 1,000 Hz were observed for one of these patients. Tone decay testing was not completed for one of these 19 patients. Curiously, excess tone decay was observed at 500 and 1,000 Hz for one of the patients in this group, even though acoustic reflexes were elicited at all three test frequencies and reflex decay was not found at either 500 or 1,000 Hz. Altogether, excess tone decay was found for 17 of the 27 patients in this group for whom tone decay testing was completed. These results indicate that tone decay tests such as described by Carhart (1957) and by Olsen and Noffsinger (1974) identified fewer of the subsequently confirmed eighth nerve lesions than did acoustic reflex and reflex decay testing. Results that were suggestive of retrocochlear involvement were observed less frequently from tone decay tests than from acoustic reflex tests for the ears with cochlear lesions (5 percent vs. 21 percent).

The findings of this study are in agreement with the observations of Anderson et al. (1969) and Jerger et al. (1974) with regard to the sensitivity of acoustic reflex and reflex decay tests for identifying eighth nerve lesions. However, on the basis of our study it would appear that approximately 20 percent of ears having cochlear lesions due to noise trauma or to Ménière disease may also fail to yield acoustic reflexes or show reflex decay that is suggestive of retrocochlear involvement.

ACKNOWLEDGMENT

This study was supported by the Mayo Foundation, and by National Institute of Neurological Disorders and Stroke grant NSO7791.

REFERENCES

Alberti, P. W., Kristensen, R. Stapedial reflex threshold and decay: A normal study in clinical practice, in Rose, D. E., Keating, L. W. (compilers): *Impedance Symposium,* Rochester, Minn., Mayo Foundation, 1972, pp. 237–251.

Anderson, H.; Barr, B.; Wedenberg, E. Intraaural reflexes in retrocochlear lesions, in Hamberger, C. A., Wersäll, J. (eds.), *Disorders of the Skull Base Region,* Nobel Synposium 10. Stockholm, Almqvist & Wiksell, 1969, pp. 49–55.

Carhart, R. Clinical determination of abnormal auditory adaptation. *Arch. Otolaryngol.,* **65:** 32–39, 1957.

Chiveralls, K., FitzSimons, R. Stapedial reflex action in normal subjects. *Br. J. Audiol.,* **7:** 105–110, 1973.

Colletti, V. Some stapedius reflex parameters in normal and pathological conditions. *J. Laryngol. Otol.,* **88:** 127–137, 1974.

Habener, S. A., Snyder, J. M. Stapedius reflex amplitude and decay in normal hearing ears. *Arch. Otolaryngol.,* **100:** 294–297, 1974.

Hoshino, T., Paparella, M. M. Middle ear muscle anomalies. *Arch. Otolaryngol.,* **94:** 235–239, 1971.

Jerger, J., Jerger, S. Audiological comparison of cochlear and eighth nerve disorders. *Ann. Otol. Rhinol. Laryngol.,* **83:** 275–285, 1974.

Jerger, J.; Jerger, S.; Mauldin, L. Studies in impedance audiometry: I. Normal and sensorineural ears. *Arch. Otolaryngol.,* **96:** 513–523, 1972.

Jerger, J.; Harford, E.; Clemis, J., et al. The acoustic reflex in eighth nerve disorders. *Arch. Otolaryngol.,* **99:** 409–413, 1974.

Lidén, G. The stapedius muscle reflex used as an objective recruitment test: A clinical and experimental study, in Wolstenhome, G. W., Knight, J., (eds.), *Sensorineural Hearing Loss.* London, J. & A. Churchill, 1970, pp. 295–308.

Metz, O. Threshold of reflex contractions of muscles of middle ear and recruitment of loudness. *Arch. Otolaryngol.,* **55:** 536–543, 1952.

Olsen, W. O., Noffsinger, D. Comparison of one new and three old tests of auditory adaptation. *Arch. Otolaryngol.,* **99:** 94–99, 1974.

Sanders, J. W.; Josey, A. F.; Glasscock, M. E. III. Audiologic evaluation in cochlear and eighth nerve disorders. *Arch. Otolaryngol.,* **100:** 283–289, 1974.

part VI

IDENTIFICATION (SCREENING) AUDIOMETRY

The term *identification audiometry* assumed prominence after publication of the American Speech and Hearing Association (ASHA) monograph that summarized the proceedings and recommendations of ASHA's 1960 conference on identification audiometry (American Speech and Hearing Association, 1961). Those who favor *identification* over the more conventional term, *screening,* apparently want to emphasize the principle that the primary goal of hearing screening tests is to find (i.e., identify) persons who have significant or potentially significant hearing problems. On the other hand, in most medical and public health publications," "screening" is the adjective that has usually been used to describe brief tests applied to large populations in an effort to locate individuals who may have specific disorders.

A remarkable amount of research on the efficiency of hearing screening procedures has been conducted with incomplete or misconceived research paradigms that have diminished or negated the validity or usefulness of reported data. The most common problem has been the assumption that air-conduction screening tests are designed to identify middle ear disease efficiently (particularly in school children) when, in fact, air-conduction screening tests are relatively inefficient at this task (Eagles, 1963).[1] On the other hand, they are very useful for their intended purpose (to identify hearing impairment). Nonetheless, medical diagnosis of middle ear disease has persisted as a primary validity criterion for evaluating the effectiveness of hearing screening tests. There is, in fact, no way in which a substantial percentage (on the order of 50 percent) of cases of middle ear disease would not be missed by a pure-tone screening test, even if the ambient noise in the screening environment were quiet enough to allow screening within 5 or 10 dB of audiometric zero.

The advent of impedance audiometry has compounded the conceptual problem discussed above. Professionals who see middle ear disease as the primary target of all screening tests in hearing conservation programs, or who assume (incorrectly) that all children with middle ear diseases have significant hearing deficits, have tended to see impedance audiometry as the ultimate screening test for children. This preoccupation has even spawned a number of studies pitting impedance screening (tympanometry or tympanometry plus a reflex test) against air-conduction hearing screening tests. The goals of specific screening tests are sometimes confused with the broader goals of screening or identification programs. Both types of tests discussed above or either one alone might be used in a program, depending on the program's scope and resources. This distinction is crucial when the efficiency of programs or tests is evaluated.

The foregoing comments reflect concerns that preoccupied us as we evaluated articles for this section. At times we considered excluding the section entirely because of the apparent reduction of articles on hearing screening *per se.* Instead, we decided to emphasize research reports and didactic articles concerning the efficiency of screening tests, with special emphasis on principles relevant to interpretation and research evaluation of screening tests. The principles are the same for the researcher and the clinician because each must be concerned with a test's *sensitivity* (proportion of impaired persons identified correctly) and *specificity* (proportion of normal or unaffected persons correctly passed). These screening-test indexes, combined with their complementary *false positive* and *false negative* rates, are commonplace in research reports concerning conditions other than hearing or ear disease, but are rare in audiologic research reports. It is noteworthy that the most common audiologic research paradigm for evaluating the efficiency of hearing screening tests does not include evaluation of specificity, and consequently no assessment of false negative classifications, the most costly form of screening error.

The first selection in this section is Thorner and Remein's monograph on screening theory, screening variables, and procedures for evaluating the efficiency of screening tests. Their treatment of these topics provides a firm background for applying, interpreting, and analyzing screening test results. Although none of Thorner and Remein's examples or discussion deal specifically with hearing loss or ear disease, the principles involved are generic and directly applicable to tests designed to identify hearing loss or middle ear pathology.

The next two selections, ASHA's guidelines for identification audiometry (1975) and for acoustic immittance screening (1977) set forth research-based recommendations concerning procedures for identifying hearing impairment and middle ear disorders. The guidelines represent important anchor points for strengthening screening programs and for improving inter- and intraprofessional communication in this area. Students should find the guidelines useful illustrations of the interdependence of research and clinical practice.

The Melnick, Eagles, and Levine selection, which appeared in the first edition, reports a well-controlled research evaluation of the screening recommendations of ASHA's 1960 conference on identification audiometry. A companion piece to the Melnick et al. study is Wilson and Walton's field study of the efficiency of the 1975 ASHA guidelines for identification audiometry. In the earlier study, data were gathered under ideal sound-isolated conditions that allowed threshold data and otoscopic examinations to be obtained on the same day. The Wilson and Walton study, by contrast, simulates the more typical delay between a screening test and follow-up diagnostic evaluation. Together these studies provide an excellent opportunity for the reader to consider the effects of screening variables such as test conditions, face validity of pass-fail criteria, and follow-up strategies. Since neither study employed the type of sensitivity-specificity analysis described by Thorner and Remein, it is instructive to reanalyze the data in terms of sensitivity and specificity. The apparent efficiency of the procedures changes with reanalysis but the differences provide an opportunity to consider problems such as the long-term status of initial failures who pass the rescreen recommended by both studies and by the ASHA Guidelines (i.e., do those who pass only on rescreen have the same characteristics as those who pass on the initial screen?) or the potential difficulties associated with assigning false positive status to persons who fail a screening test at 20 dB HL but "pass" a follow-up threshold test with thresholds no better than 20 dB.

The article on openended tympanometric screening for middle ear disease by Lewis, Dugdale, Canty, and Jerger emphasizes the importance of selecting failure criteria that minimize the number of unnecessary referrals (false positives), thus increasing sensitivity of the tympanometric screening process. Orchik, Morff, and Dunn's article in Part V (Impedance Audiometry) provides additional data and discussion concerning the efficiency of tympanometry and acoustic reflex tests in the diagnosis of serous otitis media.

The next selection is a case report by Holm and Thompson that serves as a vivid reminder of the unfortunate consequences of failing to consider marked high-frequency sensorineural hearing loss as an important category of impairment that must be identified in a screening program. A comprehensive treatment of marked high-frequency loss is available in a study by Matkin (1968). One of Matkin's most prominent findings was that parents of such children often found medical professionals frustratingly resistant to acknowledging the possibility of significant hearing impairment in their young patients.

The final selection in this section is Dixon and Newby's study of the characteristics of children with nonorganic (functional) hearing problems. A high proportion of Dixon and Newby's subjects were referred to them on the basis of failing a school hearing screening test. Although such cases do not represent a high percentage of screening failures, they are not rare, and when mismanaged the consequences can be serious. The existence of such cases underlines the importance of prompt audiologic follow-up as the procedure of choice to assess whether a child who has failed a school screening test does, indeed, have a valid sensitivity deficit.

ENDNOTE

1. Some of the other common problems have been (1) use of one screening test as a validity criterion for another screening test, (2) follow-up threshold tests in inappropriate environments, (3) unskilled screeners; (4) inadequate sample size, and (5) inappropriate failure criteria.

REFERENCES AND ADDITIONAL READINGS

Eagles, E. L.; Wishik, S. M.; Doerfler, L. G.; Melnick, W.; and Levine, H. S., eds. Chapter 2, "Children with otoscopic abnormalities" in *Hearing sensitivity and related factors in children; Laryngoscope,* Monograph (June 1963).

Eisenberg, R. B. Auditory behavior in the human neonate: Methodologic problems and the logical design of research procedures. *J. Aud. Res.,* **5,** 159–177 (1965).

Eisner, V., and Oglesby, A. Health assessment of school children, II: Screening tests. *J. School Health,* **41,** 341–346 (1971).

Goldstein, R., and Tait, C. Critique of neonatal hearing evaluation. *J. Speech Hearing Dis.,* **36,** 3–18 (1971).

Gullen, W. H., and Bearman, J. E. Observations on the diagnostic capabilities of laboratory tests. *Minn. Med.,* **50,** 681–685 (1967).

Matkin, N. The child with a marked high-frequency hearing impairment. *Ped. Clin. of North Amer.,* **15,** 677–690 (1968).

Simmons, F. B., and Russ, F. N. Automated newborn hearing screening, the crib-o-gram. *Arch. Otolaryng.,* **100,** 1–7 (1974).

47

Principles and Procedures in the Evaluation of Screening for Disease

Robert M. Thorner, B.S., M.B.A, M.P.H.
Associate Chief of Operational Methods in the Health Services for Long Term Illness Branch, U.S. Public Health Service when this monograph was prepared

Quentin R. Remein, B.A.
Assistant Chief of the Technical Development Branch, U.S. Public Health Service when this monograph was prepared

FOREWORD

The experience of the chronic disease program of the Public Health Service in aiding in the conduct of seminars concerned with screening programs, chiefly for diabetes, indicated the need for a compendium of information on screening tests. One session of these seminars is always devoted to test attributes and especially to sensitivity and specificity. Though the literature includes many papers dealing with various aspects of screening tests, up to now there has been no single source to which seminar students could be referred. The need for a work of this kind has also been expressed by teachers and students in schools of public health. While this monograph presents very little new material, it is hoped that it will fill the demand for a simple and comprehensive presentation of the aspects of screening tests that concern administrators and researchers in public health and related fields. (Wilfred D. David, *Assistant Chief, Division of Chronic Diseases*)

I. PRINCIPLES OF SCREENING FOR DISEASE

The screening of large population groups for chronic diseases may be expected to increase in scope as health departments continue to expand programs in

Public Health Monograph No. 67. Public Health Service Publication No. 846. Library of Congress Catalog Card No. 61-60094. Reprinted with permission of the Public Health Service.

the chronic disease field. The practical application of screening tests requires a basic knowledge of the attributes of these tests and an understanding of the results that may be expected when a particular test is applied to a population group at a selected screening level. This paper summarizes and presents information about screening tests for the use of program administrators and others concerned with screening tests as casefinding devices.

Screening tests may also be used as an epidemiological tool for estimating the prevalence and incidence of disease under certain circumstances. These aspects of screening are not dealt with in this monograph.

The basic purpose of screening for disease detection is to separate from a large group of apparently well persons those who have a high probability of having the disease under study, so that they may be given a diagnostic workup and, if diseased, brought to treatment.

Tests used in screening must be relatively simple. Since many of the tests are done by persons who are not physicians, involved tests requiring extensive training in medicine are not appropriate for screening. For obvious reasons the tests must also be relatively inexpensive. In addition, screening tests should be fairly sensitive, specific, precise, and accurate. These attributes of screening tests are discussed in detail.

Screening tests should be distinguished from diagnostic tests, which are usually more complex procedures used by the physician, along with the medical history, symptoms, and signs, to establish or rule out a definitive diagnosis. However, many of the aspects of screening tests discussed here also apply to diagnostic tests.

Sensitivity and Specificity

Sensitivity is the ability of a test to give a positive finding when the person tested truly has the disease under study. Specificity is the ability of the test to give a negative finding when the person tested is free of the disease under study.

The evaluation of sensitivity and specificity requires that a diagnosis for the disease under study be established or ruled out for *every person* tested by the screening procedure, *regardless of whether the person screened negative or positive.* The diagnosis should be established according to definite criteria by techniques that are independent of the screening test. For example, if the sensitivity and specificity of a urine sugar testing technique as a screening test for diabetes are to be evaluated, the diagnosis of diabetes may be established on the basis of a glucose tolerance test and clinical examination, but not on the basis of the urine sugar test.

The results of the screening and diagnostic examinations in an evaluative study can be examined most conveniently by use of the fourfold classification in Table 47–1.

Sensitivity is calculated by

$$\frac{a}{a+c} \times 100.$$

This is the percentage of persons with the disease who were detected by the test. Specificity is calculated by

$$\frac{d}{b+d} \times 100.$$

This is the percentage of nondiseased persons who were negative to the test.

TABLE 47–1.

Screening test results	Diagnosis Diseased	Not diseased	Total
Positive	a	b	a+b
Negative	c	d	c+d
Total	a+c	b+d	a+b+c+d

NOTE: a—diseased persons detected by the test.
b—false positives to the test.
c—false negatives to the test.
d—nondiseased persons negative to the test.

If valid sensitivity and specificity figures are to be obtained, the group of persons selected for an evaluative study of a screening test should closely approximate the type of population to which the test will be applied. The selection of a group of persons composed only of advanced cases of the disease and young, healthy persons who are almost sure to be free of the disease will yield data which may not be typical of the populations encountered in the usual screening situations because of the small probability of such persons falling into categories b and c of the fourfold classification table. Populations of this type may be useful, however, for pilot studies of the effectiveness of new techniques, or may be the only type of population available. Results of studies in populations of this type should be interpreted with caution.

Theory of Overlapping Distributions

Many aspects of the sensitivity and specificity of screening tests may be explained by the theory of overlapping population distributions. According to this theory the population being screened in reality consists of a diseased and a nondiseased group (as defined by the diagnostic criteria), both possessing the attribute being measured by the screening test with different frequencies at various test values. For some values of the test, the distributions overlap, and it is not possible to assign persons with these values to the normal or diseased group on the basis of the screening test alone.

Such a situation is illustrated by Figure 47–1. Hypothetical population A, with nonglaucomatous eyes is much larger than population B, with glaucomatous eyes, as indicated by the relative areas of the A and B distributions. Population A has a lower average intraocular pressure, with pressures ranging from approximately 14 to 26 millimeters of mercury. Population B has a higher average intraocular pressure, and pressures range from about 22 to 42 millimeters of mercury. The range of intraocular pressures from approximately 22 to 26 millimeters of mercury includes both glaucomatous and nonglaucomatous eyes. For any individual case in this range, it is not possible to assign the eye to the glaucomatous or the nonglaucomatous group on the basis of this test alone.

Similar situations can be postulated for many tests based on biological measurements that may indicate a physiological or pathological condition—for ex-

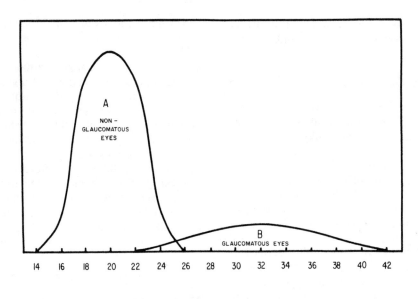

INTRAOCULAR PRESSURE IN MM HG

FIGURE 47-1. Hypothetical distribution of intraocular pressures in glaucomatous and nonglaucomatous eyes, measured by tonometer.

ample, blood sugar, blood pressure, white cell counts, and similar measurements used for screening and diagnostic tests.

For tests based on antigen-antibody systems, population A may be thought of as being composed of persons free of the disease under study, of whom some possess antibodies associated with antigenic stimuli which give cross reaction to the antigenic stimulus used for the test. An example of this is the tuberculin reaction in persons sensitized by organisms antigenically related to the tubercle bacillus.

The pattern of combinations of sensitivity and specificity associated with various screening levels of a particular test is defined by the shapes and range of overlap of the two distributions.

For purposes of illustration, a screening level of 25 millimeters of mercury has been selected and the two distributions of Figure 47-1 have been separated in Figure 47-2. Sensitivity is the shaded area of curve B divided by the total area of curve B; specificity is the shaded area of curve A divided by the total area of curve A. Changing the shapes of the curves or their overlap area would change the relationships and thus alter the sensitivity-specificity pattern. Curves based on real situations may not be the symmetrical

curves of these illustrations; instead they may be quite skewed (distorted), or have other shapes such as the J, reverse J, or U. Also, since the prevalence of most chronic illness is small, the area of curve B frequently is only about 1 or 2 percent of the area of curve A, and if the two populations are combined into a single distribution, the effect of curve B on the shape of the resulting combined curve will be negligible. For this reason, a combined curve frequently is not bimodal.

Stability of Sensitivity and Specificity

Since the sensitivity-specificity pattern of a screening test is a function of the distributions of the test attribute for diseased and nondiseased persons, the stability of these measures from area to area and from time to time depends on the stability of the distributions of test attributes.

Any change which affects the shape of either curve or the range of overlap will change the sensitivity-specificity pattern of the test. Changes in other characteristics of the diseased and nondiseased population may affect the shape of either or both curves if the changed characteristics are closely associated

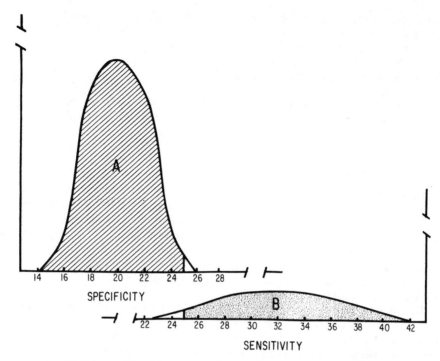

FIGURE 47-2. Graphic presentation of sensitivity and specificity.

with the test attribute. These characteristics include the age, race, and sex of the populations, exposure to antigenically related infections, and other epidemiological characteristics. The importance of a change in one of these factors will depend upon the intensity of its relationship to the attribute upon which the test is based.

For chronic diseases, age is an important characteristic, affecting such test attributes as intraocular pressure, blood sugar, blood pressure, and most physiological measurements. In test populations with similar age distributions, the sensitivity-specificity pattern is usually stable for most chronic noninfectious diseases, but it may be quite different in test populations with dissimilar age distributions.

For tests based on antigen-antibody systems, the prevalence of cross-reacting antibodies in the nondiseased group is an important factor. The tuberculin test may be cited as an example. In the southern areas of the United States where the prevalence of infection with nontuberculous acid-fast organisms is higher than in other regions of the nation, there are more cross reactions to the tuberculin test, and this tech-

nique has a lower specificity in the South than in other sections of the country (Comstock and Porter, 1959).

Prevalence, Sensitivity, and Specificity

The sensitivity-specificity pattern of a test will not be affected by a change in the prevalence of the disease if the reduction or increase in prevalence does not result in changes in the shapes of the distributions of the test attributes in the diseased and nondiseased population.

In Figure 47-1 the prevalence of glaucomatous eyes is defined by the proportion of the total area under both curves which is composed of glaucomatous eyes, or the area of curve B divided by the area of curves A + B. Any change in the prevalence of the disease will result in a change in the relative magnitude of the two curves.

The relative area of the distribution of glaucomatous eyes will increase if the prevalence of glaucoma increases. If the increase is proportionate at all levels of pressure, the relationship of the shaded area of curve B in Figure 47–2 to the total area of curve B will not change, and the sensitivity will not change. Since specificity is based on curve A, it is also not affected. It can readily be seen that under these circumstances the change in prevalence has no effect upon the sensitivity and specificity of the test.

If, however, the increase in the relative area of curve B is not proportionate at all levels of pressure, the shape of the curve will change and the sensitivity of the test will change. Thus, a change in prevalence will result in a change in the sensitivity-specificity relationship only if the general shape of either curve of test measurement is also changed.

Screening Level, Sensitivity, and Specificity

For tests which are read quantitatively or semiquantitatively, it is possible to vary the sensitivity and specificity within the established pattern by changing the level at which the test is considered positive. However, a change in the level that increases the specificity will decrease the sensitivity, and a change increasing the sensitivity will decrease the specificity. This problem is analogous to the problem of Type I and Type II errors in the selection of a significance level in tests of statistical significance.

Again referring to Figure 47–1, if the screening level is set at 26 millimeters of mercury, the test will be 100 percent specific. All of the nonglaucomatous eyes will be excluded from the positive classification at this level and will be called negative by the test. However, all of the glaucomatous eyes which are in the area of the glaucomatous curve between the values of 26 and 22 millimeters of mercury will test negative, and the sensitivity of the test will be low.

If the screening level is shifted to 22 millimeters of mercury, the test becomes 100 percent sensitive. All of the eyes which are truly glaucomatous will be positive to the test, but all of the nonglaucomatous eyes in the area under the nonglaucomatous curve between the values of 22 and 26 millimeters will also be called positive, and the test will have poor specificity. Levels between 22 and 26 millimeters will yield various combinations of sensitivity and specificity between zero and 100 percent.

For some screening tests it may not be possible to set a level low enough to achieve 100 percent sensitivity because the test technique will not permit interpretation at that level. For example, in most antigen-

antibody detection techniques the antigen is adjusted so that low levels of antibody in the blood will not be detected.

Selecting the Screening Level

The selection of the screening level is essentially an administrative decision which must be based on value judgments. Since different screening levels will result in different proportions of false negatives and false positives, the effect of false test results upon the medical and lay community must be weighed against the value of finding true negatives and positives (Packer et al., 1960). A mathematical model of this decision process has been set up by Blumberg (1957). In the same paper, Blumberg lists the following as items which help determine the value of true and false positives and negatives to the community and to the screenee:

1. What is the outlook for a person with the disease? The value of a true positive increases as the patient's chances for cure or shorter convalescense are improved by early detection. In fact, when no health benefits are attributable to the finding of cases, the advisability of screening is doubtful.

2. What facilities exist for treating cases found? The value of a true positive is reduced if inadequate facilities exist for treating those found. As far as direct benefits go, it is only profitable to find as many cases as may be treated. (In the long run, finding larger numbers of cases may lead to the provision of more adequate treatment facilities, which in turn may help the cases already found, provided they live that long.)

3. What mental status accompanies knowledge or suspicion of the disease? If suspicion of a disease is accompanied by considerable anxiety that may in turn be debilitating, then demonstration of a true negative could provide valuable reassurance and health benefits. Ordinarily, however, very little good (or harm) is done by finding a true negative. On the other hand, the fear from being falsely considered positive might very well cause undue anxiety and thus be of direct harm to those who have been placed in this category. But if the notice that directs the positives to seek further diagnostic study is tactfully and intelligently written, this danger from false positives can be minimized.

4. Who is going to do the diagnostic followup? False positives burden the diagnostic facilities. If the facilities are adequate and diagnostic study is quite inexpensive, then false positives may be less harmful. False positives also serve to discredit screening procedures and screeners in the eyes of those screened and medical practitioners. In a closed community, such as the Armed Forces, where followups are done entirely at the expense of the community and not of the individual, false positives may be less harmful.

5. What is the likelihood of repeat screening within the community? If it is unlikely that repeat screening will be carried on within a short period of time, then false negatives could be extremely detrimental. On the other hand, if screening will be repeated in a short period and the disease is not communicable or rapidly progressing, then false negatives would not be so harmful, since there may be a fair likelihood of uncovering the disease the next time.

6. Are healthy individuals being sought? Sometimes screening procedures are conducted to identify healthy rather than sick individuals. This may be the case in selecting people for certain jobs or for the armed services, as well as in screening life insurance applicants. In these cases false negatives are very costly while false positives may not be.

Factors Affecting Validity of Test Results

Since the selection of a screening level is based on the expected yield of new cases tempered by the number of false negatives and false positives associated with a particular screening level, the administrator must have some knowledge of what the frequency of false test results will be in order to be able to select the screening level that will optimize results for his particular community situation. The frequencies of false negatives and positives can be estimated easily if sensitivity and specificity data are available, and if the approximate level of prevalence and the number of persons to be screened are known.

For example, if the prevalence of unknown diabetes in a population to be screened is approximately 1.5 percent and it is assumed that 10,000 persons will be screened, an estimated 150 persons in this group will be diseased. Using the fourfold classification (Table 47–1), 10,000 constitutes $a + b + c + d$, the total persons tested; 150 is equal to $a + c$, the

total who truly have the disease; and the $b + d$ figure is 9,850 (obtained by subtraction).

Let us assume that the screening will be done by the Somogyi-Nelson method at random hours after eating with a level of 180 milligrams percent or higher considered to be positive. According to the "Diabetes Program Guide," the sensitivity percentage associated with this screening level is 22.9, and 99.8 is the specificity percentage (U.S. Public Health Service, 1960).

Since 22.9 percent of the diseased persons will be detected by the test, the number of diseased persons who will test positive (cell a) may be calculated by multiplying the number of diseased persons (150) by .229, yielding 34. The number of false negatives (cell c) is 150 minus 34, or 116.

Since the test is 99.8 percent specific, the number of true negatives that will be negative to the test is 9,850 multiplied by .998, or 9,830 (cell d). Subtracting cell d from the total negatives (9,850 minus 9,830) gives 20 as the number of false positives (cell b). The $a + b$ and $c + d$ total may then be obtained by adding across. The completed estimation is shown in Table 47–2.

The expected results of screening at a level of 180 mg. percent in this population may now be analyzed on the basis of the table. The program will yield an estimated 54 positives, which comprise the load that must be given diagnostic examinations. Of these, 20, or 37 percent, will be false positives, assuming the diagnostic criteria of the Boston Screening Evaluation Study (U.S. Public Health Service, 1960). Of the 150 diabetics in the population, 34 will be detected and 116 missed.

Suppose the administrator decides that such a program is not suitable for his community because of the large number of false negatives resulting from the use of such an insensitive screening level. He wants to examine the results expected from using a more sensitive level, knowing it will detect more cases but will result in a larger number of false positives.

TABLE 47–2.

Screening test results	True diagnosis Diabetic	Not diabetic	Total
Positive	34	20	54
Negative	116	9,830	9,946
Total	150	9,850	10,000

Let us assume a screening level of 130 milligrams percent. According to the "Diabetes Program Guide," this level has a sensitivity of 44.3 percent and a specificity of 99.0 percent. Using the techniques previously described, Table 47–3 expresses the results.

Comparing the estimated results of screening at 130 mg. with results at the previous level (180 mg.), the number of persons who would screen positive is 164 instead of 54. Under the new testing conditions, therefore, about three times as many persons will require diagnostic examinations. Of the 164 positives, 98 (compared with 20) will be false positives. This is almost a fivefold increase in false positives, and false positives now are 59.8 percent of total positives, as compared with 37.0 percent under the previous testing level. Of the 150 diabetics in the community, 66 will be detected (compared with 34), and 84 missed (instead of 116).

Next let us assume a situation in which the blood sugar distributions are similar to the previous example, but prevalence is 2.5 percent instead of 1.5 percent. The population to be tested now contains 250 diabetics instead of 150. If the screening level remains at 130 mg., the estimated results will be those presented in Table 47–4.

The number of persons testing positive is now 208, of which 97 (compared with 98) are false positives. The proportion of the positives that are false has been reduced from 59.8 to 46.6 percent. The same number of tests has yielded 111 new cases compared with 66 when the prevalence was 1.5 percent. With the sensitivity remaining constant, the gain in yield of new cases is proportional to the gain in prevalence.

Certain basic principles underlie the three illustrations. When the prevalence of a disease is low (in the order of 1.0 or 2.0 percent), as it is for many chronic diseases, most of the population will be free of the disease, and the positive results even for a highly sensitive and highly specific test will include a large proportion of false positives. A small decrease in the specificity of a test will greatly increase the number of false positives, and unless this is offset by a large gain in sensitivity, the proportion of positives that are false will increase or, at least, remain high. The effect on test results of various screening levels should, therefore, be carefully analyzed before a screening project is undertaken, especially when prevalence is low.

With a given sensitivity and specificity, a small increase in prevalence (1.0 or 2.0 percent) results in a negligible reduction in the number of false positives for the same number of tests, but the yield of new cases increases in proportion to the increase in prevalence. As a result, the proportion of false positives among persons screening positive is reduced.

By directing his screening efforts toward high prevalence groups which have been defined by epidemiological studies, the administrator can, in effect, raise prevalence in the group being screened. For example, he can limit a diabetes screening program to persons over 40 and make special efforts to screen obese persons and persons with a family history of diabetes. Screening thus becomes a two-stage process in which selection of a high prevalence group is the first stage and application of the screening test is the second.

Increasing prevalence by selection of the persons to be screened, however, may alter the distributions of the test attribute among the diseased and nondiseased populations and, likewise, the specificity-sensitivity pattern. Sensitivity-specificity data based on a general population study cannot be expected to apply in all instances to such a high prevalence population.

Chance Relationships

To be of value, a screening test must be able to select disease suspects from the screened population more frequently than would a process of purely random selection.

TABLE 47–3.

Screening test results	Diagnosis		Total
	Diabetic	Not diabetic	
Positive	66	98	164
Negative	84	9,752	9,836
Total	150	9,850	10,000

TABLE 47–4.

Screening test results	Diagnosis		Total
	Diabetic	Not diabetic	
Positive	111	97	208
Negative	139	9,653	9,792
Total	250	9,750	10,000

If the selection process were purely random with respect to diseased and nondiseased persons, the percent screening positive in the diseased group would equal the percent screening positive in the nondiseased group: in the terms of Table 47–1,

$$\frac{a}{a + c}$$

would equal

$$\frac{b}{b + d},$$

and together they would equal

$$\frac{a + b}{a + b + c + d}.$$

One can say that the results are purely random, then, if sensitivity

$$\left(\frac{a}{a + c}\right)$$

equals the percent positive

$$\left(\frac{a + b}{a + b + c + d}\right).$$

One can test whether a set of screening results differs significantly from chance by using the relatively simple statistical techniques discussed in the section on statistical evaluation.

When test results are purely random, the sensitivity percentage plus the specificity percentage add to 100 percent. This is so because the sensitivity percentage equals the percent positive in the nondiseased group when the selection process is purely random, and the percent positive and percent negative in the nondiseased group must add to 100 percent. Since the percent negative in that group is the specificity, it follows that the sensitivity plus the specificity percentages add to 100.

It also follows that if the test is perfectly selective, specificity equals 100 percent, sensitivity, 100 percent, and the two add to 200 percent. Youden has used this relationship as a basis for rating tests (Youden, 1950). Youden's index is the sensitivity proportion plus the specificity proportion minus one. This gives the index a range from zero to one.

Youden's index, however, assumes that sensitivity and specificity should be given equal weight in evaluating a screening test. For example, a test which is 40 percent sensitive and 90 percent specific has the same rating as a test which is 90 percent sensitive and 40 percent specific. This index is of limited value because, though it indicates whether test results are better than random selection, it does not evaluate sensitivity and specificity independently.

Dynamic versus Static Model

The formulations presented so far have dealt with disease in the static sense, that is, the populations have been dichotomized into diseased and nondiseased groups at some point of time. A different situation and model results if one considers the disease process as a stochastic (dynamic) process. Under this concept, the persons who fall into the overlap area of the two distributions and are assigned to the nondiseased group in the static model may actually be "pre" cases of the disease who will be assigned to the diseased category if a sufficient amount of time is allowed to pass. This is the concept of "prediabetes" or "borderline" hypertension. The development of sensitivity and specificity data for such a model requires that the persons screened be followed for a long period of time, say 5 or 10 years or longer, depending on the disease, to establish or rule out the diagnosis. Several studies of this type for the evaluation of screening tests are now in progress.

Combinations of Tests

Frequently the administrator will use a combination of screening tests to screen for a particular disease rather than a single test. The combination of tests may be used in "parallel" or in "series." When used in parallel, a screenee is considered positive if he tests positive to any one of the tests and negative if he tests negative to all tests. In series, the screenee must be positive to each successive test to be considered positive; if he is negative to any of the tests he is considered to have screened negative. The series technique is frequently used in diabetes and glaucoma screening programs and is referred to as retesting.

When used in parallel, the combination of tests is usually more sensitive but less specific (Kurlander et al., 1955). This occurs because some diseased persons are detected by one test but not the other, resulting in detection of a higher proportion of diseased persons by the combination of tests. Also, each test usually contributes independently to the combined total of false positives, thus reducing specificity.

TABLE 47-5.

Test results	Diabetic	Not diabetic
Positive to urine test, negative to blood	7	3
Positive to blood test, negative to urine	23	11
Positive to both tests	45	7
Negative to both tests	124	7,620
Total	199	7,641

Consider the hypothetical data presented in Table 47-5, assuming the test population to have been screened for diabetes using a blood sugar test and a urine sugar test.

The sensitivity of the urine test alone is computed by dividing all of the diabetic positives to this test (7 + 45) by the total diabetics (times 100) = 52/199 = 26.1 percent. The sensitivity of the blood test alone is computed by dividing all of the diabetic positives to this test (23 + 45) by the total diabetics (times 100) = 68/199 = 34.2 percent. For the combination of tests, sensitivity is computed by dividing the diabetic positives to either test alone or to both tests (7 + 23 + 45) by the total diabetics (times 100) = 75/199 = 37.7 percent. Combined sensitivity is larger than the sensitivity of either of the component tests.

By similar calculations, the specificity of the urine test is 99.9 percent, and the specificity of the blood test, 99.8 percent. However, for the combination of the two tests, specificity is calculated by dividing the figure for nondiabetics who were *negative to both tests* by the total nondiabetics (times 100). This is 7,620/7,641 = 99.7, a smaller figure than that for either test considered independently.

Similarly, it can be shown that in series, a combination of tests is usually less sensitive, but more specific. The reasoning process used by the physician in establishing a diagnosis may be conceived of as a group of test devices in a series-parallel arrangement.

Relative Sensitivity and Specificity

In some studies only persons who are positive to the screening test are given a diagnostic evaluation. Some of these positive screenees are found to be free of the disease at diagnosis, but without diagnosis it is not possible to classify persons who are negative to the test; therefore cells *c* and *d* of the fourfold classifica-

tion (Table 47-1) are indeterminate. If the assumption is made that all persons who are negative to the test are free of the disease, all of these cases will fall into cell *d,* and cell *c* will be empty. In this instance, sensitivity will be falsely stated to be 100 percent, and the specificity of the test will be overstated. A study of this type is obviously of little or no value.

In other studies, a battery of screening tests is used to screen for a disease, and persons who screen positive to any of the tests are given a diagnostic evaluation or are assumed to be truly diseased. In this type of study, some persons who are diseased are negative to one test and positive to others. For any one test, values fall into all four cells of the fourfold table if cell *d* is filled by assuming that persons negative to all of the tests are truly free of the disease. For purposes of comparison, sensitivity and specificity can be calculated for each of the tests, but these percentages should be referred to as "relative sensitivity and specificity" (Packer et al., 1960; Jolly et al., 1960). They are not true measures of sensitivity and specificity because some screenees have been incorrectly classified on the basis of the assumed diagnoses. The extent to which this procedure approximates a study of sensitivity and specificity based on diagnosis of the entire screening population depends on the ability of the battery of tests to classify screenees correctly. The procedure is a valid method for comparing techniques and is especially useful for comparing a new technique against a standard technique.

Specificity Based on a Sample

Although it was stated earlier that sensitivity and specificity should be established by a diagnostic evaluation of both negative and positive screenees, it would appear that some saving of time and money can be effected with only slight loss of reliability by establishing specificity on the basis of a sample of negative screenees.

Such a plan is undoubtedly feasible, but a fairly large sample may be required because the specificity percentage, based on a sample, should have rather narrow confidence limits to insure reliability. As illustrated previously, a small change in the specificity percentage results in a large change in the number of false positives because of the low prevalence of most chronic diseases, and the specificity percentage must be reliable to be useful. Determination of the appropriate sample size is beyond the scope of this paper.

Precision and Accuracy

Precision refers to the ability of a test to give consistent results in repeated trials, a quality also called "repeatibility" or "replicability." Any measurement of this quality is also affected by the ability of the tester to perform the test, and thus includes not only variation inherent in the test itself, but variation introduced by the skill of the tester.

Precision should be distinguished from accuracy, which is the ability of the test to give a true measurement of the item being tested.

The Folin-Wu test for blood glucose is an example of a test that can be precise but is not an accurate test for blood glucose. In the hands of a competent technician, repeated tests on paired blood samples by the Folin-Wu method can be made to yield consistent results, and the test therefore may be called precise. However, since reducing substances other than glucose are present in the blood and have the same effect on the test as glucose, the test always indicates a higher quantity of glucose than is actually present in the blood, and the test is not accurate. Because a test is inaccurate does not mean that it is useless. If the bias of a test is known, is relatively consistent, and is in one direction (plus or minus) only, an adjustment for bias can be made or a different level can be considered positive.

Measurement of Precision

In evaluating a screening test, it may be desirable to secure measurements of the precision of the test to assess the variability of the technique from person to person, laboratory to laboratory, one testing location to another, or from one period of time to another when performed by the same person, in the same laboratory, or at the same testing location. All of these situations can be evaluated by using slightly different modifications of an experimental design that consists basically of securing paired measurements of the same specimen or person.

For example, if one wishes to assess the precision of a laboratory testing blood for sugar, a number of blood specimens can be divided into paired subspecimens and submitted to the laboratory for measurement. The same technique can be used to assess the precision of the test in the hands of a particular technician. To avoid bias, it is important for the laboratory or technician not to know that an evaluation is being made, or at least to be unaware which are the paired specimens.

Caution must be exercised in conducting experiments of this type to insure that the method used to obtain a repeated measurement does not affect the test results. For example, repeated tonometric measurements tend to give progressively lower readings when made within short intervals of time because the weight of the tonometer plunger squeezes fluid from the eye, reducing the internal pressure (Goldmann, 1959). Storage of blood or other laboratory specimens may affect the results. One must also make sure that the specimens are really paired. For example, blood samples drawn from a single person at different times, or the repeating of a tonometric measurement on a single person on different days do not yield measurements that can be considered paired. Such measurements contain not only the variation inherent in the testing process, but biological variation as well.

The precision of a test can be approximated by calculating a standard deviation for each pair of measurements and pooling the standard deviations from several pairs of measurements to derive an average standard deviation.

It can be shown that where only two measurements are involved, the usual standard deviation formula reduces to

$$s = \sqrt{\frac{d^2}{2}},$$

where s is the standard deviation and d is the difference between the two measurements. The average or pooled standard deviation may be calculated by summing d^2 for the sample of paired measurements, dividing by twice the number of pairs ($2n$) and taking the square root of the answer. This formula is

$$s_p = \sqrt{\frac{\Sigma(d^2)}{2n}},$$

where s_p is the pooled standard deviation.

Table 47–6 presents hypothetical data on duplicate determinations of blood sugar in milligrams percent. There are 10 paired measurements, and $\Sigma(d^2)$ equals 236. The pooled standard deviation is

$$\sqrt{\frac{236}{2(10)}}, \text{ or } 3.44.$$

If it is assumed that there is no constant bias inherent in the measuring process, there is a 95 percent probability that a single observation varies from the true measurement by no more than 1.96 (or roughly 2) standard deviations.

TABLE 47-6.

Blood specimen	Determination I	Determination II	d	d^2
A	138	143	−5	25
B	127	123	+4	16
C	110	108	+2	4
D	122	120	+2	4
E	128	135	−7	49
F	133	139	−6	36
G	140	135	+5	25
H	152	150	+2	4
I	107	104	+3	9
J	111	119	−8	64
$n = 10$				$\Sigma(d^2) = 236$

It should be understood that this calculation measures only the precision of the test, not the accuracy (as previously defined). If a constant bias is inherent in the measuring process, this technique measures the ability of the test to give consistent measures of the true value plus (or minus) the constant bias.

This measurement of precision may be used to control the quality of output of a laboratory, testing station, or technician. On the basis of past experience or desired precision, a maximum allowable value can be assigned to the pooled standard deviation for a specified number of paired tests.

If at any time the calculated standard deviation exceeds the allowable limit, steps should be taken to determine the cause of the excessive variation, and corrective measures instituted.

Since the magnitude of the standard deviation is not independent of the mean of the values on which it is based, a further refinement of the data may be necessary where the mean values of the samples used in precision measurement for quality control can be expected to vary considerably, as in a laboratory where the blood of known diabetics may be processed on one day, and random screening samples on the next day. In situations of this type, a modified coefficient of variation should be calculated. This is the standard deviation as a percent of the mean of all of the values in the sample, or

$$c_v = \frac{s_p(100),}{\bar{\bar{X}},}$$

where c_v is the coefficient of variation, s_p the pooled standard deviation of the data, and $\bar{\bar{X}}$ the grand mean.

This calculation assumes that the magnitude of the standard deviation is directly proportional to the mean of the measurements upon which it is based. If this is true, the calculation will adjust for the differences in the magnitude of the means. This situation is rarely true over all possible mean values, and the coefficient of variation will sometimes result in only a partial correction, and in some instances in overcorrection. Use of this measure must therefore be based on a knowledge of the relationship of the magnitude of the mean to the standard deviation.

The calculation of the coefficient of variation for the precision data previously presented is shown below:

$$\text{The grand mean} = \bar{\bar{X}} = \frac{\Sigma X}{n}$$

$$\bar{\bar{X}} = \frac{2,544}{20}$$

$$\bar{\bar{X}} = 127.2$$

$$\text{The coefficient of variation} = \frac{s_p \times 100}{\bar{\bar{X}}}$$

$$c_v = \frac{3.4 \times 100}{127.2}$$

$$c_v = 2.7\%$$

The coefficient of variation may be used as a quality control measure in the same manner as the pooled standard deviation.

For tests that are read qualitatively, the calculation of precision can be made by designating all positive tests as one, and all negative tests as zero. The measure derived in this process has no meaning in terms of confidence limits, but it can be used in quality control work or for comparisons of precision.

More comprehensive presentations of quality control methods in the laboratory making use of the standard deviation and the range can be found in Benson and Freier (1960), Levey and Jennings (1950), Wernimont (1946), Freier and Rausch (1958), and others.

II. STATISTICAL EVALUATION OF SENSITIVITY, SPECIFICITY, AND PRECISION

In comparing testing techniques, problems are frequently encountered that can be handled with fairly simple statistical methods. This section reviews some of the basic techniques applicable to the more common problems and presents illustrative calculations. Since this paper is intended for use by persons who do not have extensive statistical training, the more complex methods of analysis are not illustrated.

Reliability of Sensitivity and Specificity

The standard error of a percentage based on a sample is an indication of the extent to which the sample percentage can be expected to vary from the percentage of the population from which the sample was drawn because of random variation inherent in the sampling process. The results obtained from sensitivity and specificity studies, assuming the tested population is randomly drawn from the general population, can be treated as samples from an infinite population, because the potential population to which the test may be applied is extremely large, if not infinite.

The method of assessing reliability is to compute a standard error and to place confidence limits around the sample percentage at a specified level of probability, according to an acceptable sampling distribution, by use of the standard error.

The standard error of the sensitivity or specificity proportion can be calculated by use of the formula

$$s = \sqrt{\frac{pq}{n}}$$

where s is the standard error, p is the sensitivity (or specificity) proportion, q equals $1 - p$, and n is the sample size or base of the proportion.

In most instances the normal curve may be used as the basis for confidence limits, and, as an approximation, one can say that the chances are 95 out of 100 that the true sensitivity or specificity percentage is no larger than the sample percentage plus 1.96 (or roughly 2) standard errors, or no smaller than the sample percentage minus 1.96 (or roughly 2) standard errors (95 percent confidence limits).

If the sample size (n) is small, say less than 30, more accurate confidence limits can be placed on the sample proportion by using the distribution of t found in any standard statistical text.

The n in the t table refers to "degrees of freedom" rather than sample size. In this instance the degrees of freedom are the sample size minus 1. The standard error should be multiplied by the table t value rather than by 1.96 to set the confidence limits at the appropriate significance level. For the 95 percent confidence limits use the $p = .05$ column.

If the sample percentage is close to 100 or 0, and n is small, the normal and t distributions do not apply. Confidence limits can be placed on the sample percentage indirectly by use of tables of the binomial distribution. Tables of the binomial are available from the Government Printing Office (National Bureau of Standards, 1950). A table with selected values of n given directly in percentages appears in Snedecor's "Statistical Methods" (Snedecor, 1956).

Evaluation Against a Standard

Dunn and Greenhouse have presented a method of evaluating sensitivity and specificity against an arbitrarily set standard (U.S. Public Health Service, 1950). The standard chosen for cancer tests in their presentation is a sensitivity of 90 percent and specificity of 95 percent. The method assumes that test values of the diseased and nondiseased populations are normally distributed, and that the mean test value for the diseased population is larger than the mean for the nondiseased population. The evaluation is then based on the overlap area pattern of the two curves.

To study the overlap area, the test value that will be exceeded by 5 percent of the nondiseased persons (termed the "critical" value) is determined from the mean and standard deviation of that distribution by reference to a table of area under the normal curve. The critical test value that will be exceeded by 90 percent of the diseased persons is similarly determined. If the critical test value determined for the diseased population equals or exceeds the critical test value determined for the nondiseased population, the overlap area pattern of the two curves is such that test values between the two critical values can be selected which will result in a sensitivity of at least 90 percent and a specificity of at least 95 percent for the test. If the critical value for the diseased population is lower than the critical value for the nondiseased population, there is too much overlap between the two curves to permit the selection of a test level which meets the criterion of 90 percent sensitivity and 95 percent specificity.

For the combined sensitivity-specificity standard, Dunn and Greenhouse also present a method of testing the statistical significance of obtained critical values where the results are close. Their method relies heavily on the assumption of normality for the distribution of test values, a condition frequently not met by biological data. The method should not be applied unless the distributions of diseased and nondiseased persons are approximately normal. Also, the standards of 90 percent sensitivity and 95 percent specificity have rarely been achieved in practice. However, their method can be adapted to other combinations of sensitivity-specificity as standards. An advantage of the method is that it evaluates the screening test without dependence on the selection of a test level, provided the assumption of normality holds.

An alternate approach to evaluation against a standard that does not depend upon a normal distribution is to compute the sensitivity and specificity values for various test levels and compare the observed results against the selected standard sensitivity and specificity percentages. If the observed percentages are greater than the standard, no test of statistical significance is required. If an observed percentage is less than the standard, the significance of this difference can be evaluated by setting up the hypothesis that the observed and standard percentages are truly equal and the difference is no greater than an amount compatible with sampling variation.

This hypothesis can be tested by dividing the difference between the observed and the standard percentages by the standard error of the observed percentages and making reference to a table of t. (The standard percentage has no standard error.) Since only the probability of obtaining an observed percentage as small or smaller than the standard because of sampling variation is to be tested, a "one-tailed" test is used, and the 5 percent probability is read from the 0.1 column of the t table. If the difference between the observed percentage and the standard percentage is equal to or greater than 1.645 (or the appropriate t value for the sample size) times the standard error of the observed percentage, the hypothesis that the difference is compatible with sampling variation is rejected and the observed percentage is considered significantly different from the standard. If the converse is true and the difference between the observed and standard percentages is no larger than can be expected from sampling variation, the test is considered to have met the standard.

Comparing Results of Two Test Techniques

Frequently an objective of a study is comparison of the results of one screening test against another. An approach sometimes used to make this comparison is to compute the "percentage of agreements" between the two tests—that is, the percent of test results, whether negative or positive, agreed upon by both tests. This approach has definite disadvantages. It does not evaluate the qualities of sensitivity and specificity, and since most of the population tested will not be diseased, it becomes an evaluation based chiefly on the comparability of negative results. Two widely differing tests may have a big "percentage of agreement" on the basis of negatives alone if the prevalence of the disease is small enough.

A more productive approach is to compare the sensitivity and specificity percentages of the two tests. For tests that are read quantitatively, the sensitivity percentages should be compared while specificity percentages are held constant for both tests, and the specificity percentages compared while sensitivity values are held constant. An alternative is to compare the sensitivity percentages for the maximum achievable specificity of each test, or to compare the specificity for the maximum achievable sensitivity of each test.

If, at comparable levels of specificity, one test is substantially more sensitive, and at comparable levels of sensitivity it is also more specific, it is obviously a better test. If one test has a higher sensitivity than the other at some levels of specificity and a lower sensitivity at other levels of specificity, the administrator must choose between the two tests on the basis of the size of the differences and the attribute (sensitivity or specificity) which is most important to him in his screening situation. In either case, other factors such as relative cost and ease of performance also must be considered. If one test appears to be better on the basis of a higher sensitivity or specificity, statistical techniques can be used to indicate whether the observed difference in sensitivity or specificity is probably due to chance variation inherent in the sampling process or to other causes.

It should be understood that statistical significance tests merely assess the effect of sampling variation on the screening test results; they do not indicate the superiority of one screening test over another. This is a value judgment. If a statistically significant difference is found between two test sensitivities, it merely means that the difference is probably not due to sampling. It does not mean, in itself, that the difference is of practical importance in a screening program. If the difference is not significantly different, it means that the observed difference is no larger than may be expected to occur by chance in a sample of this size. If the sample size is reasonably large, the usual interpretation is that there is essentially no difference in the percentages.

The Significance of Differences

In the comparison of sensitivity and specificity percentages for two tests, there are two situations, and each requires a different statistical approach. In the first situation, sensitivity and specificity percentages result from applying the two tests to different popu-

lations; these are "statistically independent" percentages. In the second situation, the tests are applied to the same population, that is, each person in the population is tested twice, once by each test technique, resulting in paired observations. These are "correlated," or "nonindependent" percentages.

Editors' Note: We have deleted the final four pages of text and a four-page appendix, all concerned with additional statistical evaluation of screening tests. Advanced students and professionals involved in program evaluations should consult the original version of this monograph.

REFERENCES

Benson, E. S., and Freier, E. F. Quality control. Part I. *Postgrad. Med., 28:* A–38–A–43, October 1960. Quality control. Part II. *Postgrad. Med., 28:* A–38–A–47, November 1960.

Blumberg, M. S. Evaluating health screening procedures. *Operations Research, 5:* 351–360, June 1957.

Comstock, G. W., and Porter, M. E. Tuberculin sensitivity and tuberculosis among natives of the Lower Yukon. *Pub. Health Rep., 74:* 621–634, July 1959.

Freier, E. F., and Rausch, V. L. Quality control in clinical chemistry. *Am. J. Med. Tech., 24:* 195–207, July–August 1958.

Goldmann, H. Some basic problems of simple glaucoma. *Am. J. Ophth., 48:* 213–220, September 1959.

Jolly, J. J.; White, W. V.; Portnoy, J.; and Gutridge, J. W. Blood sugar and syphilis serology using a single specimen. *Pub. Health Rep., 75:* 115–118, February 1960.

Kurlander, A. B.; Hill, E. H.; and Enterline, P. E. An evaluation of some commonly used screening tests for heart disease and hypertension. *J. Chronic Dis., 2:* 427–439, October 1955.

Levey, S., and Jennings, E. R. The use of control charts in the clinical laboratory. *Am. J. Clin. Path., 20:* 1,059–1,066, November 1950.

McNemar, Q. Psychological statistics, 2nd ed. New York: John Wiley & Sons, Inc., 1955, ch. 5, pp. 56–61, ch. 13, pp. 228–231.

National Bureau of Standards. Tables of binomial probability distribution. Washington, D.C., U.S. Government Printing Office, 1950.

Packer, H.; Ackerman, R. F.; and Hawkins, J. M. Screening for diabetes with the clinitron. *Pub. Health Rep., 75:* 1,020–1,024, November 1960.

Snedecor, G. W. Statistical methods, 5th ed. Ames, Iowa: Iowa State College Press, 1956, pp. 4–5.

U.S. Public Health Service. Cancer diagnostic tests, principles and criteria for development and evaluation. PHS Publication No. 9, Washington, D.C., U.S. Government Printing Office, 1950.

U.S. Public Health Service. Diabetes program guide. PHS Publication No. 506. Washington, D.C., U.S. Government Printing Office, revised 1960.

Wernimont, G. Use of control charts in the analytical laboratory. *Indust. Engin. & Chem., analyt. ed., 18:* 587–592, October 1946.

Youden, W. J. Index for rating diagnostic tests. *Cancer, 3:* 32–35, January 1950.

48

Guidelines for Identification Audiometry

COMMITTEE ON AUDIOMETRIC EVALUATION,
AMERICAN SPEECH-LANGUAGE-HEARING
ASSOCIATION

The set of *Guidelines for Identification Audiometry* is the second of a series developed by the Committee on Audiometric Evaluation, under the Office of Vice-President for Clinical Affairs of the American Speech and Hearing Association (ASHA).

Each of the guidelines presents a recommended set of procedures based on existing clinical practice and research findings. The spirit of these guidelines is not to mandate a single way of accomplishing the clinical process; rather the intent is to suggest standard procedures that, in the final analysis, will benefit the persons we serve. The intention is to improve interclinician and interclinic comparison of data thereby allowing for a more effective transfer of information.

The specific purpose of these guidelines is to detail procedures for accomplishing rapid and efficient identification of hearing impairment, particularly for use with young children.[1] As such, they represent an update of the procedures for identification audiometry for school-age children specified in the *Journal of Speech and Hearing Disorders* Monograph Supplement Number 9, "Identification Audiometry" (Darley, 1961). The current need for these guidelines is apparent with the development of increasing numbers of identification audiometry programs administered by state departments of education or health, the development of state mandatory special education statutes, and Medicaid guidelines for Early and Periodic Screening, Diagnosis, and Treatment (EPSDT).

Editor's Note: The set of "Guidelines for Identification Audiometry" was approved by the ASHA Legislative Council in November 1974. The following members of the ASHA Committee on Audiometric Evaluation developed these guidelines: J. B. Chaiklin, N. T. Hopkinson, J. T. Graham, Z. G. Shoeny, F. L. Sonday, V. W. Byers, R. M. McLauchlin, and W. R. Wilson, Chairman. ASHA encourages the professional community to use these guidelines in clinical practice.—K. O. J.

Reprinted by permission of the American Speech-Language-Hearing Association from *ASHA, 17,* 94–99 (1975).

For the most part, the philosophy and procedures laid out in these guidelines are based on and supported by published data. ASHA invites data-based input for future modifications of the guidelines.

SCOPE

A primary goal of identification audiometry using pure-tone air-conduction stimulation is to identify persons who have hearing impairments that interfere with or that have potential for interfering with communication. These guidelines focus on use with children of nursery-school age through grade three because early identification of communicative problems in this age group will permit maximum habilitation and avoidance of potential educational problems. Belkin, et. al. (1964) have reported successful large scale individual pure-tone screening tests with children as young as three years of age. In addition, it is this age group which, in our society, is most often involved in the formal educational process through preschools and regular schools. While these guidelines focus on use with young children, they are equally applicable for use with older children and adults.

The guidelines are designed for rapid and efficient identification of hearing impairment. A basic assumption behind the guidelines is that identification audiometry is usually conducted in the relatively poor acoustic environments of schools and offices. Consequently, the procedures recommended are designed to be robust enough to be valid in a wide range of test settings. Naturally, it would be desirable for all identification audiometry to be conducted in acoustic environments that are controlled, but such environments are seldom available.

Identification audiometry is only one component of a hearing conservation program. A well-balanced program will include screening, rescreening, threshold audiometry, referrals for audiologic and medical evaluations, education and habilitation planning, and counseling for parents and teachers. Too often the sole goal is referral for medical evaluation rather than referral for consideration of communicative needs of those who fail screening procedures. Once people have been identified by the program, they should be followed regularly to insure that their communication and medical needs are met. It is pointless to identify people who have hearing impairments unless there is a concurrent follow-up program to handle their habilitative, educational, and medical needs.

Finally, these guidelines apply only to the use of pure-tone air-conduction screening for the purpose of identifying persons who have hearing impairment that interferes with or that has the potential for interfering with communication. Research (Eagles, 1961; Eagles, Wishik, and Doerfler, 1967; Roberts, 1972) demonstrates that pure-tone air-conduction screening is inefficient for the purpose of identifying many persons who have conductive ear pathology. Thus, if the purpose of an identification audiometry program is also to identify persons with conductive ear pathology, ASHA suggests the simultaneous use of otologic screenings, or supplemental procedures such as impedance (otoadmittance) measurements or pure-tone bone-conduction measurements. However, ASHA cannot specify any standardized screening procedures that employ impedance or bone-conduction measures because sufficient research data on such procedures are unavailable at the present time.

IDENTIFICATION AUDIOMETRY

The following recommendations emphasize identification audiometry for children using a manually administered, individual, pure-tone air-conduction screening procedure.

Children to Be Screened

Individual limited-frequency screening should be administered annually to children of nursery-school age through grade three and to high-risk children.[2] The time the program saves by emphasizing the lower grades permits appropriate attention for the high-risk group and focuses the program's efforts during the years when identification of communication problems can lead to intervention that will forestall serious educational, psychological, and social problems. Some school systems may elect to screen routinely after grade three at three- or four-year intervals (Darley, 1961). Others may find that a cost vs benefit analysis does not justify routine screening beyond grade three (Downs, Doster, and Wever, 1965). To determine the merit of routine screening after grade three, more data appear to be necessary.

Procedure

Individual Screening. Individual as opposed to group screening is recommended. The Massachusetts Test (Johnston, 1948) is an example of a group pure-tone test that achieved great popularity and is still used in some states. It requires written responses and, consequently, like most group screening tests is limited to children above the second grade. Other limitations of group tests are calibration and maintenance problems of multiple earphones, increased set-up time and excessive time spent in retesting false-positive failures. All of these factors combine to increase the total time required for the screening program without increasing accuracy. Many group tests may appear to save time but the time taken to set up, check calibration, score answer sheets, and retest excessive failures may result in no saving of time.

Manual Method. A manual versus an automatic method is recommended because it is applicable with children down to three years of age. There is no known evidence that a self-recording or other type of automatic method is possible and effective with young children. Certainly, if an effective and more rapid automatic method is developed, its use should be considered.

Signal

Type. Pure-tone signals shall be used. Many different stimuli have been used to screen children and adults for the purpose of identifying persons with hearing impairment. Before audiometers were widely available, phonograph recordings were used to produce repeatable stimuli as in the Western Electric Fading Numbers Test. The Fading Numbers Test had a variety of defects: the most notable was its tendency to pass children with hearing deficits in the range above 500 Hz. Other screening tests that employ speech signals are vulnerable to the same defect.

Test Frequencies. Test frequencies shall be 1,000 Hz, 2,000 Hz, and 4,000 Hz. The Conference on Identification Audiometry (Darley, 1961) recommended the frequencies 1,000, 2,000, 4,000, and 6,000 Hz. The recommendation for 500 Hz was ambiguous but the conference's intent appears to have been to eliminate 500 Hz except for very quiet test environments.

Melnick, Eagles, and Levine (1964), in a study which tested the conference's recommendations, used 500 Hz; however, all of their tests were conducted inside double-walled audiometric rooms. Melnick, Eagles, and Levine found that the conference's recommended test was highly efficient except at 6,000 Hz, which produces too many failures. The variable interactions between earphones and ears at 6,000 Hz (Villchur, 1970) among other considerations, make 6,000 Hz a poor choice for inclusion in an identification audiometry program. The use of 500 Hz in order to assure the user that he will discover all middle ear pathologies in a group of children is contraindicated by the hard data that are available (Eagles, 1961; Eagles, Wishik, and Doerfler, 1967; Roberts, 1972).

When an inordinate number of failures is expected at 4,000 Hz, then 3,000 Hz at 20 dB HL might be considered as the alternate test signal. There are insufficient research data available at the present time to validate routine inclusion of 3,000 Hz.[3]

Screening Levels. Screening levels shall be 20 dB HL (re: ANSI-1969) at 1,000 Hz and 2,000 Hz and 25 dB HL at 4,000 Hz. It is acceptable to screen at 20 dB HL at all three frequencies, but if 4,000 Hz is not heard, output should be increased to 25 dB HL. Since most children will hear all three tones at 20 dB, the hearing level dial can remain at one setting for the entire test. It is important to remember, however, that 25 dB is the specified level at 4,000 Hz.[4]

Results

Failure Criterion. Failure to respond at the recommended screening levels at any frequency in either ear shall constitute failure.

Mandatory Rescreening. All failures should be rescreened preferably within the same session in which they failed but definitely within one week after the initial screening. Removing and repositioning the phones, accompanied by careful reinstruction, markedly reduces the number of failures. Wilson and Walton (1974) reported a 52 percent reduction in failures by rescreening. The rescreening, using the same frequencies, levels, and failure criterion, is an essential procedure for improving the efficiency of a screening program.

Disposition of Failures. Failures on rescreening should be referred for audiologic evaluation by an audiologist. Some persons, particularly young children, will fail both the screening and rescreening procedures and then yield normal thresholds on an audiometric evaluation. Therefore, a hearing impairment should not be considered identified until after receiving an audiometric evaluation by an audiologist. An example of a program employing this referral format has been described by Campanelli, Krucoff, and DiLosa (1964). The following referral priority for audiologic evaluation is recommended for those children who fail the screening and rescreening procedures:

1. Binaural loss in both ears at all frequencies
2. Binaural loss at 1,000 and 2,000 Hz only
3. Binaural loss at 1,000 or 2,000 Hz only
4. Monaural loss at all frequencies
5. Monaural loss at 1,000 and 2,000 Hz.
6. Binaural or monaural loss at 4,000 Hz only.

The constraints placed on individual programs will determine the referral format, but the hearing conservation program supervisor should be responsible for providing case management necessary to guarantee appropriate referral for audiologic and medical consultation. In addition, the supervisor should secure educational assistance, if necessary, for students during and after medical therapy or audiologic habilitation. These duties are emphasized because the primary goal of school hearing conservation programs is to reduce the negative effects of communicative problems that are secondary to hearing loss, rather than simply to identify children who pass or fail a screening test.

PROCEDURAL CONSIDERATIONS

Adherence to the following procedural recommendations should facilitate successful implementation of the ASHA guidelines for identification audiometry.

Personnel

Identification audiometry programs should be conducted or supervised by an audiologist. After appropriate training, support personnel may administer audiometric screenings and rescreenings under the supervision of an audiologist. If properly trained professionals are not involved in supervising an identification audiometry program, an inordinate number of false-positive failures and false-negative passes may occur, thus undermining the validity of the program. Without reservation, the audiologic evaluation should be administered by an audiologist.

Instructions

Instructions are critical in all audiometric procedures but particular care must be taken in instructing children. Instructions should emphasize the importance of responding "right away even when the beeps sound far away." Groups of children can be instructed at one time. Those waiting for the test profit from watching others being tested. Pantomime may have to accompany verbal instructions for the very young child or the difficult-to-test person, particularly if a conditioned play response is required rather than a hand or verbal response. Careful reinstruction is an important part of the rescreening process. Frequently children fail because they have misunderstood instructions. This is particularly true of children in the three- to six-year age range.

Time

At the third-grade level the entire screening, including earphone placement, occupies less than one minute. For younger children more time may be necessary. To avoid unnecessary failures with younger children, it is sometimes desirable to present more than one signal per frequency if there is no response. The net effect is a saving of time because the more careful screening process reduces the number of children who fail and require rescreening.

Acoustic Environment

The acoustic environment is an important variable in screening audiometry. Usually school environments are not too noisy for screening at frequencies above 1,000 Hz, but sometimes ambient noise will interfere with screening at 1,000 Hz. The 1,000-Hz to 4,000-Hz range was selected for the ASHA guidelines because it is less vulnerable to invalidation by ambient noise and because most significant hearing impairment will include failure in this range. The allowable ambient noise levels in the region of the test tone are shown in Table 48-1. Although screening at 500 Hz is not recommended, there is nothing inherently wrong in screening at 500 Hz in an appropriate environment such as double-wall test room (Melnick, Eagles, and Levine, 1964). If an individual wishes to include 500 Hz, the allowable ambient noise levels are also included in Table 48-1.

Careful snug placement of the earphones increases attenuation of ambient noise by the earphone-cushion assembly. On the other hand, ASHA does not encourage the use of large sound-attenuating circumaural earphone assemblies (for example, Auraldomes and Otocups). Below 1,000 Hz, these devices provide limited improvement in attenuation of ambient noise relative to the attenuation produced by the MX-41/AR cushion (Webster, 1954; Cox, 1955; Benson, 1971). The advantage provided above 1,000

TABLE 48-1. APPROXIMATE ALLOWABLE OCTAVE BAND AMBIENT NOISE LEVELS (SPL RE: 20 MICROPASCALS FOR THRESHOLD MEASUREMENTS AT ZERO HL (RE: ANSI-1969) AND FOR SCREENING AT THE ASHA RECOMMENDED LEVELS (RE: ANSI-1969). IN TEST ENVIRONMENTS THAT HAVE FLUCTUATING NOISE LEVELS, CAUTION MUST BE USED IN APPLYING THE MAXIMUM VALUES SHOWN IN THIS TABLE. THE COMMITTEE HAS USED THE BEST INFORMATION AVAILABLE IN THE LITERATURE TO SUPPORT THE LEVELS, AND IS BASING ITS RECOMMENDATION ON THESE LEVELS UNTIL ADDITIONAL INFORMATION IS AVAILABLE.

Test Frequency	500	1,000	2,000	4,000
Octave-Band Cutoff	300	600	1,200	2,400
Frequencies	600	1,200	2,400	4,800
Allowable ambient noise for threshold at Zero HL (re: ANSI-1969)*	26	30	38	51
Plus ASHA screening level re: ANSI-1969	20	20	20	25
Resultant maximum ambient noise allowable for ASHA screening	46	50	58	76

*The allowable ambient noise levels for ANSI-1969 Zero HL threshold measurements were calculated by subtracting from the maximum allowable noise levels specified in the ANSI standard (S3.1, 1960) the difference between the ANSI-1951 and ANSI-1969 standards for pure-tone audiometers. In effect, the lower SPLs specified at Zero HL in the 1969 standard require quieter test spaces to measure normal listeners' thresholds.

Editors' note: Although Table 48-1 shows allowable noise levels for screening at 500 Hz the Guidelines do *not* recommend 500 Hz as a screening frequency. The values shown for 500 Hz apply only in relatively quiet environments.

Hz is not needed because ambient noise is generally weak above 1,000 Hz and the MX-41/AR cushion provides relatively good attenuation of the weak high-frequency ambient noise. Furthermore, the large earphone assemblies are awkward for small children, and they increase test-retest variability in the higher frequencies.

Some persons have mistakenly assumed that sound-attenuating headsets eliminate the need for a quiet test environment, or worse, that they substitute for a sound-isolated audiometric test booth. In extremely noisy environments an audiometric test booth is often the only means of providing an environment quiet enough for screening audiometry. The sound-attenuating headsets provide the least benefit in the frequency range where it is needed most.

Audiometric Equipment and Calibration

Audiometers used for screening purposes shall meet the ANSI S3.6-1969 requirements for either a limited-range or narrow-range audiometer. Audiometers used for audiometric evaluation shall meet the ANSI S3.6-1969 requirements for a wide-range audiometer. Audiometric calibration to ANSI S3.6-1969 specifications should occur regularly, at least once every year, following the initial determination that the audiometer meets specifications.[5] All of the ANSI specifications should be met, not just sound pressure level. Frequency errors, overshoot, and transient clicks are just a few of the problems that may invalidate a screening test. The sound pressure output of each audiometer should be checked at least every three months (preferably more often) in a 6 cc coupler. In addition, a daily listening check should be performed to determine that the audiometer is grossly in calibration and that no defects exist in major components.

Reports to Parents

Recommendations for audiologic and medical evaluations should be based on local realities. The language used in notices sent to parents about screening or rescreening results should avoid diagnostic conclusions and alarming predictions. Remember that the hearing impairment is not confirmed until the audiometric evaluation is administered. Personal contact would be preferable to sending notices, if possible. Some persons become overly concerned, others express no concern, and still others would like to co-

operate but fear the expense that may be involved. If parents believe that their child can "hear," despite what a hearing screening suggests, tact and persuasion will be required to convince them that they may be in error. The word "fail" probably should be avoided in reporting screening results. The reporting aspect of programs for identification audiometry requires more time and thought than some programs have provided in the past.

SUMMARY

ASHA recommends a manually administered, individual, pure-tone, air-conduction screening procedure for accomplishing identification audiometry. The purpose of this procedure is to identify rapidly and effectively those persons with hearing impairment that interferes with communication or that has the potential for interfering with communication. The procedure is designed to be used with children as young as three years old, although it is applicable for use with adults.

The recommended identification audiometry procedure is as follows. Audiometric screening should be at 20 dB HL (re: ANSI-1969) at the frequencies of 1,000 Hz and 2,000 Hz and 25 dB HL at 4,000 Hz. Failure to respond at the screening level at one or more frequencies in either ear is the criterion for failure. An audiometric rescreening should be administered the same day or no later than within one week to all persons failing the initial screening. An audiologist should administer an audiologic evaluation to persons failing the rescreening. If a hearing impairment is identified by audiometric evaluation, referrals should be made to meet the person's habilitative, educational, and medical needs.

Several procedural considerations are vital to implementing successfully the ASHA *Guidelines for Identification Audiometry.* An audiologist should conduct or supervise an identification audiometry program, although nonprofessional support personnel may be used for the screening procedures after appropriate training. Careful instructions are very important, particularly for young children. Ambient noise levels should not exceed 50 dB SPL at 1,000 Hz, 58 dB SPL at 2,000 Hz, and 76 dB SPL at 4,000 Hz using a sound level meter with octave band filters centered on the screening frequencies. Audiometric equipment should initially meet all the ANSI S3.6-

1969 specifications and be rechecked at least annually. The sound pressure output at the phones should be checked at least every three months, and listening checks for any gross malfunctions should be made daily. Finally, appropriate reporting of screening results should avoid diagnostic conclusions and encourage further evaluation for persons not passing the screening procedures.

Note: When the following standards referred to in this document are superseded by an approved revision, the revision shall apply:

1. American National Standard Specifications for Audiometers S3.6-1969; and
2. American Standard Criteria for Background Noise in Audiometer Rooms S3.1-1960.

ENDNOTES

1. The *Guidelines for Identification Audiometry* is written with emphasis on the testing of children; however, the approach is also appropriate for use with adults. A method of identification audiometry using a tracking procedure, sometimes called self-recording monitoring audiometry, is also used with adults in military and industrial settings. ASHA considers *Guidelines for Identification Audiometry Using a Threshold Tracking Procedure* deserving of a separate document. When the writing task is undertaken ASHA recommends that representatives of military and industrial groups should be included.

2. Examples of high-risk children are those who: (1) repeat a grade, (2) require special education programs, (3) are new to the school system, (4) were absent during a previously scheduled screening exam, (5) failed a threshold test during the previous year, (6) have speech problems, language problems, or obvious difficulty in communication, (7) are suspected of hearing impairment or have a medical problem associated with hearing impairment (children with recurrent or chronic problems such as allergies may require audiometric monitoring).

Additional examples of high-risk children are given in Darley (1961, p. 36).

3. ASHA invites active research on the addition of 3,000 Hz to the screening format. Research studies also would be helpful to determine whether 3,000 Hz could be substituted for 4,000 Hz as a better predictor of subtle communicative problems among school-age children.

4. ASHA is interested in active research concerning screening levels, since there is a great deal of strong feeling expressed concerning the issue, but very little hard data are available.

5. Studies on audiometer calibration suggest that, upon receipt, most audiometers may never have been in complete calibration (Eagles and Doerfler, 1961; Thomas, et al., 1969; Walton and Williams, 1972). This information underscores the importance of initial calibration of audiometers, and indicates that they should be checked to meet ANSI specifications before they are used in a screening program. It has been shown that when specifications are met initially, the audiometers generally remain stable (Walton and Wilson, 1974).

REFERENCES

American National Standard Specifications for Audiometers (ANSI S3.6-1969). New York: American National Standards Institute, Inc. (1970).

American Standard Criteria for Background Noise in Audiometer Rooms (ANSI S3.1-1960). New York: American National Standards Institute, Inc. (1960).

American Standard Specification for Audiometers for General Diagnostic Purposes (ANSI Z24.5-1951). New York: American National Standards Institute, Inc. (1951).

Belkin, M.; Suchman, E.; Bergman, M.; Rosenblatt, D.; and Jacobziner, H. A demonstration program for conducting hearing tests in day care centers. *J. Speech Hearing Dis.,* 29, 335–338 (1964).

Benson, R. "Auraldomes" for audiometric testing. *Nat. Hearing Aid J.,* 24, 14, 42 (1971).

Campanelli, P.; Krucoff, M.; and DiLosa, L. Hearing-screening of school children. *Med. Ann Dist. of Columbia,* 33, 309–314 (1964).

Cox, J. How quiet must it be to measure normal hearing? *Noise Control,* 1, 25–29 (1955).

Darley, F. (ed.) Identification audiometry. *J. Speech Hearing Dis.,* Mono. Suppl. 9 (1961).

Downs, M.; Doster, M.; and Wever, M. Dilemmas in identification audiometry. *J. Speech Hearing Dis.,* 30, 360–364 (1965).

Eagles, E. Hearing levels in children and audiometer performance. Appendix B in *J. Speech Hearing Dis.,* Mono. Suppl. 9 (F. Darley, Ed.) 52–62 (1961).

Eagles, E. and Doerfler, L. A study of hearing in children: II. Acoustic environment and audiometer performance. *Trans. Amer. Acad. Ophthal. Otolaryng.,* 283–296 (1961).

Eagles, E.; Wishik, S.; and Doerfler, L. *Hearing Sensitivity and Ear Disease in Children: A Prospective Study.* St. Louis: The Laryngoscope, 274 pp. (Tables pp. 146 and 163) (1967).

Johnston, P. The Massachusetts Hearing Test. *J. Acoust. Soc. Amer.,* **20,** 697–703 (1948).

Jordan, R. and Eagles, E. The relation of air conduction audiometry to otological abnormalities. *Ann. Otol. Rhinol.,* **70,** 819–827 (1961).

Melnick, W.; Eagles, E.; and Levine, H. Evaluation of a recommended program of identification audiometry with school-age children. *J. Speech Hearing Dis.,* **29,** 3–13 (1964).

Roberts, J. Hearing sensitivity and related medical findings among children in the United States. *Trans., Amer. Acad. Ophthal. Otolaryng.,* 355–359 (1972).

Thomas, W.; Preslar, M.; Summers, R.; and Stewart, J. Calibration and working condition of 100 audiometers, *Pub. Hlth. Rep., Wash.,* **84,** 311–327 (1969).

Villchur, E. Audiometer-earphone mounting to improve inter-subject and cushion-fit reliability. *J. Acoust. Soc. Amer.,* **48,** 1,387–1,396 (1970).

Walton, W. and Williams, P. Stability of routinely serviced portable audiometers, *Lang. Speech Hearing Serv. Schools,* **3,** 36–43 (1972).

Walton, W. and Wilson, W. Stability of pure-tone audiometers during periods of heavy use in identification audiometry. *Lang. Speech Hearing Serv. Schools,* **5,** 8–12 (1974).

Wilson, W. and Walton, W. Identification audiometry accuracy: Evaluation of a recommended program for school-age children, *Lang. Speech Hearing Serv. Schools,* **5,** 132–142 (1974).

Webster, J. Hearing losses of aircraft repair shop personnel. *J. Acoust. Soc. Amer.,* **26,** 782–787 (1954).

49

Guidelines for Acoustic Immittance Screening of Middle-Ear Function

COMMITTEE ON AUDIOMETRIC EVALUATION, AMERICAN SPEECH-LANGUAGE-HEARING ASSOCIATION

BACKGROUND

A Committee on Audiometric Evaluation was established in 1971 by the Legislative Council for purposes of (1) studying procedural techniques and electro-acoustic characteristics of audiometric instruments used in the evaluation of auditory function, and (2) developing guidelines applicable for the practice of clinical audiometry. In 1974, the Committee's "Guidelines for Identification Audiometry" were accepted by the ASHA Legislative Council. The primary emphasis of the Guidelines was on pure-tone air conduction screening procedures with primary application to the school-age population. Although immittance* measurement was recognized as an important part of the the identification process, the Committee did not propose guidelines for this procedure due to lack of a strong research foundation. In 1975, following an increase in research and clinical data, a Subcommittee on Impedance (Immittance) Measurement was established for the purpose of preparing guidelines for acoustic immittance measure-

ment screening procedures. The guidelines that follow have been developed by the Subcommittee and present recommended procedures based on existing practice and research findings. As such, these guidelines should be considered as interim and subject to revision pending further clinical and research findings.

RATIONALE

Immittance measurements are used for the identification of conductive otologic abnormality. Conductive abnormality is usually middle-ear disease, particularly in children (Wehrs and Proud, 1958; Brownlee et al., 1969; Kaplan et al., 1973; Howie et al., 1975). Initiating screening programs for detecting middle-ear abnormality has often seemed a discouraging venture because early subtle effects of middle-ear disease may create only minimal hearing loss (less than 25 dB), the nature of the disorder can be transient in many cases, and medical management is varied.

Medical considerations have traditionally been thought to be the major reason for detecting middle-ear disease. However, Brooks (1978) reviewed pertinent literature on middle-ear disease consequences and concluded that minimal hearing loss and fluctuating middle-ear conditions have educational, social, and psychological considerations as well. Studies cited by Brooks, and additionally those cited below, support that persistent middle-ear disease can lead not only to medical complications (Bernstein, 1977; Lithicum, 1977; Mawson, 1977) but also to significant hearing impairments (Friedmann, 1970; Mawson, 1977) and educational barriers (Holm and Kunze, 1960; Ling, 1969; Menyuk, 1969; Kaplan et al., 1973; Howie, 1977; Needleman, 1977; Brooks, 1978).

Editor's Note: The set of "Guidelines for Acoustic Immittance Screening of Middle-Ear Function" was approved by the ASHA Legislative Council in November 1978. The following members of the ASHA Committee on Audiometric Evaluation Subcommittee on Impedance Measurement developed these guidelines: Quinter C. Berry, Gene A. Del Polito, Debbie Katz, Jane R. Madell, Wayne O. Olsen, Peggy S. Williams and Michael Seidemann, Chairman. ASHA encourages the professional community to use these guidelines.

*Immittance: the term used to denote either acoustic impedance or acoustic admittance. (The term is incorporated into these guidelines for the purpose of consistency with terminology used in the proposed *Standard for Aural Acoustic Immittance Instruments* being developed by the ANSI-Immittance working group.)

Reprinted by permission of the American Speech-Language-Hearing Association from *ASHA, 21,* 283–288 (1979).

These latter studies have related recurrent middle-ear disease and fluctuating hearing loss with linguistic, intellectual, social, and educational developmental lags in children. Fluctuating hearing losses and subtle middle-ear problems are often not seriously regarded at the time because they result in minimal hearing loss which is not always identified by an audiometric screening program. Of concern is that the problem remains unrecognized until the cumulative effects of serious disease of the ear or developmental lags become apparent.

The transient nature of the disease has encouraged the tendency to allow the situation to resolve without intervention, and in many cases this is successful. However, not all cases resolve, and the critical factor is the predictability of which cases will resolve and which will not. Brooks appropriately asks can we "justifiably afford to ignore a pathological condition on the assumption that in most cases it will, over a period of time, ameliorate without intervention."[1]

Although effective and necessary, present audiometry screening programs do not always identify the individual with middle-ear problems. Inconsistent relationships between hearing loss and middle-ear disease are well documented (Jordan and Eagles, 1961; Eagles et al., 1967; Cohen and Sade, 1972; Harker and Van Wagoner, 1974; Brooks, 1973; McCandless and Thomas, 1974; Northern, 1975; Cooper et al., 1976). Separate techniques for identification of hearing loss and middle-ear abnormality appear more efficient than attempting to use only one procedure for identification of both.

The development of immittance guidelines, therefore, does not imply a need for replacement of conventional pure-tone air-conduction hearing screening procedures. Acoustic immittance screening assesses middle-ear function; pure-tone audiometric screening evaluates auditory sensitivity. Thus, acoustic immittance measurements can provide supplementary information to the traditional pure-tone air-conduction screening program.

The goal of a program oriented toward immittance screening evaluations of middle-ear function is to maximize the identification of individuals who have middle-ear disorders when they exist (test sensitivity), and identify individuals who are normal when they are, in fact, normal (test specificity). Many difficulties exist in achieving test sensitivity and specificity.

Screening programs in the past have had difficulty accomplishing this goal primarily due to the use of pass/fail and referral criteria. In addition, the use of tympanometry alone (with the exclusion of the acoustic reflex) in the early screening programs limited the amount of available information on which to base such criteria. In fact, Brooks (1976) has suggested that the acoustic reflex is the more sensitive of the two. In response to immittance screening needs, most equipment manufacturers are now providing an easily accessible method of incorporating both tympanometry and the acoustic reflex into the procedure. This has allowed the capacity for obtaining more information with subsequent tightening of the pass/fail criteria.

Additional factors, however, will continue to cause difficulties when children are referred for medical evaluation following abnormal results on an immittance screening. One difficulty is the aforementioned transient nature of middle-ear disorders. Another difficulty is the occurrence of immittance measurement results which fall outside the normal range but do not constitute significant medical problems upon examination. This problem can at least be partly related to the time lag that may exist between identification and medical examination. However, the primary underlying factor is fluctuating middle-ear conditions. This recognized factor supports a need for recognition of a population that is "at risk" and may require observation and monitoring especially in the early years of educational work. Identification of these individuals, if children, may never lead to medical referral but may very well require special seating, attention and/or supplementary educational services to negate the development of educational problems.

It has also been apparent that controversies exist in the medical community as to what constitutes treatable middle-ear disease and how medical management should be conducted. While it is recognized and appreciated that there is no standard medical approach to treatment of middle-ear effusion at this time, this situation need not discourage or negate the importance of identification of middle-ear abnormalities. Identification of a problem and information on its prevalence and nature is often necessary before attempts can be made toward determining means of resolving the problem. Separate from the medical aspects, identification of children with potential fluctuating hearing loss is felt to be necessary for proper educational management. Although recognizing that further research is necessary for determining the significance and treatment of subtle middle-ear disorders, screening programs can identify potential at risk populations and, in addition, can presently identify those persons with more obvious middle-ear disease who can, in fact, benefit from medical intervention.

Since immittance measurements are objective, rapid, and efficient, a screening application for use with large populations is entirely practical. The immittance measurement has several advantages for a screening approach: sound-treated environments are not necessary, testing is rapid, no response is required from the individual being tested, the procedures are minimally limited by age, and the procedures are useful for difficult-to-test individuals.

These latter statements are neither meant to imply nor to negate a need for mass screening. Rather, they are meant to convey the practical impression that those programs wishing to incorporate middle-ear screening programs for large populations should find it possible to do so. Some large special populations, such as Eskimo children (Ling et al., 1969; Kaplan et al., 1973; Harker and Van Wagoner, 1974), children with cleft palate (Paradise, 1976; Bess et al., 1975; Bess et al., 1976), institutionalized psychotic children (Geffner and Weber, 1977), Australian aboriginal children (Lewis et al., 1975), native Indian children (Roberts, 1976), developmentally disturbed children (Bashore, 1977) and deaf children (Brooks, 1974) reportedly have a high incidence of middle-ear disorders. In such populations screening procedures may have significant application. Also, programs already undertaking pure-tone air-conduction screening of school populations should be free to consider middle-ear screening as a possible supplementary procedure which can offer added information in the achievement of a well-balanced identification program.

Thus, the early identification and treatment of middle-ear disease, especially in children and special populations, appears important. Undetected and untreated problems can lead to progression of disease, which can create irreversible changes in the conductive mechanism of the ear (Jaffe, 1977) and may additionally create unnecessary educational barriers.

PURPOSE

The purpose of these guidelines is to recommend a set of procedures and parameters for accomplishing rapid and efficient identification of middle-ear disorders using acoustic immittance screening measurements. The procedures involve evaluation of the middle-ear status using both tympanometry[2] and acoustic reflex[3] measurements and are based on existing clinical experience and research findings. The spirit of these recommendations is not to mandate a single approach for accomplishing middle-ear screening, but rather to provide an outlined procedure for guidance.

SCREENING MIDDLE-EAR FUNCTION

Procedural Considerations

Population to be Screened. The following recommendations emphasize acoustic immittance screening procedures for children since the incidence of conductive otologic abnormality is greater for children than for adults. However, these procedures may also be applied to other populations.

For school-age populations, it is recommended that screening procedures be administered annually to children of nursery-school age through grade five and to children of any higher grade who have a known history of middle-ear problems. Annual screening for children in the lower grades is appropriate because of the higher incidence of middle-ear disease in younger children (Brooks, 1968; McCandless and Thomas, 1974; Roberts, 1976) and because of the need to provide early intervention in disease processes which may create serious language, educational, psychological and social problems.

Routine screening for children younger than 7 months of age is not presently recommended since research has demonstrated inconsistent results for this group (Paradise et al., 1976).

Personnel. Screening programs should be under the direct supervision of appropriately qualified professionals. "Appropriately qualified professionals" for the purpose of these guidelines is defined as an audiologist, physician, or speech-language pathologist with appropriate training in immittance screening techniques. It is recognized that supportive personnel will often be conducting many of the activities of the screening programs under supervision. Supportive personnel should have completed an appropriate level training program for preparation.

Guidelines

The guidelines concern the parameters of measurement and do not discuss specific measurement techniques such as type of ear tips, insertion of probe-tip assembly, instructions to person being tested, color of pen recordings and so forth. These are left to the discretion of the examiner and most are usually discussed in the equipment manual provided by the manufacturer.

Equipment. Acoustic immittance instruments for screening programs should have as a minimum the capability for tympanometry and for monitoring an acoustic reflex at a specified intensity level.

The instrumentation should contain an automatic recording system which produces a permanent record of the test results.

Calibration. Pending adoption of ANSI standards for calibration of immittance instruments, electro-acoustic calibration procedures should be performed at least monthly according to the manufacturer's specifications. During active periods of screening, test cavity calibration checks should be performed daily before initial testing and once midday. The probe-unit should be checked routinely for obstructions. Further assessment of the system is necessary when immittance results appear spurious.

The acoustic reflex eliciting signal should be checked monthly and be calibrated according to the ANSI S3.6-1969 requirements for pure-tone calibration of standard earphones. For ipsilateral reflex stimuli, a 2 cc coupler must be used.

Since there is presently no available accompanying equipment provided by the manufacturer for determining accuracy of the pressure system, it is recommended that a U-tube water manometer be used at least monthly.

Calibration of the automatic recording unit should be performed according to manufacturer's specification at least monthly. Daily calibration checks of all systems should be performed during active screening periods.

Pump System. An automatic constant-rate pump system with a recording system is recommended. The instrumentation may include an automatic recording system in order to reduce screening time, reduce the possibility of recording error by nonprofessionals, and produce a permanent record of test results.

Air-Pressure Range. The recommended air-pressure range used should cover a minimum of +100 to −300 mm H_2O. The greater range in the negative direction is recommended since abnormalities in children are usually revealed in this dimension. Determining pressure status beyond −300 mm H_2O would contribute little to the screening data and would unnecessarily increase screening time. Although negative pressure status is known to fluctuate over short periods of time (Lewis et al., 1975), such pressures pose sufficient threat to the integrity of hearing (Flisberg et al., 1963; Cooper et al., 1975) to warrant rescreening and at risk classification.

Probe-Tone Frequency. A low-frequency probe-tone between 220 and 300 Hz is recommended since the bulk of screening data used the low-frequency and there is insufficient information on screening with higher frequencies. Also, the low-frequency probe-tone is the only one universally available on present screening equipment.

Rate and Direction of Air-Pressure Change. There are insufficient data to recommend guideline procedures. In the interim a consistent approach *within* each program is recommended for best test-retest comparison and reliability.

Measurement Units. ANSI guidelines for measurement units are not available at present. In the interim a consistent approach *within* each program is recommended.

Frequency for Acoustic Reflex Eliciting Signal. The recommended eliciting signal is a pure tone of 1,000 Hz. This frequency is chosen because it is less likely to be influenced by mild negative pressure affects for lower frequencies, which may elevate reflex eliciting levels, and because it is less likely to be viewed as a hearing screener for high-frequency hearing loss. In addition, this frequency appears to have a lower acoustic reflex threshold than most other pure-tone frequencies (Jepsen, 1963; DiSogra, 1978), and it was found to be the most consistent eliciting frequency (compared to 500, 2,000, 4,000 Hz) to show a reflex

TABLE 49–1. MIDDLE-EAR SCREENING CRITERIA.

Classification	Results of Initial Screen	Disposition
I. PASS	Middle-ear Pressure Normal* or Mildly positive/negative† and Acoustic Reflex Present‡	Cleared; no return
II. AT RISK	Middle-ear Pressure Abnormal§ (and Acoustic Reflex present) or Acoustic Reflex Absent (and middle-ear pressure normal or mildly positive/negative)	Retest in 3–5 weeks a. If Tymp. and AR fall into Class I, PASS b. If Tymp. or AR remain in Class II FAIL and refer.
III. FAIL	Middle-ear Pressure Abnormal and Acoustic Reflex Absent	Refer

*Normal: Pressure peak in range ± 50 mm H_2O.

†Mildly Positive/Negative: +50 to +100 mm H_2O, −50 to −200 mm H_2O.

‡Present: Pen or meter needle deflection judged to be coincident with the reflex eliciting stimulus at levels of 100 dB HL for contralateral stimulation, 105 dB SPL for ipsilateral stimulation at 1,000 Hz.

§Abnormal peak outside the ranges described for Classification I.

in a screening program with children ages 6–14 years (DiSogra, 1978).

Level of Acoustic Reflex Eliciting Signal. Levels recommended are a 100 dB HL signal for contralateral stimulation or a 105 dB SPL signal for ipsilateral stimulation.

The acoustic reflex in normal ears is elicited between 75–95 dB HL for pure-tones (Peterson and Liden, 1972). Negative pressure levels are known to elevate acoustic reflex thresholds (Peterson and Liden, 1972; Skinner et al., 1977). Skinner et al. (1977) found the mean reflex threshold elevated by 2.5 dB for ipsilateral stimulation and 5 dB for contralateral stimulation. Although wishing to compensate for negative pressure effects, the use of unusually high intensity levels can lead to artifact and may create a startle response. Therefore, it is recommended that a level at the upper limits of the normal range with an additional compensating level for mild negative pressure effects be used.

Pressure for the Acoustic Reflex Test. The acoustic reflex test should be administered at the tympanogram peak pressure point when it is identified in order to maximize the possibility of obtaining a response, or at ambient air pressure when no pressure peak can be identified.

Criteria for Pass-Fail. For screening purposes, middle-ear pressure, and presence or absence of the acoustic reflex, are the only factors involved in referral critera. Static immittance values are not included in these criteria due to the large variability in this parameter as reported in the literature (Jerger, 1970; Feldman, 1974).

Pass-fail and referral criteria are summarized in Table 49–1.

Disposition (see flow chart). Individuals demonstrating middle-ear pressure within the normal range (±50 mm H_2O) or mildly positive/negative (+50 to +100 mm H_2O, −50 to −200 mm H_2O) and presence of an acoustic reflex to a 1,000 Hz pure tone at 100 dB HL for contralateral or 105 dB SPL for ipsilateral stimulation, *pass* middle-ear screening and require no retesting (Classification I).

Individuals revealing middle-ear pressure outside this range and with absence of acoustic reflex response, *fail* the screening. These individuals are not retested as part of the screening program but are referred for audiological and medical examination (Classification III).

Individuals who have middle-ear pressure outside the normal or mildly positive/negative range with the acoustic reflex present, and individuals who have the

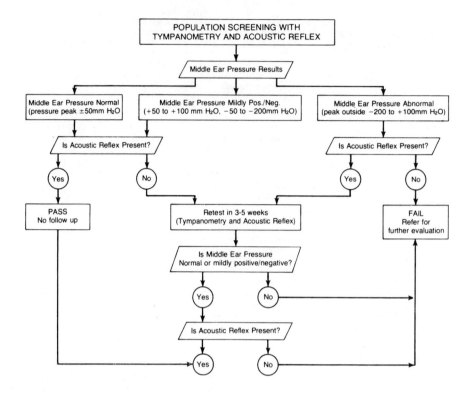

acoustic reflex absent with normal or mildly positive/negative middle-ear pressure may be considered *"at risk"* (Classification II) and should be retested in a 3–5 week period. At the time of retest the individual is passed if the tympanometry and acoustic reflex results are consistent with Classification I specifications. The individual is failed and referred if the tympanometry and the acoustic reflex results are consistent with Classification III specifications or persist in Classification II specifications.

Individuals in Classification II and III should be identified within any educational setting as to the referral disposition and to the possible presence of fluctuating hearing loss. School programs may wish to correlate results of middle-ear screening with results of hearing screening for a balanced program toward the achievement of: (1) the identification of those with educationally significant hearing problems, and (2) the identification of medically significant problems.

ENDNOTES

1. Brooks, D. N., Maico Audiological Library Series, part 1, Vol. XV, #8, p. 1, 1978.

2. Tympanometry: a procedure used to measure changes in acoustic immittance at the eardrum as air-pressure changes are artificially induced into a hermetically-sealed ear canal. The recorded results are known as a tympanogram.

3. Acoustic Reflex: a contraction of one or more muscles of the middle-ear in response to the presentation of a suprathreshold stimulus. Evidence of the presence of the reflex action is characterized by a measured change in the acoustic immittance.

REFERENCES

American National Standard Specifications for Audiometers (ANSI S3.6-1969). New York: American National Standards Institute, Inc. (1970).

Bernstein, J. Middle-ear effusions. In B. Jaffe (Ed.), *Hearing Loss in Children*. Baltimore: University Park Press, 413–415 (1977).

Bashore, S. The use of tympanometry for screening developmentally disturbed children. *Audiology and Hearing Education,* October/November, 35–40 (1976).

Bess, F.; Lewis, H.; and Cieliczka, D. Acoustic impedance measurements in cleft-palate children. *J. Speech Hearing Dis.,* **40:** 13–24 (1975).

Bess, F.; Schwartz, D.; and Redfield, N. Audiometric, impedance, and otoscopic findings in children with cleft palates. *Arch Otolaryngol.,* **102:** 465–469 (1976).

Brooks, D. An objective method of detecting fluid in the middle ear. *Int. Audiol.,* **7:** 280–286 (1968).

Brooks, D. Hearing screening—a comparative study of an impedance method and pure tone screening. *Scandinavian Audiology,* **2:** 67–72 (1973).

Brooks, D. Impedance bridge studies on normal hearing and hearing impaired children. *Acta Oto. Rhino. Laryngol. Belg.,* **28:** 140–145 (1974).

Brooks, D. School screening for middle-ear effusions. *Ann. Otol. Rhinol. Laryngol. Suppl.* 25, **85,** 223–228 (1976).

Brooks, D. Acoustic impedance testing for screening auditory function in school children, Parts I & II. *Maico Audiological Library Series,* **15** (1978).

Brownlee, R.; DeLoache, W.; Cowan, C.; and Jackson, H. Otitis media in children. *J. Pediatrics,* **75,** 636–642 (1969).

Cohen, D. and Sade, J. Hearing in secretory otitis media. *Can. J. Otolaryngol.,* **1,** 27–30 (1972).

Cooper, J.; Gates, G.; Owens, J.; and Dickson, A. An abbreviated impedance bridge for school screening. *J. Speech Hear. Dis.,* **40,** 260–269 (1975).

Cooper, J.; Langley, L.; and Meyerhoff, W. The significance of negative middle-ear pressure. *Laryngoscope,* 1976.

DiSogra, R. A comparison of two methods of stimulus presentation utilized in establishing acoustic stapedial reflex thresholds in children. Paper presented to the NYSSHA, April 1978.

Eagles, E.; Wishik, S.; and Doerfler, L. Hearing sensitivity and ear disease in children: A prospective study. *Laryngoscope,* 1–274 (1967).

Feldman, A. Eardrum abnormality and the measurement of middle ear function. *Arch. Otolaryngol.,* **99,** 172–176 (1974).

Friedmann, I. Pathology of deafness. In Wolvsevholme and Knight (Eds.), *Sensorineural Hearing Loss.* J. and A. Churchhill, London, 49 (1970).

Flisberg, K.; Ingelstedt, S.; and Ortegren, V. Controlled "ear aspiration" of air: A "physiological" test of the tubal function. *Acta Otolaryngol.* suppl., **182,** 35–68 (1963).

Geffner, D. and Weber, M. Impedance measurements of institutionalized psychotic children. Paper presented to the NYSSHA, April, 1977.

Guidelines for Identification Audiometry. *ASHA,* **17,** 94–99 (1975).

Harker, L. and Van Wagoner, R. Application of impedance audiometry as a screening instrument. *Acta Otolaryngologica,* **77,** 198–201 (1974).

Holm, V. and Kunze, L. Effect of chronic otitis media on language and speech development. *Pediatrics,* **43,** 833–839 (1969).

Howie, V. Natural history of otitis media. *Ann. Otol. Rhinol. Laryngol.,* **84,** 67–73 (1975).

Howie, V. Acute and recurrent acute otitis media. In B. Jaffe (Ed.), *Hearing Loss in Children.* University Park Press, Baltimore, 413–415 (1977).

Jaffe, B. *Hearing Loss in Children.* Baltimore: University Park Press, 378 (1977).

Jepsen, O. Middle-Ear muscle reflexes in man. In J. Jerger (Ed.), *Modern Developments in Audiology,* 193–239 (1963).

Jerger, J.; Anthony, L.; Jerger, S.; and Mauldin, L. Studies in impedance audiometry: III. Middle ear disorders. *Arch. Otolaryngol.,* **99,** 165–171 (1974).

Jordan, R. and Eagles, E. The relation of air conduction audiometry to otologic abnormalities. *Ann. Otol. Rhinol. Laryngol.,* **70,** 819–827 (1961).

Kaplan, G.; Fleshman, J.; Bender, T.; Baum, C.; and Clark, P. Long-term effects of otitis media: A ten year cohort study of Alaskan Eskimo children. *Pediatrics,* **52,** 577–585 (1973).

Lewis, H.; Dugdale, A.; Canty, A.; and Jerger, J. Open-ended tympanometric screening: A new concept. *Arch. of Otolaryngol.,* **101,** 722–725 (1975).

Ling, D.; McCoy, R.; and Levinson, E. The incidence of middle ear disorders and its educational implications among Baffin Island Eskimo children. *Canadian J. Public Health,* **60,** 385–390 (1969).

Ling, D. Rehabilitation of cases with deafness secondary to otitis media. In A. Glorig and K. Gerwin (Eds.), *Otitis Media Proceedings of the National Conference.* Springfield, Illinois: Charles C Thomas, 249–253 (1972).

Lithicum, F. Ossicular chain destruction. *Hearing Loss in Children.* University Park Press, Baltimore, 452–458 (1977).

Mawson, S. Chronic otitis media. In B. Jaffe (Ed.), *Hearing Loss in Children.* University Park Press, Baltimore, 435–438 (1977).

Menyuk, P. *Sentences Children Use.* Cambridge, Mass.: MIT Press (1969).

McCandless, G. and Thomas, G. Impedance audiometry as a screening procedure for middle ear disease. *Trans. Am. Acad. Opthalmol. Otolaryngol.,* **78,** 98–102 (1974).

Needleman, H. Effects of hearing loss from early recurrent otitis media on speech and language development. In B. Jaffe (Ed.), *Hearing Loss in Children,* 640–649 (1977).

Northern, J.; Rock, E.; and Frye, D. Tympanometry: A technique for identifying ear disease in children. *Pediatr. Nurs.,* **1,** 32–37 (1975).

Paradise, J.; Smith, C.; and Bluestone, C. Tympanometry detection of middle-ear effusion in infants and young children. *Pediatrics,* **58,** 198–210 (1976).

Paradise, J. Management of middle-ear effusions in infants with cleft palate. *Ann. Otol. Rhinol. Laryngol.,* Suppl. 25, **85,** 285–288 (1976).

Peterson, J. and Liden, G. Some static characteristics of the stapedial muscle reflex. *Audiology,* **11,** 97–114 (1972).

Roeser, R.; Soh, J.; Dunckel, D.; and Adams, R. Comparison of tympanometry and otoscopy in establishing pass/fail referral criteria. *J. Amer. Audiol. Soc.,* **3,** 20–25 (1977).

Roberts, M. Comparative study of pure tone, impedance and otoscopic hearing screening methods. *Arch. Otolaryngol.,* **102,** 690–694 (1976).

Skinner, B.; Norris, T.; and Jirsa, R. Effect of negative pressure on acoustic reflex threshold. Poster session, ASHA Convention, Chicago (1977).

Wehrs, R. and Proud, G. Conductive deafness in children. *Arch. Otolaryngol.,* **67,** 16–19 (1958).

50

Evaluation of a Recommended Program of Identification Audiometry with School-Age Children

WILLIAM MELNICK, Ph.D.
Associate Professor, Department of Otolaryngology, The Ohio State University
ELDON L. EAGLES, M.D.
Deputy Director, National Institute of Neurological Diseases and Stroke, Bethesda, Maryland
HERBERT S. LEVINE, Sc.D.
Director, Biostatistics Department, Montefiore Hospital and Medical Center, Bronx, New York

Identification audiometry refers specifically to the case-finding aspects of a hearing conservation program. It does not refer to making a specific diagnosis, to medical treatment, or to rehabilitation. An important part of such a program is early case-finding. In order to establish general guidelines to resolve the confusion regarding audiometric procedures for case-finding programs, the National Conference on Identification Audiometry was convened in Baltimore in May, 1960. The work of this conference resulted in a monograph on identification audiometry, one chapter of which presented a proposal of basic procedures in a program of identification audiometry for school-age children (Hardy, 1961, pp. 26–34). The purpose of the investigation being reported here was the evaluation of some of those procedures.[1]

Test programs for school-age children often involve testing large numbers of children by an abbreviated or screening method. From the results of one screen, children are selected for another screen from which a final selection is made of candidates for more detailed testing of hearing. The purpose of the testing program is the identification of children who should be referred to a physician for a complete diagnostic examination. These are children who have hearing less sensitive than a selected criterion hearing level as shown by the threshold hearing test.

The pure-tone sweep check, probably the most preferred screening technique, has been performed most often at a level of +15 dB for the test frequen-

cies which are routinely used during a threshold test, i.e., 125, 250, 500, 1,000, 2,000, 4,000, 6,000, and 8,000 cps. The number and choice of frequencies varies among screening programs, and there have been recommendations for using one or two frequencies for screening. The National Conference on Identification Audiometry made the following recommendations regarding screening procedures:

1. Testing should be conducted in acoustically treated test rooms.
2. The frequencies recommended for identification audiometry at the school-age level are 500, 1,000, 2,000, 4,000, and 6,000 cps.
3. The frequencies 500, 1,000, 2,000, and 6,000 cps should be screened at 10 dB and at 20 dB for the frequency 4,000 cycles.
4. The criteria for failure should be failure to respond at 10 dB at 1,000, 2,000, or 6,000 cps or at the 20-dB level at 4,000 cycles.
5. The same failure criteria should apply to both the screen and the pure-tone threshold test.

These are the recommendations that the present study attempts to evaluate. The recommended procedures differ mainly in two respects from those which have been used in testing school children. First, the screening level for the sweep check has been uniformly 15 dB re audiometric zero. Second, failure at two of the test frequencies has required the child to have a pure-tone threshold test. In some instances the child might have been tested a second time before a threshold measurement was made. Criteria for failure has specified threshold sensitivity at a level of 20

Reprinted by permission of the authors from *J. Speech Hearing Dis.*, **29**, 3–13 (1964).

dB or greater at two frequencies, or 30 dB or more for any one frequency. These levels have been based on adult test results and sensitivity norms which are themselves under question.

The recommended procedures advise a +10-dB screening level in order to identify children who begin not to hear at +15 dB, the level at which hearing impairment for speech may begin. The less stringent requirement of +20 dB at 4,000 cps suggests that a loss of this magnitude at this frequency has less significance than it would have at other frequencies.

The use of the new screen level requires testing in an environment quieter than any usually found in schools. A quiet part of a school building is no longer acceptable. The use of acoustically treated test rooms is specifically recommended.

SUBJECTS

Eight hundred and eighty children from kindergarten through the eighth grade of four elementary schools in the Pittsburgh public school system participated in the study. These children were functioning as normal public school pupils with no apparent hearing problems at the time of the test. They were participants in a larger Pittsburgh hearing study (Jordan and Eagles, 1961) and had experienced hearing testing prior to this investigation. No use was made of information from medical histories.

ENVIRONMENT

Both the screening and the threshold tests were performed in a double-walled test room, Industrial Acoustics Model 1202. Sound sampling has shown that the ambient noise levels were well below the levels described as criteria for background noise in audiometer test rooms by the American Standards Association (1960).

EQUIPMENT

Audivox 8-B audiometers with Western Electric 705A earphones and associated sponge rubber cushions were used for testing. An additional 40 dB of attenuation was provided by an auxiliary attenuator. The equipment was calibrated monthly to meet the American Standard specifications. The equipment and environment are described in more detail by Eagles and Doerfler (1961).

TECHNICIANS

Four female test technicians performed the audiometric tests. These women were trained and had considerable experience in performing the test techniques used in the Pittsburgh hearing study. Each technician was assigned a permanent school location and performed both the sweep check and the threshold examinations for children attending that school.

TEST TECHNIQUES

Sweep Check

The test frequencies were 500, 1,000, 2,000, 4,000, and 6,000 cps, and were presented in that order. The screening level was set at 20 dB for 4,000 cycles and at ten dB for the other frequencies. One ear was tested completely before shifting to the other ear. The duration of the tone varied between one and three seconds at each frequency. The criterion for failure was no response at any one of the test frequencies for either ear. Only one presentation per ear was made of a test frequency.

Threshold Test

A serial method of limits was used. The test tone was started at 40 dB and reduced in steps of ten dB until the subject failed to respond. The intensity was then increased by 5-dB steps until response was obtained. The tone was again reduced ten dB and a 5-dB ascent was presented. This procedure continued until a point was reached which produced a response in two out of three ascending trials. If there was no response at the initial 40-dB level, the tone intensity was increased until a response was obtained or until the maximum output was reached. When a response was given, the procedure continued in the way just described. Only the ascending trials were used in determining the threshold hearing levels. The thresholds at 250 and 8,000 were obtained in addition to those frequencies presented in the sweep check. In the analysis only those tones common to both types of test were investigated.

PROCEDURE

The child was instructed to raise his hand whenever he heard the tone and to keep his hand up as long as the tone was heard. This mode of response was the same for both the pure-tone sweep check and the threshold test. The child then entered the test room, the earphones were placed by the technician, and the testing was begun. The first test performed was the sweep check. If the child passed the first screen, he was immediately tested by the threshold technique. The child who failed the sweep check was dismissed at this point and scheduled for a second test session the following school day. The second test period involved another sweep check and then, regardless of whether the child failed or passed, a threshold test was performed.

All of the children who were tested by the sweep check and the threshold tests within a particular week were examined by an otolaryngologist sometime during that same week.

Although the second sweep check is not part of the recommendations of the Conference on Identification Audiometry, this procedure is often used in present hearing testing programs. It was used here in order to evaluate its effectiveness in reducing the number of false failures.

The criteria used to define a failure did not follow precisely the recommendations of the conference. Because of anticipated problems in obtaining a quiet environment and consequently of masking, the conference did not include 500 cps for consideration of failure and referral. The quiet environment was available for this study, and prior large-scale experience in testing children did not indicate a particular problem with 500 cps. Therefore, criteria were established that defined a failure as no response at 10 dB for 500, 1,000, 2,000, or 6,000 cps, and at 20 dB for 4,000 cps.

RESULTS AND DISCUSSION

A comparison of the results of the first sweep check with those of the threshold technique is shown in Table 50–1. Twenty of the participating children who could not be tested reliably were excluded from the study, and the total number of children available for analysis was thus reduced from 880 to 860. The test results were judged unreliable if the child did not per-

TABLE 50–1. COMPARISON OF THE PERFORMANCE ON THE FIRST SWEEP-CHECK SCREEN AND ON THE THRESHOLD TEST.

| | First Sweep Check | | |
	Passed	Failed	Total
Threshold Test			
Passed	666	51	717
Failed	18	125	143
Total	684	176	860

form according to test instruction and if the child's responses were inconsistent with the presentation of the test signals. The twenty unreliable subjects were distributed throughout the age range and were found to have no abnormalities upon otoscopic examination.

Table 50–1 shows that 51 children or 29 percent of the 176 who failed the initial screen, passed the threshold test. These 51 subjects represent the false positives, i.e., those who would have been needlessly referred for further audiometric testing on the basis of an initial screen and who, therefore, represent one form of inefficiency. The 18 subjects who passed the initial screen but failed the threshold test are called the false negatives. They are children who possibly might have a hearing problem but were missed by the first sweep-check screen, reflecting another type of inefficiency of screening methodology.

The number of false positives can be reduced by a second screening; but in the case where only the failures of the first sweep check are given a second screening, the number of false negatives can only be kept the same. When failures on the initial screen were rescreened and the result compared with the threshold test, Table 50–2, the number of false positives was reduced to 13, or only seven percent of the initial failures. Three of the initial failures passed the second screening but failed the threshold test. Of the

TABLE 50–2. COMPARISON OF THE PERFORMANCE ON THE SECOND SWEEP-CHECK SCREEN AND ON THE THRESHOLD TEST OF CHILDREN WHO FAILED THE FIRST SCREEN.

| | Second Sweep Check | | |
	Passed	Failed	Total
Threshold Test			
Passed	38	13	51
Failed	3	122	125
Total	41	135	176

135 who failed both screens (Table 50–2), 122 or 90.4 percent were shown to fail the threshold test also. Had only one screen been used (Table 50–1) only 71 percent of the screening failures, 125 of 176, would have failed the threshold as well. (The second screening reduced the over referrals by almost ten percent.)

A more intensive investigation of the audiometric performance of the children showed that among the 21 false negatives uncovered by both screenings, in 15 cases the child failed the threshold at only one frequency and by just one (five dB) intensity step. The six remaining children showed thresholds less sensitive than the criterion at two frequencies and again usually by five or ten dB (one or two steps).

Out of the total of 51 false positives, 38 children failed the first screen, but passed both the second screen and the threshold test (Table 50–2). Thirty-one of these 38 children failed the first sweep check at only one frequency in one ear. The difference in performance between the two screens could be attributed to variability acceptable in this type of test situation. Differences of five dB are given little significance in clinical test-retest results and yet could have produced failure of one screen with success in passing another. This much difference can result from variables other than a decrease in hearing sensitivity and could well have been an attention or a motivation problem. This is especially so when only one frequency is involved. Failure at only one frequency was seen among the remaining 13 false positives who failed both screens but passed the threshold test (Table 50–2). Nine out of the 13 who failed the first screening, and ten out of 13 who failed the second screening did so at only one frequency in one ear. In this particular sample of children, 41 of the 51 false positives, or 80 percent could have been eliminated if the criterion for failure were changed to failure at any two test frequencies in either ear rather than failure at any one frequency. Failure at 500 cycles did not contribute greatly to the number of false positives. In only three of the 51 cases was 500 cycles the sole failing frequency. In those children who failed all three of the tests, the same picture regarding performance at 500 cps was seen. Three subjects failed the first screen at 500 cycles and one child on the second screen.

The two screens showed relatively good agreement with each other. Among the 122 children who failed both, there was complete agreement in 60 cases. Thirty-two cases differed at one frequency, and the remaining 30 children differed at more than one frequency. The second screen agreed more closely with the threshold failures than the first. There was complete agreement for 71 out of 122 children, while for the first screen, this was true in only 49 cases. The greater agreement was due probably to the fact that the second screen and threshold tests were given consecutively on the same day, thus reducing the possibility of variation not only in the subjects' hearing sensitivity but in other conditions of the subject, environment, tester, and equipment.

Table 50–3 shows the number of failures for each screen as well as for the threshold examination at each frequency. Among the 122 children who failed all three tests, the greatest number of failures occurred at 6,000 cps. The larger value of the failure criterion for 4,000 cps (+20 dB) produced numbers of failures more consistent with those seen at 500, 1,000, and 2,000 cps. If a +20-dB criterion had also been adopted for 6,000 cps, the number of failures for the threshold examination at that frequency would have been reduced almost 50 percent.

The subjects varied in age from four to 15 years. It was possible that the age factor may have been an important influence in causing inconsistencies between screening and threshold test results. To investigate this possibility the failures were tabulated as a function of age. As Table 50–4 shows, however, there were no obviously consistent patterns in the age distributions which would indicate a systematic influence of the age variable for these children.

The Monograph on Identification Audiometry states that the purpose of the audiometric testing

TABLE 50–3. NUMBER OF FAILURES AT EACH FREQUENCY FOR THE 122 CHILDREN WHO FAILED* BOTH SCREENS AND THE THRESHOLD TEST. CLASSIFIED BY TEST TECHNIQUE AND EAR.

Test Technique	500	1,000	2,000	4,000	6,000
Right Ear					
First Screen	31	40	41	35	61
Second Screen	31	39	34	31	56
Threshold	28	38	37	29	60
Left Ear					
First Screen	31	40	47	33	57
Second Screen	29	38	47	36	41
Threshold	24	37	37	29	58

*Failure criteria for screening tests was no response at 10 dB re American audiometric zero for 500, 1,000, 2,000, and 6,000 cps and 20 dB at 4,000 cps. Failure on the threshold tests was indicated by a threshold higher than 10 dB at 500, 1,000, 2,000, and 6,000 cps and 20 dB at 4,000 cps.

TABLE 50-4. A COMPARISON OF PASS-FAIL PERFORMANCE ON TWO SCREENINGS USING PURE-TONE SWEEP CHECK, AND A PURE-TONE THRESHOLD TEST FOR CHILDREN CLASSIFIED BY AGE.

| Year Age of Child | Total | | Passed First Screen* | | | | Failed First Screen but Passed Second | | | | Failed Both Screens | | | |
| | | | Passed Threshold | | Failed Threshold | | Passed Threshold | | Failed Threshold | | Passed Threshold | | Failed Threshold | |
	No.	Pct.	No.	Pct.	No.	Pct.	No.	Pct.	No.	Pct.	No.	Pct.	No.	Pct.
4	2	0.2	2	0.3	—	—	—	—	—	—	—	—	—	—
5	28	3.3	20	3.0	—	—	—	—	—	—	1	7.7	7	5.7
6	131	15.2	111	16.7	3	16.7	1	2.6	—	—	3	23.1	13	10.6
7	116	13.5	87	13.1	2	11.1	6	15.8	1	33.3	1	7.7	19	15.6
8	106	12.3	82	12.3	2	11.1	2	5.3	1	33.3	1	7.7	18	14.8
9	75	8.7	51	7.6	4	22.2	6	15.8	—	—	2	15.4	12	9.8
10	101	11.7	78	11.7	1	5.6	4	10.5	—	—	2	15.4	16	13.1
11	97	11.3	77	11.6	2	11.1	3	7.9	—	—	1	7.7	14	11.5
12	116	13.5	95	14.3	2	11.1	9	23.7	—	—	1	7.7	9	7.4
13	60	7.0	43	6.4	1	5.6	6	15.8	1	33.3	—	—	9	7.4
14	25	2.9	17	2.6	1	5.6	1	2.6	—	—	1	7.7	5	4.1
15	3	0.3	3	0.4	—	—	—	—	—	—	—	—	—	—
Total	860	100.0	666	100.0	18	100.0	38	100.0	3	100.0	13	100.0	122	100.0

*Not given second screen.

" . . . is to lead to the final identification of those who should be referred to an otologist, or other physician, for a complete diagnostic work-up" (Hardy, 1961, p. 26). "The goal is to locate children who have even minimal hearing problems so that they can be referred for medical treatment of any active ear conditions discovered to be present and so that remedial educational procedures can be instituted at the earliest possible date" (Hardy, p. 16).

Thus, the purpose of audiometric testing is twofold. Initially, it is to locate children with decreased hearing sensitivity and, secondly, to locate children with active ear conditions for medical treatment. It has been assumed that the group with decreased hearing sensitivity would contain those children in need of medical attention.

To evaluate this second function of the identification program, an otolaryngological examination was given to all the children who participated, regardless of audiometric test results. The results of the otoscopic portion of the examination are shown in Tables 50-5 and 50-6.

TABLE 50-5. DISTRIBUTION OF PASS-FAIL PERFORMANCE BY CHILDREN ON THE SCREENING AND THRESHOLD TESTS, CLASSIFIED BY TYPE OF OTOSCOPIC FINDING.

| Otoscopic Finding in One or Both Ears | Total | | Passed First Screen* | | | | Failed First Screen but Passed Second | | | | Failed Both Screens | | | |
| | | | Passed Threshold | | Failed Threshold | | Passed Threshold | | Failed Threshold | | Passed Threshold | | Failed Threshold | |
	No.	Pct.	No.	Pct.	No.	Pct.	No.	Pct.	No.	Pct.	No.	Pct.	No.	Pct.
No Abnormality	610	70.9	497	74.6	10	55.6	24	63.2	1	33.3	11	84.6	67	54.9
Unsatisfactory Visibility	123	14.3	89	13.4	3	16.7	6	15.8	1	33.3	0	0.0	24	19.7
Evidence of Active Pathology	27	3.1	10	1.5	2	12.5	2	5.3	0	0.0	0	0.0	13	10.6
Evidence of Past Pathology	100	11.6	70	10.5	3	16.7	6	15.8	1	33.3	2	15.4	18	14.8
Total	860	100.0	666	100.0	18	100.0	38	100.0	3	100.0	13	100.0	122	100.0

*Not given second screen.

TABLE 50–6. CHILDREN WITH DIFFERENT TYPES OF OTOSCOPIC FINDINGS CLASSIFIED BY PERFORMANCE ON THE SCREENING AND THRESHOLD TESTS.

Otoscopic Findings in One or Both Ears	Total		Passed First Screen*				Failed First Screen				Failed Both Screens			
			Passed Threshold		Failed Threshold		Passed Threshold		Failed Threshold		Passed Threshold		Failed Threshold	
	No.	Pct.	No.	Pct.	No.	Pct.	No.	Pct.	No.	Pct.	No.	Pct.	No.	Pct.
No Abnormality	610	100	497	81.5	10	1.6	24	3.9	1	0.2	11	1.8	67	11.0
Unsatisfactory Visibility	123	100	89	72.4	3	2.4	6	4.9	1	0.8	0	0.0	24	19.5
Evidence of Active Pathology	27	100	10	37.0	2	7.4	2	7.4	0	0.0	0	0.0	13	48.0
Evidence of Past Pathology	100	100	70	70.0	3	3.0	6	6.0	1	1.0	2	2.0	18	18.0
Total	860	100	666	77.4	18	2.1	38	4.4	3	0.3	13	1.5	122	14.2

*Not given second screen.

Some definition of the otoscopic categories appears in order. The category of "unsatisfactory visibility" resulted from the fact that the physicians were not permitted to remove cerumen or any other substance which may have occluded the auditory canal. The "evidence of active pathology" category consisted of those children with inflammation or discoloration of the tympanic membrane, perforation with and without discharge, bulging, and retraction if the last finding occurred in combination with other signs which were considered evidence of acute or chronic otitis media. The category called "evidence of past pathology" included instances of scars, decreased mobility, calcium plaques, and retraction of the tympanic membrane when it was a single sign.

There was a considerable proportion of each audiometric performance classification without apparent otoscopic abnormality or unsatisfactory visibility (Table 50–5). These children, if referred to an otologist, might be considered over-referrals by him. Of the 122 children who would be referred on the basis of having failed all three tests, 67 or 54.9 percent would be found with no otologic abnormality.

The category of most interest is that of active pathology. There were 27 cases in the entire group examined, only 13 of which would have been referred for a diagnostic examination because of a failure on all three tests. Thus, the 13 children with active pathology who failed the hearing tests represent 48 percent of the total, while 52 percent were falsely labelled as negative at some point in the hearing testing program and lost to referral. Even more interesting is the fact shown in Table 50–6, that 12 of the 27 cases,

or 44 percent, passed the more carefully conducted threshold test. The audiometric program would have referred for a diagnostic work-up two out of seven children observed with inflammation of the tympanic membrane, one out of two children with acute otitis media, six out of 13 children with chronic serous otitis media, and four out of five with perforation and discharge.

The children with evidence of past infection should be identified as well as possible in a hearing conservation program in order to provide these children with more careful and perhaps more frequent monitoring of their hearing sensitivity and the physical condition of their ears. Some of these children may have been identified by historical information. Since this study did not make use of medical histories, this factor cannot be evaluated. From the results solely from hearing testing, Table 50–6 shows the test program to be less successful at identifying these children. Seventy percent passed both the initial screening and the threshold test. This is not surprising since many of the children return to levels of hearing sensitivity which are considered normal from the clinical point of view.

When the more liberal criteria for failure of the threshold test which has served in past programs, i.e., two frequencies with a hearing level of 20 dB or one frequency with a level of 30 dB or more, are used, only one additional child identified as having active pathology would have been missed. The change in the failure criteria to the more stringent levels did not apparently improve the identification of the children with otologic abnormality.

Following the completion of the threshold test, each child was questioned about his status with regard to colds, earaches, and ear discharge at the time of the test. Little positive information resulted from the children's responses. The children who failed all three tests showed a slightly higher percentage of colds at the time of the test or during the preceding week than other children. It was hoped that a history of respiratory illness might account for inconsistent results between the two screens, but this had little apparent effect.

Twenty-seven of 860 children reported earaches in one or both ears, but only seven of the 27 failed the three audiometric tests. Fourteen of the 27 showed negative otoscopic findings. There were eight cases of reported ear discharge, five of which were present in the failing group. Out of the eight, four were reported to have no abnormality by the otolaryngologists. The reliability of the cold, earache, and ear discharge information is questionable.

The results of this study show that the recommended screening program was successful in characterizing the hearing sensitivity of the participating public school children. Of the 860 children, 96 percent were correctly identified as having either normal or decreased hearing sensitivity when a threshold test was used for validation. The screening test incorrectly indicated normal hearing sensitivity in 2.5 percent of the children who subsequently were shown to have some hearing loss by the threshold measurement. The remaining 1.5 percent were falsely identified as having decreased hearing sensitivity by the screenings.

A second screening for those children who failed, reduced the number of children incorrectly labelled as failures by about 74 percent. The screening program was made more effective by using failure on two sweep checks as an indication for more thorough threshold testing.

The use of the audiometric test results to identify those children with otologic problems was not adequate. Almost half of the cases with active pathology and probably in need of immediate medical attention were missed. Seventy percent of the children with evidence of past otological difficulty were not identified. These findings are similar to those reported by Jordan and Eagles (1961). Changes in the criteria for failure of the sweep check and threshold tests to lower hearing levels did not rectify the situation.

The frequency most often failed by the children was 6,000 cps. Changing the criterion for failure to the more liberal 20 dB on the threshold test would keep the number of failures at 6,000 cps consistent with those at the other test frequencies. A similar change in the failure criterion for this frequency on the screening tests would probably produce the same effect, although this is not known since it was not done. In the quiet environment used for testing in this study, 500 cycles did not present any particular problem for the children who were tested. This study was not designed to evaluate a one- or two-frequency screen; and, therefore, no speculation concerning this aspect was made.

SUMMARY

The recommended program of the National Conference on Identification Audiometry for identification audiometry with the school-age child was applied to 860 children in four public elementary schools. The test program was successful in finding those children with a reduced hearing sensitivity. The hearing test results, both for the screening and the threshold test procedures, did not adequately identify children with otoscopic evidence of active or past ear pathology.

ENDNOTE

1. This investigation was supported in part by Grant B-2375 from the National Institute of Neurological Diseases and Blindness to the Subcommittee on Hearing in Children, Committee on Conservation of Hearing of the American Academy of Ophthalmology and Otolaryngology. Additional support was provided by a grant from the U.S. Children's Bureau through the Commonwealth of Pennsylvania Department of Health to the University of Pittsburgh.

REFERENCES

American Standard Criteria for Background Noise in Audiometer Rooms, S 3.1. New York Amer. Standards Assoc., 1960.

Eagles, E. L., and Doerfler, L. G. Acoustic environment and audiometer performance. *J. Speech Hearing Res.,* **4,** 1961, 149–163.

Hardy, W. G. (General Chairman). National Conference on Identification Audiometry Committee, Identification audiometry. *J. Speech Hearing Dis.,* Monograph Suppl. **9,** 1961.

Jordan, R. E., and Eagles, E. L. The relation of air conduction audiometry to otological abnormalities. *Ann. Otol. Rhin. and Laryng.,* **70,** 1961, 819–827.

51

Identification Audiometry Accuracy: Evaluation of a Recommended Program for School-Age Children

WESLEY R. WILSON, Ph.D.
Associate Professor, Department of Speech and Hearing Science, University of Washington, Seattle, Washington
WENDEL K. WALTON, Ph.D.
Consultant, State of Connecticut Department of Education

The purpose of identification audiometry in the schools is to detect children who may be educationally handicapped by hearing loss.[1] It is the cornerstone on which a school district's hearing conservation program is built and involves considerable expenditure of professional time and equipment. In spite of this, little effort has been devoted to studying the accuracy of identification audiometry procedures.

The accuracy of identification audiometry is stated in terms of the number of correct identifications. Incorrect identifications take two forms: children who fail the procedure yet actually have normal hearing (false positives or overreferrals) and children who pass the procedure but have educationally significant hearing losses (false negatives or underreferrals).

Melnick, Eagles, and Levine (1964) studied the accuracy of the identification audiometry procedures developed in 1960 by the National Conference on Identification Audiometry (Darley, 1961). The applicability of the results reported by Melnick et al. to most identification audiometry programs is limited by the fact that their screening testing was conducted in sound-treated test rooms. Most school districts do not have sound-treated rooms in each school building and very few have a mobile test van so that they may move the test environment from school to school. Consequently, identification audiometry usually is accomplished at best in a quiet part of the school building.

Recognition of the fact that sound-treated rooms generally are not available led to the development of a proposed new standard set of procedures for identification audiometry by the Committee on Audiometric Evaluation of the American Speech and Hearing Association (ASHA). A working paper, entitled *Guidelines for Identification Audiometry* (ASHA, 1972) was endorsed by ASHA for distribution for critical comment before final adoption of the guidelines. The main points detailed in the guidelines are as follows:

1. Test frequencies shall be 1,000, 2,000, and 4,000 Hz.
2. Screening levels shall be 20 dB HL (ANSI, 1969) at 1,000 and 2,000 Hz and 25 dB at 4,000 Hz.
3. Failure criterion shall be failure to respond at the recommended screening level at one or more frequencies in either ear.
4. Mandatory rescreening shall occur within one week for all screen failures.
5. Audiologic evaluations are to be accomplished for individuals failing the rescreening.
6. Medical referrals should be based on the results of audiologic evaluations.
7. Screening personnel should have professional preparation in screening young children.

These recommendations differ from those suggested by the National Conference on Identification Audiometry in the following ways: (1) there is no recommendation that testing be conducted in acoustically treated test rooms, (2) the frequencies of

Reprinted by permission of the authors from *Lang., Speech, Hearing Serv. in Schools*, **5**, 132–142 (1974).

500 and 6,000 Hz are excluded, and (3) rescreening of all failures is mandatory.

The purpose of this study was to investigate the accuracy of the identification audiometry method described in the *Guidelines for Identification Audiometry* (American Speech and Hearing Association, 1972) as they were applied in a public school district. The method of evaluation involved a comparison of a screening test result and a threshold test result for a large sample of children and, using a second group of children, a comparison of the result of a second screening test and the result of the first screening test for those failing the first screening.

METHOD

Subjects

Two groups of subjects were chosen from 7,800 children screened in the Renton, Washington, public elementary schools. One group consisted of 411 children who failed the first screening test and then were screened again to estimate the reduction in false positives resulting from a second screening. Of this total, 54.7 percent were males and 45.3 percent were females. Approximately 22 percent were in kindergarten and the second grade and 19 percent were in the first, third, and fifth grades.

The other group consisted of 1,168 children, each of whom had received both the screening and threshold tests. This group was used in answering the method accuracy questions. Fifteen percent of these children were in kindergarten, approximately 21 percent were in the first, second, third, and fifth grades, and distribution by sex was approximately equal. With the exception of fourth-graders, who were excluded by district policy, all children in kindergarten through fifth grade who were present on the day of screening were included in the study.

Audiometrists

The audiometrists who performed the screening tests were undergraduate and graduate students who had completed at least one course in audiology and one in audiometry. They attended a two-day training session during which each student practiced the desired screening procedures to criterion. The threshold tests were performed by graduate students and faculty, most of whom hold the Certificate of Clinical Competence in Audiology.

Test Environments and Noise Levels

Screening tests were administered in each of the schools in the same rooms that had been used in previous years. Threshold tests were administered in School 01 in a district-owned IAC 1200 room and in Schools 02 and 03 in IAC 400 rooms installed at the sites for the purpose of the study.

Frequent measures were made of the noise levels present in both the screening and threshold environments. Noise levels were within allowable limits for the screening levels (American Speech and Hearing Association, 1972) and the minimum threshold levels chosen (ANSI, 1960).

Screening Procedures

The children were admitted to the screening areas in groups of eight to 16 (depending on grade level) and were arbitrarily assigned to one of the four testing stations. Each child was screened individually at 1,000, 2,000, and 4,000 Hz. The initial level was 20 dB HL (ANSI, 1969); if the child did not pass at 4,000 Hz, the level was raised to 25 dB HL, since the recommended screening levels are 20 dB at 1,000 and 2,000 Hz and 25 dB at 4,000 Hz. Several tone presentations were used at each ear-frequency combination. Whether the subject passed or failed was recorded at each frequency for each ear.

Threshold Procedures

Each child screened in the second group ($N = 1,168$) received an individual threshold evaluation following the screening. The median elapsed time between the screening and threshold tests was seven calendar days. The threshold procedures employed an ascending presentation sequence with testing conducted at the octave frequencies of 250 through 8,000 Hz for each ear. All threshold testing began at 1,000 Hz and was followed by sequential presentation of higher and then lower octaves. The testers, who were different individuals from those who had done the screening, were unaware of the screening results for any child.

Equipment and Calibration

Eleven portable audiometers representing three makes and five models were used in the study. They were calibrated to all facets of the S3.6-1969 ANSI specification (American National Standards Institute, 1970) before the start of the study, and a complete check on all aspects of calibration of each was completed daily (see Walton and Wilson [1974] for details).

RESULTS

Screening-Rescreening Results

The first analysis considered the number of children who failed the first screening but passed a rescreening. Table 51-1 presents these data by grade and for the total sample ($N = 411$). As shown, slightly over one half of the total sample passed the rescreening. Comparison by grades demonstrates fewer overreferrals for threshold testing in the fifth grade with no clear trend in the lower grades except for first-graders, who apparently are more prone to give false positive results than are other primary grade children.

TABLE 51-1. RESCREENING RESULTS FOR 411 CHILDREN WHO FAILED THE FIRST SCREENING.

Grade	N	Rescreening Results Pass (%)	Rescreening Results Fail (%)
K	90	53	47
1	78	62	38
2	89	51	49
3	76	51	49
5	78	45	55
Total	411	52	48

Screening-Threshold Results

To determine the overall accuracy of the screening method, the sum of the individuals passing both screening and threshold tests or failing both screening and threshold tests was compared to the number passing one test and failing the other. For those who performed differently on the two tests, the threshold test was used as the validity criterion; a false positive meant that the child failed the screening and passed the threshold test, and a false negative meant the opposite. For the purpose of this study, a child was said to have passed the threshold test if his hearing level was equal to or better than the screening level. Each frequency was considered independently. The data are reported for three different definitions of the target group: (1) children failing the threshold test when only the screening frequencies are considered, (2) children failing the threshold test when only the speech frequencies are considered, and (3) children failing the threshold test at any test frequency.

Threshold Test Failure at Screening Frequencies. Table 51-2 presents a comparison of screening and threshold test results with threshold data when only the screening frequencies are considered. Including the correction for reduction in false positives by means of a second screening test, an overall screening accuracy of 94.7 percent is achieved for this target group. A smooth progression of increased accuracy by grade is noted except for the reversal at

TABLE 51-2. SCREENING METHOD ACCURACY FOR TARGET GROUP 1 DEFINITION: CHILDREN FAILING THE THRESHOLD TEST WHEN ONLY THE SCREENING FREQUENCIES ARE CONSIDERED.

Grade	N	Screening and Threshold Results Same Pass* (%)	Screening and Threshold Results Same Fail (%)	Screening and Threshold Results Different False Positive* (%)	Screening and Threshold Results Different False Negative (%)	Screening Accuracy (%)	Screening Error (%)
K	179	90.1	3.4	3.2	3.4	93.5	6.6
1	243	89.9	2.5	4.7	2.9	92.4	7.6
2	260	91.8	3.5	3.9	0.8	95.3	4.7
3	242	92.4	4.5	0.2	2.9	96.9	3.1
5	244	94.1	2.9	2.3	0.8	97.0	3.1
Total	1,168	91.4	3.3	3.2	2.0	94.7	5.2

*Computed figures based on first screening results plus correction for second screening (from data in Table 51-1).

(*Editors' note:* The number of subjects represented in columns 3–6 is provided here to facilitate further analysis: Passed screening and threshold tests (column 3) = 1,068; failed screening and threshold tests (column 4) = 39; false positive classifications (column 5) = 37; and false negative classifications (column 6) = 23. There were 62 hearing-impaired subjects (sum of columns 4 and 6) and 1,105 normal-hearing subjects (sum of columns 3 and 5). The number of subjects for each column entry is a percentage of the appropriate base figure (1,105 normal or 62 hearing impaired). The small discrepancy between the study N (1,168) and the N calculated from the sum of columns 3–6 (1,167) is attributable to rounding error. The number of subjects for each column entry in Table 51-3 may be derived in the same way.)

Grade 1 where, as previously noted, the highest percentage of false positives occurs. The false negatives for the total sample comprise 2.0 percent of the children tested, and the false positives comprise 3.2 percent. The combination of these two figures (5.2 percent) is the inaccuracy or error figure for the method as applied to this target group.

Threshold Test Failures at Speech Frequencies. A second method of analyzing the data compares the screening results to the thresholds developed in the speech frequencies 500, 1,000, and 2,000 Hz. The rationale for this analysis rests on the fact that the purpose of identification audiometry in the schools is to identify children who have educationally handicapping hearing losses. Losses in the speech frequencies are considered to meet this criterion for target group children.

The overall accuracy factor for this comparison is 95.0 percent (Table 51-3). Thus, either of the first

two definitions of target group results in a similar accuracy value. However, the error figure of 5.0 percent for the second target group definition includes only 1.9 percent false positives and 3.1 percent false negatives. The increase in false negatives is attributed to the large number of first-graders in this category, again calling attention to this grade level as being more difficult to test accurately, and the inclusion of a frequency not screened (500 Hz) in the definition of threshold failure.

Threshold Test Failures at Any Test Frequency. The third analysis considers the target group to be children with hearing losses at any frequency (250 to 8,000 Hz) in either ear, and an overall accuracy of 90.3 percent (Table 51-4) is recorded. Again, the first grade demonstrates the lowest accuracy and the fifth grade the highest. Whereas the identification audiometry method was equally accurate in defining either of the first two target groups, it was substan-

TABLE 51-3. SCREENING METHOD ACCURACY FOR TARGET GROUP 2 DEFINITION: CHILDREN FAILING THE THRESHOLD TEST WHEN ONLY THE SPEECH FREQUENCIES ARE CONSIDERED.

| Grade | N | Screening and Threshold Results Same | | Screening and Threshold Results Different | | Screening Accuracy (%) | Screening Error (%) |
		Pass* (%)	Fail (%)	False Positive* (%)	False Negative (%)		
K	179	91.2	3.9	2.7	2.2	95.1	4.9
1	243	86.0	3.3	3.7	7.0	89.3	10.7
2	260	91.1	4.2	3.2	1.5	95.3	4.7
3	242	92.1	2.9	1.7	3.3	95.0	5.0
5	244	93.1	3.7	1.5	1.6	96.8	3.1
Total	1,168	91.4	3.6	1.9	3.1	95.0	5.0

*Computed figures based on first screening results plus correction for second screening (from data in Table 51-1).

TABLE 51-4. SCREENING METHOD ACCURACY FOR TARGET GROUP 3 DEFINITION: CHILDREN FAILING THE THRESHOLD TEST AT ANY TEST FREQUENCY.

| Grade | N | Screening and Threshold Results Same | | Screening and Threshold Results Different | | Screening Accuracy (%) | Screening Error (%) |
		Pass* (%)	Fail (%)	False Positive* (%)	False Negative (%)		
K	179	82.8	5.6	1.0	10.6	88.4	11.6
1	243	83.1	4.9	2.1	9.9	88.0	12.0
2	260	85.3	5.4	2.0	7.3	90.7	9.3
3	242	86.6	4.5	0.2	8.7	91.1	8.9
5	244	89.4	4.1	1.1	5.3	93.5	6.4
Total	1,168	85.4	4.9	1.6	8.2	90.3	9.8

*Computed figures based on first screening results plus correction for second screening (from data in Table 51-1).

tially less accurate in defining this third target group, as would be expected.

DISCUSSION

It was expected that a rescreening of all children who fail an initial screening would reduce the number of overreferrals. Although a second screening test was not part of the recommendations of the Conference on Identification Audiometry, Melnick et al. (1964) included a second screening, and computations based on their data yield a reduction figure of 23 percent. The reduction figure of 52 percent found in our study was not anticipated and obviously represents a substantial reduction in overreferrals. The difference in results between these studies might be explained on the basis of test environment. In the Melnick et al. study, screening tests were completed in sound-treated test rooms with only one child present, whereas screening tests in our study were completed in the regular school environment room with several children present. Rescreenings then were accomplished with only one child in the test room at a time, and the noise level or other interfering factors were reduced for the retest. Because rescreening reduced overreferrals by approximately one half, inclusion of this procedure in identification audiometry seems mandatory, as suggested in *Guidelines for Identification Audiometry* (American Speech and Hearing Association, 1972).

The method accuracy figures developed in our study also may be compared to those developed by Melnick et al. (1964). They reported an accuracy figure of 92 percent for comparison of the first screening test to the threshold test. By including the reduction in false positives that they found by using a second screening test, a corrected overall accuracy figure of 96 percent is computed. These two values may be compared to 88 percent accuracy for the first screening-threshold comparison and 95 percent for the second screening-threshold comparison in the present study. Thus, the accuracy figure obtained in our study for identification of children with educationally significant losses (Target Group 2) compares favorably with the figure reported for the earlier recommended procedures, in spite of the fact that sound-treated test rooms were used in the earlier study but not in the present one.

Perhaps the most critical accuracy indicator in screening is the number of false negatives, since this represents the children who were not identified by the test as having hearing problems. Melnick et al. (1964) reported a value of 2.5 percent, while we reported 2.0 percent for the Target Group 1 comparison and 3.1 percent for the Target Group 2 comparison. If one excludes testing at 500 Hz, yet uses the screening to predict losses in the speech frequencies (Target Group 2), the number of false negatives increases by 1.1 percent. However, as Melnick et al. and Darley (1961) have noted, provision of an adequate acoustic environment to allow testing at 500 Hz usually will demand special acoustical treatment.

Our data suggest that giving more attention to first-grade children during testing may improve the accuracy figure even more. Without exception, first-graders presented the highest inaccuracy figures for each of the analyses. The tester may expect a kindergarten child to need special instructions for the task and take the time necessary to accomplish this, whereas he may expect the first-grade child to remember the task from his kindergarten test period. Our results suggest that the first-grade child may need the same attention typically provided the kindergarten child if we are to expect equivalent accuracy.

CONCLUSIONS

The identification audiometry procedures detailed in *Guidelines for Identification Audiometry* (American Speech and Hearing Association, 1972) were tested in a field experiment and found to be highly accurate when the complete methodology is included and the target group is children with hearing losses in the speech frequencies. The second screening is extremely important to this procedure.

ACKNOWLEDGMENT

We appreciate the cooperation and assistance of the administrators of the Renton, Washington, Public School District and the staff of each of the schools in the district. Special thanks are due the members of the district's Speech and Hearing Program, Addison Ames, head.

ENDNOTE

1. For the purpose of this study, hearing loss is defined as a shift in hearing sensitivity. We neither exclude nor include the concept of a medically significant loss in this definition, since air-conduction audiometry has been demonstrated to be a very inefficient means of identifying middle ear pathology (see Melnick et al., 1964; Jordan and Eagles, 1961; and Hildyard, Stool, and Valentine, 1963) and this study deals with an air-conduction identification audiometry procedure.

REFERENCES

American National Standards Institute. *American Standard Criteria for Background Noise in Audiometer Rooms (S3.1-1960).* New York: American National Standards Institute (1960).

American National Standards Institute. *American National Standard Specifications for Audiometers (S3.6-1969).* New York: American National Standards Institute (1970).

American Speech and Hearing Association. *Guidelines for Identification Audiometry. ASHA,* 17, 94–99 (1975).

Darley, F. L. (Ed.) Identification Audiometry. *J. Speech Hearing Dis. Monogr. Suppl. 9* (1961).

Hildyard, V. H.; Stool, S. E.; and Valentine, M. A. Tuning fork tests as aid to screening audiometry. *Arch. Otolaryng.,* 78, 151–154 (1963).

Jordan, R. E., and Eagles, E. L. The relation of air conduction audiometry to otological abnormalities. *Ann. Otol. Rhinol. Laryng.,* 70, 819–827 (1961).

Melnick, W.; Eagles, E. L.; and Levine, H. S. Evaluation of a recommended program of identification audiometry with school-age children. *J. Speech Hearing Dis.,* 29, 3–13 (1964).

Walton, W. K., and Wilson, W. R. Stability of pure-tone audiometers during periods of heavy use in identification audiometry. *Lang. Speech Hearing Serv. Schools,* 5, 8–12 (1974).

52

Open-Ended Tympanometric Screening: A New Concept

NEIL LEWIS, M.A.
Reader in Audiology, University of Queensland, Brisbane, Australia
ALLEN DUGDALE, M.D., FRACP
Reader, Department of Child Health, University of Queensland, Brisbane, Australia
ANTHONY CANTY, M.D., FRCS
Consultant ENT Surgeon, Royal Children's Hospital, Brisbane, Australia
JAMES JERGER, Ph.D.
Professor of Audiology, Baylor College of Medicine, Houston, Texas

We introduce the concept of open-ended, succesive-day tympanometric screening. In impedance screening of children for middle ear disorders, there is a serious risk of over-referral if decisions are made on the basis of a single tympanogram. Serial tympanometric studies of Australian aboriginal children show that, whereas the type B tympanogram is usually stable, type A and type C patterns are prone to vary from day to day, inviting inappropriate referral decisions unless the classifications are confirmed by tests on successive days.

The electro-acoustic impedance bridge is widely esteemed as a diagnostic aid for hearing and ear disorders (Jerger, 1970; Alberti and Kristensen, 1970; Jerger et al., 1972). Considerable interest is now being shown in the use of modified impedance audiometry as a screening device for the identification of middle ear disorders in young children. In advocating its use for this purpose, Brooks (1971, 1973) has stressed that the impedance method is easy to administer and is not greatly influenced by either environmental or motivational factors. Moreover, it is capable of yielding accurate and reproducible results that permit more confident identification of abnormality than is possible from either visual otoscopy or pure-tone audiometry. Cooper et al. (1975) also attest to the superiority of impedance audiometry in screening children for middle ear disorders, but

express some concern that it appears to generate a fairly high rate of over-referrals.

In auditory screening programs, it has been customary to assign individuals to a "pass" or "fail" category on the basis of a single, brief examination. Accordingly, an effective screening device is regarded as one that neither "fails" too many ears that are normal nor "passes" too many ears that are abnormal. Most investigators, however, accept a liberal tolerance of false-positive screening errors as preferable to possible misidentification of any case that might stand in genuine need for medical follow-up.

During the past several years, we have made extensive use of impedance audiometry in screening programs for Australian aboriginal children who suffer an unusually high prevalence of serous otitis media and other middle ear diseases (Stuart et al., 1972; Lewis et al., 1974).

Our experience leads us to believe that impedance audiometry senses the presence of middle ear disease long before the appearance of otoscopic or audio-

Reprinted by permission of the authors from *Arch. Otolaryng.*, **101**, 722–725 (1975). Copyright 1975, American Medical Association.

metric manifestations. In the case of serous otitis media, early detection followed by prompt medical treatment would seem to afford the best prospects of successful intervention into the course of a disease that is singularly resistant to treatment once it has progressed to a chronic stage. To take full advantage of the exquisite sensitivity of impedance audiometry in detecting incipient disease processes, however, it may be necessary to develop new concepts of auditory screening. The proposals set forth herein have been inspired primarily by the results of two studies of the day-to-day variability in the tympanometric patterns of Australian aboriginal children who live on a government reservation in Queensland.

SUBJECTS AND METHODS

An electro-acoustic impedance bridge was used to derive individual tympanograms of each ear of each child. These functions, relating middle ear compliance change to induced pressure variation in the internal ear canal, were classified into types A, B, or C in accordance with Jerger's widely accepted nomenclature (1972).

Calibration checks of the instrument before and after each test session established that the manometer unit of the impedance bridge consistently gave readings within ± 10 mm H_2O of the pressures developed in a simple water manometer over a range of -300 mm H_2O to $+300$ mm H_2O. The compliance scale of the instrument gave readings within .05 cu cm of the known volumes of 1 cu cm and 2 cu cm hard-walled cavities.

Prior to the tympanometric evaluation, each child was examined otoscopically by a medical otologist, and audiometrically by a qualified audiologist.

The first study examined short-term variations in the tympanogram. For this purpose, a group of ten Australian aboriginal children (age 5 to 6 years) was selected to represent a variety of ear conditions. These children were tested tympanometrically on each of five consecutive days.

In the second study, 38 children from the same community were examined on two occasions with a two-month separation between tests. The age range in this sample was 4 to 14 years. Quite by chance, none of these children received treatment for ear disorders during the test-retest interval.

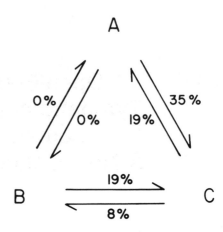

Changes in tympanometric patterns on successive daily testing. Percentages indicate probabilities of change at next test.

RESULTS

Short-Term Variations

The audiometric, otoscopic, and daily tympanometric findings of the ten children are shown in Table 52–1. Two findings are strikingly apparent. First, the incidence of an abnormal tympanogram (types B and C) was unexpectedly high. Second, the tympanometric status of ears changed frequently from day to day. These changes have been tabulated in Table 52–2. If an ear showed a type A response on any one day, there was a 35 percent chance that it would show a different response on the following day. The change was always to type C, never to type B. Ears that gave a type B response showed much greater consistency. Only 19 percent of these could be expected to change on a succeeding day, the changes always being to type C. Ears with a type C response had a 27 percent chance of changing within a day, the change usually going to type A, and only occasionally to type B. The directions and probabilities of change are summarized in the Figure.

Long-Term Variations

Table 52–3 displays the test-retest variations in the tympanograms of 76 ears (38 children) that were tested on two occasions, two months apart. In 32 percent of the untreated ears, the second tympanogram reversed the indications of the first. Type C tym-

TABLE 52–1. DAY-TO-DAY TYMPANOMETRIC CHANGES IN TEN ABORIGINAL CHILDREN.

				LEFT EAR									RIGHT EAR					
			Tympano-metric Findings	Test Day								Tympano-metric Findings	Test Day					
CASE	AHL* (dB)	Otoscopic Findings		1	2	3	4	5		AHL (dB)	Otoscopic Findings		1	2	3	4	5
1	40	TM† retracted	Type MEP‡	B ...	B ...	B ...	C −200	C −360	27		Normal	Type MEP	B ...	B ...	B ...	B ...	B ...
2	19	Normal	Type MEP	A −20	A 0	C −140	A 0	A −40	21		Normal	Type MEP	A −30	A −30	A −60	A −30	A −60
3	25	TM retracted, scarred	Type MEP	C −240	C −300	C −300	B ...	C −340	17.5		TM retracted, scarred	Type MEP	C −340	C −300	C −380	B ...	C −300
4	17.5	Normal	Type MEP	C −200	C −200	C −120	C −130	C −140	22		Normal	Type MEP	C −100	A −30	A −20	C −280	A −60
5	...	Normal	Type MEP	C −120	C −120	A −40	C −300	A −40	...		TM retracted, scarred	Type MEP	A −80	C −240	C −240	C −240	C −140
6	17	Normal	Type MEP	C −220	C −160	C −160	C −140	C −160	16		Normal	Type MEP	C −160	C −160	C −200	C −200	C −180
7	32.5	TM retracted	Type MEP	B ...	B ...	B ...	B ...	B ...	31		Normal	Type MEP	C −360	B ...	B ...	B ...	B ...
8	13	Healed perforation	Type MEP	A −50	C −100	A −10	A −40	C −100	23		Normal	Type MEP	C −140	C −300	C −140	C −200	C −200
9	16	Normal	Type MEP	A −60	A −40	A −80	C −100	A −80	12.5		Normal	Type MEP	A −60	A −60	A −60	A −60	A −80
10	22	TM retracted	Type MEP	C −220	C −320	... ...	C −380	C −380	21		TM retracted	Type MEP	A −40	C −250	... ...	C −200	A −60

*AHL, average hearing level.
†TM, tympanic membrane.
‡MEP, middle ear pressure (mm H_2O).

TABLE 52–2. DAY-TO-DAY TYMPANOMETRIC CHANGES.

Tympanometric Status on Successive Daily Tests (Type)	No. of Occurrences
A to A	15
A to B	0
A to C	8
B to A	0
B to B	13
B to C	3
C to A	7
C to B	3
C to C	27

TABLE 52–3. TEST-RETEST VARIABILITY IN THE TYMPANOMETRIC PATTERNS OF 76 EARS.

Type	No. of Ears
A to A	22
A to B	1
A to C	5
B to A	1
B to B	5
B to C	6
C to A	17
C to B	3
C to C	16

panograms showed the most variability, shifting frequently to type A on retest, and sometimes to type B. Fewer ears attracted abnormal classifications on the second test. Only one ear that was initially classified as type B showed spontaneous recovery to type A.

COMMENT

Previous studies of clinical tympanometry have suggested that the method yields highly repeatable test-retest data in otologically normal ears. Brooks (1971) retested one individual on nine separate occasions during an 18-month period, and reported remarkable consistency in the pressure-compliance functions. Lidén et al. (1970) obtained similar consistency in repeated tympanograms of three otologically normal subjects who were tested 20 times during a ten-hour period.

The tympanogram has no such stable expression, however, for the children in our study, who belong to a population that is exceptionally vulnerable to serous otitis media. Although little knowledge exists about the cause of this disease, faulty middle ear ventilation has been implicated as a predisposing factor (Fagan, 1973). In children, the course of the disease appears to be characterized by frequent remission and recidivation. Some ears appear to recover spontaneously, but others develop a "glue ear" stage that often requires surgery.

The capricious nature of serous otitis media that is evident in our studies creates serious difficulties for conventional screening philosophies that stipulate that a pass-fail designation should be made after a single examination. As Cooper et al. (1975) have shown, there is a real danger of over-referral in abbreviated impedance audiometry, especially in regard to type C tympanograms, which often reflect a transitional phase of pathologic features. Adding otoscopy and pure-tone audiometry to the screening battery is not likely to solve the problem, since the day-to-day variations in middle ear status that are exposed by serial tympanometry are too subtle to produce visually discernible changes or substantial shifts in hearing sensitivity (Lewis et al., 1974). Two cases that are described in Table 52–1 highlight the problem.

In one patient (Table 52–1, case 5), otoscopy revealed that the left ear was normal; the right ear had a retracted drum with scarring. On the third test day, the left tympanogram changed from type C to type A. On the following day (day 4), it reverted to type C, with a middle ear pressure registration of −300 mm H_2O. On day 5, the tympanogram returned to type A (middle ear pressure, 40 mm H_2O; compliance, 0.65 cu cm). If this ear had been tested only on day 3 or day 5, it would have passed the screen despite an obvious Eustachian tube dysfunction.

In another patient (Table 52–1, case 2), otoscopic and audiometric assessment gave "pass" classification on both ears. Tympanometric findings were normal (type A) on each day except day 3, when the classification shifted to type C (middle ear pressure, 140 mm H_2O). On this one day, the child would have failed the tympanometric screen, possibly on the basis of a transient and clinically insignificant pressure variation.

OPEN-ENDED SUCCESSIVE-DAY SCREENING

Our findings show a clear need for open-ended tympanometric screening on successive days for children in high-risk populations. In many instances, responsible referral decisions should be possible after two such tests, although transitional patients, whose results fluctuate between type A and type C tympanograms, can require as many as four successive tests. Specific recommendations in illustrative cases have been tabulated in Table 52–4 in the form of a decision matrix. The recommendations in each case are based exclusively on serial tympanometric configurations. It should be noted that a type B tympanogram always dictates a "fail" designation, whereas initial type A and type C tympanograms always require further testing.

TABLE 52–4. ILLUSTRATIVE DECISION MATRIX USED IN OPEN-ENDED, SUCCESSIVE-DAY SCREENING CONCEPT.*

Case	Day 1 (Type)	Day 2 (Type)	Decision	Day 3 (Type)	Day 4 (Type)	Decision
1	A	A	Pass	...	...	...
2	A	C	Retest	A	A	Pass
3	C	A	Retest	C	C	Fail
4	C	C	Fail	...	...	...
5	C	B	Fail	...	...	...
6	C	A	Retest	A	C	Fail
7	B	B	Fail	...	...	...

*Serial tympanogram results are shown for seven hypothetical cases.

The proposal calls for a heavier investment of time and money than is customary in conventional screening procedures. We believe, however, that screening strategies should be consonant with the character of the disorder under investigation. It is unrealistic to expect more than token validity from single-occasion screening of populations that suffer from a disease that is intrinsically labile. Our results show that serous otitis media in young children varies its expression from day to day. During a longer time span, the disease appears to follow a hesitant course, frequently leading to a state of chronic middle ear effusion that might persist for months or even years (Stuart et al., 1972). Its intermittencies are monitored accurately and reliably by serial tympanometry, which shows systematic changes from types A to C to B during progression, and from types B to C to A during remission.

Successive-day tympanometry would be wasteful, of course, in screening situations in which the target disorders are intrinsically stable; it would be no more wasteful, perhaps, than inappropriate use of pure-tone audiometry or visual otoscopy in populations that are known to have a high prevalence of serous otitis media. Over-referral in screening programs adds a considerable cost burden in the form of unnecessary medical follow-up. Under-referral penalizes any child whose auditory inefficiency passes unnoticed during the years in which he is acquiring linguistic and educational competence. In this context, the additional expenditures of successive-day screening might be a small price to pay for a more exact definition of middle ear status at the time that a referral decision must be made.

ACKNOWLEDGMENT

The Department of Aboriginal and Island Affairs, Queensland, and the Department of Aboriginal Affairs, Canberra, Australia, cooperated in this study.

REFERENCES

Alberti, P., and Kristensen, R. The clinical application of impedance audiometry. *Laryngoscope,* **80:** 735–746, 1970.

Brooks, D. A new approach to identification audiometry. *Audiology* **10:** 334–339, 1971.

Brooks, D. Electro-acoustic impedance bridge studies on normal ears of children. *J. Speech Hear. Res.,* **14:** 247–253, 1971.

Brooks, D. Hearing screening: A comparative study of an impedance method and pure tone screening. *Scand. Audiol.,* **2:** 67–72, 1973.

Cooper J.; Gates, G.; Owen, J. et al. An abbreviated impedance bridge technique for school screening. *J. Speech Hear. Dis.,* **40:** 260–269, 1975.

Fagan, P. Glue ear: An unnecessary problem. *Med. J. Aust.,* **1:** 501–506, 1973.

Jerger, J. Clinical experience with impedance audiometry. *Arch. Otolaryngol.,* **92:** 311–324, 1970.

Jerger, J. Suggested nomenclature for impedance audiometry. *Arch. Otolaryngol.,* **96:** 1–3, 1972.

Jerger, J.; Jerger, S.; Mauldin, L. Studies in impedance audiometry: I. Normal and sensorineural ears. *Arch. Otolaryngol.,* **96:** 513–523, 1972.

Lewis, A.; Barry, M.; Stuart, J. Screening procedures for the identification of hearing and ear disorders in Australian aboriginal children. *J. Laryngol. Otol.,* **88:** 335–347, 1974.

Lidén, G.; Petersen, J.; Björkman, G. Tympanometry. *Arch. Otolaryngol.,* **92:** 248–257, 1970.

Stuart, J.; Quayle, C.; Lewis, A. et al. Health, hearing and ear disease in aboriginal school children. *Med. J. Aust.,* **1:** 855–859, 1972.

53

Marked High-Frequency Hearing Loss: Clues to Early Identification*

Vanja A. Holm, M.D.

Assistant Professor of Pediatrics, Department of Pediatrics; Child Development and Mental Retardation Center, University of Washington, Seattle, Washington

Gary Thompson, Ph.D.

Associate Professor, University of Washington, Child Development and Mental Retardation Center, Seattle, Washington

Children who are deaf or hard of hearing often are not referred for audiological evaluation as early as possible (Luterman and Chasin, 1970). As a consequence, medical, audiological, and educational remediation may be delayed beyond the optimum time for intervention.

Among hearing-impaired children, one of the most difficult to identify is the child with selective hearing loss (Matkin, 1968). Selective hearing loss implies normal hearing for some frequencies and a substantial loss for others. If the loss occurs at frequencies which are important for hearing speech, the deleterious effect on speech and language development may be substantial. The following case report of a child with selective high-frequency hearing loss illustrates the confusion experienced by parents, physicians, teachers, and other professional persons when this kind of hearing handicap goes unidentified for a long time. It is presented in order to emphasize factors aiding the physician in the early identification of the child whose hearing is impaired with a partial loss.

CASE HISTORY

Matthew, a 5¼-year-old Caucasian boy, was referred to the Clinical Training Unit of the Child De-

velopment and Mental Retardation Center at the University of Washington for an evaluation of suspected brain damage. Hyperactive and distractible behavior were noted in his Head Start class and at home; inconsistent, spotty and inappropriate verbal responses were observed during a speech and language evaluation performed elsewhere.

M.'s mother was 44 years of age at the time of his birth. One episode of vaginal bleeding is reported during the second trimester of the 44-week pregnancy. Birth weight was 2,825 gm. The infant was meconium stained and described as dysmature. One minute Apgar was 6. Tracheal aspiration and positive pressure breathing for 15 to 20 seconds was followed by spontaneous respirations.

At a few hours of age episodes of apnea with cyanosis and clonic seizures began. A high pitched cry was noted. Hypoglycemia was diagnosed (blood glucose levels of 24, 20, and 11 mg per 100 ml) and treated with intravenous glucose and cortisone. Phenobarbital and paraldehyde were also given to control the seizures. Lumbar puncture was within normal limits. Subdural taps gave no fluid. Because of suspected sepsis, penicillin and kanamycin were administered. Of the latter, a total of 60 mg were given over a 3-day period. No more seizures were observed after the third day of life. Glucose and cortisone treatment were continued for 6 weeks. Several glucose profiles were normal. He was discharged at 7 weeks of age doing well.

M.'s subsequent medical and developmental history is typical for a child with high frequency hearing loss. What follows are selected excerpts from his medical records coupled with mother's and the authors' retrospective comments:

*The title of this article has been modified to facilitate cross-referencing to other literature concerning high-frequency hearing loss. Originally published under the title "Selective Hearing Loss: Clues to Early Identification" the article is reprinted with the permission of the authors from *Pediatrics,* 47, 447–451 (1971).

Six Months: Physician: "Laughs, hears, reaches. Normal development."

Fourteen Months: Walking.

Two Years: Physician: "Beginning to speak. Jabbers continually. Aggressive behavior. Anxious mother."

Mother: "I knew he was not talking like he should at two."

Twenty-eight Months: Physician: "Still doesn't say words clearly. Mental retardation? Appointment for psychological testing."

Psychologist's report: "Social Quotient on the Vineland Social Maturity Scale 97. Enunciation unclear. IQ 97 on Merrill Palmer Scale of Mental Tests."

(It is interesting to note that all verbal items starting at the 18 to 23 months level were marked "refused," but that he passed one puzzle item that required no language at 36 to 41 months level. This report was interpreted to rule out mental retardation as a cause for delayed language development.)

Mother: "I was concerned about the way he talked, but I was told he would outgrow it."

Thirty-three Months: Physician: "Routine physical normal." Eight days later mother returns.

Physician: "(1) Not talking in sentences but makes all needs known. (2) Stools and urinates in pants. Impression: (1) Mother has infantalized this child for symbiotic reasons (2) Manipulative child. Plan: Preschool. Counseling."

Mother: "I kept taking him back to the doctors. I wondered if he didn't pay attention or if he could not hear; but then sometimes he heard me when I whispered. His speech was so garbled. I *knew* something was wrong."

Thirty-three Months to 3½ Years: Several visits for minor complaints.

Mother: "I quit mentioning about his speaking, nobody seemed concerned."

Three and three-fourths Years: Follow-up on otitis media.

Physician: "TM's normal. Not speaking properly. Should have audio, but too resistive."

Mother: "He could hear very low noises, so everybody thought his hearing was all right."

Four Years: Physical examination for Head Start.

Physician: "In good health. Visual acuity 20/20 R-L. Audiometry at 30 dB, 500 cps R-L." (The only frequency recorded is a low tone where his hearing happens to be intact. The mild deficit noted was attributed to resolving otitis media.)

Four and one-fourth Years: M. was referred to a special program after 2 months' attendance in a regular Head Start class. Teacher observation: "Indistinct speech and poor language skills, short attention span, difficulty in following directions. Works constructively with all classroom materials."

Five Years: M. was seen for a speech evaluation on a referral by his physician concerned about his retarded language development following several bouts of otitis media.

Speech therapist: "Normal milestones except speech. Peers cannot understand him. Difficulty in distinguishing and repeating consonant sounds. Volume not a primary factor. Articulation errors not consistent. Responses often inappropriate. Recommend special resource for further evaluation."

At age 5¼ years, when M. was seen at the Clinical Training Unit, the routine pure tone screening by an audiologist revealed a marked high-frequency hearing loss (Figure 53–1). Speech audiometry showed M. to have awareness of speech within normal limits. For example, when his name was called as softly as at the 10 dB level, he responded appropriately. However, when asked to discriminate between words, his responses were erratic. A ball, airplane, truck, and cup were placed in front of him and he was instructed to point to the one named over the loudspeaker. He consistently identified "ball" and "airplane" correctly at 10 dB. In contrast, he had difficulty discriminating between "truck" and "cup" even at moderate to loud voice levels (40 to 60 dB Hearing Level ISO 1964).

Speech and language evaluation showed that M. was functioning at approximately the 3-year level in both receptive and expressive language. He had difficulty articulating consonant sounds, especially s, th, f, and sh.

Psychological testing confirmed that his nonverbal intellectual function was within normal limits (mental age 5 ²⁄₁₂ years on the Leiter International Performance Scale: IQ 90), but that when no allowance was made for speech and hearing deficits,

Audiogram

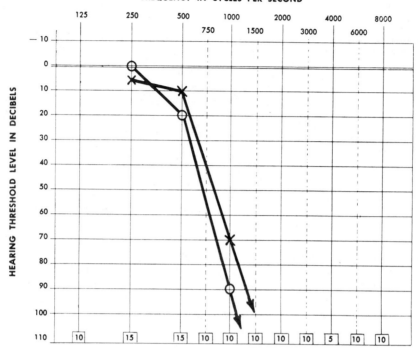

FIGURE 53-1. Audiogram showing good hearing for low frequencies and poor hearing for middle and high frequencies.

he fell in the borderline range of intellectual functioning (mental age 4 4/12 years on the Stanford-Binet, Form L-M: IQ 73).

DISCUSSION

The birth history and neonatal course of M. would indicate a child with "high risk" of physical and mental handicaps, including hearing deficit (Oppé, 1967). Many high risk factors are associated with congenital hearing loss: family history of hearing handicap; maternal rubella; complicated birth accompanied by cerebral anoxia; hyperbilirubinemia and exposure to ototoxic drugs (neomycin, streptomycin, kanamycin) in the neonatal period; and encephalitis and meningitis during the first few months of life. In this case the amount of kanamycin

given probably was too small to be ototoxic, but there were complications during the neonatal period which could have caused the hearing deficit. It is interesting to note that neonatal cerebral anoxia has been found as a common etiology for high frequency hearing loss (Matkin, 1968).

The type and extent of hearing loss to a large degree determine speech and language development in the hearing handicapped child. The frequency and intensity range of normal conversational speech is shown in Figure 53-2. A child with a "flat" hearing loss (loss for all frequencies) in excess of 60 dB would hear little or no speech unless it was made more intense by means of a hearing aid. In contrast, a child with selective hearing loss of the type experienced by M. (Figure 52-3) is aware of speech but does not always understand what is being said. He can hear vowel sounds which contain energy mainly in the

Audiogram

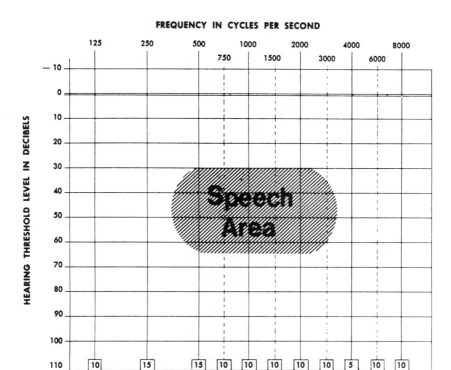

FIGURE 53-2. Conversational level speech plotted as a function of frequency (cps) and intensity (dB).

lower frequencies. He cannot hear many of the consonants, which are necessary for speech clarity, because they have their primary energy in the higher frequencies. The net effect is a distortion of speech perception. This poor understanding of language may go unnoticed at an early age because gestures and circumstantial cues often allow young children to give proper responses. When a child with this type of hearing loss starts to imitate the garbled language he hears, poor pronunciation and jargon are the result. Often he adds gestures to make himself understood.

When a child shows signs of language deficiency, further investigation, including hearing assessment, is warranted. A significant language delay from whatever cause usually becomes evident to parents by 24 to 30 months of age or earlier. They are likely to view abnormal language development with alarm and to bring their concern to the physician. He can con-

firm the presence of language delay by performing developmental assessment. For example, the Denver Developmental Screening Test, now widely used by pediatricians, lists several language items which 90 percent of children 2½ years of age should be able to pass. (Frankenburg and Dodds, 1967).

A number of informal hearing tests suitable for children of different ages are available to physicians and are useful for screening (Rupp and Wolski, 1969). However, a child with a selective hearing loss might respond to having his name whispered from behind, the crumbling of cellophane, or other informal tests, as they contain energy in many frequencies. The child in this report had responded often enough, even though erratically, to informal testing to convince his mother and the professional people concerned with him that his hearing was intact. Unfortunately, when, at 4 years, a pure tone audio-

Audiogram

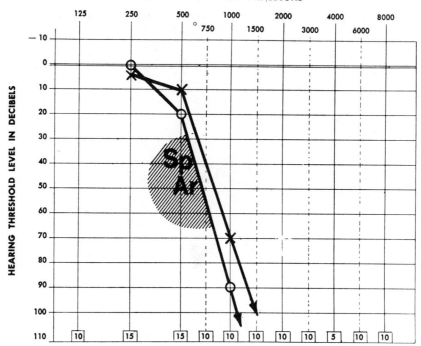

FIGURE 53-3. The expected effect of high frequency hearing loss on the perception of conversational level speech.

metric screening was done, only one frequency was tested, a dubious practice. A child with a language delay deserves a more precise audiological evaluation than can be obtained by gross screening.

An audiologist specializing in evaluation of children can make a reasonable estimate of a child's hearing at less than 1 year of age (Hoversten and Moncur, 1969). The preciseness of threshold measurement is related to the general developmental level of the child. Referral for audiological testing is appropriate for any child whose hearing is questionable regardless of age, functional level, and behavior. It is the physician's responsibility to familiarize himself with facilities for testing hearing available in his community. The audiologist is the one to determine the degree of testing accuracy that can be obtained with an individual child.

When M.'s hearing loss was discovered a remediation program was instituted. It consisted of appropriate audiological management, parental guidance with interpretation of the nature of his handicap, and proper educational placement. Unfortunately, by the time this youngster's hearing handicap was identified crucial years for normal language development had already passed.

SUMMARY AND CONCLUSIONS

The child in this report was thought at various times to be mentally retarded, emotionally disturbed, and brain damaged before his selective hearing loss was discovered at age 5¼ years. He had developed puzzling behavior secondary to the confusing verbal messages he received and his unpredictability in turn had had a disturbing effect on his environment.

Physicians will assist in the early identification of these children if they:

1. Recognize conditions in infancy associated with high risk of hearing handicap.
2. Listen to parents' observations about their child's language development and take their concerns seriously.
3. Pay attention to language development in the 2-year old; delay can easily be demonstrated on the Denver Developmental Screening Test.

4. Remember that prolonged jargoning, poor enunciation, and excessive use of gestures are suspicious symptoms of hearing loss.
5. Are aware of the fact that informal hearing screen may fail to identify partial hearing loss.
6. Refer the child suspected of hearing impairment to the audiologist regardless of the child's age, developmental level, and behavior. The audiologist is the professional best qualified to determine the degree of testing accuracy that can be obtained.

REFERENCES

Frankenburg, W. K., and Dodds, J. B. The Denver Developmental Screening Test. *J. Pediat.,* **71:** 181, 1967.

Hoversten, G. and Moncur, J. Stimuli and intensity factors in testing infants. *J. Speech Hearing Res,* **12:** 687, 1969.

Luterman, D. M., and Chasin, J. The pediatrician and the parent of the deaf child. Pediatrics, **45:** 115, 1970.

Matkin, N. D. The child with a marked high frequency hearing impairment. *Pediat. Clin. N. Amer.,* **15:** 677, 1968.

Oppé, T. E. Risk registers for babies. *Develop. Med. Child Neurol.,* **9:** 13, 1967.

Rupp, R. R., and Wolski, W. Hearing testing in young children: Simple technics adaptable to pediatric office practice for screening neonates, infants and young children. *Clin. Pediat.,* **8:** 263, 1969.

54

Children with Nonorganic Hearing Problems

RICHARD F. DIXON, Ph.D.
*Director, Division of Communication Disorders,
University of North Carolina at Greensboro*
HAYES A. NEWBY, Ph.D.
*Professor of Audiology at Stanford University
when this article was prepared.*

INTRODUCTION

Hearing problems which are not correlated with actual pathology of the hearing mechanism have been referred to variously as "functional" losses of hearing, "psychogenic" losses, or "malingering." From the audiologist's point of view, none of these terms is completely satisfactory. "Functional" is frequently used in other contexts to refer to a loss of function which may be on an organic basis, and thus it is probably not the proper term to apply to a hearing problem which may have no organic correlate. "Psychogenic" and "malingering" refer to the presumed absence or presence of a conscious element of feigning as a part of the symptom-picture. While the psychiatrist may be able to differentiate between an unconscious variety of hearing loss, which might be considered as a conversion reaction or so-called hysterical deafness, and the conscious type of assumed loss, which is properly termed malingering, the audiologist is usually in no position to make this kind of judgment. From the audiologist's—and perhaps the otologist's—standpoint, a better term to encompass all forms of assumed hearing loss would be "nonorganic." Such a term obviously means that the pathological condition of the hearing mechanism is in doubt, and it does not attempt to identify the hearing problem as being of the conscious or the unconscious variety. As a matter of fact, to be strictly accurate, the audiologist should probably refer to nonorganic hearing *problems* rather than to nonorganic hearing *losses,* because some patients appear to have no hearing handicap except in the examination situation.

In recent years, as audiologic diagnostic methods have been refined, it has become apparent that nonorganic hearing problems are more prevalent among the adult population than had previously been assumed. Audiology centers concerned with the testing of veterans for compensation purposes are required to employ a battery of tests designed to discover the presence of nonorganic problems and to enable the examiner to determine the true organic threshold of each individual patient. In such centers, the incidence of nonorganic problems among the veteran population tested has been estimated at from 20 percent to 40 percent. Johnson, Work, and McCoy (1956) have reviewed the literature and discussed the increase in the incidence of nonorganic hearing problems in military and veteran populations as familiarity with this type of difficulty has become more widespread. A nonorganic hearing problem, however, may range from a situation in which all of the patient's assumed hearing loss is nonorganic in nature to the situation in which a genuine loss exists but the patient exaggerates the true extent of his hearing problem.

As more audiologists and otologists have become involved in examining claimants in medicolegal cases, the presence of nonorganic hearing problems in nonveteran populations is also being discovered to a greater degree. While there are instances of such problems among adults which are not concerned with monetary compensation, these cases are relatively rare. It is commoner to find financial considerations closely tied in with the individual patient's misleading performance on certain auditory tests.

Reprinted by permission of the authors from *Arch. Otolaryng.,* **70,** pp. 619–623 (1959). Copyright 1959, American Medical Association.

Nonorganic hearing problems may exist in children as well as in adults. In the case of children, the motivation for assuming a hearing loss is almost never associated with monetary compensation. In fact, without considerable additional study of a psychodiagnostic nature, it is not possible to establish in most cases just what motivates children to behave in the test situation as if they were hard of hearing. It behooves school audiometrists, school psychologists, teachers, administrators, and others who are concerned with the health programs in the schools to be aware of the possibility of the existence of nonorganic hearing problems in children of school age.

Over the past two years, some 40 children with significant nonorganic hearing problems have been examined at the San Francisco Hearing and Speech Center. The purpose of this paper is to discuss some findings pertaining to these 40 children and to describe the procedures which seemed to be the most effective in demonstrating true acuity.

DESCRIPTION OF SUBJECTS

The 40 children who constitute the subjects of this discussion ranged in age from 6 to 18 years, with a mean of 10.9 years. Thirty-one of the children were female and nine were male. In all 40 cases the audiogram furnished by the referral source indicated a suspected marked bilateral hearing impairment when, in fact, our examination eventually revealed the hearing to be within normal limits in each ear.

Twelve children had a history suggesting previous disease of the middle ear and, perhaps, previous hearing loss of an organic nature. Fourteen were receiving special help in school, such as lip-reading instruction, auditory training, and preferential seating. Two children were in special classes for the hard of hearing, and one was in a class for the deaf. One child had been furnished with a hearing aid. It should be noted that in the case of most of these children there was no indication in the referral information to suggest that the hearing loss was not as represented on the accompanying audiograms. In fact, 16 of the children were referred to the Hearing and Speech Center specifically for a hearing aid evaluation.

Most of the children seemed to be performing well academically, to be intellectually normal, and were without noticeable emotional disturbances. Nine children displayed symptoms which might be related to their "hearing problems." These symptoms included functional articulatory speech disorders, and—according to parental reports—strong sibling rivalry, persistent enuresis, anxiety reactions, possible nonorganic visual difficulties, and lack of satisfactory academic progress. It should be reemphasized, however, that children with any symptoms or history of psychological significance were definitely in the minority—less than 25 percent of the total group. On the basis of our own observations, we cannot state why these children performed as they did on hearing tests. We can only report how they did behave, and how we were able to establish that their hearing was normal.

TESTING PROCEDURES

It was noted that during their initial interview, 39 of the 40 children were able to follow normal conversation with no difficulty. Typically, parents reported that in their observations the children usually did not behave as if they were hard of hearing. In almost every case, poor hearing had not been suspected by the parents until this possibility had been pointed out to them by the results of pure-tone tests, usually performed in the school situation. Apparently it was only in a testing situation that all of the children demonstrated hearing problems. It was curious that only a few previous examiners had noted inconsistencies between the children's responses to conversation and their hearing test results.

At the Hearing and Speech Center, pure-tone tests routinely precede speech audiometry. In the case of these 40 children, it became apparent very quickly that their responses to the pure-tone stimuli were grossly inconsistent with their behavior in a conversational situation. Typically, these children would profess average threshold levels between 40 and 60 dB at all frequencies. Their audiograms tended to be "flat" in configuration and with equal losses by air and by bone conduction. Figure 54-1 is a typical initial audiogram. Note that this loss pattern bears a striking resemblance to the curve of the most comfortable listening level for normal ears.

At this point, it should be mentioned that serial pure-tone audiograms, even widely spaced in time,

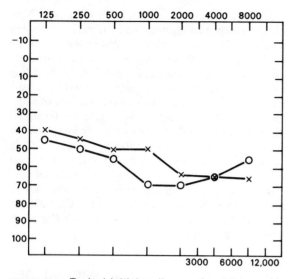

FIGURE 54-1. Typical initial audiogram for children with nonorganic hearing problems.

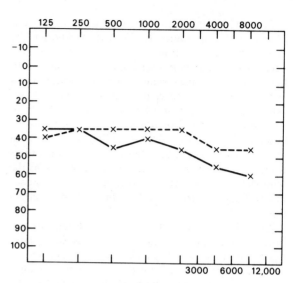

FIGURE 54-2. Test-retest reliability for the same ear of one child later found to have normal hearing.

do not necessarily provide sufficient variation to make one suspect a nonorganic hearing problem. Although we had no opportunity to estimate the ability of these children to give consistent erroneous thresholds from day to day, we were frequently provided with medical and school records indicating good test-retest reliability, sometimes over a long period of time. Figure 54-2 illustrates one child's ability to maintain consistent false thresholds over an interval of six weeks. The thresholds of the opposite ear showed equally small variations. This child was later found to have normal hearing in each ear.

After examining a few of these children, it became apparent that the speech reception threshold (SRT) was almost always closer to normal levels than the pure-tone thresholds. We recommend, therefore, that at the first indication one may be dealing with a nonorganic problem in a child—for example, the impression gained in the initial interview—monaural, live-voice speech audiometry be employed. The method by which one obtains the child's SRT is important. We found that best results were obtained when the SRT was approached from below, that is, by use of an ascending technique. The use of a descending or an ascending-descending method usually resulted in establishing a false SRT, and the task of

measuring the true organic threshold became more difficult.

It is usually necessary to spend considerable time—and to exercise a great deal of patience—in obtaining the child's SRT. Starting at maximum attenuation, the examiner presents 6 to 10 spondee words, interspersed with such comments as, "I know it's very soft, but you must try hard to repeat these words." If the child fails to respond, the intensity of the signal is increased by 5 dB and the examiner tries again, coaxing the child to respond at almost every word. Occasionally, the examiner may insert a question, such as, "Will you take off the earphones now?" to see if any reaction is observed to indicate that the child heard the question. Also, it may be possible to engage the child in a conversation on a topic that the examiner knows is of particular interest to the child. Thus, one child who would not repeat a spondee word at any sensation level was willing to talk about her pet dog and answer the examiner's questions when the hearing-loss dial was set at 5 dB.

With the use of an ascending method and considerable urging of one kind and another, we were able to establish SRT's of 10 dB or better in each ear in 33 of the 40 children. Thus, for most of the children, it was possible to rule out any marked hearing loss by the use of speech-reception measurements. Incidentally, it was unusual to find one of these children manifesting any significant loss of speech discrimination ability. Thirty-four of the children scored 90 percent or better in each ear on discrimination tests administered at levels well above previously established thresholds.

In a few of the children, normal hearing could not be shown by either speech audiometry or conventional pure-tone techniques. It was then necessary to use such special tests as PGSR and delayed feedback measurements to obtain valid estimates of organic thresholds. But even in these cases, before any special testing was done, there were indications of normal hearing. These were usually found in the subject's responses to conversational voice when he was not aware that he was being tested.

At the conclusion of each examination session, after normal hearing had been established by one method or another, a final attempt was made to secure valid pure-tone thresholds, that is, pure-tone thresholds which would agree reasonably well with the speech audiometric results, or the results of special tests such as PGSR and delayed feedback. The subjects were told that the pure-tone test was being repeated because it was obvious that they had misunderstood the directions on earlier tests, or had made a mistake in judging why they should respond. Sometimes they were told they would hear a different kind of tone which would be easier to hear than the previous ones used. Then, either a warbled tone or a pulsed tone would be employed. Valid final audiograms were obtained in the case of 33 of the children. It was possible to obtain valid thresholds with some children even when they did not respond *correctly* to the number of pulses presented. These children, after being instructed to count the number of tones they heard, would wait until a series of pulses had been presented and then blandly respond with the wrong number. But the very consistency of their responding with a number after each series of pulses, even though the intervals between presentations were widely varied, argued for the fact that they were hearing the tones. Although, as stated earlier, it is not within the audiologist's province to determine the relative consciousness of motivation in patients displaying nonorganic problems in hearing-test situations, there does seem adequate reason to believe that some of these children willfully and deliberately attempted to deceive the examiner.

In some respects children with nonorganic hearing problems are similar in their behavior to adults with such problems, and in some respects they are dissimilar. Both children and adults tend to respond to incidental conversation in a manner that is inconsistent with their test results. Both may present a history of previous middle ear problems, but pure-tone test results that are characteristic of perceptive losses. In the test situation, however, the adult will generally exhibit some degree of loss for speech stimuli, even though the speech audiometric results may not be reasonably consistent with the pure-tone results, whereas most children will respond with valid thresholds to speech audiometry, provided the techniques suggested earlier are employed.

SUMMARY AND CONCLUSIONS

In discussing our experience at the San Francisco Hearing and Speech Center with 40 children who had nonorganic hearing problems, it has been our intention to point out that children with normal hearing, like adults, will sometimes perform on hearing tests as if a hearing loss were present. We found this tendency to be considerably more marked in girls. Children with such problems typically do not show difficulty in understanding conversational speech. While they are likely to exhibit grossly erroneous pure-tone responses, most of them will give normal speech-reception scores when time-consuming modifications of standard speech audiometric procedures are employed. A child's consistency on serial pure-tone audiograms in itself does not rule out the possibility that he has a nonorganic hearing problem. While speech audiometry will yield valid results in most cases, in some instances it will be necessary to resort to special test procedures, such as PGSR and delayed feedback, in order to obtain valid organic thresholds. In most cases it is possible to obtain a final pure-tone audiogram which represents the child's actual hearing levels. The reasons why a child will demonstrate a nonorganic hearing problem in a test situation are obscure but apparently are not, as with adults, associated with pecuniary gain.

It is our hope that audiometrists, educators, and health authorities who deal with hearing-impaired children will be alert to observe that some children who fail school hearing tests may actually be exhibiting hearing problems of a nonorganic nature. On the basis of our observations, we recommend that children who fail school hearing tests not be placed in special classes or be regarded in any way as hearing-impaired children until the organicity of their hearing problems has been established through proper audio-logical study. We also suggest that nonorganic hearing problems deserve the attention of psychiatrists and psychologists in order to determine why some children behave in an aberrant fashion while having their hearing assessed.

REFERENCE

Johnson, K. O.; Work, W. P.; and McCoy, G. Functional Deafness, *Ann. Otol. Rhin. & Laryng.,* **65**: 154–170 (March) 1956.